Prevention, Diagnosis and Treatment of Parasitic Infections

Prevention, Diagnosis and Treatment of Parasitic Infections

Editor: Gregory Hamilton

MURPHY & MOORE
www.murphy-moorepublishing.com

www.murphy-moorepublishing.com

MURPHY & MOORE

Cataloging-in-Publication Data

Prevention, diagnosis and treatment of parasitic infections / edited by Gregory Hamilton.
p. cm.
Includes bibliographical references and index.
ISBN 978-1-63987-449-1
1. Parasitic diseases. 2. Parasitic diseases--Diagnosis. 3. Parasitic diseases--Treatment.
4. Parasitic diseases--Prevention. 5. Communicable diseases. 6. Medical parasitology. I. Hamilton, Gregory.
RC119 .P74 2022
616.96--dc23

Murphy & Moore Publishing,
1 Rockefeller Plaza,
New York City, NY 10020, USA

ISBN 978-1-63987-449-1 (Hardback)

Contents

Preface

This book has been a concerted effort by a group of academicians, researchers and scientists, who have contributed their research works for the realization of the book. This book has materialized in the wake of emerging advancements and innovations in this field. Therefore, the need of the hour was to compile all the required researches and disseminate the knowledge to a broad spectrum of people comprising of students, researchers and specialists of the field.

Parasites are the organisms that live in a symbiotic relationship with other organisms. The organism on or inside which the parasite lives is known as the host. The size of a parasite can vary from microscopic to large enough to be seen with naked eyes. Parasites survive by feeding from the host. Giardia infection, Chagas disease and tapeworm are some of the examples of parasitic infections. The signs of parasitic infections depend on the parasite. Symptoms of giardiasis are diarrhea, nausea, abdominal cramping and bloating, fatigue, and weight loss. People having Chagas disease may not develop symptoms for few weeks. Its symptoms are low fever, skin rash, nausea and vomiting, diarrhea, etc. The topics covered in this extensive book deal with the core subjects of parasitic infections. It provides significant information of this discipline to help develop a good understanding of the prevention and treatment of parasitic infections. A number of latest researches have been included to keep the readers up-to-date with the global concepts in this area of study.

At the end of the preface, I would like to thank the authors for their brilliant chapters and the publisher for guiding us all-through the making of the book till its final stage. Also, I would like to thank my family for providing the support and encouragement throughout my academic career and research projects.

Editor

1

Translational Rodent Models for Research on Parasitic Protozoa

Totta Ehret[1,2], Francesca Torelli[1], Christian Klotz[1], Amy B. Pedersen[3] and Frank Seeber[1]*

[1] FG16 – Mycotic and Parasitic Agents and Mycobacteria, Robert Koch Institute, Berlin, Germany, [2] Department of Molecular Parasitology, Humboldt-Universität zu Berlin, Berlin, Germany, [3] School of Biological Sciences, University of Edinburgh, Edinburgh, United Kingdom

Edited by:
Kenneth Fields, University of Kentucky, United States

Reviewed by:
Aaron Conrad Ericsson, University of Missouri, United States
Luciana Oliveira Andrade, Universidade Federal de Minas Gerais, Brazil

***Correspondence:**
Frank Seeber
seeberf@rki.de

Rodents, in particular *Mus musculus*, have a long and invaluable history as models for human diseases in biomedical research, although their translational value has been challenged in a number of cases. We provide some examples in which rodents have been suboptimal as models for human biology and discuss confounders which influence experiments and may explain some of the misleading results. Infections of rodents with protozoan parasites are no exception in requiring close consideration upon model choice. We focus on the significant differences between inbred, outbred and wild animals, and the importance of factors such as microbiota, which are gaining attention as crucial variables in infection experiments. Frequently, mouse or rat models are chosen for convenience, e.g., availability in the institution rather than on an unbiased evaluation of whether they provide the answer to a given question. Apart from a general discussion on translational success or failure, we provide examples where infections with single-celled parasites in a chosen lab rodent gave contradictory or misleading results, and when possible discuss the reason for this. We present emerging alternatives to traditional rodent models, such as humanized mice and organoid primary cell cultures. So-called recombinant inbred strains such as the Collaborative Cross collection are also a potential solution for certain challenges. In addition, we emphasize the advantages of using wild rodents for certain immunological, ecological, and/or behavioral questions. The experimental challenges (e.g., availability of species-specific reagents) that come with the use of such non-model systems are also discussed. Our intention is to foster critical judgment of both traditional and newly available translational rodent models for research on parasitic protozoa that can complement the existing mouse and rat models.

Keywords: wild rodent, protozoa, parasite, model organism, mouse, rat, translational research

INTRODUCTION

Gregor Mendel introduced the basic concept of a "model organism" when he reported his experiments on plant hybrids. He picked peas as a model because they had clear experimental advantages for addressing his question: "*At the very outset special attention was devoted to the* Leguminosae *on account of their peculiar floral structure (...) this led to the result that the genus*

Pisum *was found to possess the necessary qualifications.*" (Mendel, 1866) Since then this approach for model selection for a particular purpose is widely used, meaning that a model organism should be accessible, experimentally tractable, have short generation times, be affordable to maintain and breed, possess clearly identifiable features that are to be studied, and more recently be genetically tractable (which includes access to a sequenced genome), to name a few (Rand, 2008). Given the importance of model systems in biology, the history and diversity of model organisms has been extensively reviewed (Conn, 2008; Hunter, 2008; Müller and Grossniklaus, 2010; Ankeny and Leonelli, 2011; Bolker, 2012; Alfred and Baldwin, 2015).

The available model organisms span a great taxonomic range, and for many questions single-celled organisms such as bacteria (*Escherichia coli*) or yeasts (*Saccharomyces cerevisiae*) are sufficient. However, in many biomedical studies which aim to translate findings to humans, non-mammals are not applicable as translational models (Hau, 2008). Yet, shorter phylogenetic distances and anatomical similarities are no guarantee for translational success, as research on primates has demonstrated (detailed in section The CD28 Superagonist Antibody "Disaster"). Given the high relevance of protozoa for human and animal health and our own scientific interests in these parasites, we will concentrate on such infections in rodents. While their value as translational models is not without dispute (see section Protozoan Parasites) they have been, still are, and will continue to be, invaluable for both basic biological questions in host-parasite interactions as well as pre-clinical studies. Their importance for scientific progress is demonstrated, for example by the essential role laboratory mice played in the discovery of dendritic cells (see references in Steinman, 2012) and macrophages (reviewed by Gordon, 2007). The value of rodents, and mice in particular, has also been highlighted for leading to fundamental insights in infection biology (Buer and Balling, 2003; Vidal et al., 2008; Douam et al., 2015). Given the historical and current importance of rodents, we here explore benefits and limitations of, e.g., inbred or outbred mice, lab rodents, or rodents from the wild, etc., as well as possible external confounders, such as breeding conditions in lab facilities or interactions in an ecosystem, that might have great impact on research results. With this review, we encourage experimentalists, particularly in translational medicine, to consider a broad set of potential rodent models in order to identify and use the best available system for specific studies. We aim to provide a foundation and useful references for such decisions.

PROTOZOAN PARASITES

Infections with protozoan parasites cause substantial illness and economic loss in humans worldwide (see **Tables 1, 2** for details; Fletcher et al., 2012; Murray et al., 2012; Andrews et al., 2014; Robertson et al., 2014; Kassebaum et al., 2016). These parasites with high impact on humans mostly are the Amoeba, e.g., *Entamoeba* spp.; the flagellates, e.g., *Trichomonas* spp., *Giardia* spp., *Leishmania* spp., and *Trypanosoma* spp., and the large group of Apicomplexans, which contain, e.g., *Plasmodium* spp., *Toxoplasma gondii*, and *Cryptosporidium* spp. They are most often transmitted to their host either via ingestion of contaminated food, water, or via a vector (e.g., mosquitoes or flies; see **Table 2**). Here we provide a brief overview of some parasitic protozoa which substantially impact humans, and of which many are referred to in our examples used in following sections.

The significance of protozoan infections for global human health is here exemplified by data (see **Table 1**) where the impact of infections by the most devastating protozoan parasites is expressed as "disability-adjusted life-years" (DALYs, used by the World Health Organization (WHO) and others as a measure of disease impact). These diseases ranked second in importance across all infectious diseases, behind lower respiratory infections, and before AIDS and tuberculosis. The great majority of this impact can be attributed to malaria alone (85% caused by *Plasmodium* spp.). However, the collective disease burden of the other protozoa evaluated was also substantial and in the range of influenza (Murray et al., 2012). While many of these figures, including those for malaria, are fortunately on the decline, this disease was still ranked among the top 20 leading diseases as identified by the WHO worldwide in 2015 (Kassebaum et al., 2016). In addition to these human health concerns, protozoan parasites cause significant losses in many species of domestic animals (Perry and Grace, 2009; Torgerson and Macpherson, 2011; Fitzpatrick, 2013; Torgerson, 2013) and are in some cases a conservation concern for wildlife (Pedersen et al., 2007).

While many of these parasites have a very restricted host range (infecting a single host species and/or tissue), other extremes such as *T. gondii*, a zoonotic parasite assumed to infect all nucleated cells in all warm-blooded animals, exist. Consequently, there is a mixture of more or less natural relationships between the parasites and the rodent hosts when the latter are used as translational models for human infections (see **Table 2**). Many parasite genera contain species which naturally infect rodents (e.g., *Plasmodium, Giardia, Cryptosporidium*), although in most cases the very same species do not also infect humans. For other parasite species, the rodent model has been made susceptible, frequently by genetic means, to human relevant parasites (e.g., *P. falciparum* or *C. parvum/C. hominis*). In malaria research, rodents have been successfully used as models, but the suitability of the mouse to mimic severe human malaria has been questioned (Langhorne et al., 2011). In leishmaniasis research, rodents are acknowledged for contributing to a better understanding of the immune response to the parasite (Lipoldová and Demant, 2006) but other authors point out limitations and the lack of suitability of certain mouse strains to study specific parasite genotypes (Mears et al., 2015). Research on human sleeping sickness (*T. brucei*) has benefitted largely from mouse models (Antoine-Moussiaux et al., 2008; Giroud et al., 2009; Magez and Caljon, 2011) but criticism has been raised that more suitable animal models should be applied to address sleeping sickness in livestock (*T. congolense* and *T. vivax;* Morrison et al., 2016).

TABLE 1 | Global "Disability-Adjusted Life-Years," DALYs, for high impact infectious diseases, with several examples from protozoan parasites.

	DALYs (*1,000) 2010[a]	DALYs (*1,000) 2015[b]
Lower respiratory infections	115,227 (95,983)[c]	142,384
Influenza	19,244	nr[d]
Diarrhoeal diseases	89,513 (78,904)[e]	84,928
HIV/AIDS	81,547	62,759
Tuberculosis	49,396	56,037
Protozoan diseases, total	97,884 (15,199)[f]	40,695
Malaria	82,685	38,520
Leishmaniasis	3,317	1,357
African trypanosomiasis	560	372
Chagas disease	546	253
Trichomoniasis	167	194
Cryptosporidiosis	8,372	nr[d]
Amoebiasis	2,237	nr[d]

Data shown for 2010 and 2015. For causative agents of protozoan diseases see ***Table 2****.*
[a]*Murray et al. (2012).*
[b]*Kassebaum et al. (2016).*
[c]*Number in brackets, without influenza.*
[d]*nr, not reported.*
[e]*Number in brackets, without cryptosporidiosis and amoebiasis.*
[f]*Number in brackets, without malaria.*

WHY ARE MICE AND RATS SUCH POPULAR MODELS?

Biomedical research depends heavily on model organisms and the majority of these are rodents, particularly in infectious disease and immunological research. A few numbers illustrate this impressively. For example, in the European Union alone, 75% of all animals used for "experimental and other scientific purposes" in 2011 were house mice (*Mus* spp. 61%) and rats (*Rattus* spp. 14%; The Commission to the Council and the European Parliament, 2013). Other rodents (gerbils, hamsters, different species of mice, and other rodents) only constitute 0.47% of animals used (**Figure 1A**). In Germany, 91.5% of animals used in research on infectious diseases were rodents, with the vast majority being *Mus musculus* (88.6%; **Figure 1B**). Similar numbers are reported in the United Kingdom, with 82% of all research using rodents, again dominated by *M. musculus* (74.6%; UK Home Office, 2015). While these numbers also include animals that were used as donors, e.g., for blood or organs and thus for *in vitro* experimentation these data nevertheless illustrate the dominance and importance of rodents, in particular laboratory inbred mice, as model organisms.

Another informative figure shows that the number of publications where mice and rats were mentioned in the title dominates all other model organisms included (**Figure 2**), e.g., *Arabidopsis, Drosophila, S. cerevisiae, Caenorhabditis elegans, Xenopus*, zebrafish, *Neurospora*, and *Dictyostelium discoideum.* It is presumably no coincidence that a sharp increase in these "mouse publications" was seen in the 1990s, given that it was when embryonic stem cell manipulation met homologous recombination of the mouse genome. This resulted in the generation of defined gene knock-out mice (**Figure 2**), a finding which was later rewarded with the Nobel Prize in Physiology (Mak, 2007). The importance of this discovery for scientific progress in infection biology cannot be overestimated. However, in rats no such methods were available until relatively recently (Tong et al., 2010; van Boxtel and Cuppen, 2010), which is reflected in the drastic increase of mouse models and a relatively stable use of rats from 1990s until now. It is likely due to the highly developed genetic tools in mice, together with the more than 450 inbred mouse strains established since the first strain (DBA/2) was developed by Clarence Cook Little, that mice, and in particular the C57BL/6 strain, are the most popular animal model (Beck et al., 2000; Festing and Fisher, 2000). However, with the advent of CRISPR/Cas9 gene modifications in rats this will likely change (Hu et al., 2013; Li D. et al., 2013; Li W. et al., 2013), since this method has worked so far in almost all organisms tried and it can most likely also be applied to wild rodents. The historic establishment of tools for mice combined with the fact that 99% of genes are conserved between the human and the mouse genomes (Waterston et al., 2002) has made and will continue to make the mouse an obvious choice for translational efforts, i.e., research to understand the basics of and find treatments for human diseases. In addition, it will be exciting to see contributions from so far poorly explored model systems.

The Mice We Use in Experiments — Who Are They and How Do They Live?

Here we will briefly cover definitions of nomenclature for referring to different types of mice, from laboratory to "wild" rodents.

Classical inbred mice are defined as either being "produced using at least 20 consecutive generations of sister x brother or parent x offspring matings" or "traceable to a single ancestral pair in the 20th or subsequent generation." ("Nomenclature of Inbred Mice," defined by the Mouse Genomic Nomenclature Committee). However, it can be noted that 20 generations of inbreeding does not lead to fixed alleles in the entire genome, although for most phenotypes no differences are detected after this threshold (Chia et al., 2005). Different inbred populations exist and are referred to as strains (whereas outbred populations are often referred to as stocks). Inbred strains are genetically highly homogenous, well-defined, and often with genomes and SNP data available. In addition, extensive descriptions of (mutant) strains are available in the Mouse Phenome Database (Grubb et al., 2014) or the International Mouse Phenotyping Consortium database (Koscielny et al., 2014; see Table S1 for links) and should be consulted when planning experiments.

Wild-derived inbred strains are "descendants of mice captured in wild populations during the mid to late 20th century and represent several different *Mus* species from around the world" (Lutz et al., 2012). These mice are considered suitable for, e.g., evolutionary studies and gene mapping, but notably do not represent the genetic diversity of wild animals.

Outbred stocks are defined as "a closed population (for at least four generations) of genetically variable animals that is bred to maintain maximum heterozygosity" (Chia et al., 2005), meaning

TABLE 2 | The diseases caused, transmission routes, and suitability of rodents as models for human disease are listed for selected protozoan parasites.

Parasite species	Disease (organ(s) mainly affected)	Transmission route	Suitability of rodent model for human infectious species	References
Plasmodium spp.	Malaria (blood and liver)	Vector	(yes)	Cowman et al., 2016
Toxoplasma gondii	Acute and congenital toxoplasmosis (brain, heart, systemic)	Food, water, congenital	yes	Schluter et al., 2014
Cryptosporidium spp.	Cryptosporidiosis (intestine)	Food, water	(yes)	Checkley et al., 2015
Trichomonas vaginalis	Trichomoniasis (urogenital tract)	Sexual	(yes)	Kusdian and Gould, 2014
Giardia duodenalis	Giardiasis (intestine)	Food, water	(yes)	Ankarklev et al., 2010
Entamoeba spp.	Amoebiasis (intestine, liver, other organs)	Food, water	(yes)	Stanley, 2003
Leishmania spp.	Cutaneous and visceral leishmaniasis (skin; several organs)	Vector	(yes)	Stuart et al., 2008; Akhoundi et al., 2016
Trypanosoma brucei (gambiense and *rhodesiense)*	African trypanosomiasis/sleeping sickness (blood, lymphatics, brain)	Vector	(yes)	Matthews, 2015
Trypanosoma cruzi	Chagas disease (heart, systemic)	Vector	(yes)	Messenger et al., 2015

Reference is given to a single article describing the basic biology of the respective protozoan to serve as starting point for further reading.
(yes), adopted to model.

that each individual is genetically different from the others. Once established, the goal is to keep the genetic variability between generations to a minimum which is achieved by using, e.g., a certain number of breeding pairs (Chia et al., 2005). We onwards refer to inbred and outbred *M. musculus* models as lab mice, if nothing else is specified.

Recombinant Inbred Strains, RIS, are a collection of mice established by inbreeding two existing inbred strains into a set of strains (often called set or panel). Each such strain is genetically homogenous, but "parallel" strains produced from the same two well-defined ancestral strains are genetically more different from each other than either of the two ancestors (Chia et al., 2005). One advantage of using a RIS set compared to pure inbred strains is that phenotypic differences (e.g., pathogen or drug susceptibility) can be fairly easily assigned to specific genotypes (Guénet et al., 2015), and obtaining high-quality quantitative data on transcripts and proteins is feasible (Chick et al., 2016). Other options for lab mice, such as genetic crosses, will be covered in the section Humanized Mice: Rodents Which Mimic the Human Immune System.

We refer to **wild rodents** (including wild mice, e.g., species of *Mus*) as rodents which breed without direct intervention or manipulation by humans, in their natural habitats, e.g., farmland, forests or cities (Singleton and Krebs, 2007). Such populations may in some cases be under experimental study and manipulated, for example by regular trapping, diet manipulations and drug treatment, and will here still be considered as wild populations.

Mouse Housing Influences Experimental Outcome

Almost all animal research facilities can house rodents in specific pathogen-free, SPF, barrier facilities. This standard includes regular screening for a large set of common pathogens (in order to detect contamination), and commonly autoclaving cages, bedding, water, food and other housing related materials to assure hygienic and controlled housing, as well as controlled light/dark cycles (Hedrich and Nicklas, 2012). For details see respective lab manuals (Ayadi et al., 2011; Hedrich, 2012). Animal psychological status has been shown to influence variability in experimental studies, including examples of more reproducible results from "happier" mice, which display less anxiety or depression-associated behavior as a result of increased animal welfare (Bayne and Würbel, 2012). Although, wild mice can run several 100 m per night (Latham and Mason, 2004) including a means for physical activity (e.g., running wheels) is not standard in animal housing. Moreover, it is debated whether such so-called enrichment of housing is always required, beneficial, or adequate for the outcome of an experiment (Bayne and Würbel, 2012), given that after decades of breeding and selection lab mice in many respects show different behaviors to wild mice (Latham and Mason, 2004).

Recent publications highlight the important role of microbiota in rodents (and humans). Even though SPF animals are the most commonly used rodents in experiments (Fiebiger et al., 2016), gut microbiota are not homogenous (e.g., in composition or bacterial numbers) in such research settings and the extent of this variation has only recently emerged. Microbiota differ between vendors and mouse strains (Hufeldt et al., 2010; Ericsson et al., 2015; Hilbert et al., 2017), different shipments from the same vendor (Hoy et al., 2015), between research animal facilities (Rausch et al., 2016) and even between rooms in the same breeding facility (Rogers et al., 2014). Determining factors for gut microbiota differences under SPF housing conditions without experimental perturbations have been analyzed, and apart from vendor, the fodder and treatment thereof is important (Rausch et al., 2016). Therefore, housing conditions strongly influence mouse microbiota. Data also suggest a general difference between inbred lab mice and wild mice in that the proportion of *Firmicutes* vs. *Bacteroides* vary, with wild rodents being dominated by *Firmicutes* and vice versa (Weldon et al., 2015).

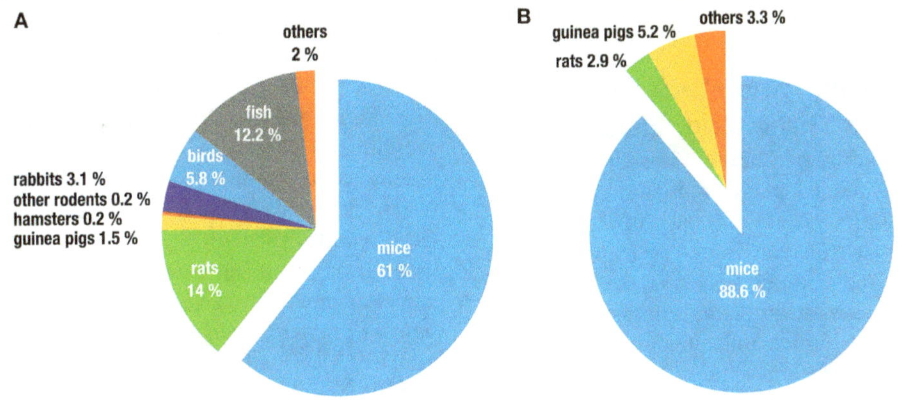

FIGURE 1 | Animal classes used in experiments for **(A)** all life sciences disciplines in the 27 EU member states (2011 in %). Data taken from (The Commission to the Council and the European Parliament, 2013), and **(B)** research on infection biology only, in Germany (2011 in %). Data taken from (German Federal Ministry of Food and Agriculture, 2011).

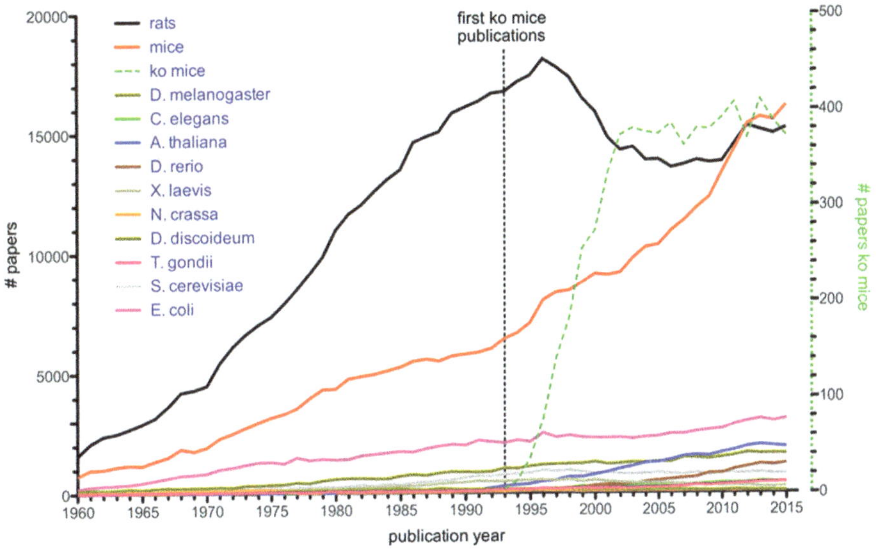

FIGURE 2 | Number of citations with organism's name in title (Dietrich et al., 2014), based on Web of Science entries for a given year. Numbers for single-celled model organisms like *T. gondii, S. cerevisiae,* and *E. coli* are given for comparison. Green dashed line (with corresponding y-axis on the right) illustrates articles mentioning knock-out mice, with first papers appearing in the early 1990s.

MISLEADING RESULTS DUE TO INAPPROPRIATE ANALYSIS OR AN INAPPROPRIATE MODEL

"If you have cancer and you are a mouse, we can take good care of you" (Kolata, 1998). This famous sentence from Judah Folkman (the "father" of tumor angiogenesis) makes this point: any model - animal or even mathematical - only returns the output it is capable of producing. A translational mouse model that lacks human feature X will never give a response in X, no matter how important that particular feature is in the context of a human disease. While the mouse model has been very successful for understanding the general principles of the mammalian immune system and infectious disease (e.g., Buer and Balling, 2003), it is important to be aware of, and acknowledge, the intrinsic benefits and limitations in any model chosen for a specific experiment. However, before we focus on biological confounders we want to consider that failures in the transition from preclinical studies to humans may also be due to poorly designed or performed studies (see Couzin-Frankel, 2013; Justice and Dhillon, 2016). To illustrate that problems of very different character can challenge the suitability of translational rodent models, we will first discuss two past examples from different disciplines (sepsis and immunology) that caused vibrant discussions in the scientific community and were subsequently analyzed in great detail. They can thus provide valuable insights of general importance for scientists with different research interests. In the section Non-genetic Confounders in Rodent Infections with Protozoan

Parasites we will then turn to confounders in translational rodent models of infections with protozoan parasites.

Analysis, Re-Analysis and Meta-Analysis – Three Studies and Three Conclusions

Due to its importance for human health, research on sepsis in mouse models is heavily funded, but its translational success has so far been disappointing (van der Worp et al., 2010). Few papers in biomedical research have therefore raised such an excitement and storm of replies and counter-replies as the Seok et al. (2013) study on sepsis. They analyzed transcriptomic data from various mouse models of human inflammatory diseases, and human samples in particular from septic shock, and concluded that "genomic responses in mouse models poorly mimic human inflammatory diseases" (Seok et al., 2013). However, re-analysis of the very same data subsequently concluded the opposite, and these authors simply replaced "poorly" with "greatly" in the article's title of their reply (Takao and Miyakawa, 2015). This discussion is still ongoing, with a recent paper (Weidner et al., 2016) pointing out that the data from Seok et al. *per se* are good enough to compare the transcriptional responses of certain (but not all) mouse models to humans, but that the analytical tools used in the two first papers were inappropriate. The authors' conclusions were that gene set enrichment analysis (GSEA) is more appropriate than gene-to-gene comparisons, which require setting an arbitrary threshold for the determination of differentially expressed genes (as opposed to identification by statistical means). Those tools were used differently by various authors for re-analyses of the original data sets, thus leading to opposite conclusions (Seok et al., 2013; Shay et al., 2013; Takao and Miyakawa, 2015; Warren et al., 2015). A further level of complexity that makes conclusions derived from transcriptomic comparisons challenging is that for many genes there is no correlation between mRNA levels and protein quantities (see section Transcriptomes Do Not Necessarily Predict Protein Levels). Although transcriptome analysis is a fairly easily accessible and promising technique, these examples illustrate that such relatively young tools require close evaluation of the entire work-flow. Understanding and considering the physics or chemistry behind the method and to critically assess appropriate analysis methods is a community task when new scientific methods are being established.

The CD28 Superagonist Antibody "Disaster"

It is well known that substantial differences between the mouse and human immune systems exist (Mestas and Hughes, 2004; Zschaler et al., 2014; Sellers, 2017) and that they need to be considered when using mice as preclinical models of human disease (e.g., Beura et al., 2016). In 2006, a small human phase I clinical trial aimed at alleviating rheumatoid arthritis tested a humanized monoclonal antibody, TGN1412, directed against the human T cell receptor CD28. However, instead of improving the autoimmune condition, it resulted in devastating consequences (reviewed by Hunig, 2016). It was anticipated from laboratory mouse studies that injection of the antibody would result in the preferential production of regulatory T cells, followed by a downregulation of active T cells. However, all six volunteers had to be hospitalized and at least four of them suffered multiple organ dysfunctions. TGN1412 had caused an immediate "cytokine storm" in these patients due to substantial TNF-α release, followed by dramatically increased plasma concentrations of several cytokines. This "cytokine release syndrome" (CRS) was caused by a strong activation of $CD4^+$ effector memory T cells, which eventually caused severe tissue damage. But why had preclinical studies in primate models, namely cynomolgus and rhesus monkeys, not indicated any signs of problems? What was unknown in 2006 was that those primates' $CD4^+$ effector memory T-cells do not express CD28 whereas humans do (Eastwood et al., 2010). In this particular case, the monkeys were a poor model for humans, despite their phylogenetically close relationship.

And why had the human response not been seen in the numerous rodent experiments performed prior to the trial? Interestingly, later experiments have demonstrated that at least two drastically modified lab mouse models can indeed be good models for the TGN1412 experiments. The first example is linked to the fact that, as is the case for most immunological experiments, mice in the initial studies had been raised and kept under SPF conditions. Thereby, they had no exposure to microbial antigens that would elicit $CD4^+$ memory T cells. Thus, CRS was not initiated upon TGN1412 treatment as it was in humans. Consequently, when TGN1412 was later given to non-laboratory "dirty" mammals (including rodents, see section Getting the Rodent Model "Dirty") exposed to prior environmental microbial stimuli, they experienced similar syndromes as the human volunteers (Eastwood et al., 2010). The second alternative model consists of humanized mice (see section Humanized Mice: Rodents Which Mimic the Human Immune System). A recent study made use of mice which had been reconstituted with human peripheral blood mononuclear cells. Injecting TGN1412 into those animals recapitulated a number of the disastrous immunological outcomes also seen in the initial human trial (Weissmuller et al., 2016). Importantly, the transplanted human cells also included a small amount of effector memory cells. Therefore, both the use of "dirty" and humanized mice better mimicked human biology than the rodent models which were used in the pre-clinical studies (although both these models have gained interest more recently and were, if at all, very new ideas at that time).

NON-GENETIC CONFOUNDERS IN RODENT INFECTIONS WITH PROTOZOAN PARASITES

Lab rodent models have been essential for understanding molecular, cellular, and immunological responses; however, most of the variability inherent in natural populations is not captured by them (Pedersen and Babayan, 2011; Beura et al., 2016). Even so, sources of variation which influence experimental outcomes in lab experiments have also been identified in these very models. Reports based on lab experiments have often not accounted for such variability and instead ascribed differences between experimental groups to the aspect under study.

Microbiota as a General Confounder for Rodent Experiments

Recently, the role of microbiota as a confounder for experimental outcomes in various scientific fields has gained increasing interest (Servick, 2016), largely due to the development of next-generation sequencing and related methods. Common approaches to study microbiota include sequencing fecal content from lab mice and germ-free mice (discussed in detail in Fiebiger et al., 2016), fecal transplants, antibiotics treatment, probiotics, addition of a specific bacterium, and infectious agents. For biomedical research it is noteworthy that microbiota influences host susceptibility to drugs. One example are proteins encoded by drug processing genes, DPGs, which are responsible for uptake, distribution, metabolism, and excretion of xenobiotics such as drugs (Aplenc and Lange, 2004; Klaassen et al., 2011). DPGs in mouse liver display different expression patterns depending on the microbiota status of the animal (Fiebiger et al., 2016). Some authors have linked microbiota differences to subsequent variation in brain activity and changes in social behavior, a concept referred to as the gut-brain axis (e.g., Foster and McVey Neufeld, 2013; Mayer et al., 2015; Gacias et al., 2016) which is proposed to depend on several factors, including the immune system. Variation in microbiota is known to influence both local and systemic immune function by altering the balance of Th1/Th2 cell composition, influencing re-localization of neutrophils, or affecting macrophage polarization (Denny et al., 2016; Lopes et al., 2016). Taken together, it is therefore not surprising that differences in microbiota can have a substantial impact on protozoan parasite infections in the gut and elsewhere. It is also easy to imagine a situation in which genetically modified mice obtained from one breeder or lab and control mice from other sources leads to unintended differences in microbiota composition with resulting influence on the outcome of infection experiments.

Protozoan Infection Experiments Are Influenced by Microbiota

One early study pointing to the importance of microbiota for the establishment of a protozoan infection used germ-free mice which were infected with the intestinal parasite *G. duodenalis* (Torres et al., 1992). The authors demonstrated that the microbiota influences the establishment and nature of intestinal infection with regards to severity and parasite reproductive success. A later study showed that female mice with the same genetic background were either susceptible or resistant to *G. duodenalis* infection (Singer and Nash, 2000). Differences were due to the origin (vendor) of the animals, and the same was true for immunodeficient mice. Co-housing led to resistance in all animals, whereas treatment with antibiotics made all animals equally susceptible to intestinal infection. It was therefore concluded that the microbiota determined the outcome of infection. These studies have recently been complemented with more in-depth investigations of the microbial community, showing changes in the amount of microbiota and its composition upon *G. duodenalis* infection in mice (Barash et al., 2016). Hence, not only do microbiota influence infection outcome but the parasite in turn alters the gut microbiota. These studies emphasize the complexity of gastrointestinal parasite infections. Further analysis of microbiota-parasite-host cohabitation will likely reveal interactions such as competition for nutrients or synergies in metabolism.

The complexity of microbiome influences is not limited to gut microbiota. Skin microbiota has also been shown to influence the outcome of cutaneous leishmaniasis in mice. Its causative agent, *L. major*, differently induced skin lesions, edema, and necrosis in germ-free mice compared to SPF mice upon intradermal infection (Naik et al., 2012). Germ-free mice displayed less disease severity, but also reduced levels of IFN-γ and IL-17A from αβ T cells in the infected skin area compared to SPF reared animals. By orally administering antibiotics, the gut microbiota, but not skin microbiota, changed without influencing cytokine production. However, introduction of a skin commensal bacterium, *Staphylococcus epidermis*, did rescue IL-17A production in the skin. The authors concluded that local cytokine production was specifically linked to skin microbiota. In a different study, *L. major* infection altered the gut microbiota of infected animals (but differently depending on mouse strain) (Lamour et al., 2015). Infection changed how gut microbiota correlated with systemic functions such as urine metabolites, plasma metabolites, and the immune system. Such findings also highlight that simple correlations between microbiota and protozoan parasites may not be adequate to elucidate the dynamic role of microbiota during infection.

Interestingly, the microbiota does not only affect the site of infection but can also influence how host and parasite interact at other sites. Recent work provided evidence that the severity of malaria infection with rodent *Plasmodium* spp. can also depend on vendor. Differences in disease severity correlate with differences in microbiota composition (Villarino et al., 2016) or bacterial transcription profiles (Stough et al., 2016), demonstrating systemic effects by the microbiota. A study from 2014 also reported a mechanism for such correlations, describing production of anti-*Plasmodium* spp. antibodies in response to gut colonization, specifically by *E. coli* O86:B7 but not by the reference *E. coli* K12 (Yilmaz et al., 2014). These studies demonstrate that infections in specific compartments which are not colonized by commensal bacteria are nevertheless influenced and such effects must be considered in planning experiments and interpreting results.

Excursion 1: A Reductionist *In vitro* Approach Using Organoids

Protozoa-host interaction studies have largely been restricted to more or less suitable rodent models, cell lines (often cancer-derived), and short-lived primary tissue cultures from biopsy or surgery. Recent advances in stem cell research have paved the way for the development of self-renewing and complex tissue-like culture systems, so-called organoids, which mimic organs in their main functions and structural features (Willyard, 2015). Major advantages include that host-parasite interactions can be investigated in a primary, long-lived, organ-like tissue from the organism of choice, including humans, in real time (Klotz et al., 2012). Organoids have been developed from the gastro-intestinal tract (GIT), including stomach, gut and liver, and also from kidney and brain (Clevers, 2016). Importantly, organoids lack tissue-specific immune cells and in the GIT the microbiota, and therefore complexity is low compared to *in vivo* settings. However, this feature allows the researcher to construct an experimental setup with exactly the desired level of complexity, adding for instance the Mouse Intestinal Bacterial Collection (Lagkouvardos et al., 2016), human microbiota from biopsies, and/or a set of cytokines or immune cells of interest. For elucidating the role of individual actors during a parasitic infection, organoids are promising alternatives to animal models, cell culture systems, and the use of human biopsy material.

Sex and Age

Two long-known factors that influence infection success by parasites are sex and age. The most obvious differences between the sexes are hormones (Roberts et al., 2001; Klein, 2004; Bernin and Lotter, 2014) but X chromosome-linked mutations (van Lunzen and Altfeld, 2014; Garenne, 2015) and sex-specific behavior can also affect the outcome of infectious diseases. A prominent example in protozoan infections is glucose-6-phosphate dehydrogenase (G6PD) deficiency, which protects humans of both sexes to different extents from clinical outcomes of infections with *P. falciparum* (Shah et al., 2016). A previously developed humanized mouse model of G6PD deficiency (Rochford et al., 2013) has recently been used in screening efforts to identify malaria transmission-blocking drugs (Wickham et al., 2016). A second example involves X-linked immunodeficiency in the B-cell responses due to mutations in the Bruton's tyrosine kinase. The mutation causes a sex-specific effect which leads to X-linked agammaglobulinaemia (XLA). Human patients and mice bearing a similar mutation (CBA/N) are more prone to develop chronic giardiasis (Skea and Underdown, 1991; Van der Hilst et al., 2002).

In rodent models of, e.g., *Plasmodium* spp., *Cryptosporidium* spp., and *Leishmania* spp. infection age significantly influences susceptibility (Adam et al., 2003), parasite reproductive success (Rhee et al., 1999), and severity of disease (Muller et al., 2008). In the case of *Cryptosporidium* (Rhee et al., 1999), hamsters displayed age-dependent differences (within the first 2 months of life) in infection persistence measured by time for shedding oocysts, whereas mice did not. The results demonstrate that rodents can be used to study cryptosporidosis, but simultaneously suggest that generalizations of these results to other species are difficult, and translational success is not obvious. For leishmaniasis, recent work showed mouse age-specific differences in the induction of adaptive immunity. Animals were exposed to a vaccine candidate based on genetically modified *L. donovani* and aged mice (~16 months) had a less pronounced adaptive immune response compared to young mice (~2 months) upon *L. major* challenge after vaccination (Bhattacharya et al., 2016). In *Babesia microti* infection of lab mice between the ages of 2 and 18 months (Vannier et al., 2004), one of three strains (DBA/2 mice) mimicked patterns seen in humans in which susceptibility and an inability to clear infection increased with age. The other two strains displayed smaller differences in susceptibility and no change in infection clearance, illustrating possibilities to use rodents as models for human babesiosis, but alerting to possible issues with interpretation and translation of results.

Given these examples it seems obvious to consider age and sex aspects when planning rodent experiments. However, it is not unusual to use only male or only female mice (Flórez-Vargas et al., 2016) based on convenience, local availability, costs, legal issues (more animals required when both sexes are examined; Clayton and Collins, 2014) or research area. In particular in infectious disease research there is a strong bias toward using female mice (Flórez-Vargas et al., 2016). One reason for this is presumably that they are less aggressive and thus cheaper since they can be housed in (experimental) groups in a single cage whereas this is challenging for male mice. Likewise, younger mice are cheaper to obtain since housing cost are lower. Thus, convenience rather than scientific reasoning might influence the choice of sex or age in many studies.

MODELS FOR ALL PURPOSES – FROM FIXED ALLELES TO COMPLEX ECOLOGY

Even before the first draft of the mouse genome was published in 2002 (Waterston et al., 2002), scientists were aware of the relative genetic homogeneity of the lab mouse compared to wild mouse populations (Guenet and Bonhomme, 2003). Inbreeding over almost a century fixed alleles in currently available lab mice, which now represent just a fraction of the genetic variability found in nature. Although a desirable feature for some questions, this variability can be of great importance in studies of host-parasite interactions. Genetic variability might be the reason for different host susceptibility together with, e.g., the confounders discussed above (see section Non-genetic Confounders in Rodent Infections with Protozoan Parasites). In many cases allelic variations of a gene involved in immune responses were identified as the cause of infection outcome.

When Immune Responses Depend on Genetics – Selected Examples

Allelic variation at Lsh and H2 loci is involved in the opposite outcome of the acquired immune response in *L. donovani* infection between e.g., CBA and BALB/c mice (Loeuillet et al., 2016). Another emerging example is the role that the inflammasome has in sensing protozoan infections (reviewed in Zamboni and Lima-Junior, 2015). During *T. gondii* infection in rodents, sequence differences in the pathogen sensor *Nlrp1* accounts for species-specific inflammasome induction - and thus outcome - in lab mice (Ewald et al., 2014) and rat strains (Cirelli et al., 2014). Phenotypic differences between model animals can also be due to polymorphisms in the inflammasome pathway effectors, e.g., IL-18 and IL-1β. A study on a wild, natural population of field voles (*Microtus agrestis*) found associations with polymorphisms of IL-1β, IL-2, and IL-12β and differential susceptibility to pathogen infection (Turner et al., 2011), with the impact on susceptibility being comparable to parameters like sex and body weight. The parasites considered in the study were mostly nematodes, cestodes, and *B. microti*, making the influence of these cytokines' polymorphisms in other protozoan parasite infections a likely scenario.

Recently, polymorphisms in immunity-related GTPases (IRGs) affecting the rodent immune responses to *T. gondii* were described in a study comparing the DNA sequences of several inbred and wild-derived mice (Lilue et al., 2013). Remarkably, the authors showed that while the sequences of all the examined lab mice were highly conserved, genes in the wild-derived mice were extremely diverse, comparable to the diversity of MHC genes. One of those genes, the highly polymorphic *Irgb2-b1* from a wild-derived *M. musculus*, when expressed in C57BL/6 fibroblasts, was sufficient to confer resistance (i.e., prevent cell lysis) to so-called virulent strains of *T. gondii*. While 1–10 parasites of these strains can kill a lab mouse, IRG-polymorphic wild-derived mice are resistant to infection by much higher numbers of the same *T. gondii* strain. Apart from highlighting extensive sequence variability of wild-derived but not classical inbred laboratory strains in these gene loci, this work emphasizes that the definition of virulence is heavily dependent on the animal of choice and that its definition should always be accompanied by stating the experimental conditions. In the following section we move from traditional, genetically homogenous and inbred mice to mice manipulated to resemble aspects of the human immune system, and then to genetic crosses between inbred and wild-derived mice. Lastly, we will turn our attention to "dirty mice" and wild rodents in natural settings.

Humanized Mice: Rodents Which Mimic the Human Immune System

Designing an immune system with human features within the mouse—generating humanized mice—has recently emerged as an approach to expand the areas where lab mice can be used to model disease. Generation of humanized mice is based on immunodeficient animals (e.g., SCID, $Rag2^{-/-}$) whose innate and adaptive immune systems are severely compromised and the animals are instead characterized by increased survival of transplanted human hematopoietic cells (Kaushansky et al., 2014; Good et al., 2015), which produce a large number of different human immune cells in the mouse. Depending on further needs, these mice can be populated with, for example human red blood cells and/or $CD34^+$ hematopoietic stem cells that further give rise to T cells and antigen presenting cells (APC). Recent advances in the development of humanized mice offer the possibility to study human infectious diseases which could previously not be investigated in mice, in the mouse model (Brehm et al., 2013). Even though the use of rodent-infecting *Plasmodium* spp. such as *P. berghei* has greatly contributed to understanding the parasite's biology and general principles of protective immune mechanisms in mammals (Craig et al., 2012), it is promising that human-infecting *P. falciparum* now can be researched in lab mice (Kaushansky et al., 2014). The basic strategy for generating humanized mice, and adaptations of it lead to the generation of mice in which the blood stages of human malaria parasite life cycles could be established (Kaushansky et al., 2014; Good et al., 2015).

More advanced models with engrafted human hepatocytes (FRG-NOD huHep) have been further used to establish the complete development of the pre-erythrocytic liver stage of *P. falciparum* after mosquito bite, including formation of exo-erythrocytic merozoites, subsequently infectious to human red blood cells in the same mouse (Vaughan et al., 2012). Although, the development of the mature sexual stages (gametocytes) that are necessary to complete the parasite life cycle is still inefficient, it seems possible that complete *P. falciparum* (and other human *Plasmodium* spp.) life cycles could be routinely maintained using humanized mice. Recently, such mice were also used to conduct a genetic cross between two *P. falciparum* strains in those animals, something that so far was only possible in non-human primates, including chimpanzees (Vaughan et al., 2015).

These examples and others from several other infectious agents (Ernst, 2016) suggest that humanized mice will continue to contribute to a new repertoire of mouse translational models. Understanding host specificity factors for a given human pathogen is crucial for the design of susceptible humanized mice, and methods to identify such factors are described in detail by Douam et al. (2015). However promising, the establishment of these mice is relatively new and already several limitations are known (described in more detail in Ernst, 2016), which limit the extent to which the models actually mimic the human immune system. For instance, several mouse cytokines differ largely in their sequences between mouse and human, and IL-13 has no effect on human cells. This might explain the low proportions of certain human immune cell types in humanized mice. In addition, signaling and adhesion molecules are different between humans and mice and, importantly, the expression of murine and not human major histocompatibility complexes impairs the function of T cells. Attempts have been made to account for some of these limitations (Ernst, 2016) but so far humanized mice are probably best considered as a promising, but yet developing, tool in translational research.

Even so, host-specificity has limited the choice of model systems for studying protozoan parasites. The *Plasmodium* spp. examples and initial attempts with *L. major* infection in humanized mice (Wege et al., 2012) hold promise for future possibilities to investigate also other human-specific protozoan parasite species in lab mice.

Mixing the Known — Recombinant Inbred Strains and the Collaborative Cross

In order to document an influence of genetic heterogeneity on experimental results, models beyond inbred animals are required (Phifer-Rixey and Nachman, 2015; Chow, 2016). This is also true in translational research, where humans represent a genetically diverse population. When the aim is to find differences across the genome, as in genome-wide association studies (GWAS) where a given phenotype is thought to be linked to genetics, outbred stocks of mice or rats are not a solution since they are "a genetically ill-defined set of laboratory mice that are often used erroneously in toxicology, pharmacology and basic research" (Chia et al., 2005). In addition, their usefulness is limited for practical reasons, e.g., individual phenotypic variability requires larger sample sizes than necessary with inbred strains, or the study will lack statistical power to correlate experimental differences with certain genotypes (see Chia et al., 2005; Festing, 2014). In order to address the problem of limited genetic diversity but avoid the ill-defined genetic composition of wild animals, numerous mouse collections besides the RIS (see section The Mice We Use in Experiments — Who Are They and How Do They Live) have been established.

The concept for producing RIS sets has been extended by the Complex Traits Consortium to produce more genetically variable sets (Chia et al., 2005). These are known as Collaborative Crosses (CC) and are based on a set of 8 defined and sequenced founder strains, including three wild-derived strains of *Mus* and five traditional inbred strains. Although the set of strains is genetically diverse, each CC strain is at least 90% homogenous and hence genetically well-defined. The CCs were designed specifically for complex trait analysis (Churchill et al., 2004; Threadgill and Churchill, 2012) and the derived Diversity Outbred (DO) population (Churchill et al., 2012) has resulted in an even more genetically diverse mouse population (see **Figure 3**). Other derivatives of CC's concept exist, like the Heterogeneous Stock mice (Valdar et al., 2006) or the Hybrid Mouse Diversity Panel (Bennett et al., 2010). Besides GWAS studies, which map determinants for non-infectious diseases, CC animals have recently been used to map susceptibility or pathogenesis determinants in bacterial and viral infection models (Durrant et al., 2011; Ferris et al., 2013; Rasmussen et al., 2014; Vered et al., 2014; Gralinski et al., 2015; Lore et al., 2015; Smith et al., 2016). However, no data for parasite infections have been reported so far, and their large potential for exploring how host genotype influences infections needs to be explored in the future. Nevertheless, CC and DO mice also have limitations (Phifer-Rixey and Nachman, 2015). They are all derived from subspecies, which limits the genetic variation and may cause partial hybrid sterility in crosses. This, in turn, might have resulted in the elimination of genetic variation at these genomic loci. However, it is expected that further crosses will improve these models on the genetic level.

Yet, these mice will never approach the genetic diversity found in the human population or wild animal populations. In addition, individuals in natural populations encounter seasonal and spatial variability in the environment, as well as differences in climate and food availability. Wild animals are also exposed to and infected with a vast array of parasites and other pathogens, harbor different microbiota, and individuals vary in their demography, behavior and genetic composition. While it is possible to add key elements of natural variation into the above described rodent model systems, there is an increasing interest in moving beyond the controlled laboratory setting to a more realistic scenario.

Excursion 2: Metabolic Disease in Lab Mice and Humans — Is Ecological Complexity Better than SPF Facilities?

Around 25% of the world population has a metabolic syndrome, defined by the International Diabetes Federation as either diabetes / prediabetes, abdominal obesity, high cholesterol or high blood pressure. Animal studies provide important information on these conditions (Bäckhed et al., 2004; Turnbaugh et al., 2006). The role of microbiota has gained interest also in this field because of potential new treatments which can manipulate the microbiome community and function (Borody and Khoruts, 2012). Of interest here are the large numbers of studies conducted in rodents which demonstrate, for instance, alterations in body weight and insulin sensitivity which correlate with changes in microbiota upon antibiotics treatment in these model rodents (Bäckhed et al., 2004; Turnbaugh et al., 2006). Although similar data also exists from human studies and therefore support that translation of results from rodent models to humans in this case is possible, a recent contribution to this topic questions the rodent model to mimic metabolic disease and microbiota correlations in humans. In a study performed on 57 overweight and obese adult men, the systemic effects of two antibiotic treatments compared to placebo were investigated (Reijnders et al., 2016). Changes in microbiota composition (detected by 16S rRNA microarray analysis) were observed for specific antibiotics against gram-positive bacteria, but no differences were seen with the broad-spectrum antibiotic. On most other readouts, the authors did not see significant responses to antibiotics treatment. Hence, changes in microbiota composition did not correlate with changes in systemic functions in humans (e.g., insulin sensitivity, energy metabolism and gut permeability; Reijnders et al., 2016), which is in contrast with rodent data (Bäckhed et al., 2004; Turnbaugh et al., 2006). Reijnders et al. (2016) discuss hypotheses for these discrepancies, mentioning treatment duration and the method of antibiotic intake (capsules or in water). In addition, a possibly important difference between the described rodent studies and the human study is the fact that humans are a "wild" population. The genetic heterogeneity and environmental influences in the human population of 57 men are indeed different from the SPF bred rodents. The effects of both previous and current microbe colonization and/or infections do influence immune responses in an individual and constitute an important difference between wild and controlled laboratory populations (reviewed in Tao and Reese, 2017). Possibly, the use of a "dirty" or wild rodent population would be a more suitable choice when the aim is to investigate correlations in a highly complex biological system.

Getting the Rodent Model "Dirty"

In the continuum of approaches that can be employed to better understand protozoan parasite infection and immunity, "dirty" animals taken from the wild or laboratory animals exposed to wild cage-mates have emerged as a promising model (Maizels and Nussey, 2013). Arguing for such translational models, recent results demonstrate that inbred mice reared in SPF conditions have the immunological phenotype of neonatal humans, lacking

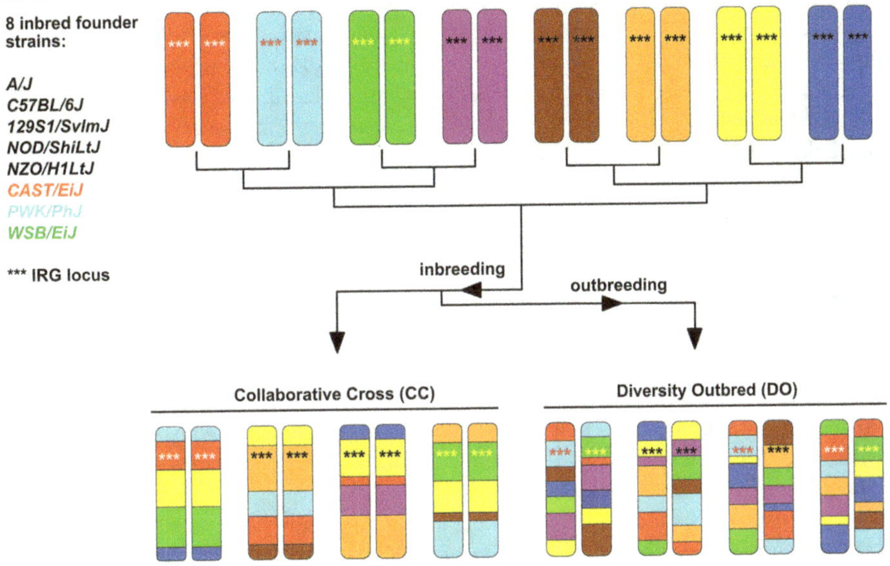

FIGURE 3 | Scheme explaining the principle of Collaborative Cross (CC) and Diversity Outbred (DO) sets (based on Chick et al., 2016). Initially, they all derived from 8 inbred founder strains. Chromosome 11 is given as an example, with the IRG locus (see section When immune responses depend on genetics – selected examples) indicated by ***. The locus is highly homogenous in 5 of the 8 founder strains (black ***) but highly polymorphic in the 3 wild-derived strains CAST, PWK, and WSB, indicated by differently colored *** in the chromosomes.

effector-differentiated and mucosally distributed memory T cells (Beura et al., 2016). In contrast, "dirty" *M. musculus* brought in from either a pet shop or from feral barn populations had immune responses more similar to adult humans, with high levels of memory CD8$^+$ cells, likely due to diverse microbial exposure and infection. These changes in both the innate and adaptive immune cellular responses and immune gene expression could also be recapitulated by co-housing previously SPF inbred mice with pet shop mice. While about 20% of the SPF mice died due to microbial infection, the immune response of those that survived also resembled adult humans within 4–8 weeks, with effector-differentiated and mucosal memory T cells. In addition, within that short time frame, co-housed mice responded similarly to the wild-caught pet shop mice in terms of infection, such that they were significantly more resistant, amongst other pathogens, to challenge with the cerebral malaria model *P. berghei* (Beura et al., 2016). Another research group has aimed to make their inbred laboratory mouse strains "dirty" by giving them sequential infection with mouse herpes virus, influenza and an intestinal helminth in order to test how this more natural pattern of exposure to pathogens may affect immune variation and expression after vaccination (Reese et al., 2016). They found that co-infected mice had different immune gene signatures, cytokine expression and antibody levels in the blood both before and after yellow fever virus vaccination compared with their SPF lab mice controls. These expression patterns resembled those of pet store-raised mice. While getting the traditional sterile laboratory mouse models dirty may pose logistical challenges, such results should encourage researchers to revisit abandoned vaccine candidates as well as to establish different routines for testing new ones.

Benefits of Using Wild Mice

Studies on dirty mice with the benefits described above still lack other aspects of natural variation that are important (Pedersen and Babayan, 2011). Thus, there is a need for wild model organisms that permit robust studies of the individual and environmental variation inherent in natural populations (including humans). Populations of wild mice vary in many of the same ways as humans (e.g., age, sex, condition, resources, parasite exposure, infection/co-infection, genetics, etc.), yet can provide a tractable, experimental system to test the importance of natural variability on infection, immunity and disease control. There are several key epidemiological features in wild mouse populations that closely resemble human infection dynamics, such as having great variation in infection probability, burdens and disease severity across individuals. Moreover, wild mice are commonly found chronically infected with parasites, suggesting either a high frequency of re-infection, long-lasting infections, or both (Pedersen and Babayan, 2011; Knowles et al., 2013).

One approach to start a research program on wild rodents is to study the traditional laboratory mouse species (*M. musculus*) in the wild (Potter et al., 1986; Viney et al., 2015). Abolins et al. (2011) found that the immune function of wild-caught *M. musculus* was significantly greater than lab-reared C57BL/6 mice, such that after immunization with a novel antigen wild-caught mice had higher concentrations of total IgG and IgE, produced higher and more avid concentrations of antigen-specific IgG, and had greater activation of T helper cells, macrophages and dendritic cells than lab-reared mice. While wild *M. musculus* offer a great parallel to lab-reared mice and can serve as comparisons for protozoan infection in the laboratory, many studies do not exhaustively sample for ectoparasites and protozoans and their true infection status is not well described. Commonly, wild *M. musculus* are reported to be infected with mainly ectoparasites and a few nematodes (mostly *Syphacia spp.* pinworms; e.g., Weldon et al., 2015); however there are records of natural infections with *Giardia muris*, *Spironucleus muris*, and *Encephalitozoon cuniculi* (Baker, 1998), *Eimeria* spp. (Ball and Lewis, 1984), *Cryptosporidium* spp. (Backhans et al., 2013), and *T. gondii* (Kijlstra et al., 2008).

Rodents beyond Wild Mice Are Natural Hosts of a Wide Variety of Protozoa

Beyond *M. musculus,* there are several well-studied wild rodents that are both commonly infected with protozoan parasites and also offer tractable wild model systems for both longitudinal and experimental studies of infection and immunity. In North America, much work has focused on white-footed mice and deer mice (*Peromyscus leucopus* and *P. maniculatus*), both because they are very abundant and widespread, but also because they are competent reservoirs of important emerging zoonotic pathogens (e.g., Hantavirus and *Borrelia* spp.; Bedford and Hoekstra, 2015). In Europe, wood mice (*Apodemus sylvaticus*; e.g., Knowles et al., 2013), yellow-necked mice (*A. flavicollis*; e.g., Ferrari et al., 2004), bank voles (*Myodes glareolus*; e.g., Withenshaw et al., 2016), and field voles (*M. agrestis;* Smith et al., 2005; Turner et al., 2014) have been commonly studied as models for wild host-pathogen interactions and are all regularly infected with protozoan parasites. For example, wild populations of *A. sylvaticus* in the United Kingdom have been found to be infected with *C. parvum*, *C. muris* (Chalmers et al., 1997); > five species of *Eimeria* (Ball and Lewis, 1984; Higgs and Nowell, 2000); *Babesia* sp. and *Hepatozoon* sp. (Turner, 1986); two species of *Trypanosoma* (Noyes et al., 2002), *Frenkelia microti* (Svobodova et al., 2004) and *T. gondii* (Jackson and Siim, 1986). It is very likely that this list is a far from exhaustive.

The benefits of using wild rodent-parasite models to better understand protozoan infection dynamics include the ability to: (i) conduct longitudinal field experiments which follow marked individuals throughout their lives while measuring infection status, physiological and demographic metrics (Knowles et al., 2013; Pedersen and Antonovics, 2013; Turner et al., 2014), and crucially (ii) test the efficacy of disease control interventions at the individual and population level in an ecologically relevant environment (Knowles et al., 2013; Pedersen and Antonovics, 2013). For example, in a population of wild field voles (*M. agrestis*) the researchers repeatedly treated one population with a standard insecticide to reduce the prevalence of fleas, and in turn, found that this reduced the prevalence of vector-transmitted *Trypanosoma* spp. by ~33% (Smith et al., 2005). In addition, in experimental field studies of both *P. maniculatus* and *P. leucopus* in the US, and *A. sylvaticus* in the UK, anthelmintic treatment was used to reduce nematode burdens within specific, marked animals. The treatment was found to unexpectedly increase the prevalence and/or intensity of co-infecting *Eimeria* spp. suggesting strong antagonistic within-host interactions between a worm and a protozoon (Knowles et al., 2013; Pedersen and Antonovics, 2013).

Research on wild rodents benefit from the extensive immunological toolbox developed in lab mice (Pedersen and Babayan, 2011). In wild populations of *A. sylvaticus*, innate immune responsiveness, as measured by splenocyte tumor necrosis factor responses to toll-like receptor (TLR) agonists, was found to correlate positively with *Eimeria* spp. fecal oocysts counts, most strongly with receptors TLR7 and TLR9 (Jackson et al., 2009). More recently, the availability of genomes for wild rodents has enabled the ability to measure immunological expression in wild rodent populations. A recent investigation of wild field voles measured expression of a wide range of innate and adaptive responses by cultured and stimulated splenocytes. Importantly, repeated measures from peripheral blood samples of IFN-y, Gata3 and IL-10 expression enabled the authors to test for correlations with specific parasite infections (Jackson et al., 2014). Taken together, wild rodents reach large sample sizes, can be repeatedly recaptured using live traps, marked and followed before and after interventions, and are commonly infected with protozoan parasites. Studying the dynamics of protozoan infections in wild rodents is a valuable resource for expanding our knowledge in infection biology and might thus be a useful addition for translational research on human protozoan infections.

A Case for Going Wild: Do *T. gondii*-Induced Behavioral Changes Exist in Natural Habitats?

How relevant are findings which suggest parasite influences on lab mouse behavior when performed in lab environments? The so-called "manipulation hypothesis" of a *T. gondii* infection in rodents suggests that infection leads to subsequent changes in the animal's behavior, with one consequence being that they lose their fear for feline odor (e.g., fur or urine). Cats and other felids are the only definite hosts where sexual reproduction of *T. gondii* can take place. Therefore, at first sight it makes sense that such "manipulated" infected rodents would experience more fatal encounters with a cat than non-infected ones, thereby increase the chance for *T. gondii* to sexually reproduce with another strain from a second subsequent infected prey.

The advantage or necessity of this scenario for parasite sexual reproduction in the wild has been called into question (Worth et al., 2013), but here we focus on the fact that all reported experiments were done exclusively in lab animals (Worth et al., 2014). At first sight this might not seem problematic since *M. musculus* and *T. gondii* naturally occur together. However, it is well known, but not necessarily well appreciated, that behavioral studies of rodents can be influenced by the methods used, housing conditions, genetic background and whether they are lab or wild-derived animals (Wolff, 2003; Beckers et al., 2009; Fonio et al., 2012; Chalfin et al., 2014; Newman et al., 2015). Even differences in the microbiota can have profound effects (Hsiao et al., 2013; see section Microbiota as a General Confounder for Rodent Experiments). Moreover, lab mice have been selected for decades for docile behavior, while wild mice show anxious behavior under natural conditions (Latham and Mason, 2004;

Yoshiki and Moriwaki, 2006; Fonio et al., 2012; Chalfin et al., 2014).

How well does the manipulation hypothesis apply to the natural situation of predator (cat) and prey (*T. gondii*-infected mouse or rat)? Ecological observations might explain some of the observed discrepancies, i.e., no behavioral differences were found in one study but were indeed found in another (Worth et al., 2014). Several studies indicate that predation risk of wild or wild-derived small rodents depends more on habitat characteristics (e.g., ability to hide) than on whether the rodent senses a present predator by its odor or even by its physical presence (Orrock, 2004; Powell and Banks, 2004; Verdolin, 2006). Aversive responses to predator odor can also differ dramatically between individual lab rats (Hogg and File, 1994) and, importantly, between lab mice and wild mice (Coulston et al., 1993; Hebb et al., 2004). Thus, experiments with "fearless" lab mice in non-natural terrains may not accurately reflect the behavioral changes induced by a parasite like *T. gondii* under natural conditions.

EXPERIMENTAL CHALLENGES AND AVAILABLE RESOURCES FOR NON-TRADITIONAL RODENT MODELS

Having provided a number of reasons for considering wild rodents as alternatives, we will briefly address the experimental challenges. Approaching studies on non-model rodents is demanding but the toolbox has improved significantly compared to a decade ago (Pedersen and Babayan, 2011; Zimmerman et al., 2014). Method development in the fields of genomics, transcriptomics and proteomics together with increasing affordability provide better prerequisites for research on non-model alternatives (Jackson, 2015). Next-generation sequencing has led to constantly expanding genomic data. This is demonstrated by the nearly 4,000 eukaryotic genomes available on NCBI Genome (February, 2017) as compared to around 650 in 2013 (Ellegren, 2014).

Database Resources for Wild Rodent Genomes

Any resources available for lab mice are to varying extents useful starting-points for work on wild rodents. The Mouse Genomes Project is the biggest collection of genomic data on rodents (Table S1). Currently it consists of whole-genome assemblages and strain-specific gene annotations of 16 inbred and wild-derived mouse strains. A goal of this project is the classification of sequence variations between common laboratory strains compared to the reference strain C57BL/6J (Adams et al., 2015; Doran et al., 2016). All sequence reads, variants and assemblages can be useful references for highly recombinant outbred strains (Nicod et al., 2016) or wild rodent genomes. There are also increasing numbers of genomes and/or transcriptomes available for wild rodents (e.g., *A. sylvaticus*, *M. glareolus*, and *M. agrestis*; see **Figure 4**), with most of them being "work-in-progress" considering assemblage status and annotations (for details see Table S1 and links therein). The quality and coverage of these genomes vary and there is for instance no clear definition of a required coverage for referring to DNA sequences as a "genome" (Ellegren, 2014). However, they do provide a good source for homology searches for a gene-of-interest, primer design for PCR applications etc. Naturally, purification of DNA, RNA or proteins and functional PCR protocols may require protocol optimization when applied to new species but otherwise follow established schemes. Some database resources and other initiatives to promote such development are discussed below and summarized in Table S1.

While reference genomes are not a prerequisite for some studies they are, for instance, indispensable as a template in quantitative gene expression studies with high-throughput sequencing of RNA (RNA-seq; Vijay et al., 2013). However, bioinformatics pipelines are often developed for established model organisms and may require considerable adjustments for non-model organisms (Ekblom and Wolf, 2014). Although such limitations may hamper the speed of omics applications to non-model organisms, genomes of non-model rodents will serve as excellent resources for developing species-specific tools to measure, for example, expression of immunological responses to infection. Readers that are interested in considering genome sequencing for their own non-model organism are referred to a recent step-by-step introduction of the required workflows (Ekblom and Wolf, 2014) and to the Generic Model Organism Database (GMOD) initiative, which provides software tools and data models for subsequent representation of their annotated genomes and curated data of their model organism (O'Connor et al., 2008).

Transcriptomes Do Not Necessarily Predict Protein Levels

It should be emphasized that genomic and transcriptomic data, as valuable as they are, provide only indirect means with regards to proteomic output in response to infection. In general, the relationship between the concentration of a given transcript and its encoded protein(s) is difficult to predict just by RNA-seq or qPCR data (Liu et al., 2016). For example, Chick et al. (2016) used the currently most sensitive technology for abundance determination of both transcripts and proteins and applied them to CC and DO mice (see section Humanized Mice: Rodents Which Mimic the Human Immune System and **Figure 3**). They showed that for many genes the levels of the corresponding protein varied substantially in genetically divergent mice. Sex also influenced protein amounts within a given species (Chick et al., 2016). These recent data emphasize the importance of quantitative proteomic measures in general to complement or validate transcriptomic data, but also highlight that genetic diversity within mice influences the results.

Antibodies, Cytokines, and Protein Quantification

Antibody-based assays are still the cornerstone for qualitative and quantitative determination of immunological parameters like chemokines or cytokines but also other proteins of interest. Numerous well-defined and evaluated reagents exist for lab mice and rats but their usefulness for wild rodents with respect to

Species	Genome ID	Common name
Apodemus sylvaticus	40375	European woodmouse
Castor canadensis	9723	American beaver
Cavia aperea	31959	Brazilian guinea pig
Cavia porcellus	231	domestic guinea pig
Chinchilla lanigera	10466	long-tailed chinchilla
Cricetulus griseus	2791	Chinese hamster
Dipodomys ordii	772	Ord's kangaroo rat
Ellobius lutescens	45549	Transcaucasian mole vole
Ellobius talpinus	45550	Northern mole vole
Fukomys damarensis	16808	Damara mole-rat
Heterocephalus glaber	6965	naked mole-rat
Ictidomys tridecemlineatus	472	thirteen-lined ground squirrel
Jaculus jaculus	10766	lesser Egyptian jerboa
Marmota marmota	36409	European marmot
Mesocricetus auratus	11998	golden hamster
Microtus agrestis	40376	short-tailed field vole
Microtus ochrogaster	10848	prairie vole
Mus musculus	52	house mouse
Mus spretus	12818	western wild mouse
Myodes glareolus	12837	Bank vole
Nannospalax galili	12743	Upper Galilee mountains blind mole rat
Neotoma lepida	16657	desert woodrat
Octodon degus	11848	degu
Peromyscus maniculatus	11397	North American deer mouse
Phodopus sungorus	13189	Djungarian hamster
Rattus norvegicus	73	Norway rat

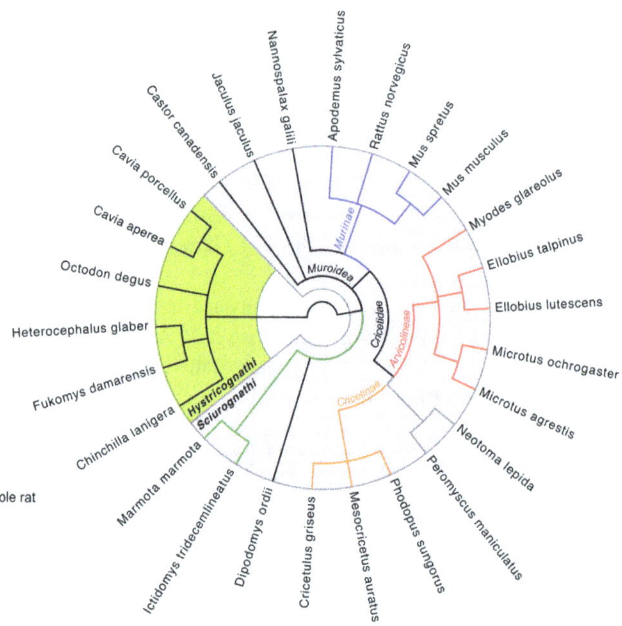

FIGURE 4 | Names of rodents (with links in Table S2 to their available genome sequences at NCBI), together with their phylogenetic relationship (tree computed at https://www.ncbi.nlm.nih.gov/Taxonomy/CommonTree/wwwcmt.cgi).

cross-reactivity is largely unexplored and presumably quite low in many cases. The same applies to immunological effector molecules like cytokines, for which IFN-γ is a good example. IFN-γ is known to be highly species-specific, which made the production of a recombinant protein active with *M. glareolus* or *Microtus* spp. cell lines a prerequisite (Torelli et al, in preparation). Starting from genomic sequences and going to the purification of active recombinant protein from *E. coli* required less than half a year and will now provide the scientific community with this important cytokine.

Developing antibodies that (cross)react with wild rodents is certainly much more time and resource-consuming, but feasible. An alternative could be parallel (or selective) reaction monitoring (PRM, SRM) which are mass spectrometry-based methods that quantify unique, specific peptide sequences of a given protein (Rauniyar, 2015; Bourmaud et al., 2016). The method was recently used to quantify several cytokines and chemokines from human cells (Muqaku et al., 2015). The appealing aspect of this admittedly demanding method lies in the fact that by carefully selecting peptide sequences conserved between rodent species, they could be used across those species at relatively low cost, once established (Hüttenhain et al., 2009). Ideally, it could thus be regarded as a community effort. A database with corresponding peptides from human and mouse proteomes does exist (see Table S1) and constitutes a useful starting point (Peptide Atlas; Deutsch et al., 2008).

Given the availability of published genomic and transcriptomic data of wild rodent species (Table S2), work similar to the studies mentioned will hopefully expand the current toolbox for non-model rodents in the near future. A dedicated web site with information on such shared resources, but also on cross-reacting reagents such as polyclonal or monoclonal antibodies or commercial cytokines and other proteins tested in non-model rodents, although not yet existing, would greatly boost the interest and ease of use of non-model organisms in future studies.

CONCLUDING REMARKS

We are convinced that rodents will continue to be important translational models for research on protozoan parasites, given that appropriate considerations are made during experimental design. By providing some examples where translation from rodent disease models to human medicine has failed, and, more importantly, by pointing at identified reasons for inconclusive or misleading data, we wish to inspire readers to consider more than the most convenient model for future experiments. Making use of rich database-resources that are available for investigating, e.g., expected phenotypes of mice, will aid in this respect. We also hope that readers are encouraged to consider and control for various confounders such as microbiota influences and housing conditions in their experimental designs. While wild models pose some challenges, we have pointed out that these rodents possess distinct advantages with regards to genetic variability and environmental exposures that can reflect immunological responses to parasites in humans more adequately than current lab models. The increasing availability of genome and transcriptome datasets as well as improved methods for quantitative proteomics already show their impact on wild infection biology.

AUTHOR CONTRIBUTIONS

TE, FT, CK, AP, and FS contributed to the text and approved its final version.

FUNDING

TE and FT are supported by and TE, FT, CK, and FS are members of the Research Training Group 2046 "Parasite Infections: From Experimental Models to Natural Systems," funded by the Deutsche Forschungsgemeinschaft. Own cited work from FS and CK was supported by the Robert Koch Institute. AP is supported by a Chancellors Fellowship from the University of Edinburgh, and her cited work was supported by a NERC grant (NE/G006830/1 and NE/G007349/1) and a Wellcome Trust Centre for Infection, Immunity and Evolution Advanced Fellowship (no. 095831).

ACKNOWLEDGMENTS

The authors thank Toni Aebischer and Ankur Midha for valuable comments and suggestions on the manuscript.

REFERENCES

Abolins, S. R., Pocock, M. J., Hafalla, J. C., Riley, E. M., and Viney, M. E. (2011). Measures of immune function of wild mice, Mus musculus. *Mol. Ecol.* 20, 881–892. doi: 10.1111/j.1365-294X.2010.04910.x

Adam, E., Pierrot, C., Lafitte, S., Godin, C., Saoudi, A., Capron, M., et al. (2003). The age-related resistance of rats to Plasmodium berghei infection is associated with differential cellular and humoral immune responses. *Int. J. Parasitol.* 33, 1067–1078. doi: 10.1016/s0020-7519(03)00176-0

Adams, D. J., Doran, A. G., Lilue, J., and Keane, T. M. (2015). The Mouse Genomes Project: a repository of inbred laboratory mouse strain genomes. *Mamm. Genome* 26, 403–412. doi: 10.1007/s00335-015-9579-6

Akhoundi, M., Kuhls, K., Cannet, A., Votypka, J., Marty, P., Delaunay, P., et al. (2016). A historical overview of the classification, evolution, and dispersion of Leishmania parasites and sandflies. *PLoS Negl. Trop. Dis.* 10:e0004349. doi: 10.1371/journal.pntd.0004349

Alfred, J., and Baldwin, I. T. (2015). The natural history of model organisms: new opportunities at the wild frontier. *Elife* 4:e06956. doi: 10.7554/eLife.06956

Andrews, K. T., Fisher, G., and Skinner-Adams, T. S. (2014). Drug repurposing and human parasitic protozoan diseases. *Int. J. Parasitol. Drugs Drug Resist.* 4, 95–111. doi: 10.1016/j.ijpddr.2014.02.002

Ankarklev, J., Jerlstrom-Hultqvist, J., Ringqvist, E., Troell, K., and Svard, S. G. (2010). Behind the smile: cell biology and disease mechanisms of Giardia species. *Nat. Rev. Microbiol.* 8, 413–422. doi: 10.1038/nrmicro2317

Ankeny, R. A., and Leonelli, S. (2011). What's so special about model organisms? *Stud. Hist. Phil. Sci.* 42, 313–323. doi: 10.2307/40985626

Antoine-Moussiaux, N., Magez, S., and Desmecht, D. (2008). Contributions of experimental mouse models to the understanding of African trypanosomiasis. *Trends Parasitol.* 24, 411–418. doi: 10.1016/j.pt.2008.05.010

Aplenc, R., and Lange, B. (2004). Pharmacogenetic determinants of outcome in acute lymphoblastic leukaemia. *Br. J. Haematol.* 125, 421–434. doi: 10.1111/j.1365-2141.2004.04932.x

Ayadi, A., Ferrand, G., Cruz, I. G. D., and Warot, X. (2011). Mouse breeding and colony management. *Curr. Protoc. Mouse Biol.* 1, 239–264. doi: 10.1002/9780470942390.mo100214

Backhans, A., Jacobson, M., Hansson, I., Lebbad, M., Lambertz, S. T., Gammelgard, E., et al. (2013). Occurrence of pathogens in wild rodents caught on Swedish pig and chicken farms. *Epidemiol. Infect.* 141, 1885–1891. doi: 10.1017/s0950268812002609

Bäckhed, F., Ding, H., Wang, T., Hooper, L. V., Koh, G. Y., Nagy, A., et al. (2004). The gut microbiota as an environmental factor that regulates fat storage. *Proc. Natl. Acad. Sci. U.S.A.* 101, 15718–15723. doi: 10.1073/pnas.0407076101

Baker, D. G. (1998). Natural pathogens of laboratory mice, rats, and rabbits and their effects on research. *Clin. Microbiol. Rev.* 11, 231–266.

Ball, S. J., and Lewis, D. C. (1984). Eimeria (Protozoa: Coccidia) in wild populations of some British rodents. *J. Zool.* 202, 373–381. doi: 10.1111/j.1469-7998.1984.tb05089.x

Barash, N. R., Maloney, J. G., Singer, S., and Dawson, S. C. (2016). Giardia alters commensal microbial diversity throughout the murine gut. *bioRxiv*. doi: 10.1101/087122

Bayne, K., and Würbel, H. (2012). "Mouse enrichment," in *The Laboratory Mouse, 2nd Edn.*, ed H. J. Hedrich (Boston, MA: Academic Press), 547–566.

Beck, J. A., Lloyd, S., Hafezparast, M., Lennon-Pierce, M., Eppig, J. T., Festing, M. F., et al. (2000). Genealogies of mouse inbred strains. *Nat. Genet.* 24, 23–25. doi: 10.1038/71641

Beckers, J., Wurst, W., and de Angelis, M. H. (2009). Towards better mouse models: enhanced genotypes, systemic phenotyping and envirotype modelling. *Nat. Rev. Genet.* 10, 371–380. doi: 10.1038/nrg2578

Bedford, N. L., and Hoekstra, H. E. (2015). Peromyscus mice as a model for studying natural variation. *Elife* 4:e06813. doi: 10.7554/eLife.06813

Bennett, B. J., Farber, C. R., Orozco, L., Kang, H. M., Ghazalpour, A., Siemers, N., et al. (2010). A high-resolution association mapping panel for the dissection of complex traits in mice. *Genome Res.* 20, 281–290. doi: 10.1101/gr.099234.109

Bernin, H., and Lotter, H. (2014). Sex bias in the outcome of human tropical infectious diseases: influence of steroid hormones. *J. Infect. Dis.* 209(Suppl. 3), S107–S113. doi: 10.1093/infdis/jit610

Beura, L. K., Hamilton, S. E., Bi, K., Schenkel, J. M., Odumade, O. A., Casey, K. A., et al. (2016). Normalizing the environment recapitulates adult human immune traits in laboratory mice. *Nature* 532, 512–516. doi: 10.1038/nature17655

Bhattacharya, P., Dey, R., Dagur, P. K., Joshi, A. B., Ismail, N., Gannavaram, S., et al. (2016). Live attenuated Leishmania donovani centrin knock out parasites generate non-inferior protective immune response in aged mice against visceral leishmaniasis. *PLoS Negl. Trop. Dis.* 10:e0004963. doi: 10.1371/journal.pntd.0004963

Bolker, J. (2012). Model organisms: there's more to life than rats and flies. *Nature* 491, 31–33. doi: 10.1038/491031a

Borody, T. J., and Khoruts, A. (2012). Fecal microbiota transplantation and emerging applications. *Nat. Rev. Gastroenterol. Hepatol.* 9, 88–96. doi: 10.1038/nrgastro.2011.244

Bourmaud, A., Gallien, S., and Domon, B. (2016). Parallel reaction monitoring using quadrupole-Orbitrap mass spectrometer: principle and applications. *Proteomics* 16, 2146–2159. doi: 10.1002/pmic.201500543

Brehm, M. A., Jouvet, N., Greiner, D. L., and Shultz, L. D. (2013). Humanized mice for the study of infectious diseases. *Curr. Opin. Immunol.* 25, 428–435. doi: 10.1016/j.coi.2013.05.012

Buer, J., and Balling, R. (2003). Mice, microbes and models of infection. *Nat. Rev. Genet.* 4, 195–205. doi: 10.1038/nrg1019

Chalfin, L., Dayan, M., Levy, D. R., Austad, S. N., Miller, R. A., Iraqi, F. A., et al. (2014). Mapping ecologically relevant social behaviours by gene knockout in wild mice. *Nat. Commun.* 5, 4569. doi: 10.1038/ncomms5569

Chalmers, R. M., Sturdee, A. P., Bull, S. A., Miller, A., and Wright, S. E. (1997). The prevalence of Cryptosporidium parvum and C. muris in Mus domesticus, Apodemus sylvaticus and Clethrionomys glareolus in an agricultural system. *Parasitol. Res.* 83, 478–482. doi: 10.1007/s004360050283

Checkley, W., White, A. C. Jr., Jaganath, D., Arrowood, M. J., Chalmers, R. M., Chen, X. M., et al. (2015). A review of the global burden, novel diagnostics, therapeutics, and vaccine targets for cryptosporidium. *Lancet Infect. Dis.* 15, 85–94. doi: 10.1016/s1473-3099(14)70772-8

Chia, R., Achilli, F., Festing, M. F. W., and Fisher, E. M. C. (2005). The origins and uses of mouse outbred stocks. *Nat. Genet.* 37, 1181–1186. doi: 10.1038/ng1665

Chick, J. M., Munger, S. C., Simecek, P., Huttlin, E. L., Choi, K., Gatti, D. M., et al. (2016). Defining the consequences of genetic variation on a proteome-wide scale. *Nature* 534, 500–505. doi: 10.1038/nature18270

Chow, C. Y. (2016). Bringing genetic background into focus. *Nat. Rev. Genet.* 17, 63–64. doi: 10.1038/nrg.2015.9

Churchill, G. A., Airey, D. C., Allayee, H., Angel, J. M., Attie, A. D., Beatty, J., et al. (2004). The Collaborative Cross, a community resource for the genetic analysis of complex traits. *Nat. Genet.* 36, 1133–1137. doi: 10.1038/ng1104-1133

Churchill, G. A., Gatti, D. M., Munger, S. C., and Svenson, K. L. (2012). The Diversity Outbred mouse population. *Mamm. Genome* 23, 713–718. doi: 10.1007/s00335-012-9414-2

Cirelli, K. M., Gorfu, G., Hassan, M. A., Printz, M., Crown, D., Leppla, S. H., et al. (2014). Inflammasome sensor NLRP1 controls rat macrophage susceptibility to Toxoplasma gondii. *PLoS Pathog.* 10:e1003927. doi: 10.1371/journal.ppat.1003927

Clayton, J. A., and Collins, F. S. (2014). Policy: NIH to balance sex in cell and animal studies. *Nature* 509, 282–283. doi: 10.1038/509282a

Clevers, H. (2016). Modeling development and disease with organoids. *Cell* 165, 1586–1597. doi: 10.1016/j.cell.2016.05.082

Conn, P. M. (2008). *Sourcebook of Models for Biomedical Research.* Totowa, NJ: Humana Press.

Coulston, S., Stoddart, D. M., and Crump, D. R. (1993). Use of predator odors to protect chick-peas from predation by laboratory and wild mice. *J. Chem. Ecol.* 19, 607–612. doi: 10.1007/bf00984995

Couzin-Frankel, J. (2013). When mice mislead. *Science* 342, 922–925. doi: 10.1126/science.342.6161.922

Cowman, A. F., Healer, J., Marapana, D., and Marsh, K. (2016). Malaria: biology and disease. *Cell* 167, 610–624. doi: 10.1016/j.cell.2016.07.055

Craig, A. G., Grau, G. E., Janse, C., Kazura, J. W., Milner, D., Barnwell, J. W., et al. (2012). The role of animal models for research on severe malaria. *PLoS Pathog.* 8:e1002401. doi: 10.1371/journal.ppat.1002401

Denny, J. E., Powell, W. L., and Schmidt, N. W. (2016). Local and long-distance calling: conversations between the gut microbiota and intra- and extra-gastrointestinal tract infections. *Front. Cell. Infect. Microbiol.* 6:41. doi: 10.3389/fcimb.2016.00041

Deutsch, E. W., Lam, H., and Aebersold, R. (2008). PeptideAtlas: a resource for target selection for emerging targeted proteomics workflows. *EMBO Rep.* 9, 429–434. doi: 10.1038/embor.2008.56

Dietrich, M. R., Ankeny, R. A., and Chen, P. M. (2014). Publication trends in model organism research. *Genetics* 198, 787–794. doi: 10.1534/genetics.114.169714

Doran, A. G., Wong, K., Flint, J., Adams, D. J., Hunter, K. W., and Keane, T. M. (2016). Deep genome sequencing and variation analysis of 13 inbred mouse strains defines candidate phenotypic alleles, private variation and homozygous truncating mutations. *Genome Biol.* 17, 167. doi: 10.1186/s13059-016-1024-y

Douam, F., Gaska, J. M., Winer, B. Y., Ding, Q., von Schaewen, M., and Ploss, A. (2015). Genetic dissection of the host tropism of human-tropic pathogens. *Annu. Rev. Genet.* 49, 21–45. doi: 10.1146/annurev-genet-112414-054823

Durrant, C., Tayem, H., Yalcin, B., Cleak, J., Goodstadt, L., de Villena, F. P., et al. (2011). Collaborative Cross mice and their power to map host susceptibility to Aspergillus fumigatus infection. *Genome Res.* 21, 1239–1248. doi: 10.1101/gr.118786.110

Eastwood, D., Findlay, L., Poole, S., Bird, C., Wadhwa, M., Moore, M., et al. (2010). Monoclonal antibody TGN1412 trial failure explained by species differences in CD28 expression on $CD4^+$ effector memory T-cells. *Br. J. Pharmacol.* 161, 512–526. doi: 10.1111/j.1476-5381.2010.00922.x

Ekblom, R., and Wolf, J. B. W. (2014). A field guide to whole-genome sequencing, assembly and annotation. *Evol. Appl.* 7, 1026–1042. doi: 10.1111/eva.12178

Ellegren, H. (2014). Genome sequencing and population genomics in non-model organisms. *Trends Ecol. Evol.* 29, 51–63. doi: 10.1016/j.tree.2013.09.008

Ericsson, A. C., Davis, J. W., Spollen, W., Bivens, N., Givan, S., Hagan, C. E., et al. (2015). Effects of vendor and genetic background on the composition of the fecal microbiota of inbred mice. *PLoS ONE* 10:e0116704. doi: 10.1371/journal.pone.0116704

Ernst, W. (2016). Humanized mice in infectious diseases. *Comp. Immunol. Microbiol. Infect. Dis.* 49, 29–38. doi: 10.1016/j.cimid.2016.08.006

Ewald, S. E., Chavarria-Smith, J., and Boothroyd, J. C. (2014). NLRP1 is an inflammasome sensor for Toxoplasma gondii. *Infect. Immun.* 82, 460–468. doi: 10.1128/iai.01170-13

Ferrari, N., Cattadori, I. M., Nespereira, J., Rizzoli, A., and Hudson, P. J. (2004). The role of host sex in parasite dynamics: field experiments on the yellow-necked mouse Apodemus flavicollis. *Ecol. Lett.* 7, 88–94. doi: 10.1046/j.1461-0248.2003.00552.x

Ferris, M. T., Aylor, D. L., Bottomly, D., Whitmore, A. C., Aicher, L. D., Bell, T. A., et al. (2013). Modeling host genetic regulation of influenza pathogenesis in the collaborative cross. *PLoS Pathog.* 9:e1003196. doi: 10.1371/journal.ppat.1003196

Festing, M., and Fisher, E. (2000). Mighty mice - Clarence Little's brainwave gave biomedical researchers their best friend. *Nature* 404, 815–815. doi: 10.1038/35009167

Festing, M. F. W. (2014). Evidence should trump intuition by preferring inbred strains to outbred stocks in preclinical research. *ILAR J.* 55, 399–404. doi: 10.1093/ilar/ilu036

Fiebiger, U., Bereswill, S., and Heimesaat, M. M. (2016). Dissecting the interplay between intestinal microbiota and host immunity in health and disease: lessons learned from germfree and gnotobiotic animal models. *Eur. J. Microbiol. Immunol.* 6, 253–271. doi: 10.1556/1886.2016.00036

Fitzpatrick, J. L. (2013). Global food security: the impact of veterinary parasites and parasitologists. *Vet. Parasitol.* 195, 233–248. doi: 10.1016/j.vetpar.2013.04.005

Fletcher, S. M., Stark, D., Harkness, J., and Ellis, J. (2012). Enteric protozoa in the developed world: a public health perspective. *Clin. Microbiol. Rev.* 25, 420–449. doi: 10.1128/cmr.05038-11

Flórez-Vargas, O., Brass, A., Karystianis, G., and Bramhall, M. (2016). Bias in the reporting of sex and age in biomedical research on mouse models. *Elife* 5:e13615. doi: 10.7554/eLife.13615

Fonio, E., Golani, I., and Benjamini, Y. (2012). Measuring behavior of animal models: faults and remedies. *Nat. Methods* 9, 1167–1170. doi: 10.1038/nmeth.2252

Foster, J. A., and McVey Neufeld, K. A. (2013). Gut-brain axis: how the microbiome influences anxiety and depression. *Trends Neurosci.* 36, 305–312. doi: 10.1016/j.tins.2013.01.005

Gacias, M., Gaspari, S., Santos, P. M. G., Tamburini, S., Andrade, M., Zang, F., et al. (2016). Microbiota-driven transcriptional changes in prefrontal cortex override genetic differences in social behavior. *Elife* 5:e13442. doi: 10.7554/eLife.13442

Garenne, M. (2015). Demographic evidence of sex differences in vulnerability to infectious diseases. *J. Infect. Dis.* 211, 331–332. doi: 10.1093/infdis/jiu448

German Federal Ministry of Food and Agriculture (2011). *Versuchstierzahlen 2011.* Available online at: http://www.bmel.de/DE/Tier/Tierschutz/_texte/TierschutzTierforschung.html?docId=8596776#doc8596776bodyText11

Giroud, C., Ottones, F., Coustou, V., Dacheux, D., Biteau, N., Miezan, B., et al. (2009). Murine models for Trypanosoma brucei gambiense disease progression—from silent to chronic infections and early brain tropism. *PLoS Negl. Trop. Dis.* 3:e509. doi: 10.1371/journal.pntd.0000509

Good, M. F., Hawkes, M. T., and Yanow, S. K. (2015). Humanized mouse models to study cell-mediated immune responses to liver-stage malaria vaccines. *Trends Parasitol.* 31, 583–594. doi: 10.1016/j.pt.2015.06.008

Gordon, S. (2007). The macrophage: past, present and future. *Eur. J. Immunol.* 37(Suppl. 1), S9–S17. doi: 10.1002/eji.200737638

Gralinski, L. E., Ferris, M. T., Aylor, D. L., Whitmore, A. C., Green, R., Frieman, M. B., et al. (2015). Genome wide identification of SARS-CoV susceptibility loci using the Collaborative Cross. *PLoS Genet.* 11:e1005504. doi: 10.1371/journal.pgen.1005504

Grubb, S. C., Bult, C. J., and Bogue, M. A. (2014). Mouse phenome database. *Nucleic Acids Res.* 42, D825–D834. doi: 10.1093/nar/gkt1159

Guénet, J. L., Benavides, F., and Panthier, J. J. (2015). "The different categories of genetically standardized populations of laboratory mice," in *Genetics of the Mouse,* eds J. L. Guénet, F. Benavides, J. J. Panthier, and X. Montagutelli (Berlin Heidelberg: Springer-Verlag), 319–359.

Guenet, J. L., and Bonhomme, F. (2003). Wild mice: an ever-increasing contribution to a popular mammalian model. *Trends Genet.* 19, 24–31. doi: 10.1016/S0168-9525(02)00007-0

Hau, J. (2008). "Animal models for human diseases: an overview," in *Sourcebook of Models for Biomedical Research,* ed P. M. Conn (Totowa, NJ: Humana Press), 3–8.

Hebb, A. L., Zacharko, R. M., Gauthier, M., Trudel, F., Laforest, S., and Drolet, G. (2004). Brief exposure to predator odor and resultant anxiety enhances mesocorticolimbic activity and enkephalin expression in CD-1 mice. *Eur. J. Neurosci.* 20, 2415–2429. doi: 10.1111/j.1460-9568.2004.03704.x

Hedrich, H. J. (2012). *The Laboratory Mouse, 2nd Edn.* Boston, MA: Academic Press.

Hedrich, H. J., and Nicklas, W. (2012). "Housing and Maintenance," in *The Laboratory Mouse, 2nd Edn.*, ed H. J. Hedrich (Boston, MA: Academic Press), 521–545.

Higgs, S., and Nowell, F. (2000). Population biology of Eimeria (Protozoa: Apicomplexa) in Apodemus sylvaticus: a capture/recapture study. *Parasitology* 120(Pt 4), 355–363. doi: 10.1017/S0031182099005545

Hilbert, T., Steinhagen, F., Senzig, S., Cramer, N., Bekeredjian-Ding, I., Parcina, M., et al. (2017). Vendor effects on murine gut microbiota influence experimental abdominal sepsis. *J. Surg. Res.* 211, 126–136. doi: 10.1016/j.jss.2016.12.008

Hogg, S., and File, S. E. (1994). Responders and nonresponders to cat odor do not differ in other tests of anxiety. *Pharmacol. Biochem. Behav.* 49, 219–222.

Hoy, Y. E., Bik, E. M., Lawley, T. D., Holmes, S. P., Monack, D. M., Theriot, J. A., et al. (2015). Variation in taxonomic composition of the fecal microbiota in an inbred mouse strain across individuals and time. *PLoS ONE* 10:e0142825. doi: 10.1371/journal.pone.0142825

Hsiao, E. Y., McBride, S. W., Hsien, S., Sharon, G., Hyde, E. R., McCue, T., et al. (2013). Microbiota modulate behavioral and physiological abnormalities associated with neurodevelopmental disorders. *Cell* 155, 1451–1463. doi: 10.1016/j.cell.2013.11.024

Hufeldt, M. R., Nielsen, D. S., Vogensen, F. K., Midtvedt, T., and Hansen, A. K. (2010). Variation in the gut microbiota of laboratory mice is related to both genetic and environmental factors. *Comp. Med.* 60, 336–342.

Hunig, T. (2016). The rise and fall of the CD28 superagonist TGN1412 and its return as TAB08: a personal account. *FEBS J.* 283, 3325–3334. doi: 10.1111/febs.13754

Hunter, P. (2008). The paradox of model organisms - The use of model organisms in research will continue despite their shortcomings. *EMBO Rep.* 9, 717–720. doi: 10.1038/embor.2008.142

Hüttenhain, R., Malmström, J., Picotti, P., and Aebersold, R. (2009). Perspectives of targeted mass spectrometry for protein biomarker verification. *Curr. Opin. Chem. Biol.* 13, 518–525. doi: 10.1016/j.cbpa.2009.09.014

Hu, X., Chang, N., Wang, X., Zhou, F., Zhou, X., Zhu, X., et al. (2013). Heritable gene-targeting with gRNA/Cas9 in rats. *Cell Res.* 23, 1322–1325. doi: 10.1038/cr.2013.141

Jackson, J. A. (2015). Immunology in wild nonmodel rodents: an ecological context for studies of health and disease. *Parasite Immunol.* 37, 220–232. doi: 10.1111/pim.12180

Jackson, J. A., Friberg, I. M., Bolch, L., Lowe, A., Ralli, C., Harris, P. D., et al. (2009). Immunomodulatory parasites and toll-like receptor-mediated tumour necrosis factor alpha responsiveness in wild mammals. *BMC Biol.* 7:16. doi: 10.1186/1741-7007-7-16

Jackson, J. A., Hall, A. J., Friberg, I. M., Ralli, C., Lowe, A., Zawadzka, M., et al. (2014). An immunological marker of tolerance to infection in wild rodents. *PLoS Biol.* 12:e1001901. doi: 10.1371/journal.pbio.1001901

Jackson, M. H., and Siim, J. C. (1986). Toxoplasmosis in a wild rodent population of central Scotland and a possible explanation of the mode of transmission. *J. Zool.* 209, 549–557. doi: 10.1111/j.1469-7998.1986.tb03610.x

Justice, M. J., and Dhillon, P. (2016). Using the mouse to model human disease: increasing validity and reproducibility. *Dis. Model. Mech.* 9, 101–103. doi: 10.1242/dmm.024547

Kassebaum, N. J., Arora, M., Barber, R. M., Bhutta, Z. A., Brown, J., Carter, A., et al. (2016). Global, regional, and national disability-adjusted life-years (DALYs) for 315 diseases and injuries and healthy life expectancy (HALE), 1990–2015: a systematic analysis for the Global Burden of Disease Study 2015. *Lancet* 388, 1603–1658. doi: 10.1016/s0140-6736(16)31460-x

Kaushansky, A., Mikolajczak, S. A., Vignali, M., and Kappe, S. H. I. (2014). Of men in mice: the success and promise of humanized mouse models for human malaria parasite infections. *Cell. Microbiol.* 16, 602–611. doi: 10.1111/cmi.12277

Kijlstra, A., Meerburg, B., Cornelissen, J., De Craeye, S., Vereijken, P., and Jongert, E. (2008). The role of rodents and shrews in the transmission of Toxoplasma gondii to pigs. *Vet. Parasitol.* 156, 183–190. doi: 10.1016/j.vetpar.2008.05.030

Klaassen, C. D., Lu, H., and Cui, J. Y. (2011). Epigenetic regulation of drug processing genes. *Toxicol. Mech. Methods* 21, 312–324. doi: 10.3109/15376516.2011.562758

Klein, S. L. (2004). Hormonal and immunological mechanisms mediating sex differences in parasite infection. *Parasite Immunol.* 26, 247–264. doi: 10.1111/j.0141-9838.2004.00710.x

Klotz, C., Aebischer, T., and Seeber, F. (2012). Stem cell-derived cell cultures and organoids for protozoan parasite propagation and studying host-parasite interaction. *Int. J. Med. Microbiol.* 302, 203–209. doi: 10.1016/j.ijmm.2012.07.010

Knowles, S. C., Fenton, A., Petchey, O. L., Jones, T. R., Barber, R., and Pedersen, A. B. (2013). Stability of within-host-parasite communities in a wild mammal system. *Proc. Biol. Sci.* 280:20130598. doi: 10.1098/rspb.2013.0598

Kolata, G. (1998, May 3). A special report: a cautious awe greets drugs that eradicate tumors in mice. *The New York Times.*

Koscielny, G., Yaikhom, G., Iyer, V., Meehan, T. F., Morgan, H., Atienza-Herrero, J., et al. (2014). The International Mouse Phenotyping Consortium Web Portal, a unified point of access for knockout mice and related phenotyping data. *Nucleic Acids Res.* 42, D802–D809. doi: 10.1093/nar/gkt977

Kusdian, G., and Gould, S. B. (2014). The biology of Trichomonas vaginalis in the light of urogenital tract infection. *Mol. Biochem. Parasitol.* 198, 92–99. doi: 10.1016/j.molbiopara.2015.01.004

Lagkouvardos, I., Pukall, R., Abt, B., Foesel, B. U., Meier-Kolthoff, J. P., Kumar, N., et al. (2016). The Mouse Intestinal Bacterial Collection (miBC) provides host-specific insight into cultured diversity and functional potential of the gut microbiota. *Nat. Microbiol.* 1:16131. doi: 10.1038/nmicrobiol.2016.131

Lamour, S. D., Veselkov, K. A., Posma, J. M., Giraud, E., Rogers, M. E., Croft, S., et al. (2015). Metabolic, immune, and gut microbial signals mount a systems response to Leishmania major infection. *J. Proteome Res.* 14, 318–329. doi: 10.1021/pr5008202

Langhorne, J., Buffet, P., Galinski, M., Good, M., Harty, J., Leroy, D., et al. (2011). The relevance of non-human primate and rodent malaria models for humans. *Malar. J.* 10:23. doi: 10.1186/1475-2875-10-23

Latham, N., and Mason, G. (2004). From house mouse to mouse house: the behavioural biology of free-living Mus musculus and its implications in the laboratory. *Appl. Anim. Behav. Sci.* 86, 261–289. doi: 10.1016/j.applanim.2004.02.006

Li, D., Qiu, Z., Shao, Y., Chen, Y., Guan, Y., Liu, M., et al. (2013). Heritable gene targeting in the mouse and rat using a CRISPR-Cas system. *Nat. Biotechnol.* 31, 681–683. doi: 10.1038/nbt.2661

Li, W., Teng, F., Li, T., and Zhou, Q. (2013). Simultaneous generation and germline transmission of multiple gene mutations in rat using CRISPR-Cas systems. *Nat. Biotechnol.* 31, 684–686. doi: 10.1038/nbt.2652

Lilue, J., Müller, U. B., Steinfeldt, T., and Howard, J. C. (2013). Reciprocal virulence and resistance polymorphism in the relationship between Toxoplasma gondii and the house mouse. *Elife* 2:e01298. doi: 10.7554/eLife.01298

Lipoldová, M., and Demant, P. (2006). Genetic susceptibility to infectious disease: lessons from mouse models of leishmaniasis. *Nat. Rev. Genet.* 7, 294–305. doi: 10.1038/nrg1832

Liu, Y., Beyer, A., and Aebersold, R. (2016). On the dependency of cellular protein levels on mRNA abundance. *Cell* 165, 535–550. doi: 10.1016/j.cell.2016.03.014

Loeuillet, C., Banuls, A. L., and Hide, M. (2016). Study of Leishmania pathogenesis in mice: experimental considerations. *Parasit. Vectors* 9, 144. doi: 10.1186/s13071-016-1413-9

Lopes, M. E. M., Carneiro, M. B. H., Dos Santos, L. M., and Vieira, L. Q. (2016). Indigenous microbiota and Leishmaniasis. *Parasite Immunol.* 38, 37–44. doi: 10.1111/pim.12279

Lore, N. I., Iraqi, F. A., and Bragonzi, A. (2015). Host genetic diversity influences the severity of Pseudomonas aeruginosa pneumonia in the Collaborative Cross mice. *BMC Genet.* 16:106. doi: 10.1186/s12863-015-0260-6

Lutz, C. M., Linder, C. C., and Davisson, M. T. (2012). "Strains, Stocks and Mutant Mice," in *The Laboratory Mouse, 2nd Edn.*, ed H. J. Hedrich (Boston, MA: Academic Press), 37–56.

Magez, S., and Caljon, G. (2011). Mouse models for pathogenic African trypanosomes: unravelling the immunology of host-parasite-vector interactions. *Parasite Immunol.* 33, 423–429. doi: 10.1111/j.1365-3024.2011.01293.x

Maizels, R. M., and Nussey, D. H. (2013). Into the wild: digging at immunology's evolutionary roots. *Nat. Immunol.* 14, 879–883. doi: 10.1038/ni.2643

Mak, T. W. (2007). Gene targeting in embryonic stem cells scores a knockout in Stockholm. *Cell* 131, 1027–1031. doi: 10.1016/j.cell.2007.11.033

Matthews, K. R. (2015). 25 years of African trypanosome research: from description to molecular dissection and new drug discovery. *Mol. Biochem. Parasitol.* 200, 30–40. doi: 10.1016/j.molbiopara.2015.01.006

Mayer, E. A., Tillisch, K., and Gupta, A. (2015). Gut/brain axis and the microbiota. *J. Clin. Invest.* 125, 926–938. doi: 10.1172/JCI76304

Mears, E. R., Modabber, F., Don, R., and Johnson, G. E. (2015). The current *in vivo* models for the discovery and utility of new anti-leishmanial drugs targeting cutaneous leishmaniasis. *PLoS Negl. Trop. Dis.* 9:e0003889. doi: 10.1371/journal.pntd.0003889

Mendel, G. (1866). *Versuche über Pflanzen-Hybriden. Verhandlungen des Naturforschenden Vereines in Brünn* Vol. 4, 3–47. English version available online at: http://www.esp.org/foundations/genetics/classical/gm-65.pdf (May, 2017).

Messenger, L. A., Miles, M. A., and Bern, C. (2015). Between a bug and a hard place: Trypanosoma cruzi genetic diversity and the clinical outcomes of Chagas disease. *Expert Rev. Anti Infect. Ther.* 13, 995–1029. doi: 10.1586/14787210.2015.1056158

Mestas, J., and Hughes, C. C. W. (2004). Of mice and not men: differences between mouse and human immunology. *J. Immunol.* 172, 2731–2738. doi: 10.4049/jimmunol.172.5.2731

Morrison, L. J., Vezza, L., Rowan, T., and Hope, J. C. (2016). Animal African trypanosomiasis: time to increase focus on clinically relevant parasite and host species. *Trends Parasitol.* 32, 599–607. doi: 10.1016/j.pt.2016.04.012

Müller, B., and Grossniklaus, U. (2010). Model organisms — a historical perspective. *J. Proteomics* 73, 2054–2063. doi: 10.1016/j.jprot.2010.08.002

Muller, I., Hailu, A., Choi, B. S., Abebe, T., Fuentes, J. M., Munder, M., et al. (2008). Age-related alteration of arginase activity impacts on severity of leishmaniasis. *PLoS Negl. Trop. Dis.* 2:e235. doi: 10.1371/journal.pntd.0000235

Muqaku, B., Slany, A., Bileck, A., Kreutz, D., and Gerner, C. (2015). Quantification of cytokines secreted by primary human cells using multiple reaction monitoring: evaluation of analytical parameters. *Anal. Bioanal. Chem.* 407, 6525–6536. doi: 10.1007/s00216-015-8817-9

Murray, C. J., Vos, T., Lozano, R., Naghavi, M., Flaxman, A. D., Michaud, C., et al. (2012). Disability-adjusted life years (DALYs) for 291 diseases and injuries in 21 regions, 1990-2010: a systematic analysis for the Global Burden of Disease Study 2010. *Lancet* 380, 2197–2223. doi: 10.1016/s0140-6736(12)61689-4

Naik, S., Bouladoux, N., Wilhelm, C., Molloy, M. J., Salcedo, R., Kastenmuller, W., et al. (2012). Compartmentalized control of skin immunity by resident commensals. *Science* 337, 1115–1119. doi: 10.1126/science.1225152

Newman, A. E. M., Edmunds, N. B., Ferraro, S., Heffell, Q., Merritt, G. M., Pakkala, J. J., et al. (2015). Using ecology to inform physiology studies: implications of high population density in the laboratory. *Am. J. Physiol. Regul. Integr. Comp. Physiol.* 308, R449–R454. doi: 10.1152/ajpregu.00328.2014

Nicod, J., Davies, R. W., Cai, N., Hassett, C., Goodstadt, L., Cosgrove, C., et al. (2016). Genome-wide association of multiple complex traits in outbred mice by ultra-low-coverage sequencing. *Nat. Genet.* 48, 912–918. doi: 10.1038/ng.3595

Noyes, H. A., Ambrose, P., Barker, F., Begon, M., Bennet, M., Bown, K. J., et al. (2002). Host specificity of Trypanosoma (Herpetosoma) species: evidence that bank voles (Clethrionomys glareolus) carry only one T. (H.) evotomys 18S rRNA genotype but wood mice (Apodemus sylvaticus) carry at least two polyphyletic parasites. *Parasitology* 124(Pt 2), 185–190. doi: 10.1017/S0031182001001019

O'Connor, B. D., Day, A., Cain, S., Arnaiz, O., Sperling, L., and Stein, L. D. (2008). GMODWeb: a web framework for the Generic Model Organism Database. *Genome Biol.* 9:R102. doi: 10.1186/gb-2008-9-6-r102

Orrock, J. L. (2004). Rodent foraging is affected by indirect, but not by direct, cues of predation risk. *Behav. Ecol.* 15, 433–437. doi: 10.1093/beheco/arh031

Pedersen, A. B., and Antonovics, J. (2013). Anthelmintic treatment alters the parasite community in a wild mouse host. *Biol. Lett.* 9:20130205. doi: 10.1098/rsbl.2013.0205

Pedersen, A. B., and Babayan, S. A. (2011). Wild immunology. *Mol. Ecol.* 20, 872–880. doi: 10.1111/j.1365-294X.2010.04938.x

Pedersen, A. B., Jones, K. E., Nunn, C. L., and Altizer, S. (2007). Infectious diseases and extinction risk in wild mammals. *Conserv. Biol.* 21, 1269–1279. doi: 10.1111/j.1523-1739.2007.00776.x

Perry, B., and Grace, D. (2009). The impacts of livestock diseases and their control on growth and development processes that are pro-poor. *Philos. Trans. R. Soc. Lond. B. Biol. Sci.* 364, 2643–2655. doi: 10.1098/rstb.2009.0097

Phifer-Rixey, M., and Nachman, M. W. (2015). Insights into mammalian biology from the wild house mouse Mus musculus. *Elife* 4:e05959. doi: 10.7554/eLife.05959

Potter, M., Nadieau, J. H., and Cancro, M. P. (1986). *The Wild Mouse in Immunology.* Berlin Heidelberg: Springer

Powell, F., and Banks, P. B. (2004). Do house mice modify their foraging behaviour in response to predator odours and habitat? *Anim. Behav.* 67, 753–759. doi: 10.1016/j.anbehav.2003.08.016

Rand, M. S. (2008). "Selection of biomedical animal models," in *Sourcebook of Models for Biomedical Research*, ed P. M. Conn (Totowa, NJ: Humana Press), 9–16.

Rasmussen, A. L., Okumura, A., Ferris, M. T., Green, R., Feldmann, F., Kelly, S. M., et al. (2014). Host genetic diversity enables Ebola hemorrhagic fever pathogenesis and resistance. *Science* 346, 987–991. doi: 10.1126/science.1259595

Rauniyar, N. (2015). Parallel reaction monitoring: a targeted experiment performed using high resolution and high mass accuracy mass spectrometry. *Int. J. Mol. Sci.* 16, 28566–28581. doi: 10.3390/ijms161226120

Rausch, P., Basic, M., Batra, A., Bischoff, S. C., Blaut, M., Clavel, T., et al. (2016). Analysis of factors contributing to variation in the C57BL/6J fecal microbiota across German animal facilities. *Int. J. Med. Microbiol.* 306, 343–355. doi: 10.1016/j.ijmm.2016.03.004

Reese, T. A., Bi, K., Kambal, A., Filali-Mouhim, A., Beura, L. K., Bürger, M. C., et al. (2016). Sequential infection with common pathogens promotes human-like immune gene expression and altered vaccine response. *Cell Host Microbe* 19, 713–719. doi: 10.1016/j.chom.2016.04.003

Reijnders, D., Goossens, G. H., Hermes, G. D. A., Neis, E. P., van der, Beek, C. M., Most, J., et al. (2016). Effects of gut microbiota manipulation by antibiotics on host metabolism in obese humans: a randomized double-blind placebo-controlled trial. *Cell Metab.* 24, 63–74. doi: 10.1016/j.cmet.2016.06.016

Rhee, J. K., So, W. S., and Kim, H. C. (1999). Age-dependent resistance to Cryptosporidium muris (strain MCR) infection in golden hamsters and mice. *Korean J. Parasitol.* 37, 33–37.

Roberts, C. W., Walker, W., and Alexander, J. (2001). Sex-associated hormones and immunity to protozoan parasites. *Clin. Microbiol. Rev.* 14, 476–488. doi: 10.1128/cmr.14.3.476-488.2001

Robertson, L. J., Sprong, H., Ortega, Y. R., van der Giessen, J. W., and Fayer, R. (2014). Impacts of globalisation on foodborne parasites. *Trends Parasitol.* 30, 37–52. doi: 10.1016/j.pt.2013.09.005

Rochford, R., Ohrt, C., Baresel, P. C., Campo, B., Sampath, A., Magill, A. J., et al. (2013). Humanized mouse model of glucose 6-phosphate dehydrogenase deficiency for *in vivo* assessment of hemolytic toxicity. *Proc. Natl. Acad. Sci. U.S.A.* 110, 17486–17491. doi: 10.1073/pnas.1310402110

Rogers, G. B., Kozlowska, J., Keeble, J., Metcalfe, K., Fao, M., Dowd, S. E., et al. (2014). Functional divergence in gastrointestinal microbiota in physically-separated genetically identical mice. *Sci. Rep.* 4:5437. doi: 10.1038/srep05437

Schluter, D., Daubener, W., Schares, G., Gross, U., Pleyer, U., and Luder, C. (2014). Animals are key to human toxoplasmosis. *Int. J. Med. Microbiol.* 304, 917–929. doi: 10.1016/j.ijmm.2014.09.002

Sellers, R. S. (2017). Translating mouse models. *Toxicol. Pathol.* 45, 134–145. doi: 10.1177/0192623316675767

Seok, J., Warren, H. S., Cuenca, A. G., Mindrinos, M. N., Baker, H. V., Xu, W., et al. (2013). Genomic responses in mouse models poorly mimic human inflammatory diseases. *Proc. Natl. Acad. Sci. U.S.A.* 110, 3507–3512. doi: 10.1073/pnas.1222878110

Servick, K. (2016). Of mice and microbes. *Science* 353, 741–743. doi: 10.1126/science.353.6301.741

Shah, S. S., Rockett, K. A., Jallow, M., Sisay-Joof, F., Bojang, K. A., Pinder, M., et al. (2016). Heterogeneous alleles comprising G6PD deficiency trait in West Africa exert contrasting effects on two major clinical presentations of severe malaria. *Malar. J.* 15, 64. doi: 10.1186/s12936-015-1045-0

Shay, T., Jojic, V., Zuk, O., Rothamel, K., Puyraimond-Zemmour, D., Feng, T., et al. (2013). Conservation and divergence in the transcriptional programs of the human and mouse immune systems. *Proc. Natl. Acad. Sci. U.S.A.* 110, 2946–2951. doi: 10.1073/pnas.1222738110

Singer, S. M., and Nash, T. E. (2000). The role of normal flora in Giardia lamblia infections in mice. *J. Infect. Dis.* 181, 1510–1512. doi: 10.1086/315409

Singleton, G. R., and Krebs, C. J. (2007). "The secret world of wild mice," in *The Mouse in Biomedical Research, 2nd Edn.*, eds M. T. Davisson, F. W. Quimby, S. W. Barthold, C. E. Newcomer, and A. L. Smith (Burlington, NJ: Academic Press), 25–51.

Skea, D. L., and Underdown, B. J. (1991). Acquired resistance to Giardia muris in X-linked immunodeficient mice. *Infect. Immun.* 59, 1733–1738

Smith, A., Telfer, S., Burthe, S., Bennett, M., and Begon, M. (2005). Trypanosomes, fleas and field voles: ecological dynamics of a host-vector-parasite interaction. *Parasitology* 131(Pt 3), 355–365. doi: 10.1017/S0031182005007766

Smith, C. M., Proulx, M. K., Olive, A. J., Laddy, D., Mishra, B. B., Moss, C., et al. (2016). Tuberculosis susceptibility and vaccine protection are independently controlled by host genotype. *MBio* 7:e01516. doi: 10.1128/mBio.01516-16

Stanley, S. L. Jr. (2003). Amoebiasis. *Lancet* 361, 1025–1034. doi: 10.1016/s0140-6736(03)12830-9

Steinman, R. M. (2012). Decisions about dendritic cells: past, present, and future. *Annu. Rev. Immunol.* 30, 1–22. doi: 10.1146/annurev-immunol-100311-102839

Stough, J. M. A., Dearth, S. P., Denny, J. E., LeCleir, G. R., Schmidt, N. W., Campagna, S. R., et al. (2016). Functional characteristics of the gut microbiome in C57BL/6 mice differentially susceptible to plasmodium yoelii. *Front. Microbiol.* 7:1520. doi: 10.3389/fmicb.2016.01520

Stuart, K., Brun, R., Croft, S., Fairlamb, A., Gürtler, R. E., McKerrow, J., et al. (2008). Kinetoplastids: related protozoan pathogens, different diseases. *J. Clin. Invest.* 118, 1301–1310. doi: 10.1172/JCI33945

Svobodova, M., Vorisek, P., Votypka, J., and Weidinger, K. (2004). Heteroxenous Coccidia (Apicomplexa: Sarcocystidae) in the populations of their final and intermediate hosts: European buzzard and small mammals. *Acta Protozool.* 43, 251–260.

Takao, K., and Miyakawa, T. (2015). Genomic responses in mouse models greatly mimic human inflammatory diseases. *Proc. Natl. Acad. Sci. U.S.A.* 112, 1167–1172. doi: 10.1073/pnas.1401965111

Tao, L., and Reese, T. A. (2017). Making mouse models that reflect human immune responses. *Trends Immunol.* 38, 181–193. doi: 10.1016/j.it.2016.12.007

The Commission to the Council and the European Parliament (2013). *Seventh Report on the Statistics on the Number of Animals Used for Experimental and Other Scientific Purposes in the Member States of the European Union*. Available online at: http://ec.europa.eu/environment/chemicals/lab_animals/reports_en.htm

Threadgill, D. W., and Churchill, G. A. (2012). Ten years of the Collaborative Cross. *Genetics* 190, 291–294. doi: 10.1534/genetics.111.138032

Tong, C., Li, P., Wu, N. L., Yan, Y., and Ying, Q. L. (2010). Production of p53 gene knockout rats by homologous recombination in embryonic stem cells. *Nature* 467, 211–213. doi: 10.1038/nature09368

Torgerson, P. R. (2013). One world health: socioeconomic burden and parasitic disease control priorities. *Vet. Parasitol.* 195, 223–232. doi: 10.1016/j.vetpar.2013.04.004

Torgerson, P. R., and Macpherson, C. N. (2011). The socioeconomic burden of parasitic zoonoses: global trends. *Vet. Parasitol.* 182, 79–95. doi: 10.1016/j.vetpar.2011.07.017

Torres, M. R., Silva, M. E., Vieira, E. C., Bambirra, E. A., Sogayar, M. I., Pena, F. J., et al. (1992). Intragastric infection of conventional and germfree mice with Giardia lamblia. *Braz. J. Med. Biol. Res.* 25, 349–352.

Turnbaugh, P. J., Ley, R. E., Mahowald, M. A., Magrini, V., Mardis, E. R., and Gordon, J. I. (2006). An obesity-associated gut microbiome with increased capacity for energy harvest. *Nature* 444, 1027–1131. doi: 10.1038/nature05414

Turner, A. K., Begon, M., Jackson, J. A., Bradley, J. E., and Paterson, S. (2011). Genetic diversity in cytokines associated with immune variation and resistance to multiple pathogens in a natural rodent population. *PLoS Genet.* 7:e1002343. doi: 10.1371/journal.pgen.1002343

Turner, A. K., Beldomenico, P. M., Bown, K., Burthe, S. J., Jackson, J. A., Lambin, X., et al. (2014). Host-parasite biology in the real world: the field voles of Kielder. *Parasitology* 141, 997–1017. doi: 10.1017/s0031182014000171

Turner, C. M. (1986). Seasonal and age distributions of Babesia, Hepatozoon, Trypanosoma and Grahamella species in Clethrionomys glareolus and Apodemus sylvaticus populations. *Parasitology* 93(Pt 2), 279–289.

UK Home Office (2015). *Annual Statistics of Scientific Procedures of Living Animals Great Britain 2015*. Available online at: https://www.gov.uk/government/uploads/system/uploads/attachment_data/file/537708/scientific-procedures-living-animals-2015.pdf

Valdar, W., Solberg, L. C., Gauguier, D., Burnett, S., Klenerman, P., Cookson, W. O., et al. (2006). Genome-wide genetic association of complex traits in heterogeneous stock mice. *Nat. Genet.* 38, 879–887. doi: 10.1038/ng1840

van Boxtel, R., and Cuppen, E. (2010). Rat traps: filling the toolbox for manipulating the rat genome. *Genome Biol.* 11:217. doi: 10.1186/gb-2010-11-9-217

Van der Hilst, J. C., Smits, B. W., and van der Meer, J. W. (2002). Hypogammaglobulinaemia: cumulative experience in 49 patients in a tertiary care institution. *Neth. J. Med.* 60, 140–147.

van der Worp, H. B., Howells, D. W., Sena, E. S., Porritt, M. J., Rewell, S., O'Collins, V., et al. (2010). Can animal models of disease reliably inform human studies? *PLoS Med.* 7:e1000245. doi: 10.1371/journal.pmed.1000245

van Lunzen, J., and Altfeld, M. (2014). Sex differences in infectious diseases-common but neglected. *J. Infect. Dis.* 209(Suppl. 3), S79–S80. doi: 10.1093/infdis/jiu159

Vannier, E., Borggraefe, I., Telford, S. R. III, Menon, S., Brauns, T., Spielman, A., et al. (2004). Age-associated decline in resistance to Babesia microti is genetically determined. *J. Infect. Dis.* 189, 1721–1728. doi: 10.1086/382965

Vaughan, A. M., Mikolajczak, S. A., Wilson, E. M., Grompe, M., Kaushansky, A., Camargo, N., et al. (2012). Complete Plasmodium falciparum liver-stage development in liver-chimeric mice. *J. Clin. Invest.* 122, 3618–3628. doi: 10.1172/jci62684

Vaughan, A. M., Pinapati, R. S., Cheeseman, I. H., Camargo, N., Fishbaugher, M., Checkley, L. A., et al. (2015). Plasmodium falciparum genetic crosses in a humanized mouse model. *Nat. Methods* 12, 631–633. doi: 10.1038/nmeth.3432

Verdolin, J. L. (2006). Meta-analysis of foraging and predation risk trade-offs in terrestrial systems. *Behav. Ecol. Sociobiol.* 60, 457–464. doi: 10.1007/s00265-006-0172-6

Vered, K., Durrant, C., Mott, R., and Iraqi, F. A. (2014). Susceptibility to Klebsiella pneumonaie infection in collaborative cross mice is a complex trait controlled by at least three loci acting at different time points. *BMC Genomics* 15:865. doi: 10.1186/1471-2164-15-865

Vidal, S. M., Malo, D., Marquis, J. F., and Gros, P. (2008). Forward genetic dissection of immunity to infection in the mouse. *Annu. Rev. Immunol.* 26, 81–132. doi: 10.1146/annurev.immunol.26.021607.090304

Vijay, N., Poelstra, J. W., Kunstner, A., and Wolf, J. B. (2013). Challenges and strategies in transcriptome assembly and differential gene expression quantification. A comprehensive in silico assessment of RNA-seq experiments. *Mol. Ecol.* 22, 620–634. doi: 10.1111/mec.12014

Villarino, N. F., LeCleir, G. R., Denny, J. E., Dearth, S. P., Harding, C. L., Sloan, S. S., et al. (2016). Composition of the gut microbiota modulates the severity of malaria. *Proc. Natl. Acad. Sci. U.S.A.* 113, 2235–2240. doi: 10.1073/pnas.1504887113

Viney, M., Lazarou, L., and Abolins, S. (2015). The laboratory mouse and wild immunology. *Parasite Immunol.* 37, 267–273. doi: 10.1111/pim.12150

Warren, H., Tompkins, R., Moldawer, L., Seok, J., Xu, W., Mindrinos, M., et al. (2015). Mice are not men. *Proc. Natl. Acad. Sci. U.S.A.* 112, E345. doi: 10.1073/pnas.1414857111

Waterston, R. H., Lindblad-Toh, K., Birney, E., Rogers, J., Abril, J. F., Agarwal, P., et al. (2002). Initial sequencing and comparative analysis of the mouse genome. *Nature* 420, 520–562. doi: 10.1038/nature01262

Wege, A. K., Florian, C., Ernst, W., Zimara, N., Schleicher, U., Hanses, F., et al. (2012). Leishmania major infection in humanized mice induces systemic infection and provokes a nonprotective human immune response. *PLoS Negl. Trop. Dis.* 6:e1741. doi: 10.1371/journal.pntd.0001741

Weidner, C., Steinfath, M., Opitz, E., Oelgeschläger, M., and Schönfelder, G. (2016). Defining the optimal animal model for translational research using gene set enrichment analysis. *EMBO Mol. Med.* 8, 831–838. doi: 10.15252/emmm.201506025

Weissmuller, S., Kronhart, S., Kreuz, D., Schnierle, B., Kalinke, U., Kirberg, J., et al. (2016). TGN1412 induces lymphopenia and human cytokine release in a humanized mouse model. *PLoS ONE* 11:e0149093. doi: 10.1371/journal.pone.0149093

Weldon, L., Abolins, S., Lenzi, L., Bourne, C., Riley, E. M., and Viney, M. (2015). The gut microbiota of wild mice. *PLoS ONE* 10:e0134643. doi: 10.1371/journal.pone.0134643

Wickham, K. S., Baresel, P. C., Marcsisin, S. R., Sousa, J., Vuong, C. T., Reichard, G. A., et al. (2016). Single-dose primaquine in a preclinical model of glucose-6-phosphate dehydrogenase deficiency: implications for use in malaria transmission-blocking programs. *Antimicrob. Agents Chemother.* 60, 5906–5913. doi: 10.1128/aac.00600-16

Willyard, C. (2015). The boom in mini stomachs, brains, breasts, kidneys and more. *Nature* 523, 520–522. doi: 10.1038/523520a

Withenshaw, S. M., Devevey, G., Pedersen, A. B., and Fenton, A. (2016). Multihost Bartonella parasites display covert host specificity even when transmitted by generalist vectors. *J. Anim. Ecol.* 85, 1442–1452. doi: 10.1111/1365-2656.12568

Wolff, J. O. (2003). Laboratory studies with rodents: facts or artifacts? *Bioscience* 53, 421–427. doi: 10.1641/0006-3568(2003)053[0421:LSWRFO]2.0.CO;2

Worth, A. R., Andrew Thompson, R. C., and Lymbery, A. J. (2014). Reevaluating the evidence for Toxoplasma gondii-induced behavioural changes in rodents. *Adv. Parasitol.* 85, 109–142. doi: 10.1016/B978-0-12-800182-0.00003-9

Worth, A. R., Lymbery, A. J., and Thompson, R. C. A. (2013). Adaptive host manipulation by Toxoplasma gondii: fact or fiction? *Trends Parasitol.* 29, 150–155. doi: 10.1016/j.pt.2013.01.004

Yilmaz, B., Portugal, S., Tran, T. M., Gozzelino, R., Ramos, S., Gomes, J., et al. (2014). Gut microbiota elicits a protective immune response against malaria transmission. *Cell* 159, 1277–1289. doi: 10.1016/j.cell.2014.10.053

Yoshiki, A., and Moriwaki, K. (2006). Mouse phenome research: implications of genetic background. *ILAR J.* 47, 94–102. doi: 10.1093/ilar.47.2.94

Zamboni, D. S., and Lima-Junior, D. S. (2015). Inflammasomes in host response to protozoan parasites. *Immunol. Rev.* 265, 156–171. doi: 10.1111/imr.12291

Zimmerman, L. M., Bowden, R. M., and Vogel, L. A. (2014). A vertebrate cytokine primer for eco-immunologists. *Funct. Ecol.* 28, 1061–1073. doi: 10.1111/1365-2435.12273

Zschaler, J., Schlorke, D., and Arnhold, J. (2014). Differences in innate immune response between man and mouse. *Crit. Rev. Immunol.* 34, 433–454. doi: 10.1016/j.freeradbiomed.2015.04.015

2

Strain- and Dose-Dependent Reduction of *Toxoplasma gondii* Burden in Pigs is Associated with Interferon-Gamma Production by CD8+ Lymphocytes in a Heterologous Challenge Model

Malgorzata Jennes[1†], Stéphane De Craeye[2†], Bert Devriendt[1], Katelijne Dierick[2], Pierre Dorny[3,4] and Eric Cox[1]*

[1] Laboratory for Immunology, Faculty of Veterinary Medicine, Ghent University, Merelbeke, Belgium, [2] National Reference Laboratory for Toxoplasmosis, Operational Direction Communicable and Infectious Diseases, Scientific Institute of Public Health, Security of Food Chain and Environment, Brussels, Belgium, [3] Department of Biomedical Sciences, Institute for Tropical Medicine, Antwerp, Belgium, [4] Laboratory for Parasitology, Faculty of Veterinary Medicine, Ghent University, Merelbeke, Belgium

Edited by:
Anton Aebischer,
Robert Koch-Insitute, Germany

Reviewed by:
Susan M. Bueno,
Pontificia Universidad Católica de Chile, Chile
Anthony P. Sinai,
University of Kentucky, United States
Anja Joachim,
Veterinärmedizinische Universität Wien, Austria

***Correspondence:**
Eric Cox
eric.cox@ugent.be

† These authors have contributed equally to this work.

Toxoplasma gondii is a worldwide prevalent parasite of humans and animals. The global infection burden exceeds yearly one million disability-adjusted life years (DALY's) in infected individuals. Therefore, effective preventive measures should be taken to decrease the risk of infection in humans. Although human toxoplasmosis is predominantly foodborne by ingestion of tissue cysts in meat from domestic animals such as pigs, the incidence risk is difficult to estimate due to the lack of screening of animals for infection and insights in location and persistence of the parasite in the tissues. Hence, experimental infections in pigs can provide more information on the risk for zoonosis based on the parasite burden in meat products intended for human consumption and on the immune responses induced by infection. In the present study, homo- and heterologous infection experiments with two distinct *T. gondii* strains (IPB-LR and IPB-Gangji) were performed. The humoral and cellular immune responses, the presence of viable parasites and the parasite load in edible meat samples were evaluated. In homologous infection experiments the parasite persistence was clearly strain-dependent and inversely correlated with the infection dose. The results strongly indicate a change in the amount of parasite DNA and viable cysts in porcine tissues over time. Heterologous challenge infections demonstrated that IPB-G strain could considerably reduce the parasite burden in the subsequent IPB-LR infection. A strong, however, not protective humoral response was observed against GRA7 and TLA antigens upon inoculation with both strains. The *in vitro* IFN-γ production by TLA-stimulated PBMCs was correlated with the infection dose and predominantly brought about by $CD3^{+}CD4^{-}CD8\alpha^{bright}$ T-lymphocytes. The described adaptive cellular and humoral immune responses in pigs are in line with the induced or natural infections in mice and humans.

Previous studies underscored the heterogeneity of *T. gondii* strains and the corresponding virulence factors. These findings suggest the potential of the IPB-G strain to elicit a partially protective immune response and to reduce the parasite burden upon a challenge infection. The IPB-G strain could be used as a promising tool in limiting the number of viable parasites in edible tissues and, hence, in lowering the risk for human toxoplasmosis.

Keywords: ***Toxoplasma gondii*, infection, pigs, IFN-γ, T lymphocytes, immunity**

INTRODUCTION

Toxoplasmosis is a parasitic infection caused by the intracellular protozoa *Toxoplasma gondii*. This parasite has a complex lifecycle and affects its definitive host as well as various intermediate hosts, among which domestic and wild animals and humans (Dubey, 2010). During its distinct developmental phases, the parasite manifests itself as a tachyzoite, a bradyzoite or a sporozoite in the oocyst. The sexual multiplication proceeds only within the definitive hosts (domestic or wild members of the family *Felidae*), wherein five morphologically different generations of the gamonts develop in the enterocytes, leading to formation of the gametocytes. Following the fertilization of the micro- and the macrogamete and the rupture of the infected cell, the unsporulated oocysts are discharged into the intestinal lumen. The final hosts are responsible for the extensive shedding of oocysts in the environment (Dubey, 1995; Afonso et al., 2008). The sporulated oocysts containing eight sporozoites show a high resistance to different environmental factors and under convenient circumstances may remain infectious for 1.5 years (Dubey, 2010). On average, the final host sheds at least one million oocysts in the acute phase of the infection, resulting in a massive contamination of the environment. This explains the persistence of the parasite in wild reservoir and livestock (Black and Boothroyd, 2000; Afonso et al., 2008; Innes, 2010; Opsteegh et al., 2016). The sporulated oocysts release the sporozoites upon ingestion by the intermediate host, followed by a differentiation to tachyzoites, several cell divisions in the enterocytes, and eventually dissemination to the peripheral tissues. There, the fast-multiplying tachyzoites convert into tissue cysts with the slowly dividing bradyzoites, and remain there as the dormant stage of the infection. The predation of the intermediate host or its tissues by the Felidae leads to the new sexual reproduction cycle, in which the bradyzoites transform back to tachyzoites and merozoites (Dubey, 1995; Afonso et al., 2008).

Several infection routes have been described for the different hosts of *T. gondii*; the majority of the herbivorous animals acquires the infection through ingestion of water or plants contaminated with oocysts. The predation of other mammals or birds or ingestion of the placenta and/or the aborted offspring of small ruminants facilitates the transmission of toxoplasmosis to carnivores and omnivores (Black and Boothroyd, 2000; Innes, 2010). In humans, foodborne toxoplasmosis mainly results from the consumption of raw or undercooked meat from infected animals, like domestic pigs. The global prevalence of this parasite includes one third of the human population and as such represents one of the most common parasitic zoonosis worldwide (Tenter et al., 2000; Ajzenberg et al., 2002; Aspinall et al., 2002; Bosch-Driessen et al., 2002; Kijlstra and Jongert, 2008; Innes, 2010; Robert-Gangneux and Dardé, 2012; Torgerson and Mastroiacovo, 2013). Consequently, infection in human has a severe short- and long-term impact, ranging from congenital or adult toxoplasmosis in healthy individuals to *T. gondii*-induced encephalitis in immune-compromised patients. In particular congenital toxoplasmosis in seronegative pregnant women has a very severe clinical relevance for the fetus, since the infection may result in abortion, intracranial calcifications, mental retardation or chorioretinitis in the newborn (Peyron et al., 2017). Finally, acquired toxoplasmosis has recently been associated with an increase in suicide rates or Parkinson's disease (Israelski and Remington, 1993; Holland, 2003; Lester, 2010; Miman et al., 2010; Wang et al., 2017). Therefore, numerous preventive measures are recommended in an attempt to decrease the global infection burden in the human population. The commonly applied precautions include hygienic processing of water and meat, such as boiling of surface water and avoiding the consumption of raw or undercooked meat, as only long term freezing at $-12°C$ or baking above $67°C$ can effectively deactivate tissue cysts. Especially, pork is often consumed undercooked and is processed in many other meat products, reaching on average 300 consumers per pig (Fehlhaber et al., 2003; Belluco et al., 2016). Additionally, direct contact with contaminated soil, plants or cat feces should be avoided by wearing gloves when gardening or emptying the litter box, and by thoroughly washing fresh vegetables and fruits. Providing clear information on these preventive measures to seronegative pregnant women, in combination with a frequent serological screening to detect the acute infection during pregnancy, has proven to be successful in decreasing the infection rate (Breugelmans et al., 2004; Peyron et al., 2017). In livestock, the preventive measures are predominantly focused on strictly indoor housing, preventing access for cats, rodent control and the appropriate carcass disposal (Jones and Dubey, 2012; Robert-Gangneux and Dardé, 2012). Whereas environmental contamination as well as the prevalence of toxoplasmosis in sheep is overall high, the situation in regard to pigs may vary per country or the farm management. Consequently, the lack of uniform validation of the variety of serological assays, and the missing gaps in the correlation between the persistence of antibodies and parasite in pork are still to be improved. Nevertheless, the estimated average prevalence in the pig population seems to be very low in European countries (2.2%)

and the USA (2.7%), presumably due to a shift from small and less strictly confined to large scale facilities, implementing all-in-all-out or farrow-to-finish models (Hill et al., 2008; EFSA, 2012; Guo et al., 2015). However, the recent rise of organic or free-range farming in order to improve animal welfare seems to contribute to an increase in infection rate in pig livestock and, as such, to the incidence of foodborne human toxoplasmosis (Kijlstra et al., 2004; Dubey et al., 2012; EFSA, 2012). The risk for humans to become infected by consumption of undercooked or raw pork is also not clear. The knowledge of the parasite persistence in edible tissues of naturally infected pigs is limited, as are the role of strain or dose in the parasite survival in the host. Such information might be of pivotal importance for vaccine development.

In the last decades numerous potential vaccine candidates have been experimentally tested mainly in mice and to a lesser extent in pigs. The formulations varied between a single recombinant parasitic protein or a combination of antigens, among which surface antigens (SAGs) or excretion/secretion proteins (GRAs, ROPs, MICs), but also DNA vaccines encoding B or T cell epitopes have been evaluated. However, the degrees of success were variable and did not led to a commercial vaccine (Vercammen et al., 2000; Letscher-Bru et al., 2003; Jongert et al., 2008; Li et al., 2011; Cao et al., 2015; Wagner et al., 2015). Vaccination did move forward by the use of attenuated viable strains, which resulted with a single commercially available vaccine for sheep, but their efficiency is tested under experimental circumstances and strictly species-dependent, and cannot yet be extrapolated to other livestock species or humans (Katzer et al., 2014; Burrells et al., 2015). Nevertheless, several experimental data in pigs reported reduction in parasite burden in infected and subsequently heterologous challenged pigs, in which the choice of the strain had an important effect on the viability of the parasite (Solano Aguilar et al., 2001; Dawson et al., 2004, 2005; Kringel et al., 2004; Garcia et al., 2005; Verhelst et al., 2011, 2015). In these studies, the involvement of the innate and acquired immune system was observed, dominated by antibodies production against the parasitic antigens, and by the Th1-type of the immune response. Depending on the experimental model, high levels of anti-GRA7 alone or anti-GRA1, -GRA7 and –TLA IgG's were detected upon an inoculation with IPB-G strain or a DNA GRA1-GRA7 cocktail vaccination, followed by the RH-strain or IPB-G challenge, respectively (Jongert et al., 2008; Verhelst et al., 2011), whereas a challenge with heterologous M4-strain oocysts after an experimental inoculation with viable S48-strain tachyzoites elicited a high TLA-specific IgG production (Burrells et al., 2015). In addition to the enhanced humoral immunity, a polarized Th1-immune response was observed after inoculation with a variety of the infectious *T. gondii* strains (Solano Aguilar et al., 2001; Dawson et al., 2004, 2005; Jongert et al., 2008; Verhelst et al., 2015). The significantly increased IFN-γ protein concentration in serum and the supernatant from the cultured PBMCs, and IFN-γ mRNA or DNA expression in PBMCs and intestinal lymphoid tissues, appeared positively correlated with the duration of the experiments (Solano Aguilar et al., 2001; Dawson et al., 2004, 2005; Jongert et al., 2008; Verhelst et al., 2015). In parallel with IFN-γ, also other cytokines were involved in the immune response against the parasite, as shown in the infection with the VEG-strain oocysts and the increased secretion of IL-15 and TNF-α (Dawson et al., 2005). Subsequently, a Th-2 response profile with predominantly IL-10 as anti-inflammatory cytokine was observed after the early phase of the infection, dominated by IFN-γ production, as mentioned earlier (Solano Aguilar et al., 2001; Aliberti, 2005). In contrast, IL-12 (IL-12p35 and IL-12p40) mRNA expression was not detected in PBMCs shortly after inoculation (7 and 14 dpi) in another study in pigs (Dawson et al., 2005). Nonetheless, even an excessive production of parasite-specific antibodies or Th-1/Th2-response cytokines did not provide a full protection during the acute phase of the infection, preventing from the cysts formation. Despite the active role the different components of the host's immune system play in the early stage of *T. gondii* infection, it remains a subject of discussion and ongoing research, whether the intermediate host can clear the tissues from the cysts on long term. It is noteworthy, however, that several studies in pigs notified reduced or undetectable counts of the parasite DNA in multiple porcine tissues, and a decline in viability of the cysts, as tested by bio-assay in mice (Jongert et al., 2008; Verhelst et al., 2011, 2015; Burrells et al., 2015). Taking into account the lack of an obligatory screening of pigs or pork meat to prevent transmission to humans, knowledge on the pig as an intermediate host for *T. gondii*, and in particular strategies to reduce the amount of viable parasites in tissues, may contribute to diminishing the risk of zoonosis by consumption of porcine meat (EFSA, 2007, 2012; Opsteegh et al., 2016). In light of these data, the aim of this study was to confirm differences between *T. gondii* strains in persistence of the parasite in tissues of experimentally infected pigs and to relate the dose and strain to the immune responses in the pigs upon a single infection or a heterologous challenge.

MATERIALS AND METHODS

T. gondii Strains

Two *T. gondii* strains were used for the experimental infections: the IPB-Gangji (IPB-G) strain and the IPB-LR strain. The first one was isolated from the placenta of a patient with congenital toxoplasmosis and is highly virulent in mice. It produces a large number of tissue cysts and has an atypical mixed type I and type II genotype (Ajzenberg et al., 2002). The latter was isolated from pigs and belongs to genotype II, which is less pathogenic and commonly present in the European pig population (Dubey, 2009; Dubey et al., 2012). Both strains are maintained at the National Reference Laboratory for Toxoplasmosis (Scientific Institute for Public Health, Brussels, Belgium) by passage in Swiss female mice, since there is no alternative available to obtain a sufficient number of tissue cysts for the inoculation experiments than via bio-assay, as approved by the Ethical Committee (no. 20140704-01) and conform the European legislation (2010/63/EU). Tissue cysts from both strains were isolated from homogenized brain tissue, counted by phase-contrast microscopy and suspended in 10 ml of sterile phosphate buffered saline (PBS) solution at the desired concentration (700 cysts for the low dose and 6,000 for the high dose). The animals were inoculated within 8 h after cysts isolation. The inoculum for the negative control group was prepared identically from naive Swiss mice.

Animals and Experimental Design

Two-week-old Belgian Landrace piglets were tested for the presence of anti-*T. gondii* serum antibodies (IgM and IgG) with an indirect immunofluorescence assay (IFA) as described previously (Verhelst et al., 2015). For the infection experiments, 3-week-old newly weaned, seronegative piglets were selected and randomly assigned to 10 groups of 3 animals (**Table 1**). These groups were housed in isolation units (Biosafety permit no, AMV/11062013/SBB219.2013/0145) at the Faculty of Veterinary Medicine, Ghent University, Belgium. All experiments were approved by the Ethical Committee of the faculties Veterinary Medicine and Bioscience Engineering at Ghent University (EC 2009/149).

In a first experiment we aimed to study the effect of a low or high infection dose of two different *T. gondii* strains on the humoral and cellular immune responses and tissue cyst persistence until 120 days after inoculation (**Table 1**). In a second experiment we focused on the effect of a subsequent challenge with a heterologous strain at 60 dpi and the persistence of the parasite in the tissues at 120 dpi (**Table 1**). In study 3 we compared kinetics of the IFN-γ producing porcine T cell subsets following infection with high doses of the IPB-G or the IPB-LR strain until 98 dpi (**Table 1**). In each experiment the peripheral blood monomorphonuclear cells (PBMCs) were sampled at regular intervals for the detection of cytokine mRNA by RT-qPCR, and for the quantification of the IFN-γ producing T cell subsets, respectively. At euthanasia, PBMCs and lymphocytes from the peripheral lymph nodes and spleen were isolated for further *in vitro* assays, whereas heart, diaphragm, skeletal muscles and brain were collected to determine the parasite load as explained further. The experimental timeline presenting the collected samples and the sampling intervals is shown in **Figure 1**.

Humoral Immune Response

For each experiment the seroconversion was monitored during the first 2 weeks after inoculation (wpi) by daily and subsequently weekly blood collection from the vena jugularis until 120 days post infection (dpi).

Antibody ELISA's with Recombinant GRA7 and Native TLA Antigens

As dense granule protein 7 (GRA7) is considered as a marker of an active infection, being expressed by all *T. gondii* stages, recombinant GRA7 is frequently used to demonstrate the immune response during acute and chronic toxoplasmosis in humans and animals (Jacobs et al., 1999). GRA7 was prepared as previously described (Jongert et al., 2007). Briefly, GRA7 was produced as a His-tagged fusion protein by *Escherichia coli* (*E. coli*) TOP 10 cells (Life Technologies, Ghent, Belgium) and purified under denaturing conditions (8 M urea, 0.1% SDS) using nickel-nitrilotriacetic acid (Ni-NTA) chelate affinity column chromatography (Ni-NTA Superflow, Qiagen, Venlo, The Netherlands). GRA7 was then eluted from the Ni-NTA column using 250 mM imidazole and further purified by sequential dialysis steps reducing the urea and SDS concentration to 0.1 M and 0.01%, respectively.

T. gondii total lysate antigen (TLA) from tachyzoites of the RH-strain was prepared as previously described (Jongert et al., 2007) in the biosafety level 2 laboratory (Biosafety permit no, 415240), as approved by the Ethical Committee (no. 20140704-01) at the National Reference Laboratory for Toxoplasmosis (Scientific Institute for Public Health, Brussels, Belgium). TLA-based assays show a high reactivity due to a broad range of antigens in the lysate, however, differences in the production method can affect the composition of the lysate (Gamble et al., 2005; Ferra et al., 2015). Concisely, tachyzoites were diluted with PBS and then purified by differential centrifugation and filtration through a 5 μm syringe filter (MilleX®SV, Merck KGaA, Darmstadt, Germany). The tachyzoite suspension was

TABLE 1 | Experimental design: G, IPB-G strain; LR, IPB-LR strain.

Study no.	Strain	Dose of tissue cysts	Group	Number of animals	Duration (dpi)	Heterologous challenge (y/n)
1	G	700	G_{low}	3	120	No
	G	6000	G_{high}	3	120	No
	LR	700	LR_{low}	3	120	No
	LR	6000	LR_{high}	3	120	No
2	G	6000	G_{high}/ LR_{high}	3	120	Yes (at 60 dpi)
	G	6000	$G_{high1/2t}$	3	60	No
	LR	6000	LR_{high}/ G_{high}	3	120	Yes (at 60 dpi)
3	G	6000	G_{high}	3	98	No
	LR	6000	LR_{high}	3	98	No
Control	/	0	$G+LR_{cltr}$	7	120	No

Groups, a single low or high dose of the IPB-G strain (G_{low} and G_{high}); a single low or high dose of the IPB-LR strain (LR_{low} and LR_{high}); a high dose of the IPB-G strain, followed 60 dpi by a high dose of the IPB-LR strain (G_{high}/LR_{high}); a high dose of the IPB-G strain 60 dpi ($G_{high1/2t}$); a high dose of the IPB-LR strain, followed 60 dpi by a high dose of the IPB-G strain (LR_{high}/G_{high}).

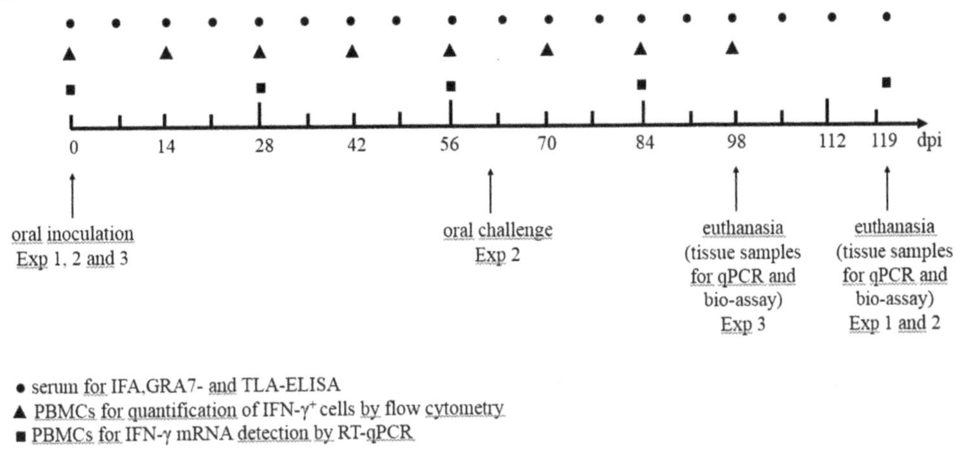

FIGURE 1 | The timeline of the experiments from the inoculation (day 0 dpi) until euthanasia (day 120 dpi). Exp, experiment; • serum for IFA, GRA- and TLA-ELISA; ▲ PBMCs for the quantification of IFN-γ^+ T-lymphocytes by flow cytometry; ■ PBMCs for IFN-γ mRNA detection by qPCR.

then lysed by alternating sonication with cooling cycles using an Ultrasonic disintegrator (MSE, Leicester, United Kingdom). To evaluate the protein content of the lysate, the bicinchoninic acid (BCA) reaction (Thermo Scientific Pierce BCA protein Assay Kit, Erembodegem, Belgium) was used. Finally, the TLA was aliquoted and stored at −20°C until further use.

Both TLA and GRA7 were used in indirect Enzyme-Linked Immunosorbent Assays (ELISA's) at 10 μg/ml to detect *T. gondii*-specific IgM and IgG antibodies in serum samples diluted 1/50 with the goat anti-pig IgM- and IgG-Horse Radish Peroxidase (HRP) conjugate (Bethyl Laboratories Inc., Montgomery, Texas, USA), respectively, and 2,2′-azino-bis(3-ethylbenzothiazoline-6-sulphonic acid (ABTS) as substrate-chromogen solution (Verhelst et al., 2015). On each plate previously collected sera from one positive and three negative control animals as established by IgM and IgG immunofluorescence assay (IFA) were included and diluted 1/50 in dilution buffer (0.05% Tween-20 in PBS). The absorbance was measured at 405 nm (TECAN Spectra Fluor, Tecan Group Ltd., Männedorf, Switzerland) and the obtained data were analyzed in Microsoft Excel. Serum samples from infected animals were considered positive when exceeding the cut-off value calculated using the formula: mean OD_{405} negative controls + 3 x its standard deviation (SD).

Immunofluorescence Assay

The presence of IgM and IgG antibodies against *T. gondii* was also evaluated by IFA using slides coated with formaline-fixed tachyzoites from the *T. gondii* RH-strain (Toxo-Spot IF, Biomérieux, Marcy-l'Etoile, France). Briefly, serum samples, diluted 1/50 in PBS, were applied to the slides for 30 min at 37°C, followed by washing with PBS. After drying, a second incubation with fluorescein isothiocyanate (FITC)-conjugated goat anti-swine IgM(μ) or IgG (H+L) (KPL, Maryland, USA) antibody (diluted 1/25 in PBS with Evans Blue as counter dye) was performed for 30 min at 37°C. After washing, drying and mounting with PBS-buffered glycerol, the slides were observed by fluorescence microscopy (Carl Zeiss, Germany). The cut-off read-out was established with positive and negative reference sera at a 1/50 dilution.

Detection of the Cellular Immune Response

PBMCs were isolated from 20 ml heparinized blood (LEO Pharma, Ballerup, Denmark) by density gradient centrifugation (800 × g at 18°C, 25 min) using Lymphoprep™ (Axis-Shield, Oslo, Norway) (Sonck et al., 2010). Subsequently, the cell pellets were resuspended in leukocyte medium [RPMI-1640 (GIBCO BRL, Life Technologies, Merelbeke, Belgium), supplemented with fetal calf serum (10%) (Greiner, Bio-One, Merelbeke Belgium), non-essential amino acids (100 mM) (Gibco), Na-pyruvate (100 μg/ml), L-glutamine (292 μg/ml) (Gibco), penicillin (100 IU/ml) (Gibco), streptomycin (100 μg/ml) (Gibco), and kanamycin (100 μg/ml) (Gibco)]. The cells (10^6 cells/well) were cultured for 6 and 72 h upon stimulation with either TLA (10 μg/ml) as a heterologous challenge or the mitogen concanavalin A (ConA, Sigma-Aldrich, USA; 5 μg/ml) as a positive control.

Cytokine mRNA Quantification by RT-qPCR

After 6 h of incubation with TLA, ConA or medium, the cells were lysed by adding 350 μl of RLT-buffer (Qiagen) supplemented with 1% β-mercaptoethanol (99%, Thermo Fisher Scientific, Aalst, Belgium) and stored at −80°C until RNA isolation. Total RNA extraction and conversion into cDNA was performed using the RNeasy kit (Qiagen) and the iScript kit (Biorad, Hercules, CA, USA), respectively. The purity of the RNA was assessed by an on-column DNase digestion step as recommended by the supplier. The amount of cytokine cDNA was then tested by quantitative polymerase chain reaction (qPCR). The qPCR reaction mix consisted of 12.5 μl iQ SYBR Green Supermix (Biorad), 0.5 μl of each primer set at a concentration of 20 μM, 1.5 μl PCR grade water and 10 μl of the 1/100 diluted cDNA. Interleukin (IL)-10, IL-12A, IL-17A, and interferon-gamma (IFN-γ) cDNA was amplified with the primer sets presented in **Table 2**. In order to normalize the cytokine expression, β-actin, glyceraldehyde phosphate dehydrogenase (GAPDH) and the ribosomal 18S gene were used as reference genes (**Table 2**). Special care was taken to choose a set of primers on different exons or spanning exon-exon junctions to exclude the amplification of genomic DNA. The qPCR amplification protocol consisted of an initial denaturation at 95°C for 3 min, followed by 45 cycles of 95°C for 15 s and 61°C for 20 s. After each run, a melt curve analysis was performed to confirm the presence of the correct amplicon and to exclude false positives due to the formation of primer dimers. The cDNA was tested in duplicate for each cytokine and the three reference genes (GADPH, β-actin, r18S), showing a stable expression. The mRNA expression in PBMCs was calculated with the CFX96 Manager™ Software v3.1 (Biorad), using a mathematical model (delta-delta Ct method). The mean value was determined for the target cytokines and normalized relative to the geometric mean of the reference genes (Verhelst et al., 2015).

Flow Cytometric Detection of IFN-γ Production

The flow cytometric detection of IFN-γ-producing proliferating lymphocytes was performed on cultured PBMCs 72 h after heterologous stimulation with TLA (10 μg/ml). First, the cell division marker Violet Proliferation Dye 450 (VPD450, BD Biosciences, Erembodegem, Belgium) was added to the isolated mononuclear cells, showing a diminishing fluorescence after each cell division. At the end of the incubation period, a protein transport inhibitor, Golgi Plug™, was added and the cells were fixed and permeabilized using the Cytofix/Cytoperm™ kit (both from BD Biosciences). Subsequently, cells were stained using murine monoclonal antibodies (Mab) against CD3 (IgG1, clone PPT3), CD4 (IgG2b, clone 72-14-4), and CD8 (IgG2a, clone 11/295/33) and anti-isotype-specific conjugates (goat anti-mouse IgG1-PerCP-Cy5.5; Santa Cruz Biotechnology, Dallas, Texas, USA), goat anti-mouse IgG2b-FITC (Southernbiotech, Birmingham, Alabama, USA) and goat anti-mouse IgG2a-Alexa Fluor®647 (Invitrogen™, Merelbeke, Belgium). Finally, phycoeryrthrin (PE)-conjugated mAb against porcine IFN-γ (Mouse IgG1, BD Biosciences) was added to identify the lymphocyte subsets producing IFN-γ. A minimum of 10,000 events was recorded within the proliferating cell gate (Appendix 1). The IFN-γ secretion in the different lymphocyte subsets was determined and compared with the results of the isotype-matched control (Mouse IgG1-PE, Abcam, Cambridge, UK) using a FACSAria III and FACSDIVA™ software (both from BD). The gating strategy is included in the supplementary data (Appendix 1).

Animals were euthanized at 98 dpi and the splenocytes and lymphocytes from the peripheral lymph nodes (mediastinal, mesenteric and popliteal) were isolated as previously described (Verhelst et al., 2011). Subsequently, the cells were stimulated with the same antigens as the PBMCs for 6 h and 72 h, whereafter the same staining occurred for flow cytometric analysis as for the PBMCs.

TABLE 2 | List of primers for qPCR.

Target	Sequence	Length amplicon (bp)
IL-10	F: CCTGGGTTGCCAAGCCTT	240
	R: GCTTTGTAGACACCCCTCTCTT	
IL-12A	F: ACCAGCACAGTGGAGGC	95
	R: CGAATGAGAGTTGCCTGGCT	
IL-17A	F: GGACAAGAACTTCCCTCAGCA	124
	R: CTCGTTGCGTTGGAGAGTC	
IFN-γ	F: GAGCCAAATTGTCTCCTTCTACTT	262
	R: CTGACTTCTCTTCCGCTTTCT	
GAPDH	F: CCATCACTGCCACCCAGAA	130
	R: CAGGGATGACCTTGCCCA	
B-actin	F: GGCATCCTGACCCTCAAGTA	137
	R: GCCTCGGTCAGCAGCA	
r18S	F: GTTGATTAAGTCCCTGCCCTTT	141
	R: GATAGTCAAGTTCGACCGTCTT	

Detection of the Parasite: Bio-Assay and qPCR

In experiments 1 and 2, all animals were euthanized at 120 dpi and the parasite load was determined in brain (Br), heart (He), spleen, diaphragm (Di) and skeletal muscles (m. gastrocnemius (Mg), mm. intercostales (Ic), m. longissimus dorsi (Ld), and m. psoas major (Mp) by qPCR and a bio-assay. For this, 100 g of each tissue was homogenized in 10 ml 0.85% sodium chloride (NaCl) and digested with pepsin [0.8 g/l pepsin in 7 ml/l hydrogen chloride (HCl)] for 1 h for brain and 2 h for the other tissues, while stirring in a water bath at 37°C. The obtained suspension was filtered and centrifuged for 15 min at 1,180 × g, the supernatant removed and the pellet resuspended in 10 ml PBS supplemented with 40 IU/ml gentamicin. For the bio-assay, 1 ml of the tissue suspension was inoculated intraperitoneally into 5 naive Swiss female mice. The mice were observed frequently on a daily base for the next 5 weeks and euthanized in respect to the human end points in case of acute toxoplasmosis associated with suffering or reduced welfare. The surviving mice were euthanized and tested serologically by immunofluorescence for the presence of *T. gondii* IgG antibodies or by qPCR for lungs and ascites when pre terminated due to the ethical aspects in case of acute toxoplasmosis. To determine the parasite load by qPCR DNA was extracted from the tissue suspensions with the QIAamp DNA Mini kit (Qiagen). A 10-fold serial dilution of *T. gondii* DNA prepared from RH-strain tachyzoite suspension containing 10^6 parasites per ml was used as a standard, with a detection limit of 2–4 tissue cysts per 100 g of tissue. Real-Time PCR (RT-PCR) amplifying both the *T. gondii* repeat element (AF146527) and the ribosomal 18S rDNA of the host cells was performed as previously described (Rosenberg et al., 2009).

Statistics

The parasite-specific antibody and IFN-γ responses in different groups at different time points are presented as means ± SD. A one-way Analysis of Variance (ANOVA) was performed, followed by post hoc Bonferroni's and Dunnett's Multiple Comparison Tests for antibody production and cytokine response, respectively, to discriminate between infected and control groups (GraphPad Prism 5). A $p < 0.05$ was considered statistically significant.

RESULTS

Parasite Burden and Immune Response after Single Inoculation with a Low or a High Infection Dose of the IPB-G or IPB-LR Strain

GRA-7 and TLA-Specific Antibody Response

The GRA7-specific IgM antibodies appeared approximately at the same time in the low and the high dose group (10 and 9 dpi, respectively) upon inoculation with the IPB-G strain and declined gradually from 14 and 11 dpi, respectively, until 91 dpi (**Figure 2A**). In contrast, in the IPB-LR infected group a pronounced IgM production was detected 8 dpi in the low dose group and even a stronger response at 10 dpi in the high dose group (**Figure 2B**), but both declined to control levels around 12 dpi. GRA7-specific IgG antibodies were detected shortly after IgM, irrespective of the inoculation strain, and remained detectable until the end of the experiment (**Figures 2C,D**). Nevertheless, the high dose of the IPB-LR strain induced the highest levels of GRA7-specific IgG.

TLA-specific IgM occurred earlier than GRA7-specific IgM, namely 7 to 8 dpi in the G_{low} and G_{high} groups. In the latter, the IgM response remained present until the end of the experiment, slightly increasing in time, irrespective from the infection dose (**Figure 3A**). On the contrary, for the LR_{low} and LR_{high} groups the seroconversion to TLA-specific IgM was prominently present until 21 to 28 dpi, showing again the highest concentration in the high dose group (**Figure 3B**). The TLA-specific IgG antibodies appeared approximately 14 dpi in both dose groups inoculated with the IPB-G strain (**Figure 3C**), but already at 8 dpi in animals infected with the IPB-LR strain. There, the antibodies increased significantly starting from 28 dpi and remained elevated until

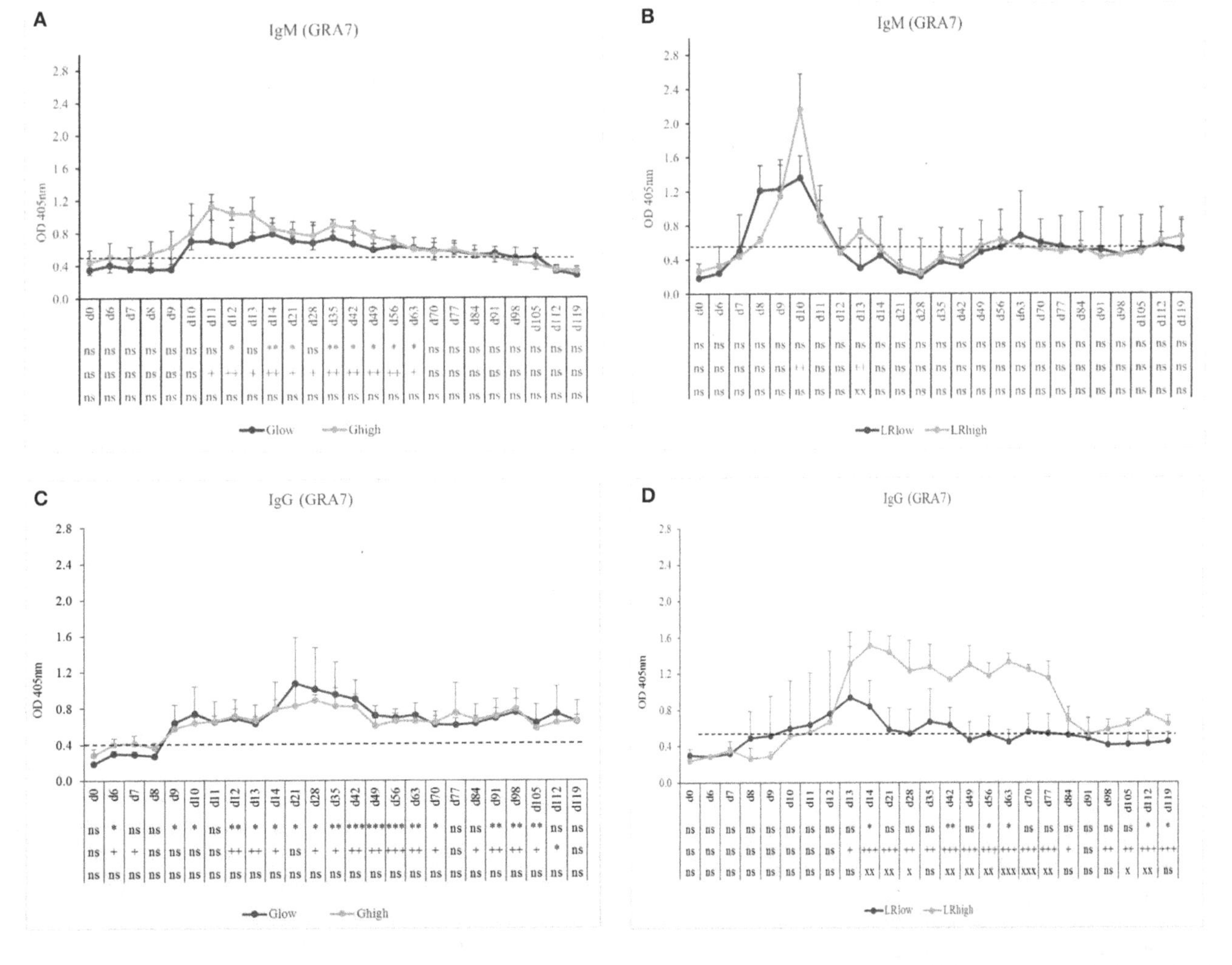

FIGURE 2 | GRA7-specific IgM and IgG responses after inoculation with IPB-G or IPB-LR *T. gondii* strain. IgM **(A,B)** and IgG **(C,D)** responses in animals inoculated with a low or a high dose of the IPB-G **(A,C)** or the IPB-LR **(B,D)** strain. Groups: G_{low}, G_{high}, LR_{low}, LR_{high}. The horizontal dashed line indicates the cut-off value based on the mean of the negative animals. The results represent a mean of the infected group ± SD; * (low dose vs. controls) or + (high dose vs. controls) or x (low dose vs. high dose): $P < 0.05$, ** or ++ or xx: $P < 0.01$; *** or +++ or xxx: $P < 0.001$; ns, not significant.

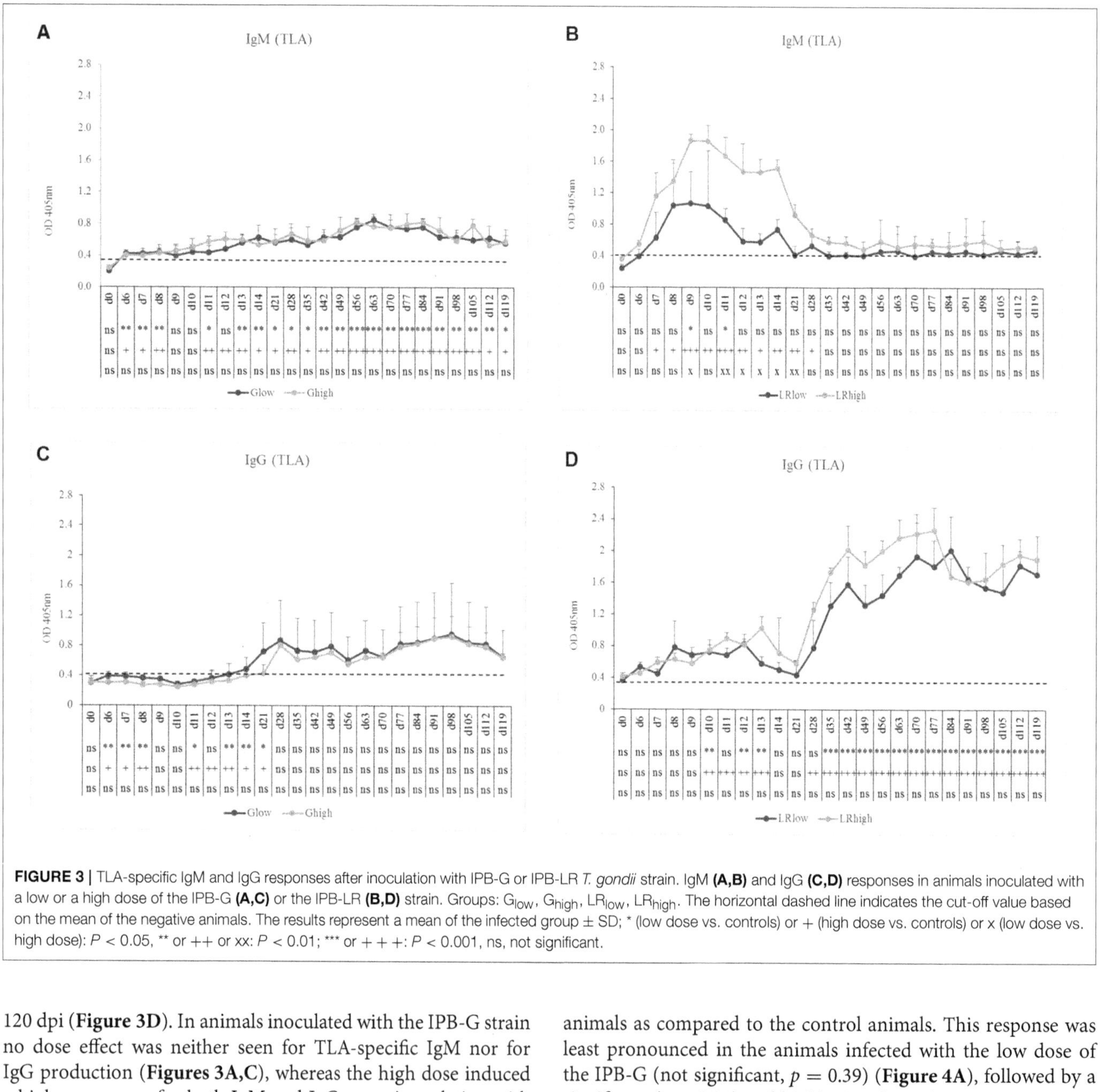

FIGURE 3 | TLA-specific IgM and IgG responses after inoculation with IPB-G or IPB-LR *T. gondii* strain. IgM **(A,B)** and IgG **(C,D)** responses in animals inoculated with a low or a high dose of the IPB-G **(A,C)** or the IPB-LR **(B,D)** strain. Groups: G_{low}, G_{high}, LR_{low}, LR_{high}. The horizontal dashed line indicates the cut-off value based on the mean of the negative animals. The results represent a mean of the infected group ± SD; * (low dose vs. controls) or + (high dose vs. controls) or x (low dose vs. high dose): $P < 0.05$, ** or ++ or xx: $P < 0.01$; *** or + + +: $P < 0.001$, ns, not significant.

120 dpi (**Figure 3D**). In animals inoculated with the IPB-G strain no dose effect was neither seen for TLA-specific IgM nor for IgG production (**Figures 3A,C**), whereas the high dose induced a higher response for both IgM and IgG upon inoculation with the IPB-LR strain (**Figures 3B,D**). The IFA results confirmed the seroconversion from *T. gondii* - negative toward IgM positive animals and the persistence of the IgG antibodies in each infection experiment (data not shown).

TLA-Specific IFN-γ mRNA Responses in PMBCs

PBMCs were restimulated *in vitro* with TLA for 6 h, where after IL-10, IL-12A, IL-17A, and IFN-γ mRNA responses were determined. No detectable IL-10, IL-12, and IL-17A mRNA production was observed (data not shown) in any infected group, irrespective of the strain or infection dose. However, a substantial increase in IFN-γ mRNA production was observed from 1 month post infection (mpi) onwards in the majority of the inoculated animals as compared to the control animals. This response was least pronounced in the animals infected with the low dose of the IPB-G (not significant, $p = 0.39$) (**Figure 4A**), followed by a significant ($p < 0.01$) and highly significant ($p < 0.001$) increase in the high dose of the IPB-G strain group (**Figure 4B**). In the low dose of the IPB-LR group we noticed a steady though not significant ($p = 0.18$) increase (**Figure 4C**). The highest IFN-γ production was observed in the animals infected with the high dose of the IPB-LR strain starting from 1 mpi ($p < 0.01$), which stayed high throughout the experiment, becoming highly significant ($p < 0.001$) at 2, 3, and 4 mpi (**Figure 4D**). No detectable IFN-γ level was detected in splenocytes from IPB-G or IPB-LR infected animals (data not shown).

Parasite Load in Tissues

At 120 dpi, the parasite load was determined in heart and striated skeletal muscles by qPCR and a bioassay, while in brain by qPCR

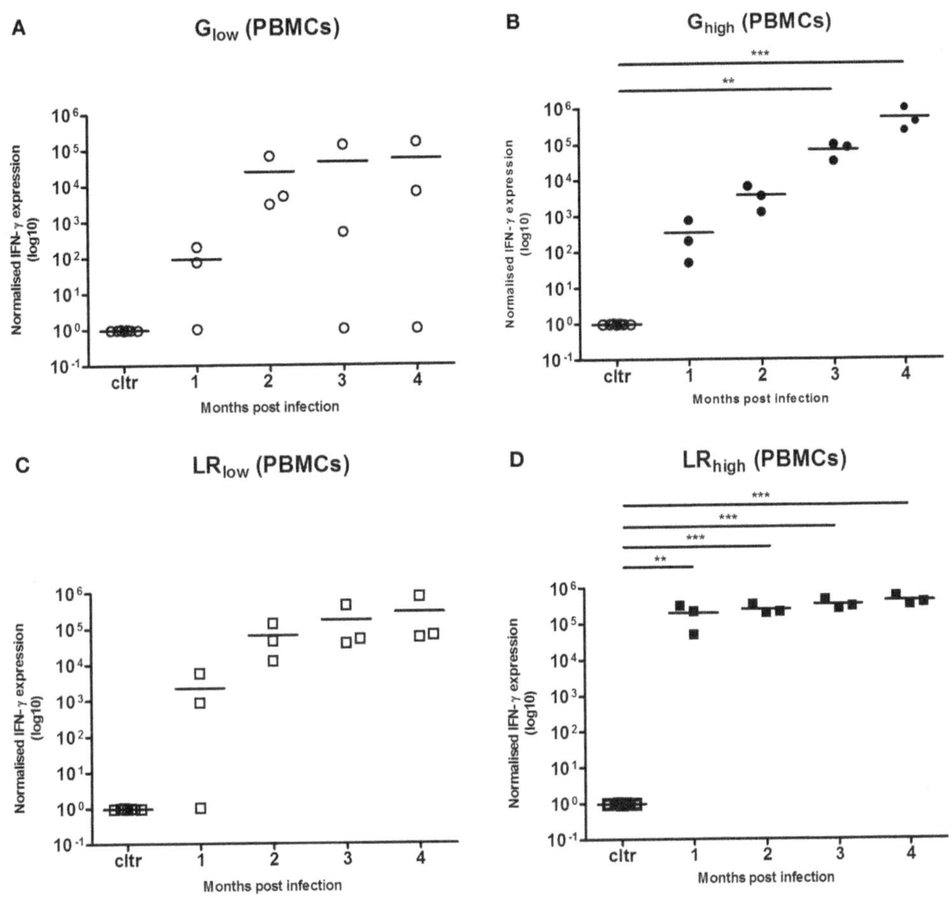

FIGURE 4 | Relative normalized IFN-γ expression in PBMCs after a single IPB-G or IPB-LR inoculation. PBMCs were isolated monthly from pigs orally infected with **(A)** a low or **(B)** a high dose of the IPB-G strain (G_{low} and G_{high}) or **(C)** a low or **(D)** a high dose of the IPB-LR strain (LR_{low} and LR_{high}). Cells were restimulated *in vitro* with TLA and IFN-γ mRNA was quantified with RT-PCR. The thick lines indicate the group mean. The significance level: $^{**}P < 0.01$; $^{***}P < 0.001$.

only. In animals infected with the IPB-LR strain, the highest parasite load was found in brain followed by heart (**Table 3**). Interestingly, the inoculation dose did not affect the distribution or load in the tissues. Besides brain and heart, also intercostal muscles and the longissimus dorsi were consistently positive in qPCR, whereas heart of all 6 animals was also positive in the bioassay.

A different pattern was seen in pigs inoculated with the IPB-G strain (**Table 3**), where a clear effect of the inoculation dose on the parasite distribution and load in the tissues was found. When inoculated with the low dose, the parasite was present in more tissues and in higher amounts than when inoculated with the high dose. However, even when inoculated with the low dose, the longissimus dorsi and psoas major remained negative in all three animals in this group. Summarizing, animals inoculated with the high dose of IPB-G showed the lowest amount of *T. gondii* DNA in their tissues. Brain, gastrocnemius and the longissimus dorsi were negative, whereas for diaphragm and psoas major only one sample was positive in the bioassay and qPCR, respectively. These results strongly suggest a dose-dependent decreased burden of the IPB-G strain in the examined tissues following inoculation, pointing toward an immune-mediated reduction of the parasite load.

Parasite Tissue Load and Immune Response in a Subsequent Infection Model with Two *T. gondii* Strains

In order to assess if the low parasite load observed in some tissues after infection with the IPB-G strain was related to an immune response, in a second experiment animals were first infected with the high dose of one strain, followed 60 days later with the high dose of the other strain (**Table 1**). Since we hypothesized an effect of the inoculation with the IPB-G strain, an additional control group was included in the study inoculated with the high dose at 60 dpi and 60 days before euthanasia.

GRA-7 and TLA-Specific Antibody Response

As in the first experiment, inoculation with the IPB-LR strain induced higher GRA7- and TLA-specific IgM production than with the IPB-G strain, independently from the order of inoculation (**Figures 5A,B**). This was most pronounced for the TLA-specific IgM response (**Figure 5B**). The presence of a clear

TABLE 3 | Parasite load (number of bradyzoites per 1E+08 cells) by qRT-PCR after inoculation with two *T. gondii* strains, in comparison with bio-assay (number of positive/total tested).

	qPCR							Bio-assay						
	Br	Ha	Di	Ic	Mg	Ld	Mp	Br	Ha	Di	Ic	Mg	Ld	Mp
G_{low}	2/3	2/3	2/3	3/3	2/3	0/3	0/3	nt	2/3	1/3	1/3	0/3	0/3	0/3
Average	1.1E+05	8.5	20.6	44.6	3.0	0.0	0.0							
SD	1.1E+05	8.4	29.9	13.4	2.7	0.0	0.0							
G_{high}	0/3	1/3	0/3	2/3	0/3	0/3	1/3	nt	2/3	1/3	0/3	0/3	0/3	0/3
Average	0.0	1.0	0.0	21.2	0.0	0.0	2.3							
SD	0.0	1.0	0.0	19.1	0.0	0.0	4.0							
LR_{low}	3/3	3/3	3/3	3/3	2/3	3/3	3/3	nt	3/3	3/3	1/3	0/3	0/3	0/3
Average	378.78	169.63	8.46	23.45	52.40	28.67	189.07							
SD	94.86	228.70	12.25	17.52	45.38	29.94	244.88							
LR_{high}	3/3	3/3	2/3	3/3	3/3	3/3	2/3	nt	3/3	1/3	1/3	0/3	1/3	1/3
Average	1339.97	592.25	7.82	29.4	35.0	72.6	67.8							
SD	322.83	281.15	11.61	30.5	8.6	28.5	68.0							
G_{high}/LR_{high}	3/3	3/3	3/3	2/3	1/3	0/3	2/3	nt	3/3	2/3	1/3	0/3	0/3	1/3
Average	489.07	70.66	19.22	16.7	8.1	0.0	66.3							
SD	614.04	51.02	17.93	22.3	14.1	0.0	102.2							
$G_{high1/2t}$	2/3	3/3	1/3	0/3	1/3	1/3	0/3	nt	2/3	1/3	0/3	0/3	0/3	0/3
Average	1742.74	16.18	5.82	0.0	2.2	6.7	0.0							
SD	1570.94	26.09	10.07	0.0	3.9	11.6	0.0							
LR_{high}/G_{high}	3/3	3/3	1/3	0/3	1/3	0/3	1/3	nt	2/3	1/3	0/3	1/3	0/3	1/3
Average	5950.50	105.32	1.67	0.0	0.8	0.0	1.6							
SD	8708.45	128.54	2.90	0.0	1.5	0.0	2.7							

Groups, a single low or high dose of the IPB-G strain (G_{low} and G_{high}) 120 dpi; a single low or high dose of the IPB-LR strain (LR_{low} and LR_{high}); a high dose of the IPB-G strain, followed 60 dpi by a high dose of the IPB-LR strain (G_{high}/LR_{high}); a high dose of the IPB-G strain 60 dpi ($G_{high1/2t}$); a high dose of the LR strain, followed 60 dpi by a high dose of the IPB-G strain (LR_{high}/G_{high}). Tissues: Br, brain; Ha, heart; Di, diaphragm; Ic, intercostal m.; Mg, gastrocnemius m.; Ld, long. dorsi m.; Pm, poas major m.; nt, not tested.

TLA-specific IgM response after the second inoculation with the IPB-LR strain was remarkable and suggests differences in antigen expression between both strains (higher immunogenicity, different antigens or other reasons), leading to the induction of a primary immune response against various TLA antigens. Interestingly, the increase in TLA-specific IgM levels in the IPB-G infected animals upon initial inoculation at day 60 ($G_{high1/2t}$) was higher in comparison with G_{high} or G_{low} groups (**Figure 3A**), suggesting maturation of the immune system. Similar to our findings of the first experiment (**Figures 2C,D, 3C,D**), the GRA7- and TLA-specific IgG antibodies appeared within 2 weeks following the primary inoculation with the IPB-G or IPB-LR strain (**Figures 5C,D**). A pronounced booster response against GRA7 occurred upon the heterologous challenge at 60 dpi in both re-infected groups, as evidenced by a much faster increase in IgG levels in contrast to animals from the $G_{high1/2t}$ group (**Figure 5C**). The TLA IgG was not boosted following the heterologous infections in both challenged groups (**Figure 5D**). However, these distinct IgG responses were more pronounced by the challenge with the IPB-LR strain than with the IPB-G strain.

TLA-Specific IFN-γ mRNA Responses in PMBCs and Spleen

IFN-γ responses after the initial inoculation with both *T. gondii* strains (**Figure 6**) were comparable with those in the first experiment (**Figure 4**). In two of the three animals receiving the IPB-G strain as a first inoculation (G_{high}/LR_{high}), IFN-γ mRNA expression could not be detected 1 mpi in the PBMCs recall assay with TLA. However, from 2 mpi all three animals showed a significantly ($p < 0.05$) to highly significant ($p < 0.001$) increased IFN-γ mRNA level (**Figure 6A**), similarly to the expression seen in animals receiving the IPB-LR strain as a first inoculum (LR_{high}/G_{high}) (**Figure 6B**), even though the latter showed a more homogenous response from 1 mpi onwards ($p < 0.01$). In both groups the IFN-γ mRNA expressions remained significantly elevated ($p < 0.05$ to $p < 0.001$) during the experiment and no additional increase was seen after inoculation with the heterologous strains. Slightly lower yet significant ($p < 0.05$) IFN-γ production was observed in group $G_{high1/2t}$, inoculated for the first time at 60 dpi (**Figure 6C**).

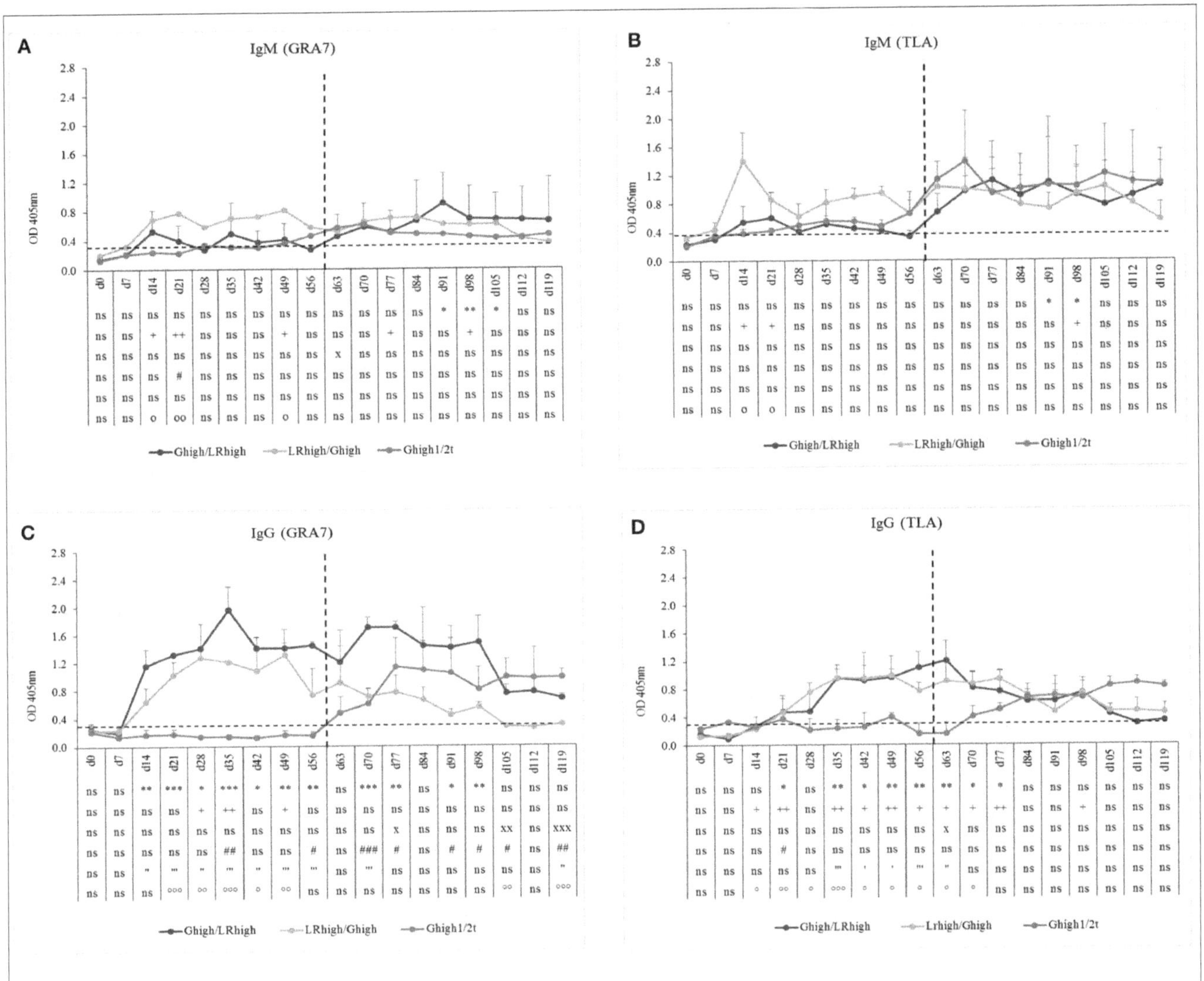

FIGURE 5 | GRA7- and TLA-specific IgM and IgG responses after inoculation with IPB-G and IPB-LR *T. gondii* strains. IgM **(A,B)** and IgG **(C,D)** antibody response toward *T. gondii* GRA7 **(A,C)** and TLA **(B,D)** in animals after a consecutive infection with a high dose of IPB-G and IPB-LR strains. Groups: G_{high}/LR_{high}, LR_{high}/G_{high}. Piglets infected after 60 days with a high dose IPB-G served as a control ($G_{high1/2t}$). The horizonthal dashed line indicates the cut-off value based on the mean of the negative animals, and the vertical one the timepoint of reinfection.The results represent a mean of the infected group ± SD; * G_{high}/LR_{high} vs. controls, + LR_{high}/G_{high} vs. controls, x $G_{high1/2t}$ vs. controls, # G_{high}/LR_{high} vs. LR_{high}/G_{high}, ' G_{high}/LR_{high} vs. $G_{high1/2t}$, ° LR_{high}/G_{high} vs. $G_{high1/2t}$: $P < 0.05$, ** or ++ or xx or ## or " or °°: $P < 0.01$; *** or xxx or ### or "' or °°°; $P < 0.001$; ns, not significant.

While no detectable cytokine production was found at 120 dpi in the spleen of animals from both infection groups in the first experiment (data not shown), in the heterologous infection model significant IFN-γ transcript levels were detected 60 days after the second infection for the G_{high}/LR_{high} ($p < 0.05$), $G_{high1/2t}$ ($p < 0.01$), and LR_{high}/G_{high} ($p < 0.001$) (**Figures 7A,B**).

Parasite Load in Tissues

To assess the parasite load in tissues animals were euthanized 60 days after a first ($G_{high1/2t}$ group) or second infection (G_{high}/LR_{high} and LR_{high}/G_{high} groups). Interestingly, animals receiving only the high dose of the IPB-G strain ($G_{high1/2t}$) showed a parasite distribution and load (13 tissue samples negative in a bioassay) in between those observed at 120 dpi with the IPB-G low dose (10 tissue samples negative in a bioassay) and the high dose (17 samples negative) in the first experiment (**Table 3**). This could suggest that the reduction in parasite load induced by the IPB-G strain was already appearing at 60 dpi upon inoculation with the high dose. The tissue distribution at 120 dpi in animals, which first received the IPB-LR high dose and 60 days later the IPB-G high dose, could also be explained by this phenomenon. At 120 dpi the animals showed a different parasite load and tissue distribution (12 samples negative) than in the first experiment (1 and 2 samples negative after infection with the low and the high dose, respectively). Animals receiving first the IPB-G high dose and 60 days later the IPB-LR high dose, showed a wider parasite tissue distribution and a higher parasite tissue load (7 samples negative), more comparable to animals receiving only the IPB-LR strain.

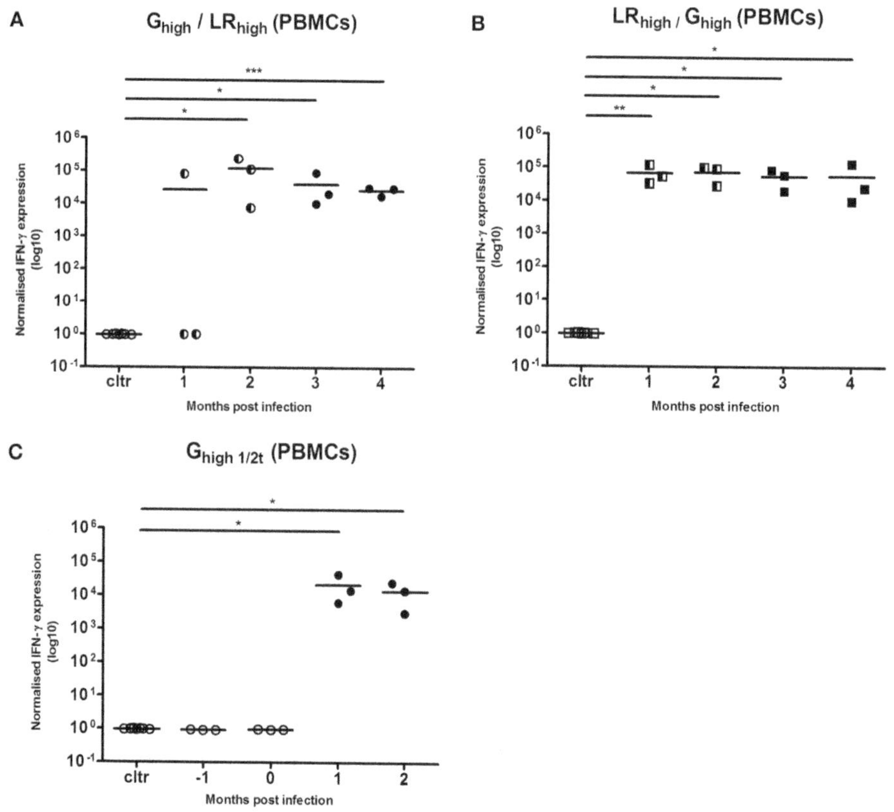

FIGURE 6 | Relative normalized IFN-γ expression in PBMCs after a consecutive IPB-G and IPB-LR inoculation. PBMCs were isolated monthly from pigs orally infected with **(A)** a high dose of the IPB-G strain followed 60 days later by a high dose of the IPB-LR strain (G_{high}/LR_{high}) or **(B)** reversed infection model (LR_{high}/G_{high}). Piglets infected with a high dose of the IPB-G strain at day 60 served as a control **(C)** ($G_{high1/2t}$). Cells were restimulated *in vitro* with TLA and IFN-γ mRNA was quantified with RT-PCR. The thick lines indicate the group mean. The significance level: $^{*}P < 0.05$, $^{**}P < 0.01$; $^{***}P < 0.001$.

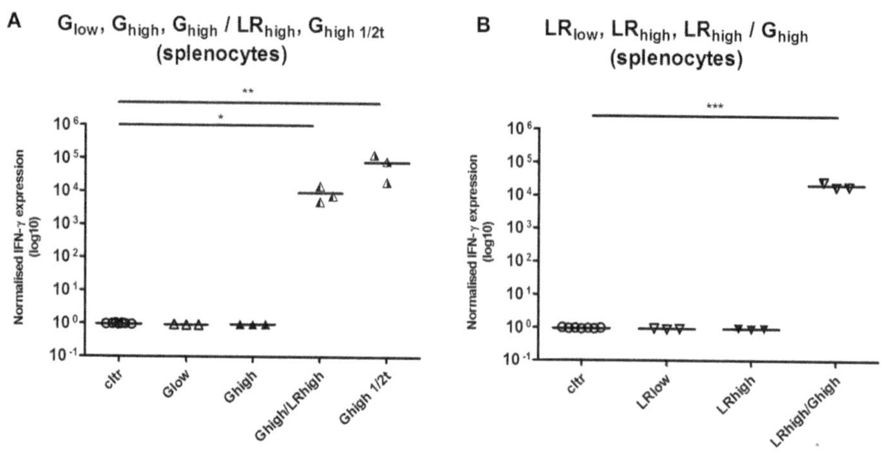

FIGURE 7 | Relative normalized IFN-γ expression in splenocytes after a single or consecutive IPB-G and IPB-LR inoculation. Splenocytes were isolated from pigs orally infected with **(A)** a low dose of the IPB-G strain (G_{low}), a high dose of the IPB-G strain (G_{high}), a high dose of the IPB-G strain followed 60 days later by a high dose of the IPB-LR strain (G_{high}/LR_{high}), a high dose of IPB-G at day 60 ($G_{high1/2t}$), or **(B)** a low dose of the IPB-LR strain (LR_{low}), a high dose of the IPB-LR strain (LR_{high}) or a high dose of the IPB-LR strain followed 60 days later by a high dose of the IPB-G strain reversed infection model (LR_{high}/G_{high}). Cells were isolated at 2 mpi (group: $G_{high1/2t}$) or 4 mpi (groups: G_{low}, LR_{low}, G_{high}, LR_{high}, G_{high}/LR_{high}, LR_{high}/G_{high}) and restimulated *in vitro* with TLA. IFN-γ mRNA was quantified with RT-PCR. The thick lines indicate the group mean. The significance level: $^{*}P < 0.05$, $^{**}P < 0.01$; $^{***}P < 0.001$.

The Involvement of CD4+ and CD8+ T Cells in the Strain-Dependent IFN-γ Production

Results of the above experiment supported our hypothesis that the IPB-G strain reduced the parasite burden. Since many studies suggested an important role for IFN-γ responses in controlling *T. gondii* infections, in a next experiment we compared the kinetics of IFN-γ producing T cell subsets in blood, following infection with the high dose of both strains in an *in vitro* TLA recall assay. Depending on the *T. gondii* strain, differences in the kinetics of circulating IFN-γ producing T cell subpopulations were observed (**Figure 8**). The $CD3^+CD4^+CD8\alpha^-$ and $CD3^+CD4^+CD8\alpha^{dim}$ represent porcine T-helper cells, while $CD3^+CD4^-CD8\alpha^{bright}$ cells are cytotoxic T cells (Gerner et al., 2015). Animals inoculated with the IPB-LR strain showed at 21 dpi a significant increase in the $CD3^+IFN\text{-}\gamma^+$ T cell subsets ($CD4^+CD8\alpha^-$, $CD4^+CD8\alpha^{dim}$, and $CD4^-CD8\alpha^{bright}$ T cells), with the $CD4^+CD8\alpha^-$ T-helper cells (up to 22.2 ± 8.3% of $CD3^+IFN\text{-}\gamma$ producing cells) being most prevalent (**Figure 8A**). This latter population remained stable, whereas the $CD4^-CD8\alpha^{bright}$ population gradually increased from 9.3 ± 0.87% of the $IFN\text{-}\gamma^+$ producing cells at 28 dpi to > 40% (41.1 ± 17.4%) at 98 dpi (**Figure 8C**). In contrast, the percentage $CD4^+CD8\alpha^{dim}IFN\text{-}\gamma^+$ cells gradually decreased from 16.4 ± 1.4% to <2.1 ± 0.8% at the end of the experiment (**Figure 8B**). In animals inoculated with the IPB-G strain, a similar increase in the percentage of $CD4^+CD8\alpha^{dim}IFN\text{-}\gamma^+$ cells at 21 dpi to 10.4 ± 0.4%, and a subsequent gradual decrease to 2.2 ± 0.5% was seen (**Figure 8B**). The $IFN\text{-}\gamma^+$ within $CD4^+CD8\alpha^-$ and $CD4^-CD8\alpha^{bright}$ T cells gradually increased, reaching significantly higher levels (22.6 ± 11.9% and 18.7 ± 9.5%, respectively) at 84 dpi as compared to 0 dpi (**Figures 8A,C**). Intriguingly, the increase of the latter T cell population was clearly less pronounced in the G_{high} ($p < 0.05$) than in the LR_{high} group ($p < 0.01$).

The difference in circulating $CD4^-CD8\alpha^{bright}$ T cell populations between both high dose groups seems to be reflected on the long term in the significantly higher ($p < 0.05$) percentage of $CD4^-CD8\alpha^{bright}$ $IFN\text{-}\gamma^+$ T cells in the popliteal lymph nodes (LN) in the LR_{high} group than in the G_{high} group at 98 dpi (**Figure 9C**). Additionally, a similar difference in the percentage of the same population between both groups can be detected in the mesenteric LN. However, in mediastinal LN, which drain heart and diaphragm, a higher percentage of $CD4^-CD8\alpha^{bright}$ $IFN\text{-}\gamma^+$ T cells was found in the G_{high} group, although not significantly different from the LR_{high} group. The distribution of the other T cell subpopulations in different lymphoid tissues shows a comparable pattern: a higher percentage of the $CD4^+CD8\alpha^-IFN\text{-}\gamma^+$ T was found in the mesenteric ($p < 0.05$) and popliteal ($p > 0.05$) LN of the LR_{high} group than in the G_{high} group (**Figure 9A**). Likewise for the $CD4^-CD8\alpha^{bright}$ T cells, a reverse situation was noticed in the mediastinal LN. Regarding the $CD4^+CD8\alpha^{dim}IFN\text{-}\gamma^+$ cells, relatively low percentages were detected in both infected groups. The highest counts were found in the mesenteric and popliteal LN in the LR_{high} group, followed by the mesenteric LN in the G_{high} group, whereas they were nearly absent in the other sampled LN (**Figure 9B**).

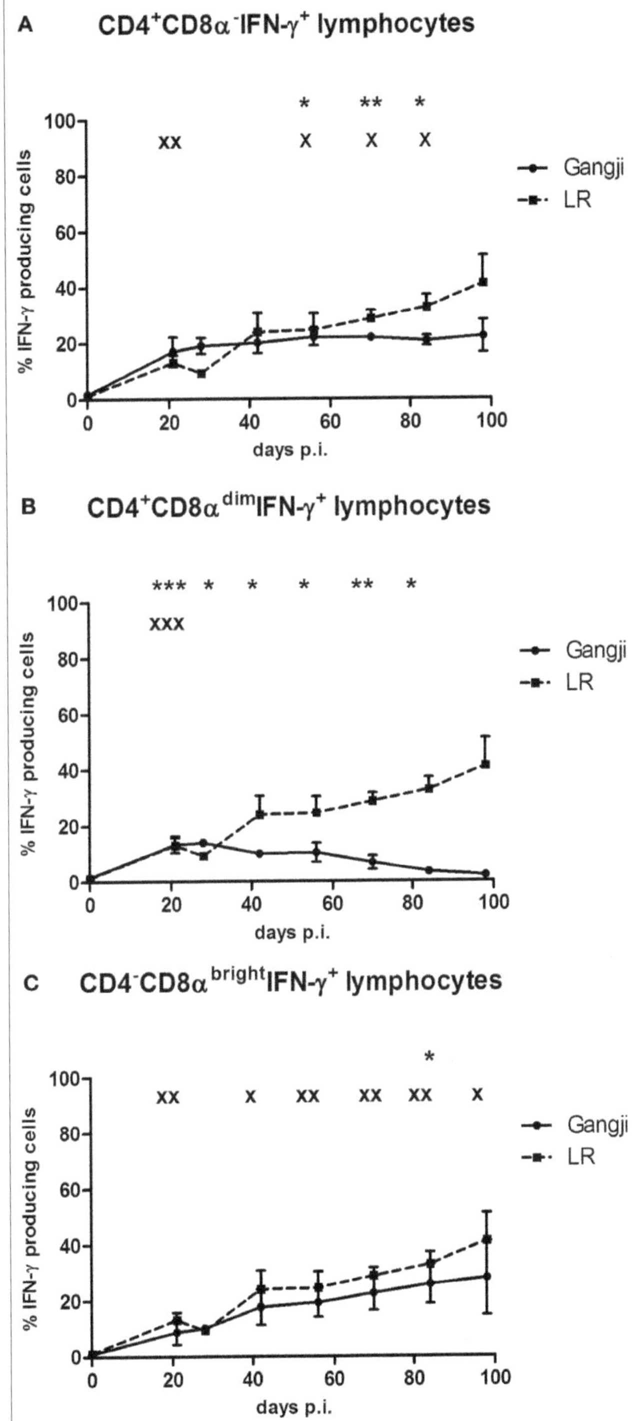

FIGURE 8 | The percentage of $IFN\text{-}\gamma^+$ T lymphocyte subsets in PBMCs after a single IPB-G or IPB-LR inoculation. $IFN\text{-}\gamma^+$ T lymphocyte subsets in PBMC's of pigs after oral infection with a high dose of the IPB-G (G_{high}) or the IPB-LR strain (LR_{high}). Cells were restimulated *in vitro* with TLA and demonstrated by flow cytometry following triple staining for IFN-γ, CD3, CD4, and CD8 **(A)**. $IFN\text{-}\gamma^+$ cell populations were identified as **(A)** $CD3^+CD4^+CD8\alpha^-IFN\text{-}\gamma^+$, **(B)** $CD3^+CD4+CD8\alpha^{dim}$ $IFN\text{-}\gamma^+$, **(C)** $CD3^+CD4^-CD8^{bright}IFN\text{-}\gamma^+$ lymphocytes. The results represent mean percentages ± SD for each group; * (IPB-G) or x (IPB-LR): $P < 0.05$, ** or xx: $P < 0.01$; *** or xxx: $P < 0.001$ in comparison with day 0.

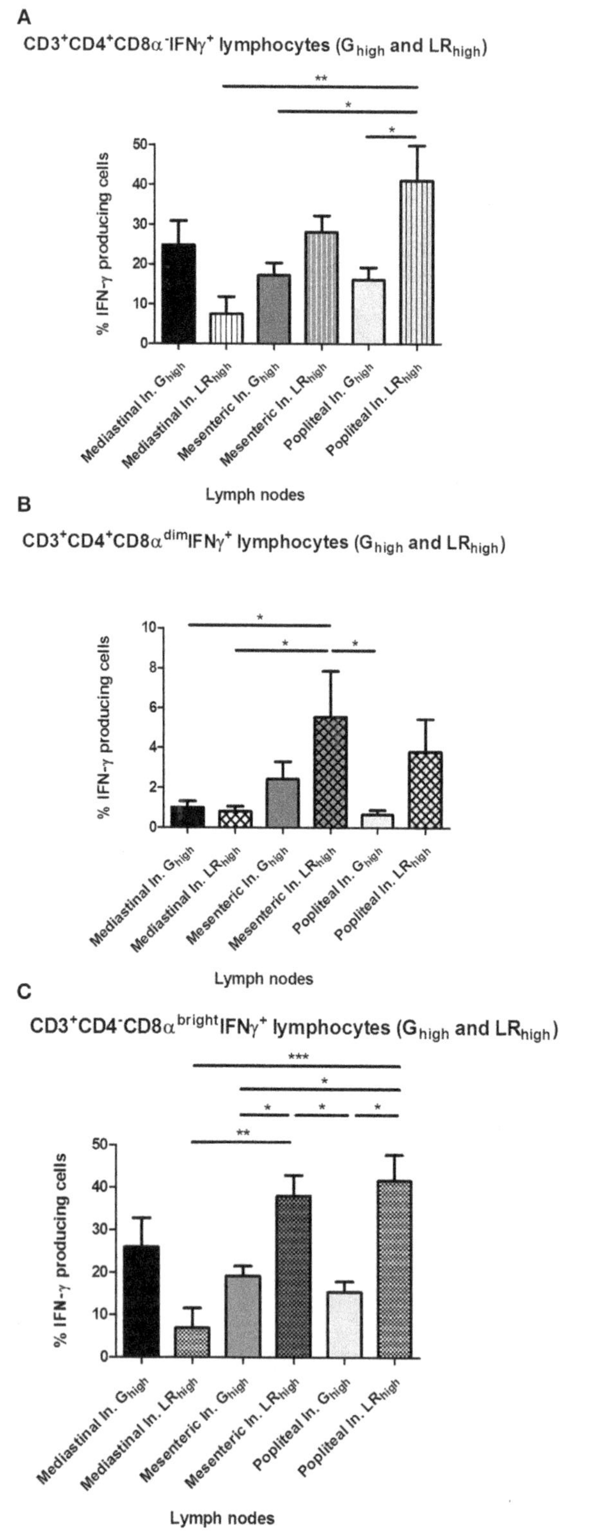

FIGURE 9 | The percentage of IFN-γ^+ T lymphocyte subsets from lymph nodes after a single IPB-G or IPB-LR inoculation. IFN-γ^+ T lymphocyte subsets in leukocytes from peripheral lymph nodes of pigs 98 dpi with a high dose of the IPB-G (G_{high}) or the IPB-LR strain (LR_{high}). Cells were restimulated *(Continued)*

FIGURE 9 | Continued
in vitro with TLA and demonstrated by flow cytometry following triple staining for IFN-γ, CD3, CD4, and CD8 **(A)**. IFN-γ^+ cell populations were identified as **(A)** $CD3^+CD4^+CD8\alpha^-$IFN-γ^+, **(B)** $CD3^+CD4+CD8\alpha^{dim}$ IFN-γ^+, **(C)** $CD3^+CD4^-CD8^{bright}$IFN-γ^+ lymphocytes. The results represent mean percentages ± SD for each group; $^*P < 0.05$, $^{**}P < 0.01$; $^{***}P < 0.001$.

DISCUSSION

In the performed experiments, we compared the single or subsequent infection in pigs inoculated with either a high or a low dose of the IPB-G and the IPB-LR strains for the tissue specific parasite load and the accompanying immune response. The IPB-G strain has a mixed type I/II genotype, while the IPB-LR strain has a classic type II genotype (Jongert et al., 2008; Dubey et al., 2012). The antibody response against GRA7 and TLA, which are frequently used in serological assays in different species, was monitored until 120 dpi to confirm the successful inoculation and persistence of the infection (**Figures 2**, **3**). Overall, for both IgM and IgG, independent from the infection dose, the GRA7-specific antibodies were detected very soon after the initial infection, starting from 10 dpi (**Figure 2**). Similar to previous results (Verhelst et al., 2015), we detected a late TLA-specific IgG response from 28 to 35 dpi onwards (**Figure 3**). However, results of the present study demonstrated that strain and dose are important factors to consider, since primary GRA7- and TLA-specific antibody responses could be detected earlier during infection and were higher upon inoculation with a high dose of the IPB-LR strain as compared to the IPB-G strain. A low dose on the other hand resulted in a later and less prominent seroconversion. Interestingly, whereas primary antibody responses were comparable in the heterologous challenge model, a clear IgM response was seen after the challenge with the heterologous strains, indicating exposure to other antigens, presumably due to the genetic diversity of both strains (**Figure 5**). Burrells et al. (2015) described a significant TLA-specific IgG increase after challenge of pigs with the heterologous strain M4 upon inoculation with the S48 strain. Strikingly, the challenge was performed with oocysts, after an initial inoculation with tachyzoites, stressing the expression of related or identical variability antigens in correlation to the parasite stage and the strain.

Together with a robust humoral response following *T. gondii* infection, a strong innate and cellular immune reaction is well described in mouse and human models, involving several populations of immune cells as well as different activation pathways (Aliberti, 2005; Miller et al., 2009; Andrade et al., 2013; Gazzinelli et al., 2014; Sturge and Yarovinsky, 2014). To date, it is well known that innate immune cells (macrophages, dendritic cells (DC's) and neutrophils) are involved in the acute stage of the infection by triggering the myeloid-differentiation primary response protein 88 (MyD88) signaling pathway after uptake and intracellular recognition of the parasite by CC-receptor 5 (CCR5) or Toll-like receptor (TLR) 11 and 12 in mice; TLR7, 8, and 9 in human and TLR7 and 9 in other mammals like pigs (Miller et al., 2009; Andrade et al., 2013; Koblansky et al., 2013; Gazzinelli et al., 2014). In particular interferon regulatory factor 8 (IRF8)$^+$ dendritic cells, activated by the uptake of the parasite's protein profilin, are crucial for the induction of IL-12 secretion in mice. Human and porcine DCs and monocytes are activated by the recognition of the parasite's ssRNA and DNA via TLR7 and TLR9, respectively, prior to their pro-inflammatory cytokine response (Uenishi et al., 2012; Andrade et al., 2013).

Consequently and irrespective of the activated TLRs, the DC-driven IL-12 production leads to the activation of T-helper 1 cells and Natural Killer (NK) cells (Sturge and Yarovinsky, 2014). The latter massively produce IFN-γ, which not only continuously activates macrophages via a positive feedback mechanism, but also elicits the expression of the GTPases. The GTPases family includes four subfamilies: the very large inducible GTPases (VLIG), the Mx proteins, the immunity-related GTPases (IRGs) such as p47 or p65, and the guanylate-binding proteins (GBPs). The p47 IRG offers a robust protection against intracellular pathogens, being recruited to the parasite attachment site at the host cell (MacMicking, 2004; Taylor et al., 2004; Liesenfeld et al., 2011). Subsequently, a lethal damage to the parasitophorus vacuole (PV) is induced, leading to the rupture of the infected cell and release of the parasite into the cytosol (Gazzinelli et al., 2014). The infected cell undergoes necrosis, simultaneously with an enhanced local immune response. It is important to mention that IFN-γ-inducible IRGs are well studied in murine models, where 23 different genes have been identified to date, but the corresponding genes are not present in the human genome, which includes only one gene and one pseudogene (Bekpen et al., 2005; Zhao et al., 2009). This implies that both species deploy other intracellular defense mechanisms against *T. gondii*. The data on the identification of porcine GTPases are scarce, but a high similarity to the human IRGs is mentioned (MacMicking, 2004). Only two porcine GBPs have been reported until now: GBP1 and GBP2, whereas in humans 7 different GBPs have been identified (MacMicking, 2004; Li et al., 2016). More IRG's have been found using Affymetrix GeneChip® Porcine Genome Array but a detailed study in pigs is lacking (Fossum et al., 2014).

Thus, the continuous production of IFN-γ seems to be necessary in maintaining a delicate balance between the host immune system and the parasite's evasion strategies. Additionally, this cytokine plays a pivotal role in controlling both the acute and chronic phase of infection, as it facilitates stage conversion from the tachyzoite to the bradyzoite in acute toxoplasmosis and suppresses the opposite conversion during chronic infection (Denkers, 1999). Likewise, we detected a significant increased IFN-γ production by PBMC's after inoculation with two different *T. gondii* strains (**Figure 4**), which corroborates our previous results when inoculating pigs with the IPB-G strain (Verhelst et al., 2015). Here, we demonstrated a time- and dose-dependent increase in IFN-γ mRNA expression upon infection with the IPB-G strain. Several studies focused on experimental infection in pigs reported a time-dependent increase of IFN-γ levels in serum, supernatant from cultured PBMCs and IFN-γ mRNA expression in PBMCs and intestinal lymphoid tissues (Solano Aguilar et al., 2001; Dawson et al., 2004, 2005; Verhelst et al., 2015).

On the contrary, the inoculation with the low dose of the IPB-LR strain was almost as potent in inducing a relatively fast and strong IFN-γ production by PBMCs as the high dose of the same strain, which resulted in high IFN-γ mRNA levels at already 2 mpi, that were maintained until 120 dpi. Interestingly, the IFN-γ mRNA production in the LR_{high} dose group did not show any increase over time, implying reaching the maximum capacity from 1 mpi onwards. In line with our findings, IL-12 (IL-12p35 and IL-12p40) mRNA expression was not detected in PBMCs in the acute phase of the infection (7 and 14 dpi) in an earlier study in pigs (Dawson et al., 2005).

Based on the results of the detection of IFN-γ and the parasite DNA in tissues (**Table 3**), a balance between the host defense mechanisms and the invasion of the parasite was probably established soon after inoculation with the IPB-LR strain. Namely, the high IFN-γ production during the infection study was associated with the high counts of parasite DNA in the animal tissues. On the contrary, in the IPB-G groups IFN-γ production was elevated in the late phase of the infection and resulted in a very low to undetectable parasite load in the tissues, implying that high IFN-γ levels can tip the balance in favor of the host. Intriguingly, based on our observations and unpublished data from the acute infection model with the same strains, we speculate that exposure to a high dose of the IPB-G strain is more effective in activating innate immunity than the low dose of the same strain or the inoculation with the IPB-LR strain. The strain-dependent differences in the IFN-γ production profile may result from the genetic and thus, biological features of the used strains, indicating expression of variable virulence factors toward the intermediate host. In our opinion and according to others (Hunter and Sibley, 2012), the IPB-LR as genotype II strain, activates other pathway than the IPB-G strain, which is of an atypical genotype (mixed genotype I and II). The virulence factors initiating a pathway would be GRA15 (via NF-κB) for the former, and ROP18 (via STAT3/STAT6 pathway) for the latter. Consequently, the IPB-LR induces Th1 type of protective immunity and remains persistent in the chronic phase. When looking at the IPB-LR infected groups, no substantial difference was noticed in the IFN-γ production pattern or in the amount of *T. gondii* DNA at the end of the experiment. In our view, the IPB-LR strain does not show an acute virulence but it is adapted to persist within the intermediate host and, as such, increase own survival. To support these speculations, we observed a much milder clinical manifestation upon inoculation with the IPB-LR strain (Jennes et al., unpublished data). We further hypothesize that resistance to the chronic infection in IPB-G model results from the high acute virulence and the subsequent fast elimination of the tachyzoites before they can successfully multiply and disseminate. Consequently, fewer parasites can survive the initial parasitemia, which eventually will lead to reduced numbers of cysts in the tissues. Importantly, we conducted the studies in a homogenous pig population in order to exclude host diversity; however, as the strains are maintained by serial passage in mice, their virulence might be altered compared to the original isolate. Therefore, it is tempting to speculate that the high IFN-γ production together with the lower parasite counts in the porcine tissues originate from a coevolution toward host tolerance and reduced virulence, as suggested earlier by others (Gazzinelli et al., 2014). Furthermore, looking at the total IFN-γ expression following reinoculation with the heterologous *T. gondii* strain in the second experiment, no obvious difference between the groups could be observed (**Figure 6**). In the G_{high}/LR_{high} group we detected an initial increase, which was followed by a steady decrease after the challenge. The IFN-γ production profile in the reversed infection model (LR_{high}/G_{high}) supports our previous findings, showing a constant IFN-γ detection over time. Interestingly, in some animals basal or low level of cytokine mRNA were detected at 1mpi, followed by a substantial increase at the later time points, similar to the single infection experiment (**Figures 4A, 6A**). However, the final IFN-γ concentration at the end of the experiment upon a heterologous challenge was 10 times lower than after a single high dose inoculation. We could speculate that the primary infection with a mixed genotype I/II strain, characterized by a high acute virulence and long-term STAT3 and STAT6 activation, partially modulates the immune response upon the challenge with genotype II strain. As the result, the initial impairment of the Th1 response after the challenge leads to a lower than in a single infection model IFN-γ production, and elimination of a certain fraction of the parasites. Consequently, a reduced amount of the tachyzoites disseminate to convert into bradyzoites. The latter has been shown by a lower parasite load 60 dpi challenge than in IPB-LR experiment (**Table 3** and **Figure 6**).

In regard to the involvement of immune cells in controlling the parasite's dissemination to the tissues and the chronic phase of toxoplasmosis, different populations seem to play a role. As described earlier and analogous to the acute infection stage, the production of IFN-γ is gradually taken over from the innate immune cells by T lymphocytes (Guan et al., 2007). Experimental infections in mice (Jongert et al., 2010; Suzuki et al., 2012) demonstrated the importance of $CD4^+$ and $CD8^+$ IFN-γ producing T cells in maintaining a chronic *T. gondii* infection, but the exact contribution of each subset remains unknown. Miller et al. (2006) describes higher production of IFN-γ by murine $CD4^+$ cells upon *in vitro* stimulation by infected macrophages or by TLA, but admits that the higher protective potential against dissemination of the parasite by $CD8^+$ or $CD4^+$ lymphocytes is not simply expressed by the amount of this cytokine. Indeed, it seems that IL-4 and IL-10 cytokines, produced by $CD4^+$ lymphocytes in addition to IFN-γ, might down regulate this protective capacity against the parasite. In line with that, due to their IFN-γ-independent cytolytic activity, the role of primed $CD8^+$ T cells in the host's immunity during chronic toxoplasmosis has been widely acknowledged (Wang et al., 2005; Suzuki et al., 2012; Sa et al., 2013). In pigs, only a few experiments identified $CD8^+$ and $CD4^+CD8^+$ cells in the acute phase of the infection as the major source of the IFN-γ production (Solano Aguilar et al., 2001; Dawson et al., 2005). The additive or synergistic effect of $CD4^+$ T cells on the activity of the $CD8^+$ T cell population should not, however, remain neglected. In our study, regardless of the strain, the $CD4^-CD8\alpha^{bright}$ T cell subset contained the most IFN-γ positive cells, followed by the $CD4^+CD8\alpha^-$ subset, whereas the $CD4^+CD8\alpha^{dim}$ T cell subset showed very few IFN-γ positive cells (**Figure 8**). Additionally, the $CD4^-CD8\alpha^{bright}$ population showed a temporal increase in IFN-γ production in animals infected with IPB-LR, while the percentage of this subset was rather declining from 4 wpi onwards, when infected with the IPB-G. The IFN-γ production resulting from the induced toxoplasmosis in pigs and the involvement of the different lymphocyte populations are in line with other studies, where the *in vitro* cytokine profile was investigated until 14 (Dawson et al., 2005), 40 (Solano Aguilar et al., 2001), or 56 dpi (Verhelst et al., 2011). However, opposite to the pig model, in murine experiments only two T lymphocyte subsets were differentiated ($CD4^+$ and $CD8^+$). Furthermore, the extent of the cellular response was positively correlated with the infection dose and the time-interval from the inoculation and was higher when induced by the strain with a greater tissue persistence. In perspective of future experiments in pigs, it would be desirable to focus on other immune cells, involved in the responses throughout the infection such as the immunosuppressive T regulatory (Treg) or Th17 cells. As recently shown in mice, the robust immune reaction expressed by the high IFN-γ levels in the acute phase of the infection severely reduces the activity of Tregs in a IL-2 dependent and IL-10 independent manner (Tenorio et al., 2011; Olguin et al., 2015). In a longitudinal clinical case study of human acquired cerebral toxoplasmosis a dual function of the Treg population was described, by simultaneous down regulation of $CD4^+$ and activation of pathogen-specific $CD8^+$ T lymphocytes (Rb-Silva et al., 2017). In human congenital infections not only $CD4^+$ Treg cell population seems to be involved in the immune reaction triggered by *T. gondii*, but also a different subset of $CD4^+$ or $CD8^+$, namely Th17. The activity of this population is independent from IFN-γ, IL-4 and perforin activation, as their migration to the inflammation sites in initiated by certain chemokines. Interestingly, the results of the *in vitro* PBMCs stimulation with tachyzoites showed a higher percentage of $CD4^+$ IL17 producing cells above the $CD8^+$ (Silva et al., 2014). By investigating the fluctuations of the activity of Tregs and Th17 cells during the acute and chronic phase of the infection, we might determine whether these populations are also involved in the persistent immunity toward the parasite.

When considering the parasite load in the tissues and the viability of the cysts in the bio-assay, a clear correlation was found between the amount of detected DNA and the dose of the used strain (**Table 3**). In general, we observed a decline in the concentration of the parasite's DNA in animals when inoculated with a high dose of the IPB-G, but not the IPB-LR strain. This dose- and time-dependent decline is prominently present in different tissues in the G_{high} group in comparison with G_{low} and $G_{high1/2t}$ groups, indicating that the effect of the high dose is particularly visible after a longer infection time. These results are in line with the findings of Verhelst et al. (2011), where neither parasite DNA nor viable parasites were detected in certain muscle tissues 6 months after initial infection with the IPB-G strain. In the same study, brain and heart of all animals remained infectious as determined by a bio-assay and qPCR. However, these findings are opposite to results obtained in rats and cats, showing that inoculation with increasing amounts of tachyzoites or bradyzoites resulted in a decreased survival rate or in a higher number of tissue cysts, respectively (De Champs et al., 1998; Cornelissen et al., 2014). In addition and similar to our results, others reported a reduction in parasite burden in strain-vaccinated and challenged pigs (Kringel et al., 2004; Garcia et al., 2005; Jongert et al., 2008; Burrells et al., 2015). In these experiments vaccination with oligonucelotides, antigens or infection with attenuated strains can enhance Th1 responses to elicit sufficient protection during the acute phase of the infection, resulting in a lower parasite burden in comparison with the infected control animals. Referring to that, the strains used in our study differ greatly in terms of genetic background and associated virulence, both in mice and in pigs. Therefore, we have grounded scientific reasons to believe that the observed differences in the parasite load upon infection with both strains, especially in the heterologous co-infection model, are not coincidental.

For most tissue samples this dose- and strain-dependent reduction in the number of the tissue cysts in qPCR is consistent with the bio-assay in mice. It is noteworthy that a few qPCR-positive samples were negative in the bio-assay, indicating that parasite DNA, but not viable parasites were present. Consequently, these results show a substantially higher sensitivity of the qPCR method used here above the bio-assay, since it has been optimized and successfully applied for the detection of the parasite in various human or animal tissues, with a detection limit of 2–4 tissue cysts in 100 g of sample (De Craeye et al., 2011). Conversely, both techniques gave positive results on all samples derived from animals upon single inoculation with the IPB-LR strain. Therefore, we can assume that the reduced parasite load occurred due to the earlier infection with the IPB-G strain in the group G_{high}/LR_{high}. This phenomenon does not seem to be limited to type II strains (Velmurugan et al., 2009; Suzuki et al., 2012), but is also common in type I strains (Burrells et al., 2015).

Summarizing, the groups infected with the IPB-LR strain can serve as a classical model of *T. gondii* persistence in its intermediate host. The prominent production of parasite-specific antibodies, consistent amounts of IFN-γ and activation of cytotoxic T lymphocytes on the one hand and well-distributed DNA concentration together with isolation of the viable parasite on the other hand, clearly prove an established balance between the host immunity and the pathogen's activity. The parasite's persistence appears to be beneficial for the two, under conditions that the immunocompetent host can resist the immunomodulation by *T. gondii*. On the contrary, as the partial or total removal of the tissue cysts was observed in the IPB-G infected animals together with the increasing IFN-γ production profile on both the mRNA and protein level, we propose that the IPB-G strain induces a robust immune reaction in the host in the early phase of the infection. This IFN-γ-mediated response in pigs can lead to the resistance of the host to parasite invasion by elimination of the tissue cysts during the chronic infection. Further experiments to unravel the nature of this resistance are warranted as it could serve an important role in vaccination strategies and in the risk assessment for food safety and human health.

ETHICS STATEMENT

This study was carried out in accordance with the recommendations of the ethical standards defined by the EU legislation on the use of laboratory animals (2010/63/EU) and in accordance with the Belgian law (the Royal Decree 29/5/2013 and the Royal Decree 30/11/2001). The protocol was approved by the Ethical Committee of the faculties Veterinary Medicine and Bioscience Engineering at Ghent University (approval number no. 176 2009/149) and by the Ethical Committee of the WIV-ISP Institute (approval no. 176 20140704-01). The Biosafety Level 2 permit for working with pathogens for Ugent, Merelbeke: AMV/11062013/SBB219.2013/0145. The Biosafety Level 2 permit for working with pathogens for WIV-IPH, Brussels: 415240.

AUTHOR CONTRIBUTIONS

MJ designed the study, acquired and analyzed the data and drafted the manuscript. SD designed the study, acquired, and analyzed data and revised the manuscript. BD helped to design the flow cytometry study and revised the manuscript. PD and KD helped to design the study, gave valuable input and revised the manuscript. EC designed the study, analyzed the data and wrote the manuscript.

ACKNOWLEDGMENTS

This study was granted by the Belgian Federal Public Service for Health, Food Chain Safety and Environment (grant RF 09/6213). The authors wish to thank A. Leremans for the technical assistance with the bio-assay and M. Boutry for her excellence laboratory skills with qPCR and cytokine RT-PCR. We also wish to thank R. Cooman for the animal management. B. Devriendt is supported by an FWO postdoctoral research grant. The Hercules Foundation supported the purchase of research equipment (AUGE035).

REFERENCES

Afonso, E., Lemoine, M., Poulle, M. L., Ravat, M. C., Romand, S., Thulliez, P., et al. (2008). Spatial distribution of soil contamination by *Toxoplasma gondii* in relation to cat defecation behaviour in an urban area. *Int. J. Parasitol.* 38, 1017–1023. doi: 10.1016/j.ijpara.2008.01.004

Ajzenberg, D., Cogne, N., Paris, L., Bessieres, M. H., Thulliez, P., Filisetti, D., et al. (2002). Genotype of 86 *Toxoplasma gondii* isolates associated with human congenital toxoplasmosis, and correlation with clinical findings. *J. Inf. Dis.* 186, 684–689. doi: 10.1086/342663

Aliberti, J. (2005). Host persistence: exploitation of anti-inflammatory pathways by *Toxoplasma gondii*. *Nat. Rev. Immunol.* 5, 162–170. doi: 10.1038/nri1547

Andrade, W. A., Souza, M. C., Ramos-Martinez, E., Nagpal, K., Dutra, M. S., Melo, M. B., et al. (2013). Combined action of nucleic acid-sensing Toll-like receptors and TLR11/TLR12 heterodimers imparts resistance to *Toxoplasma gondii* in mice. *Cell Host Microbe* 13, 42–53. doi: 10.1016/j.chom.2012.12.003

Aspinall, T. V., Marlee, D., Hyde, J. E., and Sims, P. F. (2002). Prevalence of *Toxoplasma gondii* in commercial meat products as monitored by polymerase chain reaction - food for thought? *Int. J. Parasitol.* 32, 1193–1199. doi: 10.1016/S0020-7519(02)00070-X

Bekpen, C., Hunn, J. P., Rohde, C., Parvanova, I., Guethlein, L., Dunn, D. M., et al. (2005). The interferon-inducible p47 (IRG) GTPases in vertebrates: loss of the cell autonomous resistance mechanism in the human lineage. *Genome Biol.* 6:R92. doi: 10.1186/gb-2005-6-11-r92

Belluco, S., Mancin, M., Conficoni, D., Simonato, G., Pietrobelli, M., and Ricci, A. (2016). Investigating the determinants of *Toxoplasma gondii* prevalence in meat: a systematic review and metaregression. *PLoS ONE* 11:e0153856. doi: 10.1371/journal.pone.0153856

Black, M. W., and Boothroyd, J. C. (2000). Lytic cycle of *Toxoplasma gondii*. *Microbiol. Mol. Biol. Rev.* 64, 607–623. doi: 10.1128/MMBR.64.3.607-623.2000

Bosch-Driessen, L. E., Berendschot, T. T., Ongkosuwito, J. V., and Rothova, A. (2002). Ocular toxoplasmosis: clinical features and prognosis of 154 patients. *Ophthalmology* 109, 869–878. doi: 10.1016/S0161-6420(02)00990-9

Breugelmans, M., Naessens, A., and Foulon, W. (2004). Prevention of toxoplasmosis during pregnancy–an epidemiologic survey over 22 consecutive years. *J. Perinat. Med.* 32, 211–214. doi: 10.1515/JPM.2004.039

Burrells, A., Benavides, J., Cantón, G., Garcia, J. L., Bartley, P. M., Nath, M., et al. (2015). Vaccination of pigs with the S48 strain of *Toxoplasma gondii* - safer meat for human consumption. *Vet. Res.* 46:47. doi: 10.1186/s13567-015-0177-0

Cao, A., Liu, Y., Wang, J., Li, X., Wang, S., Zhao, Q., et al. (2015). *Toxoplasma gondii*: vaccination with a DNA vaccine encoding T- and B-cell epitopes of SAG1, GRA2, GRA7 and ROP16 elicits protection against acute toxoplasmosis in mice. *Vaccine* 33, 6757–6762. doi: 10.1016/j.vaccine.2015.10.077

Cornelissen, J. B., van der Giessen, J. W., Takumi, K., Teunis, P. F., and Wisselink, H. J. (2014). An experimental *Toxoplasma gondii* dose response challenge model to study therapeutic or vaccine efficacy in cats. *PLoS ONE* 9:e104740. doi: 10.1371/journal.pone.0104740

Dawson, H. D., Beshah, E., Nishi, S., Solano-Aguilar, G., Morimoto, M., Zhao, A., et al. (2005). Localized multigene expression patterns support an evolving Th1/Th2-like paradigm in response to infections with *Toxoplasma gondii* and *Ascaris suum*. *Infect. Immun.* 73, 1116–1128. doi: 10.1128/IAI.73.2.1116-1128.2005

Dawson, H. D., Royaee, A. R., Nishi, S., Kuhar, D., Schnitzlein, W. M., Zuckermann, F., et al. (2004). Identification of key immune mediators regulating T helper 1 responses in swine. *Vet. Immunol. Immunopathol.* 100, 105–111. doi: 10.1016/j.vetimm.2004.03.006

De Champs, C., Pelloux, H., Dechelotte, P., Giraud, J. C., Bally, N., and Ambroise-Thomas, P. (1998). *Toxoplasma gondii* infection in rats by the RH strain: inoculum and age effects. *Parasite* 5, 215–218. doi: 10.1051/parasite/1998053215

De Craeye, S., Speybroeck, N., Ajzenberg, D., Dardé, M. L., Collinet, F., Tavernier, P., et al. (2011). *Toxoplasma gondii* and *Neospora caninum* in wildlife: common parasites in Belgian foxes and Cervidae? *Vet. Parasitol.* 178, 64–69. doi: 10.1016/j.vetpar.2010.12.016

Denkers, E. Y. (1999). T lymphocyte-dependent effector mechanisms of immunity to *Toxoplasma gondii*. *Microbes Infect.* 1, 699–708. doi: 10.1016/S1286-4579(99)80071-9

Dubey, J. P. (1995). Duration of immunity to shedding of *Toxoplasma gondii* oocysts by cats. *J. Parasitol.* 81, 410–415. doi: 10.2307/3283823

Dubey, J. P. (2009). Toxoplasmosis in pigs—The last 20 years. *Vet. Parasitol.* 164 89–103. doi: 10.1016/j.vetpar.2009.05.018

Dubey, J. P. (2010). *Toxoplasmosis of Animals and Humans, 2nd Edn.* Boca Raton, FL: CRC Press; Taylor and Francis Group.

Dubey, J. P., Hill, D. E., Rozeboom, D. W., Rajendrana, C., Choudharya, S., Ferreira, L. R., et al. (2012). High prevalence and genotypes of *Toxoplasma gondii* isolated from organic pigs in northern USA. *Vet. Parasitol.* 188, 14–18. doi: 10.1016/j.vetpar.2012.03.008

EFSA (2012). *European Food Safety Authority, European Centre for Disease Prevention and Control; The European Union Summary Report on Trends and Sources of Zoonoses, Zoonotic Agents and Food-borne Outbreaks in 2010.* The EFSA Journal 10:2597. 442. doi: 10.2903/j.efsa.2012.2597

EFSA (2007). Scientific Opinion of the Panel on Biological Hazards on a request from, EFSA on Surveillance and monitoring of Toxoplasma in humans, foods and animals. *EFSA J.* 583, 1–64. doi: 10.2903/j.efsa.2007.583

Fehlhaber, K., Hintersdorf, P., and Kruger, G. (2003). Study on the prevalence of *Toxoplasma gondii* in pigs of different management systems and in minced meat. *Fleischwirtschaft* 83, 97–99.

Ferra, B., Holec-Gąsior, L., and Kur, J. (2015). Serodiagnosis of *Toxoplasma gondii* infection in farm animals (horses, swine, and sheep) by enzyme-linked immunosorbent assay using chimeric antigens. *Parasitol. Int.* 64, 288–294. doi: 10.1016/j.parint.2015.03.004

Fossum, C., Hjertner, B., Ahlberg, V., Charerntantanakul, W., McIntosh, K., Fuxler, L., et al. (2014). Early inflammatory response to the saponin adjuvant Matrix-M in the pig. *Vet. Immunol. Immunopathol.* 158, 53–61. doi: 10.1016/j.vetimm.2013.07.007

Gamble, H. R., Dubey, J. P., and Lambillotte, D. N. (2005). Comparison of a commercial ELISA with the modified agglutination test for detection of Toxoplasma infection in the domestic pig. *Vet. Parasitol.* 128, 177–181. doi: 10.1016/j.vetpar.2004.11.019

Garcia, J. L., Gennari, S. M., Navarro, I. T., Machado, R. Z., Sinhorini, I. L., Freire, R. L., et al. (2005). Partial protection against tissue cysts formation in pigs vaccinated with crude rhoptry proteins of *Toxoplasma gondii*. *Vet. Parasitol.* 129, 209–217. doi: 10.1016/j.vetpar.2005.01.006

Gazzinelli, R. T., Mendonça-Neto, R., Lilue, J., Howard, J., and Sher, A. (2014). Innate resistance against *Toxoplasma gondii*: an evolutionary tale of mice, cats, and men. *Cell Host Microbe* 15, 132–138. doi: 10.1016/j.chom.2014.01.004

Gerner, W., Talker, S. C., Koinig, H. C., Sedlak, C., Mair, K. H., and Saalmüller, A. (2015). Phenotypic and functional differentiation of porcine αβT cells: current knowledge and available tools. *Mol. Immunol.* 66, 3–13. doi: 10.1016/j.molimm.2014.10.025

Guan, H., Moretto, M., Bzik, D. J., Gigley, J., and Khan, I. A. (2007). NK cells enhance dendritic cell response against parasite antigens via NKG2D pathway. *J. Immunol.* 179, 590–596. doi: 10.4049/jimmunol.179.1.590

Guo, M., Dubey, J. P., Hill, D., Buchanan, R. L., Gamble, H., Jones, J. L., et al. (2015). Prevalence and risk factors for *Toxoplasma gondii* infection in meat animals and meat products destined for human consumption. *J. Food Prot.* 78, 457–476. doi: 10.4315/0362-028X.JFP-14-328

Hill, D. E., Haley, C., Wagner, B., Gamble, H. R., and Dubey, J. P. (2008). Seroprevalence of and risk factors for *Toxoplasma gondii* in the US swine herd using sera collected during the National Animal Health Monitoring Survey (Swine 2006). *Zoonoses Public Health* 57, 53–59. doi: 10.1111/j.1863-2378.2009.01275.x

Holland, G. N. (2003). Ocular toxoplasmosis: a global reassessment. Part I: epidemiology and course of disease. *Am. J. Ophthalmol.* 136, 973–988. doi: 10.1016/j.ajo.2003.09.040

Hunter, C. A., and Sibley, L. D. (2012). Modulation of innate immunity by *Toxoplasma gondii* virulence effectors. *Nat. Rev. Microbiol.* 10, 766–778. doi: 10.1038/nrmicro2858

Innes, E. A. (2010). A brief history and overview of *Toxoplasma gondii*. *Zoonoses Public Health* 57, 1–7. doi: 10.1111/j.1863-2378.2009.01276.x

Israelski, D. M., and Remington, J. S. (1993). Toxoplasmosis in patients with cancer. *Clin. Inf. Dis.* 17(Suppl. 2), S423–S435. doi: 10.1093/clinids/17.Supplement_2.S423

Jacobs, D., Vercammen, M., and Saman, E. (1999). Evaluation of recombinant dense granule antigen 7 (GRA7) of *Toxoplasma gondii* for detection of immunoglobulin G antibodies and analysis of a major antigenic domain. *Clin. Diagn. Lab. Immunol.* 6, 24–29.

Jones, J. L., and Dubey, J. P. (2012). Foodborne toxoplasmosis. *Clin. Infect. Dis.* 55, 845–851. doi: 10.1093/cid/cis508

Jongert, E., De Craeye, S., Dewit, J., and Huygen, K. (2007). GRA7 provides protective immunity in cocktail DNA vaccines against *Toxoplasma gondii*. *Parasite Immunol.* 29, 445–453. doi: 10.1111/j.1365-3024.2007.00961.x

Jongert, E., Lemiere, A., Van Ginderachter, J., De Craeye, S., Huygen, K., and D'Souza, S. (2010). Functional characterization of *in vivo* effector $CD4^+$ and $CD8^+$ T cell responses in acute Toxoplasmosis: an interplay of IFN-gamma and cytolytic T cells. *Vaccine* 28, 2556–2564. doi: 10.1016/j.vaccine.2010.01.031

Jongert, E., Melkebeek, V., De Craeye, S., Dewit, J., Verhelst, D., and Cox, E. (2008). An enhanced GRA1-GRA7 cocktail DNA vaccine primes anti-*Toxoplasma* immune responses in pigs. *Vaccine* 26, 1025–1031. doi: 10.1016/j.vaccine.2007.11.058

Katzer, F., Canton, G., Burrells, A., Palarea-Albaladejo, J., Horton, B., Bartley, P. M., et al. (2014). Immunization of lambs with the S48 strain of *Toxoplasma gondii* reduces tissue cyst burden following oral challenge with a complete strain of the parasite. *Vet. Parasitol.* 205, 46–56. doi: 10.1016/j.vetpar.2014.07.003

Kijlstra, A., Eissen, O. A., Cornelissen, J., Munniksma, K., Eijck, I., and Kortbeek, T. (2004). *Toxoplasma gondii* infection in animal-friendly pig production systems. *Invest. Ophthalmol. Vis. Sci.* 45, 3165–3169. doi: 10.1167/iovs.04-0326

Kijlstra, A., and Jongert, E. (2008). Control of the risk of human toxoplasmosis transmitted by meat. *Int. J. Parasitol.* 2008, 1359–1370. doi: 10.1016/j.ijpara.2008.06.002

Koblansky, A. A., Jankovic, D., Oh, H., Hieny, S., Sungnak, W., Mathur, R., et al. (2013). Recognition of profiling by Toll-like receptor 12 is critical for host resistance to *Toxoplasma gondii*. *Immunity* 38, 119–130. doi: 10.1016/j.immuni.2012.09.016

Kringel, H., Dubey, J. P., Beshah, E., Hecker, R., and Urban, J. F. Jr. (2004). CpG-oligodeoxynucleotides enhance porcine immunity to *Toxoplasma gondii*. *Vet. Parasitol.* 123, 55–66. doi: 10.1016/j.vetpar.2004.01.021

Lester, D., (2010). Brain parasites and suicide. *Psychol. Rep.* 107:424. doi: 10.2466/12.13.PR0.107.5.424

Letscher-Bru, V., Pfaff, A. W., Abou-Bacar, A., Filisetti, D., Antoni, E., Villard, O., et al. (2003). Vaccination with *Toxoplasma gondii* SAG-1 protein is protective against congenital toxoplasmosis in BALB/c mice but not in CBA/J mice. *Infect. Immun.* 71, 6615–6619. doi: 10.1128/IAI.71.11.6615-6619.2003

Li, J., Huang, X., Zhang, G., Gong, P., Zhang, X., and Wu, L. (2011). Immune response and protective efficacy against homologous challenge in BALB/c mice vaccinated with DNA vaccine encoding *Toxoplasma gondii* actin depolymerizing factor gene. *Vet. Parasitol.* 179, 1–6. doi: 10.1016/j.vetpar.2011.03.003

Li, L. F., Yu, J., Li, Y., Wang, J., Li, S., Zhang, L., et al. (2016). Guanylate-binding protein 1, an interferon-induced GTPase, exerts an antiviral activity against classical swine fever virus depending on its GTPase activity. *J. Virol.* 90, 4412–4426. doi: 10.1128/JVI.02718-15

Liesenfeld, O., Parvanova, I., Zerrahn, J., Han, S.-J., Heinrich, F., Muñoz, M., et al. (2011). The IFN-γ-Inducible GTPase, Irga6, protects mice against *Toxoplasma gondii* but not against *Plasmodium berghei* and some other intracellular pathogens. *PLoS ONE* 6:e20568. doi: 10.1371/journal.pone.0020568

MacMicking, J. D. (2004). IFN-inducible GTPases and immunity to intracellular pathogens. *Trends Immunol.* 25, 601–609. doi: 10.1016/j.it.2004.08.010

Miller, C. M., Boulter, N. R., Ikin, R. I., and Smith, N. C. (2009). The immunobiology of the innate response to *Toxoplasma gondii*. *Int. J. Parasitol.* 39, 23–39. doi: 10.1016/j.ijpara.2008.08.002

Miller, R., Wen, X., Dunford, B., Wang, X., and Suzuki, Y. (2006). Cytokine production of CD8+ immune T cells but not of CD4+ T cells from *Toxoplasma gondii*-infected mice is polarized to a type 1 response following stimulation with tachyzoite-infected macrophages. *J. Interferon Cytokine Res.* 26, 787–792. doi: 10.1089/jir.2006.26.787

Miman, O., Kusbeci, O. Y., Aktepe, O. C., and Cetinkaya, Z. (2010). The probable relation between *Toxoplasma gondii* and Parkinson's disease. *Neurosci. Lett.* 475, 129–131. doi: 10.1016/j.neulet.2010.03.057

Olguin, J., Fernández, J., Salinas, N., Terrazas, L., and Saavedra, R. (2015). Reduction of regulatory T cells during acute *Toxoplasma gondii* infection is caused by IFN-γ (MPF2P.759). *J. Immunol.* 194(Suppl. 1) 63.18. Available online at: http://www.jimmunol.org/content/194/1_Supplement/63.18

Opsteegh, M., Schares, G., and van der Giessen, J., on behalf of the consortium (2016). Relationship between seroprevalence in the main livestock species and presence of *Toxoplasma gondii* in meat (GP/EFSA/BIOHAZ/2013/01). An extensive literature review. Final report. *EFSA Supporting Publication* 2016:EN-996:294.

Peyron, F., Mc Leod, R., Ajzenberg, D., Contopoulos-Ioannidis, D., Kieffer, F., Mandelbrot, L., et al. (2017). Congenital Toxoplasmosis in France and the United States: one parasite, two diverging approaches. *PLoS Negl. Trop. Dis.* 11:e0005222. doi: 10.1371/journal.pntd.0005222

Rb-Silva, R., Nobrega, C., Reiriz, E., Almeida, S., Sarmento-Castro, R., Correia-Neves, M., et al. (2017). Toxoplasmosis-associated IRIS involving the CNS: a case report with longitudinal analysis of T cell subsets. *BMC Infect Dis.* 17:66. doi: 10.1186/s12879-016-2159-x

Robert-Gangneux, F., and Dardé M.-L. (2012). Epidemiology of and Diagnostic Strategies for Toxoplasmosis. *Clin. Microbiol. Rev.* 25, 264–296. doi: 10.1128/CMR.05013-11

Rosenberg, C., De Craeye, S., Jongert, E., Gargano, N., Beghetto, E., Del Porto, P., et al. (2009). Induction of partial protection against infection with *Toxoplasma gondii* genotype II by DNA vaccination with recombinant chimeric tachyzoite antigens. *Vaccine* 27, 2489–2498. doi: 10.1016/j.vaccine.2009.02.058

Sa, Q., Woodward, J., and Suzuki, Y. (2013). IL-2 produced by CD8+ immune T cells can augment their IFN-γ production independently from their proliferation in the secondary response to an intracellular pathogen. *J. Immunol.* 190, 2199–2207. doi: 10.4049/jimmunol.1202256

Silva, J. L., Rezende-Oliveira, K., da Silva, M. V., Gómez-Hernández, C., Peghini, B. C., Silva, N. M., et al. (2014). IL-17-expressing $CD4^+$ and $CD8^+$ T lymphocytes in human toxoplasmosis. *Mediators Inflamm.* 2014:573825. doi: 10.1155/2014/573825

Solano Aguilar, G. I., Beshah, E., Vengroski, K. G., Zarlenga, D., Jauregui, L., Cosio, M., et al. (2001). Cytokine and lymphocyte profiles in miniature swine after oral infection with *Toxoplasma gondii* oocysts. *Int. J. Parasitol.* 31, 187–195. doi: 10.1016/S0020-7519(00)00159-4

Sonck, E., Stuyven, E., Goddeeris, B., and Cox, E. (2010). The effect of b-glucans on porcine leukocytes. *Vet. Immunol. Immunopathol.* 135, 199–207. doi: 10.1016/j.vetimm.2009.11.014

Sturge, C. R., and Yarovinsky, F. (2014). Complex Immune Cell Interplay in the Gamma Interferon Response during *Toxoplasma gondii* Infection. *Infect. Immun.* 82, 3090–3097. doi: 10.1128/IAI.01722-14

Suzuki, Y., Sa, Q., Gehman, M., and Ochiai, E. (2012). Interferon-gamma- and perforin-mediated immune responses for resistance against *Toxoplasma gondii* in the brain. *Expert Rev. Mol. Med.* 13:e31. doi: 10.1017/S1462399411002018

Taylor, G. A., Feng, C. G., and Sher, A. (2004). p47 GTPases: regulators of immunity to intracellular pathogens. *Nat. Rev. Immunol.* 4, 100–109. doi: 10.1038/nri1270

Tenorio, E. P., Fernández, J., Castellanos, C., Olguín, J. E., and Saavedra, R. (2011). CD4+ Foxp3+ regulatory T cells mediate *Toxoplasma gondii*-induced T-cell suppression through an IL-2-related mechanism but independently of IL-10. *Eur. J. Immunol.* 41, 3529–3541. doi: 10.1002/eji.201141507

Tenter, A. M., Heckeroth, A. R., and Weiss, L. M. (2000). *Toxoplasma gondii*: from animals to humans. *Int. J. Parasitol.* 30, 1217–1258. doi: 10.1016/S0020-7519(00)00124-7

Torgerson, P. R., and Mastroiacovo, P. (2013). The global burden of congenital toxoplasmosis: a systematic review. *Bull. World Health Organ.* 91, 501–508. doi: 10.2471/BLT.12.111732

Uenishi, H., Shinkai, H., Morozumi, T., and Muneta, Y. (2012). Genomic survey of polymorphisms in pattern recognition receptors and their possible relationship to infections in pigs. *Vet. Immunol. Immunopathol.* 148, 69–73. doi: 10.1016/j.vetimm.2011.07.019

Velmurugan, G. V., Su, C., and Dubey, J. P. (2009). Isolate designation and characterization of *Toxoplasma gondii* isolates from pigs in the United States. *J. Parasitol.* 95, 95–99. doi: 10.1645/GE-1746.1

Vercammen, M., Scorza, T., Huygen, K., De Braekeleer, J., Diet, R., Jacobs, D., et al. (2000). DNA vaccination with genes encoding *Toxoplasma gondii* antigens GRA1, GRA7, and ROP2 induces partially protective immunity against lethal challenge in mice. *Infect. Immun.* 68, 38–45. doi: 10.1128/IAI.68.1.38-45.2000

Verhelst, D., De Craeye, S., Jennes, M., Dorny, P., Goddeeris, B., and Cox, E. (2015). Interferon-gamma expression and infectivity of Toxoplasma infected tissues in experimentally infected sheep in comparison with pigs. *Vet. Parasitol.* 207, 7–16. doi: 10.1016/j.vetpar.2014.11.014

Verhelst, D., De Craeye, S., Melkebeek, V., Goddeeris, B., Cox, E., and Jongert, E. (2011). IFN-γ expression and infectivity of *Toxoplasma* infected tissues are associated with an antibody response against GRA7 in experimentally infected pigs. *Vet. Parasitol.* 179, 14–21. doi: 10.1016/j.vetpar.2011.02.015

Wagner, A., Schabussova, I., Ruttkowski, B., Peschke, R., Kur, J., Kundi, M., et al. (2015). Prime-boost vaccination with Toxoplasma lysate antigen, but not with a mixture of recombinant protein antigens, leads to reduction of brain cyst formation in BALB/c mice. *PLoS ONE* 10:e0126334. doi: 10.1371/journal.pone.0126334

Wang, X. J., Claflin, H., Kang, Y., and Suzuki (2005). Importance of $CD8^+Vbeta8^+$ T cells in IFN-gamma-mediated prevention of toxoplasmic encephalitis in genetically resistant BALB/c mice. *J. Cytokine Res.* 25, 338–344. doi: 10.1089/jir.2005.25.338

Wang, Z. D., Liu, H. H., Ma, Z. X., Ma, H. Y., Li, Z. Y., Yang, Z. B., et al. (2017). *Toxoplasma gondii* infection in immunocompromised patients: a systematic review and meta-analysis. *Front. Microbiol.* 8:389. doi: 10.3389/fmicb.2017.00389

Zhao, Y. O., Khaminets, A., Hunn, J. P., and Howard, J. C. (2009). Disruption of the *Toxoplasma gondii* parasitophorous vacuole by IFNc-Inducible Immunity-Related GTPases (IRG Proteins) triggers necrotic cell death. *PLoS Pathog.* 5:e1000288. doi: 10.1371/journal.ppat.1000288

3

Transcriptional Profiling Defines Histone Acetylation as a Regulator of Gene Expression during Human-to-Mosquito Transmission of the Malaria Parasite *Plasmodium falciparum*

Che J. Ngwa[1†], Meike J. Kiesow[1†], Olga Papst[1], Lindsey M. Orchard[2], Michael Filarsky[3], Alina N. Rosinski[1], Till S. Voss[3], Manuel Llinás[2,4] and Gabriele Pradel[1]*

[1] Division of Cellular and Applied Infection Biology, RWTH Aachen University, Aachen, Germany, [2] Department of Biochemistry and Molecular Biology, The Pennsylvania State University, University Park, PA, United States, [3] Department of Medical Parasitology and Infection Biology, Swiss Tropical and Public Health Institute, Basel, Switzerland, [4] Department of Chemistry and Huck Center for Malaria Research, The Pennsylvania State University, University Park, PA, United States

Edited by:
Kai Matuschewski,
Humboldt University of Berlin,
Germany

Reviewed by:
Richard Bartfai,
Radboud University Nijmegen,
Netherlands
Serge Ankri,
Technion—Israel Institute of
Technology, Israel

***Correspondence:**
Gabriele Pradel
pradel@bio2.rwth-aachen.de

† These authors have contributed equally to this work.

Transmission of the malaria parasite *Plasmodium falciparum* from the human to the mosquito is mediated by the intraerythrocytic gametocytes, which, once taken up during a blood meal, become activated to initiate sexual reproduction. Because gametocytes are the only parasite stages able to establish an infection in the mosquito, they are crucial for spreading the tropical disease. During gametocyte maturation, different repertoires of genes are switched on and off in a well-coordinated sequence, pointing to regulatory mechanisms of gene expression. While epigenetic gene control has been studied during erythrocytic schizogony of *P. falciparum*, little is known about this process during human-to-mosquito transmission of the parasite. To unveil the potential role of histone acetylation during gene expression in gametocytes, we carried out a microarray-based transcriptome analysis on gametocytes treated with the histone deacetylase inhibitor trichostatin A (TSA). TSA-treatment impaired gametocyte maturation and lead to histone hyper-acetylation in these stages. Comparative transcriptomics identified 294 transcripts, which were more than 2-fold up-regulated during gametocytogenesis following TSA-treatment. In activated gametocytes, which were less sensitive to TSA, the transcript levels of 48 genes were increased. TSA-treatment further led to repression of ~145 genes in immature and mature gametocytes and 7 genes in activated gametocytes. Up-regulated genes are mainly associated with functions in invasion, cytoadherence, and protein export, while down-regulated genes could particularly be assigned to transcription and translation. Chromatin immunoprecipitation demonstrated a link between gene activation and histone acetylation for selected genes. Among the genes up-regulated in TSA-treated mature gametocytes was a gene encoding the ring finger (RING)-domain protein PfRNF1, a putative E3 ligase of the ubiquitin-mediated signaling pathway. Immunochemistry demonstrated PfRNF1 expression mainly in the sexual stages of *P. falciparum* with peak expression in stage II gametocytes, where the protein localized to the nucleus and cytoplasm. *Pfrnf1* promoter and coding regions associated with acetylated histones, and TSA-treatment resulted in increased PfRNF1 levels. Our combined data point to an essential role of histone acetylation for gene regulation in gametocytes, which can be exploited for malaria transmission-blocking interventions.

Keywords: histone acetylation, gene expression, malaria, gametocyte, transmission

INTRODUCTION

The mosquito-borne disease malaria is the most devastating infectious tropical disease in the world, causing ~200 million new cases and more than 400,000 casualties annually (World Malaria Report, WHO, 2016). Malaria is caused by intracellularly living protozoa of the genus *Plasmodium*, with *P. falciparum* being the causative agent of malaria tropica, the most severe form of malaria.

The complex life-cycle of *P. falciparum* involves an initial round of replication in the human liver and subsequent 48-h replication cycles in the red blood cells (RBCs) that are pivotal for malaria pathogenesis. The virulence of *P. falciparum* is attributed to its ability to efficiently evade the host immune response, which includes molecular escape mechanisms to avoid complement and antibody recognition with the latter particularly depending on antigenic variation (reviewed in Scherf et al., 2008; Recker et al., 2011; Dinko and Pradel, 2016; Schmidt et al., 2016).

Immune evasion of *P. falciparum* is mediated by a tightly regulated transcription program with well-coordinated sequences of gene activation and silencing caused by chromatin-mediated epigenetic regulatory mechanisms (Duraisingh et al., 2005; Freitas-Junior et al., 2005; reviewed in Duraisingh and Horn, 2016). A major part of epigenetic control involves histone post-translational modifications (PTMs). Among others, these include histone acetylation and methylation, which are mediated by specialized transferase enzymes, including histone acetyltransferases (HATs), which promote DNA accessibility, as well as histone methyl transferases (HMTs) which can either act as promotors or inhibitors of DNA accessibility, dependent on the methylation site (Lopez-Rubio et al., 2007; Sautel et al., 2007). Histone PTMs can also be reversed, e.g., via histone deacetylases (HDACs) which remove the acetyl groups and thus inhibit gene expression. The genome of *P. falciparum* encodes five plasmodial HDACs; i.e., PfHDAC1 and 3, PfHda2 and the two type III silent information regulators PfSir2A and PfSir2B (Joshi et al., 1999; Gardner et al., 2002; reviewed in Cui and Miao, 2010) and four HATs, including the previously reported MYST and PfGNC5 (Cui et al., 2007a; Miao et al., 2010). Further, the genes coding for 10 SET (Su(var)3-9-'Enhancer of zeste-Trithorax)-domain-containing HMTs, termed PfSET1-10 were identified (Cui et al., 2008; Volz et al., 2010).

To date, histone PTMs were particularly studied during the expression of virulence-associated clonally variant multigene families, like the *var* gene family, which encodes the *P. falciparum* erythrocyte membrane protein PfEMP1 (Lopez-Rubio et al., 2007, 2009; Petter et al., 2011; reviewed in Llinás et al., 2008; Cui and Miao, 2010; Duffy et al., 2014; Duraisingh and Horn, 2016). Only a single *var* gene is expressed during replication of the RBC parasites at any one time, whereas all other *var* genes remain silent. Switching *var* expression and thus PfEMP1 structure alters the antigenic type of the infected RBCs and in consequence pathogenesis of the tropical disease. The expression of *var* genes relies on epigenetic mechanisms that induce dynamic changes in the chromatin structure (reviewed in Duffy et al., 2012). Only the active *var* gene copy assumes a euchromatic state characterized by both acetylated lysine 9 and tri-methylated lysine 4 of histone 3 (H3K9ac and H3K4me3, respectively; Lopez-Rubio et al., 2007; Salcedo-Amaya et al., 2009). On the other hand, *var* gene silencing is linked to H3K9 tri-methylation (H3K9me3) and further involves Sir2A and B and the class II HDAC PfHda2 (Duraisingh et al., 2005; Freitas-Junior et al., 2005; Lopez-Rubio et al., 2009; Tonkin et al., 2009; Coleman et al., 2014).

Recent work has further unveiled epigenetic control mechanisms during gametocyte commitment, when the RBC parasites enter the sexual pathway to form gametocytes, thus enabling parasite transmission from the human to the mosquito vector (reviewed in Josling and Llinás, 2015). Gametocyte commitment, which is proposed to be triggered by environmental signals (reviewed in Kuehn and Pradel, 2010; Bennink et al., 2016), is closely linked to the plasmodial heterochromatin protein PfHP1. This regulator usually binds specifically to H3K9me3 to maintain the heterochromatin state, resulting in *var* gene silencing and suppression of gametocyte commitment (Flueck et al., 2009; Pérez-Toledo et al., 2009; Brancucci et al., 2014). Conditional depletion of PfHP1 leads to hyper-induction of gametocytes caused by the de-repression of the *ap2-g* gene, which encodes the AP2-G transcription factor, a member of the apicomplexan Apetala2/ethylene response factor (AP2/ERF) DNA-binding protein family (Balaji et al., 2005; Kafsack et al., 2014; Sinha et al., 2014). Besides PfHP1, PfHda2 appears to be involved in the silencing of *ap2-g* gene expression in non-committed parasites, probably by removing acetylated histone residues allowing for their methylation leading to the binding of PfHP1 (Coleman et al., 2014). Once the *ap2-g* gene is activated and AP2-G becomes synthesized, the protein acts as a transcriptional switch that controls gametocyte differentiation by activating the transcription of early gametocyte genes (Kafsack et al., 2014; Sinha et al., 2014; reviewed in Voss et al., 2014; Josling and Llinás, 2015).

Once gametocyte commitment is induced, a total of about 20% of plasmodial genes are specifically expressed. These are needed for gametocyte maturation, but also for preparing the parasite to rapidly adjust to the mosquito midgut environment and to undergo gametogenesis, after the gametocytes are taken up by the blood-feeding female *Anopheles* (Florens et al., 2002; Lasonder et al., 2002; Le Roch et al., 2003). A suppression subtractive hybridization study identified 126 genes that changed in expression during initiation of gametogenesis, amongst others with putative functions in signaling, cell cycle, and gene expression (Ngwa et al., 2013). However, the mechanisms underlying differential gene regulation during gametocyte maturation and gametogenesis up to date have not been investigated.

The therapeutic use of epigenetic inhibitors in treatment of cancers has been known for more than a decade, and several HDAC inhibitors like vorinostat and romidepsin have meanwhile been approved for anticancer therapy (e.g., reviewed in Schobert and Biersack, 2017; Zagni et al., 2017). Also, the antimalarial effects of inhibitors targeting HAT and HDAC enzymes have been explored in the past (e.g., Cui et al., 2007b; Andrews et al., 2008, 2009, 2012a; Chaal et al., 2010; Wheatley et al., 2010; Sumanadasa et al., 2012; Engel et al., 2015; Alves Avelar et al., 2017; Chua et al., 2017). Additional studies showed that HDAC inhibitors also exhibit gametocytocidal activities *in vitro*, indicating that the enzymes are essential for gametocytogenesis (e.g., Hansen et al., 2014; Sun et al., 2014; Trenholme et al., 2014).

To date, only a few studies have investigated the transcriptional changes in *P. falciparum* following treatment with HDAC inhibitors. An initial study reported a general deregulation of gene expression following treatment with the HDAC inhibitor trichostatin A (TSA) during the erythrocytic replication cycle with up to 60% of the genome affected (Hu et al., 2010). Follow-up experiments, though, comparing the transcription profiles in blood stage parasites following treatment with three different HDAC inhibitors, could only detect an overlap for two genes with altered expression (Andrews et al., 2012b). The effect of HDAC inhibitors on gene expression in gametocytes has hitherto not been addressed, amongst others due to the technical challenge of harvesting high numbers of pure gametocyte stages.

To unveil the potential role of histone acetylation during gene expression in gametocytes, we now have carried out a microarray-based transcriptome analysis, in which we compared the transcriptomes of gametocytes treated with TSA and of untreated gametocytes. We show that TSA-treatment results in the deregulation of 453 genes, demonstrating a crucial role of histone PMTs in preparing the parasite for human-to-mosquito transmission.

MATERIALS AND METHODS

Antibodies

Primary antibodies used in this study included: rabbit anti-(tetra)-acetyl histone H4 K5, 8, 12, 16ac (H4Kac4) (Millipore; note: according the manufacturer's material data sheet this antibody may cross-react with other acetylated histones like H2B); rabbit anti-H3K9ac (Diagenode); rabbit anti-PfHP1 (Brancucci et al., 2014); rabbit IgG antibody (Millipore); mouse/rabbit anti-Pfs230 (Ngwa et al., 2013; Simon et al., 2016), rabbit anti-Pfs25 (BEI Resources); mouse anti-Pf39 (Scholz et al., 2008); rabbit anti-HA (Sigma Aldrich); mouse anti-proteasome SU $\alpha5$ (Aminake et al., 2012), and anti-PfActinI (Ngwa et al., 2013). Mouse anti-PfRNF1 was generated for this study (see below). For indirect immunofluorescence assays (IFAs), the following dilutions of the antibodies were used: anti-H4KAc4 (1:200), anti-H3K9ac (1:200), mouse/rabbit anti-Pfs230 (1:200), anti-Pfs25 (1:1,000), anti-PfRNF1 (1:20), anti-PfHP1 (1:300), and anti-proteasome SU $\alpha5$ (1:50). For Western blot (WB) analysis the following dilutions were used: anti-H4Kac4 (1:1,000), anti-H3K9ac (1:1,000), anti-Pf39 (1:1,000), anti-PfActinI (1:200), anti-PfRNF1 (1:200), rabbit anti-HA (1:1,000). For chromatin immunoprecipitation (ChIP) assays, 1 µg of each antibody (anti-H4Kac4, anti-H3K9ac, anti-PfHP1, IgG) was used.

Parasite Culture

P. falciparum strain NF54 was used in this study. The parasites were cultivated *in vitro* in RPMI 1640 medium supplemented with 10% heat-inactivated human serum as described (Ifediba and Vanderberg, 1981) and cultures were maintained at 37°C at an atmosphere of 5% O_2, 5% CO_2, and 90% N_2. Cultures were synchronized by repeated sorbitol treatment as described (Lambros and Vanderberg, 1979). To generate gametocytes, the cultures were kept at high parasitaemia and gametocytogenesis was induced following addition of lysed RBCs. As soon as stage I gametocytes started to emerge in the culture, the culture medium was supplemented with 50 mM N-acetyl glucosamine (GlcNac) for ~5 days to kill the asexual blood stages (Fivelman et al., 2007). The gametocyte culture was then maintained in normal culture medium without GlcNac until immature (stage II–IV) or mature stage V gametocytes were harvested and enriched by Percoll gradient purification (Kariuki et al., 1998). In order to obtain activated gametocytes, Percoll-enriched mature gametocytes were incubated with 100 µM xanthurenic acid (XA) for 30 min, 1 or 6 h at room temperature (RT). Giemsa-staining of purified gametocyte smears was used to confirm purity of the samples. The human erythrocyte concentrate and serum used in this study were purchased from the Department of Transfusion Medicine (University Hospital Aachen, Germany). The University Hospital Aachen Ethics commission approved all work with human blood, the donors remained anonymous, and serum samples were pooled.

Malstat Assay

To determine the antimalarial effect of the histone deacetylase inhibitor TSA (Sigma-Aldrich), a Malstat assay was performed as described previously (Aminake et al., 2011). Synchronized ring stages of *P. falciparum* strain NF54 were plated in triplicate in 96-well plates (200 µl/well) at a parasitaemia of 1% in the presence of TSA dissolved in 0.5% vol. ethanol (5 µM to 0.06 nM). Chloroquine, dissolved in double-distilled water, served as a positive control in the experiments. Incubation of parasites with ethanol alone at a concentration of 0.5% vol. was used as negative control. Parasites were cultivated *in vitro* for 72 h, resuspended, and aliquots of 20 µl were removed and added to 100 µl of the Malstat reagent in a 96-well microtiter plate. The assessment of parasite lactate dehydrogenase (pLDH) activity was obtained by adding 20 µl of a mixture of NBT (Nitro Blue Tetrazolium) and diaphorase (1:1; 1 mg/ml stock each) to the Malstat reaction, and optical densities were measured at 630 nm.

Each compound was tested four times, and the IC_{50} values were calculated from variable-slope sigmoidal dose-response curves using the GraphPad Prism program version 4.

Gametocyte Toxicity Test

P. falciparum strain NF54 parasites were grown at high parasitaemia to induce gametocyte formation. Upon appearance of stage II gametocytes, 1 ml of culture was aliquoted in triplicate in a 24-well plate in the presence of TSA at asexual blood stage IC_{50} (29 nM) and IC_{90} (0.26 μM) concentrations. Incubation of parasites with ethanol at a concentration of 0.5% vol. and chloroquine (IC_{50}), dissolved in double-distilled water, were used as negative controls. The proteasome inhibitor epoxomicin (60 nM), diluted in DMSO, served as a positive control in the experiments. The gametocytes were cultivated for 10 d with daily medium replacement. For the first 2 days of cultivation, the gametocytes were treated with the inhibitors, subsequently the medium was inhibitor-free. Every second day, Giemsa-stained blood smears were prepared and the gametocytemia was evaluated by determining the numbers of gametocytes of stages II to V in a total number of 1,000 erythrocytes in triplicate. The student's *t*-test was used to determine significant differences between TSA-treated and untreated samples.

Macrogamete and Zygote Development Assays

Equal volumes of mature gametocyte cultures were incubated with TSA at IC_{50} or IC_{90} concentrations or with 0.5% vol. ethanol for negative control for 1 h at 37°C. Subsequently, the cultures were activated with 100 μM XA and incubated for 30 min (macrogamete development assay) or 12 h (zygote development assay) at RT. An equal volume of each sample was then coated on Teflon slides and the cells were immunolabeled with anti-Pfs25 as described below. The numbers of Pfs25-positive macrogametes or zygotes, as distinguished by their round shapes, were counted for a total number of 1,000 erythrocytes, which were visualized by differential interference contrast in triplicate, using a Leica DMLS microscope at 1,000-fold magnification. Zygotes were distinguished from macrogametes by their larger nuclei through Hoechst nuclear stain 33342 (Molecular Probes). The student's *t*-test was used to determine significant differences between TSA-treated and untreated samples.

Indirect Immunofluorescence Assay

P. falciparum cultures (of the wild-type NF54 strain or the PfRNF1-HA-Strep-expressing transfectant line) were air-dried on glass slides and fixed for 10 min in a methanol bath at −80°C. For membrane permeabilization and blocking of non-specific binding, fixed cells were successfully incubated in 0.01% saponin/0.5% BSA/PBS and 1% vol. neutral goat serum (Sigma-Aldrich)/PBS each for 30 min at RT. For labeling of PfHP1, the air-dried samples were fixed with 4% paraformaldehyde/PBS, pH 7.4, for 10 min at RT and subsequently treated with 0.1% vol. Triton X-100/125 mM glycine (Carl Roth)/PBS at RT for 30 min, followed by blocking of non-specific binding sites with 3% BSA/PBS for 1 h. Preparations were then incubated with the primary antibody diluted in 0.01% saponin/0.5% BSA/PBS for 1.5 h each at 37°C. Binding of primary antibody was visualized by incubating the preparations with Alexa Fluor 488-conjugated goat anti-mouse or anti-rabbit IgG secondary antibody (Molecular Probes) diluted in 0.01% saponin/0.5% BSA/PBS for 1 h at 37°C. The different parasite stages were detected by double-labeling with stage-specific antibodies, i.e., polyclonal rabbit or mouse antisera directed against PfMSP1 for the detection of asexual blood stages and Pfs230 and Pfs25 for the detection of gametocytes and activated gametocytes, respectively. This was followed by incubation with Alexa Fluor 594-conjugated goat anti-rabbit or anti-mouse IgG secondary antibodies (Molecular Probes) diluted in 0.01% saponin/0.5% BSA/PBS for 1 h at 37°C. Nuclei were highlighted by treatment with Hoechst nuclear stain 33342 for 1 min at RT and cells were mounted with anti-fading solution AF2 (Citifluor Ltd) and sealed with nail varnish. In cases where double-labeling was not employed, counterstaining of erythrocytes was performed using 0.05% Evans Blue/PBS (Sigma-Aldrich) for 1 min. Digital images were taken using a Leica AF 6000 microscope and processed using Adobe Photoshop CS software.

Western Blot Analysis

Percoll-enriched immature (stages II–IV) and mature (stage V) gametocytes (of the wild-type NF54 strain or the PfRNF1-HA-Strep-expressing transfectant line) were harvested as described above and erythrocytes were lysed with 0.05% saponin/PBS followed by a washing step with PBS to remove the hemoglobin. The pellets were resuspended and sonicated in NP-40 lysis buffer (50 mM Tris HCl pH 8.0, 150 mM NaCl, 1% vol. NP-40) supplemented with a protease inhibitor cocktail (Roche Diagnostics, Germany). SDS-PAGE loading buffer was then added to the lysates, heat-denatured for 10 min at 95°C, and separated via SDS-PAGE and transferred to Hybond ECL nitrocellulose membrane (Amersham Biosciences) according to the manufacturer's protocol. Membranes were blocked for non-specific binding by incubation in Tris-buffered saline containing 5% skim milk and 1% BSA, followed by incubation with the respective rabbit or mouse antibody for 2 h at RT. After washing, the membranes were incubated with an alkaline phosphatase-conjugated anti-rabbit or anti-mouse IgG secondary antibody (Sigma-Aldrich) for 1 h at RT and developed in a solution of nitroblue tetrazolium chloride (NBT) and 5-bromo-4-chloro-3-indoxyl phosphate (BCIP; Sigma-Aldrich) for 5–30 min. Scanned blots were processed using Adobe Photoshop CS software.

Histone Hyper-Acetylation Assay

To investigate histone hyper-acetylation caused by TSA-treatment, hyper-acetylation assays were carried out as previously described (Andrews et al., 2012b). Percoll-enriched immature (stages II–IV) and mature (stage V) gametocytes were treated with TSA at IC_{90} concentrations or with 0.5% vol. ethanol (negative control) for 1 and 6 h at 37°C, respectively. Protein lysates were generated, employed to SDS-PAGE and histone hyper-acetylation was analyzed by WB analysis using anti-H4Kac4 and anti-H3K9ac antibodies as described above. Immunoblotting with anti-Pf39 antisera was used as loading control. Histone hyper-acetylation was quantified from three to six different experiments by measuring the band intensities via the Image J programme. When immunoblotting with anti-H4Kac4 antibody, total acetylation bands were quantified. The related band intensity was normalized to Pf39 and compared with respect to untreated samples.

Microarray Analysis

Total RNA was isolated from enriched immature (stages II–IV) and mature (stage V) gametocytes and gametocytes at 1 h post-activation following treatment with TSA at IC_{90} concentrations or with 0.5% vol. ethanol (untreated control) for 1 and 6 h, respectively, using the Trizol reagent (Invitrogen) according to the manufacturer's protocol. Quality of RNA samples were assessed using a ND-1000 (NanoDrop Technologies, Thermo Scientific) and by agarose gel electrophoresis. The microarray experiments were carried out as described previously (Kafsack et al., 2012). Briefly, synthesis of first strand amino-allyl cDNA was performed using Superscript II reverse transcriptase (Invitrogen). The amino-allyl cDNA was then cleaned and concentrated using the Zymo DNA clean and concentrator-5 column (Zymo Research) followed by coupling with Cy5 dye (GE Healthcare). The reference pool consisted of a mixture RNA from asexual blood stages and gametocytes, in which synthesis of first strand amino-allyl cDNA was performed as describe above, and coupled with the Cy3 dye. Equal amounts of Cy5-labeled samples from each treatment and the Cy3-labeled reference pool were subjected to array hybridization for 17 h at 65°C using a *P. falciparum* DNA Agilent microarray chip (Agilent Technologies AMADID #037237) containing the 5,363 coding genes (Bozdech et al., 2003). The arrays were scanned using the Agilent scanner G2600D (Agilent Technologies). Normalized intensities were extracted using the Agilent Feature Extraction Software version 11.5.1.1 and uploaded to the Princeton University Microarray Database (PUMA.princeton.edu) for analysis. After background subtraction, the log2 of the (Cy5/Cy3) intensity ratio was extracted. Raw intensity data have been submitted to the NCBI Gene Expression Omnibus (GEO; http://www.ncbi.nlm.nih.gov/geo/) under accession number GSE99223. Transcript abundance of treated samples were compared to that of untreated samples. For the selection of up- and down-regulated genes, a cut-off value of greater than 2-fold for at least one of the two time-points with a consistent up- or down-regulation for both time-points was chosen. A cut-off value of greater than 2-fold for both time points was considered significant. Data were analyzed using the database PlasmoDB (http://plasmodb.org/plasmo; Aurrecoechea et al., 2009) and Microsoft Excel 2010.

Real-Time RT-PCR

To validate the microarray data, total RNA was isolated from enriched immature (stages II–IV) and mature (stage V) gametocytes following treatment with TSA at IC_{90} concentration or with 0.5% vol. ethanol (untreated control) for 1 h as described above. One microgram of each total RNA sample was used for cDNA synthesis using the SuperScript III First-Strand Synthesis System (Invitrogen), following the manufacturer's instructions. The synthesized cDNA was first tested by diagnostic PCR for asexual blood stage contamination using primers specific for the gene encoding the apical membrane antigen AMA-1 (Peterson et al., 1989; Narum and Thomas, 1994) and for gametocyte-specificity using primers specific for the gene encoding the LCCL-domain protein PfCCp2 (Pradel et al., 2004; Ngwa et al., 2013). Controls without reverse transcriptase were also used to investigate potential genomic DNA (gDNA) contamination by using *pfccp2* primers (for primer sequences, see Table S1). Primers for quantitative real time RT-PCR to confirm the up-regulation of selected genes as identified by microarray analysis were designed using the Primer 3 software (http://frodo.wi.mit.edu/primer3/) and tested on gDNA in conventional PCR to confirm primer specificity (for primer sequences, see Table S1). Real time RT-PCR measurements were performed using the Bio-Rad iQ5 Real-Time Detection System. Reactions were performed in triplicate in a total volume of 20 μl using the maxima SyBR green qPCR master mix according to manufacturer's instructions (Thermo Scientific, Germany). Controls without template and without reverse transcriptase were included in all real time RT-PCR experiments. Transcript expression levels were calculated by the $2^{-\Delta Ct}$ method (Livak and Schmittgen, 2001) using the endogenous control gene encoding the *P. falciparum* seryl tRNA-ligase (PF3D7_0717700) as reference (Salanti et al., 2003), which was confirmed not to be affected in its transcript levels by TSA-treatment.

Chromatin Immunoprecipitation-Quantitative PCR

To provide evidence for a link between gene expression and histone acetylation for selected genes identified by microarray analysis, ChIP assays combined with subsequent-quantitative PCR (ChIP-qPCR) were carried as previously described (Flueck et al., 2009). Mature (stage V) gametocytes were enriched by Percoll gradient purification, treated with either 0.5% vol. ethanol (untreated) or TSA at IC_{90} concentrations for 6 h (TSA-treated) and then resuspended in RPMI 1640 medium containing human erythrocyte concentrate at 5% haematocrit. Crosslinking of gametocyte chromatin was triggered by incubation of the cultures with 1% formaldehyde (Sigma-Aldrich) for 10 min at 37°C and a termination of the reaction by addition of 0.125 M glycine diluted in doubled-distilled water. The RBCs were then lysed using 0.15% saponin/PBS and crosslinked nuclei harvested and separated from cytoplasmic proteins by the use of a 0.25 M cytoplasmic lysis buffer (20 nM Hepes, 10 mM KCl, 1 mM EDTA, 1 mM EGTA, 0.65% NP-40, 1 mM DTT, 1x protease inhibitor cocktail). The nuclei of 10^8 mature gametocytes were then pooled and the nuclei were sheared by sonication with UPH50 (Hielscher) on ice for 40 intervals with each interval composed of 10 s sonication and 50 s resting cycles to gain fragment sizes <500 bp. A total amount of 400–450 ng chromatin was incubated under rotation with 1 μg antibody (anti-H3K9ac, anti-H4Kac4, anti-PfHP1, and rabbit IgG antibody for negative control) overnight at 4°C in the presence of 20 μl of protein A- and G-coated magnetic beads (Diagenode). After six washing steps the immunoprecipitated chromatin was eluted by adding 1% SDS and 0.1 M $NaHCO_3$ as DNA elution buffer and decrosslinked at 65°C overnight. DNA purification was carried out using the PCR and Gel Clean Up

Kit (Macherey-Nagel). Primers for qPCR for selected genes as identified by microarrays were designed using Primer 3 software and tested on *P. falciparum* gDNA in conventional PCR to confirm primer specificity (for primer sequences, see Table S1). Quantitative PCR measurements were performed as described above. The amount of recovered target DNA gained from untreated and TSA-treated gametocyte samples was compared to associated input DNA sample (1:10) and depicted as percentage of input for each chosen gene.

Recombinant Protein Expression and Production of Mouse Antisera

A recombinant peptide, corresponding to the N-terminal region of PfRNF1 (Figure S1A), was expressed as a maltose-binding protein-tagged fusion protein using the pMAL^{TM}c5X-vector (New England Biolabs). DNA was amplified by PCR using gene-specific primers (for primer sequences, see Table S1). Recombinant protein was expressed in *E. coli* BL21(DE3)RIL cells according to the manufacturer's protocol (Invitrogen) and isolated and affinity-purified using amylose resin according to the manufacturer's protocol (New England Biolabs). Polyclonal antisera were generated by immunization of 6-weeks old female NMRI mice (Charles River Laboratories) with subcutaneous injections of 100 μg recombinant protein emulsified in Freund's incomplete adjuvant (Sigma-Aldrich) followed by a boost after 4 weeks. Mice were anesthetized at day 10 after the boost by intraperitoneal injection of a mixture of ketamine and xylazine according to the manufacturer's protocol (Sigma-Aldrich), and immune sera were collected via heart puncture. The immune sera of three mice immunized were pooled; sera of three non-immunized mice (NMS) were used as negative control. Experiments in mice were approved by the animal welfare committee of the District Council of Cologne, Germany (ref. no. 84-02.05.30.12.097 TVA).

Generation of a PfRNF1-HA-Strep-Tagged Parasite Line

To tag PfRNF1 with hemagglutinin (HA)-streptavidin (Strep) at the C-terminus, a 1,230 bp homologous gene fragment was amplified from *P. falciparum* NF54 gDNA using gene-specific primers (for primer sequences, see Table S1). Cloning was done using the pHAST vector (kindly provided by Alex Maier, ANU Canberra; Rug and Maier, 2013) with the help of the SacII/XhoI restriction sites. A *P. falciparum* strain NF54 culture with 5% ring stages was loaded with 100 μg of the pHAST-PfRNF1 construct in transfection buffer via electroporation (parameters: 310 V 950 μF, 13 ms; Bio-Rad gene-pulser) as described (Wirth et al., 2014). WR99210 was added to a final concentration of 2.5 nM, starting at 4 h after transfection. WR99210-resistant parasites appeared after 4 weeks. After 60–90 days of drug pressure, the respective cultures were investigated for plasmid-integration by diagnostic PCR. The gDNA of the transfected parasites was isolated using the NucleoSpin Blood Kit (Macherey-Nagel) according to the manufacturer's protocol and used as template in the diagnostic PCR to test for vector integration (for primer sequences, see Table S1; for primer location, see Figures S1B,C). Once integration was confirmed, a clonal dilution was carried out to select for single PfRNF1-HA-Strep-tagged parasite clones and one clone was used for characterization.

Determination of Protein Expression of PfRNF1 Following TSA-Treatment

To determine if the up-regulation of PfRNF1 transcript expression following TSA-treatment corroborates with the up-regulation of protein expression, purified mature gametocytes of the *P. falciparum* wild-type NF54 strain or the PfRNF1-HA-Strep-expressing transfectant line were splitted in two equal volumes and each was pipetted into a pre-warmed 96-well plate. One part of the culture was treated with TSA at IC_{90} concentrations and the other part was treated with 0.5% vol. ethanol (untreated control). The samples were incubated for 24 h at 37°C in an atmosphere of 5% O_2, 5% CO_2, and 90% N_2. Protein lysates were generated, separated via SDS-PAGE and protein levels were analyzed by WB analysis using anti-PfRNF1 antisera or anti-HA antibody as described above. Anti-Pf39 antisera was used as loading control. PfRNF1 levels were quantified for untreated and TSA-treated samples from six (for the wild-type) and two (for the transfectant) different experiments by measuring the band intensities by Image J. The related band intensities were normalized to Pf39 and compared with respect to untreated samples.

Parasite Sub-cellular Fractionation

Nuclear and cytosolic fractions of *P. falciparum* strain NF54 parasites were prepared as previously described (Voss et al., 2002). Enriched immature (stages II–IV) gametocytes were treated with 0.1% saponin in PBS to lyse RBCs and washed twice with PBS. The parasite pellet was then resuspended in cold lysis buffer (20 mM Hepes, pH 7.8, 10 mM KCl, 1 mM EDTA, 1 mM DTT, 1 mM PMSF, 1% Triton X100) and incubated for 5 min on ice. The nuclei were pelleted at 2,500 g for 5 min at 4°C and the supernatant containing the cytoplasmic proteins was collected. The nuclear pellet was washed three times with lysis buffer and resuspended in twice the pellet volume of the extraction buffer (20 mM Hepes, pH 7.8, 800 mM KCl, 1 mM EDTA, 1 mM DTT, 1 mM PMSF, 1x protease inhibitor cocktail). Following incubation under rotation for 30 min at 4°C, the extract was cleared by centrifugation at 13,000 g for 30 min and 4°C. The supernatant containing the nuclear fraction was then diluted with 1 volume of dilution buffer (20 mM Hepes, pH 7.8, 1 mM EDTA, 1 mM DTT, 30% vol. glycerol). The nuclear and cytoplasmic fractions were subjected to WB using anti-PfRNF1 antisera as described above.

RESULTS

TSA-Treatment Affects *P. falciparum* Blood and Sexual Stage Development

The effect of TSA on the blood and sexual stages of *P. falciparum* was tested *in vitro*. Malstat assays, which measure the pLDH activities demonstrated that TSA-treatment inhibited blood stage replication with a mean IC_{50} value of 29 nM and an estimated IC_{90} of 0.26 μM. Chloroquine-treatment was used for positive control in the assay and resulted in parasite growth inhibition with a mean IC_{50} value of 16 nM (**Table 1**).

We next tested the effect of TSA on gametocyte development. In this regard a culture of mainly stage II gametocytes was grown in 24-well plates in triplicate in the presence of TSA at IC_{50} and IC_{90} concentrations (as determined by Malstat assay) or in the presence of 0.5% vol. ethanol (untreated control) for 48 h. The parasites were subsequently cultured for another 8 days without inhibitor. The gametocytemia was determined every 2 days via Giemsa-stained blood smears. We showed that the numbers of stage IV and V gametocytes formed on day 10 were 43% less when the stage II gametocytes were treated with TSA at IC_{50} concentrations and 67% less when treated with IC_{90} concentrations as compared to controls (0.5% vol. ethanol and 16 nM of chloroquine) (**Figure 1A**). Treatment of stage II gametocytes with 60 nM epoxomicin as positive control resulted in complete elimination of stage IV and V gametocytes on day 10 (data not shown). We also investigated in detail the differentiation of gametocytes from stage II to stage V during incubation with TSA. TSA-treatment particularly affected gametocytes of stages II and III, but did not result in any delay of gametocyte maturation compared to the controls (Figure S2).

The effect of TSA on male gamete formation (termed exflagellation) has already been demonstrated for *P. falciparum* (Trenholme et al., 2014). The impairment of exflagellation by TSA is minor with IC_{50} values of 0.22 ± 0.04 mM (**Table 1**). To determine if TSA-treatment affects the formation of female macrogametes and zygotes, gametocyte cultures were incubated with TSA at IC_{50} and IC_{90} concentrations or with 0.5% vol. ethanol (untreated control) for 1 h at 37°C. The cultures were activated with 100 μM XA and further cultured for 30 min and 12 h to detect macrogametes and zygotes, respectively. Both stages were immunolabeled with anti-Pfs25 antibodies and counted for a total of 1,000 erythrocytes in triplicate. Comparative analyses demonstrated a slight reduction of macrogamete numbers, when these were treated with TSA at IC_{90} concentration, while the numbers of zygotes decreased by 21 and 24%, when treated with TSA at IC_{50} and IC_{90} concentrations, respectively (**Figures 1B,C**).

Treatment of Gametocytes with TSA Causes Histone Hyper-Acetylation

To assess the extent of histone acetylation during *P. falciparum* gametocyte development, two commercially available histone acetylation antibodies (anti-H3K9ac and anti-H4Kac4) were used to detect histone acetylation in gametocytes by IFA. Histone acetylation was detected throughout the nuclei of gametocyte stages II-V highlighted by Hoechst staining and immunolabeling of Pfs230, respectively (**Figures 2A,B**). WB analysis using the histone acetylation antibodies detected protein bands migrating at molecular weights of 15 kDa (for anti-H3K9ac) and of 11 and 13 kDa (for anti-H4Kac4). These molecular weights are in accord with the expected molecular weights of 15.4 kDa for histone H3 and 11.5 kDa for histone H4. The second protein band detected by the anti-H4Kac4 antibody might represent H2B, which has an expected molecular weight of 13.1 kDa, since the antibody also recognizes this acetylated histone as indicated in the manufacturer's material data sheet. The intensities of the protein bands increased, when the gametocytes were treated with TSA at IC_{90} concentrations, demonstrating hyper-acetylation of the histones following TSA treatment (**Figures 2C,D**). Quantitative WB analysis, measuring the protein band intensity of total acetylated histones showed a significant increase in their acetylation levels, when the immature and mature gametocytes were treated with TSA (**Figures 2E,F**).

TABLE 1 | Antimalarial activities of TSA against the *P. falciparum* blood and microgamete stages.

Assay	Inhibitor	IC_{50}	IC_{90}
Malstat assay	TSA	29 ± 3.0 *nM*	0.26 μM
	Chloroquine	16 ± 6.0 *nM*	N/A
Exflagellation assay[a]	TSA	0.22 ± 0.040 *mM*	N/A

N/A, Not applicable; [a]published in Trenholme et al. (2014).

TSA-Treatment Results in the Deregulation of Genes during Gametocyte Development

We next aimed to identify genes deregulated following treatment of gametocytes with TSA. Immature, mature and activated gametocytes were treated with TSA for 1 or 6 h, total RNA was isolated, and the RNA of untreated cultures was used for comparative controls. Beforehand, the purity of the cell samples was confirmed via Giemsa smears (Figure S3A). Following cDNA synthesis, the samples were applied to a *P. falciparum* DNA Agilent microarray chip containing DNA spots corresponding to the 5,363 coding genes of nucleus, mitochondrion and apicoplast (Bozdech et al., 2003; Kafsack et al., 2012) (Table S2). Genes with transcript levels greater (i.e., up-regulated genes) or lower (i.e., down-regulated) than 2-fold compared to the untreated control (0.5% vol. ethanol) for at least one of the two time-points combined with a consistent up- or down-regulation for both time-points were used for further analysis. Changes in transcript levels greater than 2-fold for both time points compared to the control were considered significant.

In immature and mature gametocytes a total of 219 and 214 genes, respectively, were identified by comparative transcript analysis that were more than 2-fold up-regulated in their expression levels, when these stages were treated with TSA. The up-regulations for 120 and 76 of these transcripts, respectively, were considered significant. Accordingly, transcripts of 90 and 66 genes were more than 2-fold down-regulated in TSA-treated immature and mature gametocytes with a significant down-regulation being observed for 8 and 11 genes, respectively. In activated gametocytes, which were less sensitive to TSA-treatment, the transcript levels of 48 genes were non-significantly increased and were decreased for 7 genes (**Figure 3A**, Table S3). The average up-regulation values for immature, mature and activated gametocytes were in the range of 1.3 to 3.2-fold absolute changes (immature: 1 h, 2.32; 6 h, 2.58: mature: 1 h, 2.03; 6 h, 3.16; activated: 1 h, 1,31; 6 h, 2.36), and the down-regulation values ranged between 0.7 and 0.5-fold absolute changes (immature: 1 h,

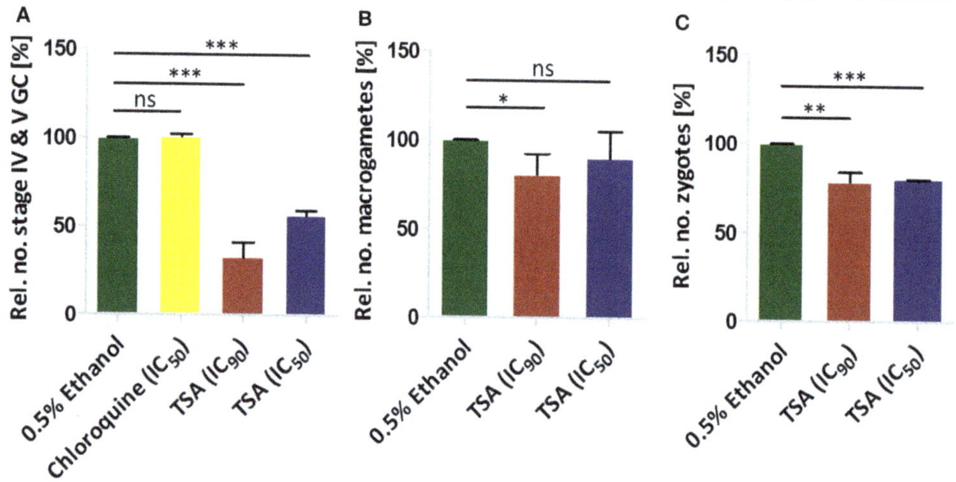

FIGURE 1 | The effect of TSA on *P. falciparum* sexual stage development. **(A)** The effect of TSA on gametocyte development. TSA at IC_{50} or IC_{90} concentrations was added to stage II gametocyte cultures for 2 days. The numbers of stage IV and V gametocytes were determined in 1,000 erythrocytes at day 10 using Giemsa-stained blood smears. Epoxomicin (60 nM) was used as a positive control (not shown), while 0.5% vol. ethanol and chloroquine (16 nM) were used as negative controls (ethanol set to 100%). **(B)** The effect of TSA on macrogamete development. A mature gametocyte culture was incubated with TSA at IC_{50} or IC_{90} concentrations or 0.5% vol. ethanol for 1 h at 37°C. The culture was then activated with 100 μM XA and further cultured for 30 min at RT for macrogamete development. Macrogametes were detected by immunolabelling with anti-Pfs25 and counted in triplicate in 1,000 erythrocytes. **(C)** Effect of TSA on zygote development. The zygote development assay was performed in the same way as the macrogamete development except for the fact that after activation the cultures were incubated for 12 h at RT. Results shown (for **A–C**) are combined from three independent experiments each performed in triplicate (mean ± SD). $^{*}P < 0.05$; $^{**}P < 0.01$; $^{***}P < 0.001$; ns, not significant; Student's *t*-test.

0.70; 6 h, 0.49; mature: 1 h, 0.62; 6 h, 0.47; activated: 1 h, 0.72; 6 h, 0.51) (**Figure 3B**). A total of 29 genes that were up-regulated in their transcript levels were shared by immature, mature and activated gametocytes, but none of the down-regulated genes were shared by the three gametocyte stages (**Figure 3C**).

For each of the identified genes, the microarray-based transcript data were compared with the transcriptomics data published in the database PlasmoDB. The comparison revealed that roughly 23 and 22% of the genes transcriptionally up-regulated in immature and mature gametocytes following TSA-treatment, respectively, have their peak expression in mature stage V gametocytes and in ookinetes (Figure S4; Table S3). Genes down-regulated in immature gametocytes following TSA-treatment were mainly expressed in gametocytes of stages II and V (25 and 23%, respectively), while for the mature gametocytes 58% of down-regulated genes showed their peak expression in gametocytes of stage V. In activated gametocytes, 42% of genes up-regulated after treatment with TSA were highly expressed in ookinetes, whereas all of the down-regulated genes exhibited peak expression profiles in gametocytes of stage V (Figure S4; Table S3).

The identified genes were grouped according to their predicted functions as indicated in PlasmoDB. The *in-silico* analyses demonstrated that in TSA-treated immature and mature gametocytes the up-regulated genes mainly associated with functions in gene expression and transcription and in antigenic variation and cytoadherence, or they code for exported proteins. Furthermore, in immature gametocytes, genes associated with RBC invasion and proteostasis were significantly up-regulated (**Figure 3D**; Figures S5A,B). The up-regulated genes mostly included ones coding for SURFINs and RIFINs, for the merozoite surface protein (MSP) family or the rhoptry neck (RON) family and for the PHIST family (Mphande et al., 2008; Proellocks et al., 2010; Beeson et al., 2016; Warncke et al., 2016). Also, genes with functions in the mosquito-specific stages were activated, when the gametocytes were treated with TSA. Down-regulated genes included ones assigned to gene expression and transcription and translation (**Figure 3D**). Furthermore, genes with assigned functions in metabolism and signaling as well as components of the cytoskeleton and the inner membrane complex were affected in their activation by TSA-treatment (Table S3).

In TSA-treated immature and mature gametocytes, several genes with more than 5-fold up-regulated transcription were identified, i.e., four genes in the immature gametocyte samples and 16 genes in the mature gametocyte samples (**Table 2**). The genes could mostly be assigned to signaling, cell cycle and DNA replication, gene expression and transcription, and proteostasis, or they included genes encoding exported proteins. Six of the genes had unknown function. One gene, encoding for the RBC invasion-related protein MSRP4 (merozoite surface protein 7-related protein 4), was identified in both immature and mature gametocytes.

To validate the microarray array data, a total 32 genes (immature gametocytes: 15 genes; mature gametocytes: 17 genes) transcriptionally up-regulated following TSA-treatment were randomly selected. The gametocyte cultures were treated with TSA at IC_{90} concentration or 0.5% vol. ethanol (untreated

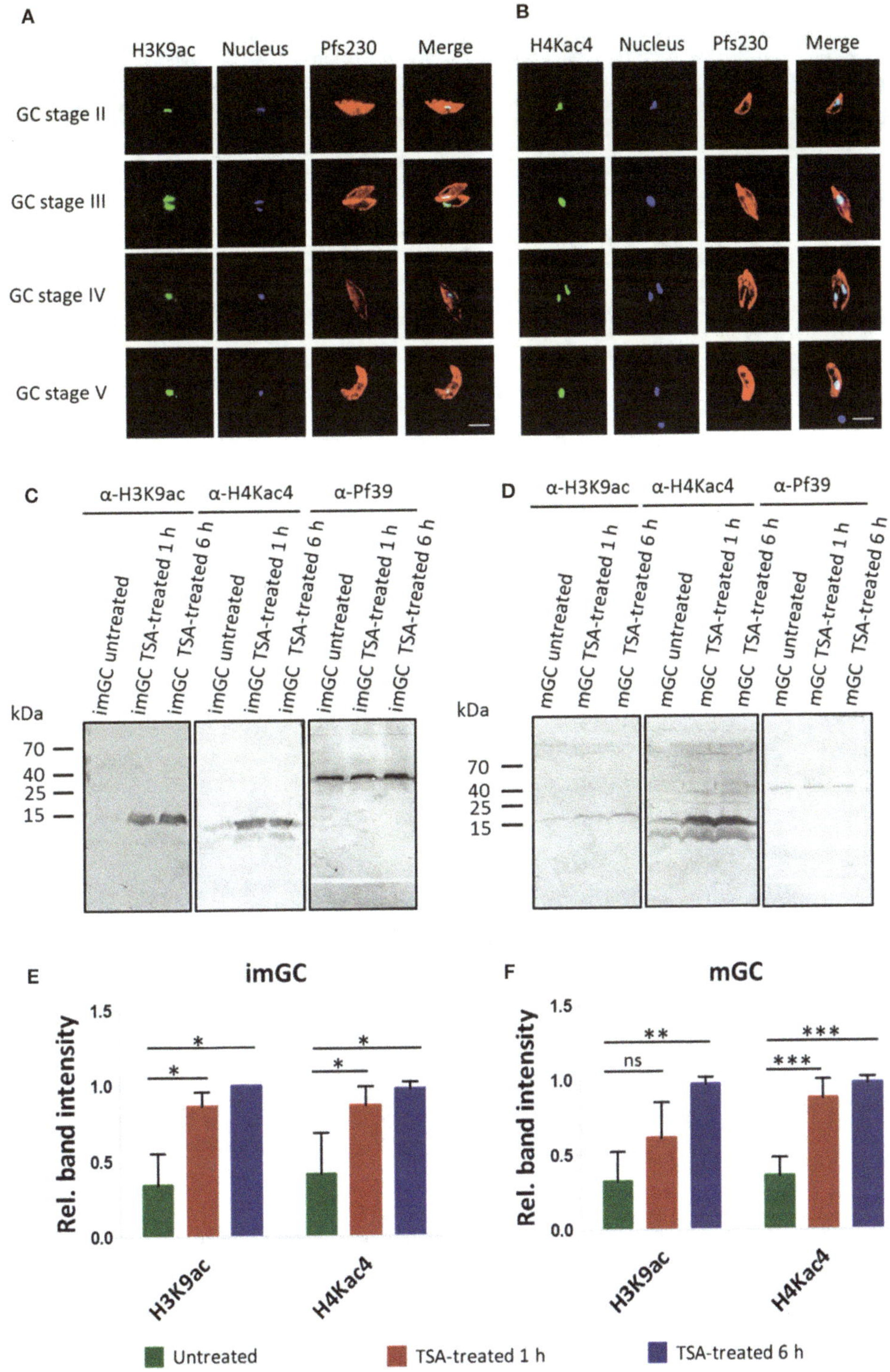

FIGURE 2 | Histone acetylation and hyper-acetylation following treatment of gametocytes with TSA. **(A,B)** Presence of acetylated histones in gametocytes. Acetylated histones were detected in the different gametocyte stages (GC stage II-V) via immunolabeling using rabbit anti-H3K9ac **(A)** and anti-H4Kac4 **(B)** antibodies (green). Gametocytes were highlighted with mouse antibodies against the gametocyte marker Pfs230 (red). Nuclei were highlighted by Hoechst nuclear stain 33342 (blue). Bar, 5 μm. **(C,D)** Histone hyper-acetylation following gametocyte treatment with TSA. Protein lysates from immature gametocytes (imGC) **(C)** and mature gametocytes (mGC) **(D)** following treatment with TSA at IC_{90} concentrations or with 0.5% vol. ethanol (untreated control) for 1 and 6 h at 37°C were subjected to WB analysis using anti-H3K9ac and anti-H4Kac4 antibodies. Results shown (for **A–D**) are representative for three to six independent experiments. **(E,F)** Quantification of histone hyper-acetylation following gametocyte treatment with TSA. Lysates of imGC **(E)** and mGC **(F)** were subjected to immunoblotting as described above and

(Continued)

FIGURE 2 | Continued
histone acetylation was quantified between TSA-treated and untreated samples by measuring the band intensities via Image J for three or more different experiments; the values were normalized with the band intensities of Pf39 used as loading control (set to 1). Since the anti-H4Kac4 detected two bands in both imGC and mGC indicating that the antibody could also detect other acetylated histones, we quantified the total histone acetylation levels from both bands. $^{*}P < 0.05$; $^{**}P < 0.01$; $^{***}P < 0.001$; ns, not significant, Student's *t*-test. According the manufacturer's material data sheet the rabbit anti-H4Kac4 antibody can cross-react with other acetylated histones like H2B.

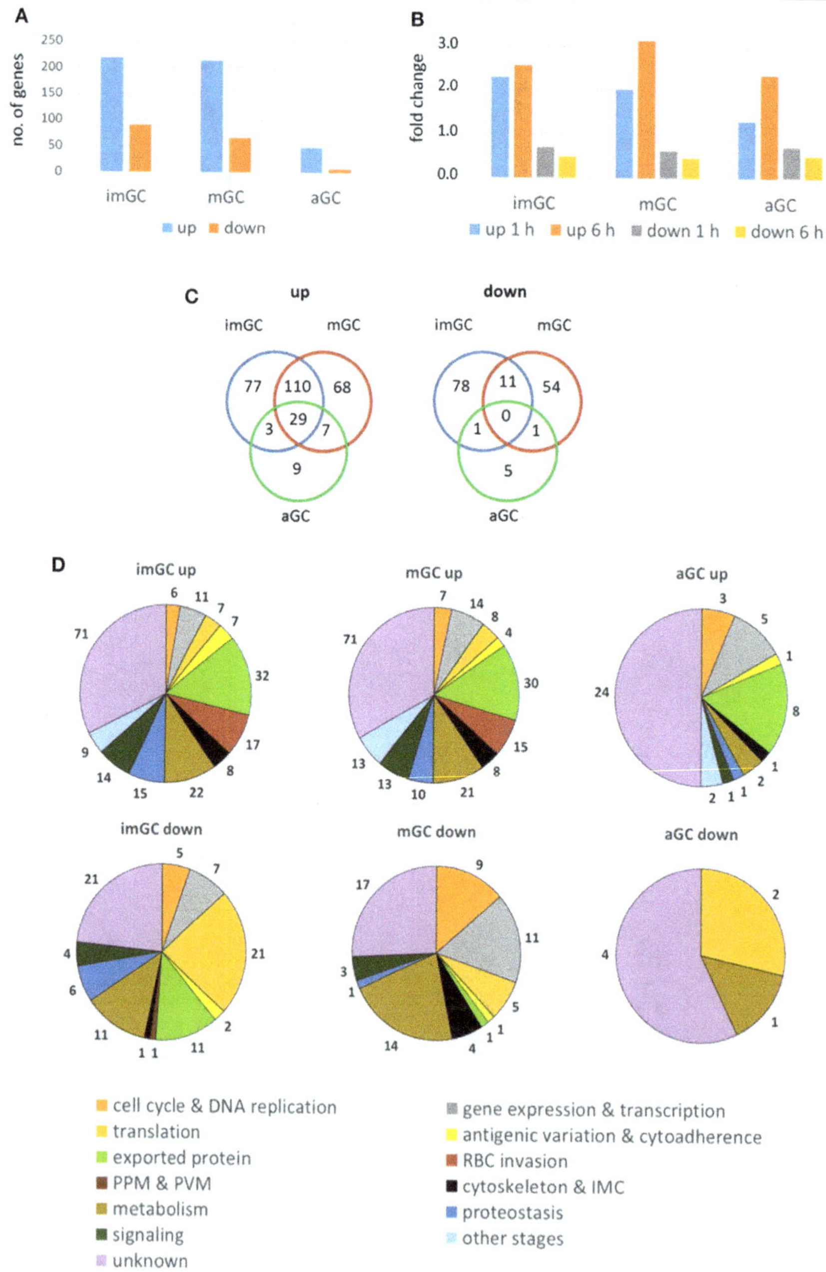

FIGURE 3 | Deregulation of gene expression following treatment of gametocytes with TSA. Immature (imGC) and mature (mGC) gametocytes as well as gametocytes at 1 h post-activation (aGC) were treated with TSA at IC_{90} concentrations or with 0.5% vol. ethanol (untreated control) for 1 and 6 h, total RNA was isolated and cDNA synthesized to be employed in microarray assays. Genes with a relative expression levels greater than 2-fold for at least one of the two time-points combined with a consistent up- or down-regulation for both time-points were used for further analysis. **(A,B)** Bar charts showing total up- and down-regulated genes in imGC, mGC and aGC **(A)**, and mean fold change of deregulated genes in imGC, mGC, and aGC **(B)** at 1 or 6 h following TSA-treatment. **(C)** Venn diagram showing the overlap among deregulated genes in imGC, mGC, and aGC after TSA-treatment. **(D)** Pie chart showing the detailed number of deregulated genes in the different gametocyte samples based on the predicted function following TSA-treatment.

TABLE 2 | Genes with more than 5-fold up-regulated transcription following TSA-treatment.

Sample	Plasmodb_ID	Gene (encoding for)	Group	Properties	Predicted function	Compartment
Immature gametocytes	PF3D7_0113600	Surface-associated interspersed protein 1.2 (SURFIN 1.2)	Antigenic variation & cytoadherence	SICA C-terminal inner membrane domain	Cytoadherence, invasion	iRBC
	PF3D7_1334400	MSP7-like protein (MSRP4)	Invasion	1 SP, MSP7-like protein C-terminal domain	RBC invasion	Merozoite PPM
	PF3D7_0902500	Serine/Threonine protein kinase, FIKK family (FIKK9.6/TSTK9F)	Signaling	Protein kinase domain profile	Protein phosphorylation	iRBC
	PF3D7_1313100	Conserved *Plasmodium* protein	Unknown	N/A	N/A	N/A
Mature gametocytes	PF3D7_0418600	Regulator of chromosome condensation	Cell cycle & DNA replication	RCC1 domain	Regulation of chromosome condensation	Nucleus, cytoplasm
	PF3D7_0613800	Transcription factor with AP2 domain(s) (ApiAP2)	Gene expression & transcription	AP2 domain	Regulation of transcription	Nucleus
	PF3D7_0424400	Surface-associated interspersed protein 4.2 (SURFIN 4.2)	Antigenic variation & cytoadherence	N/A	Cytoadherence, invasion	iRBC
	PF3D7_1102600	*Plasmodium* exported protein (GEXP14)	Exported protein	3 TMs, export domain	N/A	iRBC
	PF3D7_1148700	*Plasmodium* exported protein (PHISTc) (GEXP12)	Exported protein	1 SP, 1 TM, RESA domain, export domain	N/A	iRBC
	PF3D7_1302300	*Plasmodium* exported protein	Exported protein	1 SP, 1 TM	N/A	iRBC
	PF3D7_1334400	MSP7-like protein (MSRP4)	Invasion	1 SP, MSP7-like protein C-terminal domain	RBC invasion	Merozoite PPM
	PF3D7_0216800	Conserved *Plasmodium* membrane protein	Metabolism	1 SP, 14 TMs, CECR6/TMEM121 family domain	Cholesterol metabolism, lipid transport	PPM
	PF3D7_0207900	Serine repeat antigen 2 (SERA2)	Proteostasis	1 SP, papain family cysteine protease profile	Proteolysis; cysteine-type peptidase activity	PV
	PF3D7_0718300	Cysteine repeat modular protein 2 (CRMP2)	Signaling	1 SP, 10 TMs, 3 GCC2 and GCC3 domains, 4 epidermal growth factor-like domains	Intracellular receptor signaling pathway, intracellular transport (protein binding)	Membrane
	PF3D7_0314800	Conserved *Plasmodium* protein	Unknown	N/A	Rosetting, cytoadherence	N/A
	PF3D7_0315600	Zinc finger protein, putative	Unknown	Zinc finger C3H1-type profile	Metal ion-binding activity	N/A
	PF3D7_0507300	Conserved *Plasmodium* protein	Unknown	1 SP	N/A	N/A
	PF3D7_0720300	conserved *Plasmodium* protein	Unknown	N/A	N/A	N/A
	PF3D7_0822700	Conserved *Plasmodium* protein	Unknown	1 SP, 3 TMs, Thrombospondin type-1 (TSP1) repeat profile	Transport (cation transmembrane transporter activity)	Membrane
	PF3D7_1350600	Conserved *Plasmodium* protein	Unknown	1 SP, 2 TMs	N/A	Membrane

N/A, Not applicable; PPM, parasite plasma membrane; PV, parasitophorous vacuole; TM, transmembrane domain; SP, signal peptide.

control) for 1 h and total RNA was isolated. Complementary DNA was synthesized from each sample and purity was further assessed by diagnostic RT-PCR using stage specific markers. The tests confirmed the presence of *pfccp2* (gametocyte-specific) transcript in all the gametocyte samples while *ama1* (asexual blood stage-specific) transcript was absent (Figure S3B), confirming that the gametocyte samples were devoid of any asexual blood stage contamination. A test for gDNA contamination in sample preparations lacking reverse transcriptase using *pfccp2*-specific primers was negative.

Subsequently, the transcript expression levels of the 32 selected genes were measured via real time RT-PCR in TSA-treated and untreated samples. Transcript expression was calculated by the $2^{-\Delta Ct}$ method (Livak and Schmittgen, 2001) in which the threshold cycle number (Ct) was normalized to the Ct of the endogenous control gene encoding *P. falciparum* seryl tRNA-ligase (PF3D7_0717700) as reference gene. For TSA-treated immature gametocytes, we demonstrated a greater than 2-fold transcriptional up-regulation for 14 out of the 15 (93.3%) up-regulated genes as identified by microarray analysis (**Figure 4A**). Accordingly, 14 out of 17 (82.4%) of the identified up-regulated genes of the TSA-treated mature gametocyte samples had greater than 2-fold increased transcript levels compared to the untreated control (**Figure 4B**), which strongly validates the microarray results.

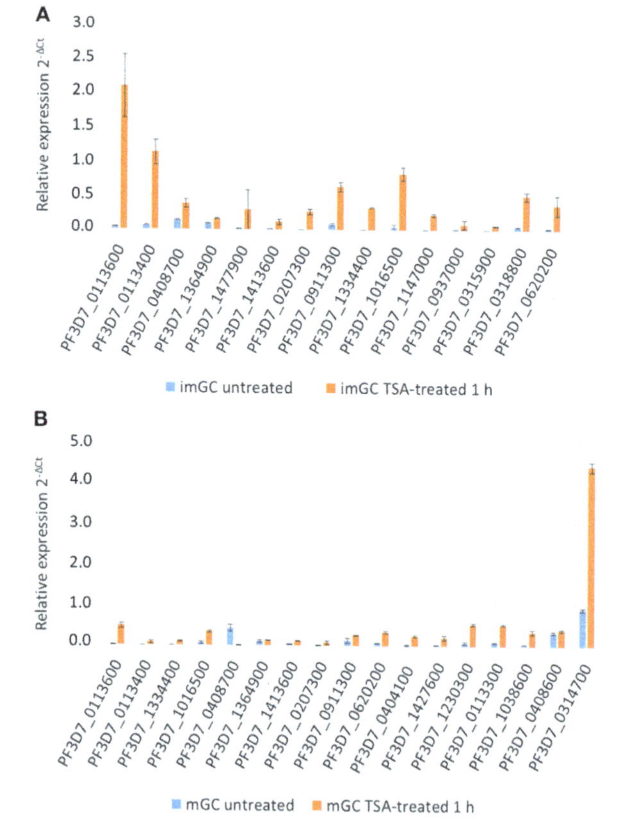

FIGURE 4 | Changes in gene expression after treatment of gametocytes with TSA. Transcript analysis for 15 up-regulated immature (imGC) **(A)** and 17 up-regulated mature (mGC) **(B)** gametocyte genes as identified by microarray via real-time RT-PCR. Transcript expression levels were calculated by the $2^{-\Delta Ct}$ method; the threshold cycle number (Ct) was normalized with the Ct of the gene encoding seryl tRNA-ligase (PF3D7_0717700) as reference. Genes were considered up-regulated when the fold changes between TSA-treated and untreated sample were greater than 2-fold. Results shown are representative for two to three independent experiments.

Genes Transcriptionally Up-Regulated Following TSA-Treatment Associate with Acetylated Histones

ChIP-qPCR assays were employed to investigate a potential link between histone acetylation and the transcriptional up-regulation of selected genes following TSA-treatment of gametocytes. Five genes transcriptionally up-regulated in TSA-treated mature gametocytes were chosen, i.e., genes encoding a putative ring finger protein (henceforth termed *pfrnf1*, 3D7_0314700), a WD40-domain protein (*pfwdtc1*, 3D7_1428400), the exported protein PHISTc (3D7_0219800) and two unknown proteins (PF3D7_0620200, PF3D7_0926600). For control a gene transcriptionally down-regulated in TSA-treated mature gametocytes was selected, i.e., *pfnep1* (PF3D7_0821500), a gene encoding the ribosomal RNA small subunit methyl-transferase NEP1 (**Figure 5A**). For further controls, the housekeeping genes coding for arginine tRNA-ligase (PF3D7_1218600) and seryl tRNA-ligase (PF3D7_0717700) were chosen. Additional controls included two genes that were previously shown to associate with chromatin bound to PfHP1, i.e., *ap2-g* (3D7_1222600) and *var* gene *upsB* (PF3D7_0426000) (Brancucci et al., 2014). For each gene, primers corresponding to the promotor and coding regions were generated (for primer locations, see **Figure 5A**). ChIP assays were performed using anti-H3K9ac and anti-H4Kac4 antibodies, which were previously used to precipitate plasmodial chromatin (Crowley et al., 2011; Gómez-Díaz et al., 2017). For negative control, an IgG antibody from non-immunized rabbit was used in the assays. For positive control, anti-PfHP1 antibody was used to precipitate *ap2-g* and *var upsB* (Flueck et al., 2009). The ChIP recovery rates of these genes following immunoprecipitation were compared between chromatin generated from mature gametocytes treated with TSA at IC_{90} concentrations for 6 h and from untreated mature gametocytes via qPCR.

Initially, the presence of PfHP1 in the nuclei of gametocytes was demonstrated via IFA and compared to PfHP1 localization in trophozoites and schizonts. As previously described, PfHP1 as a marker for heterochromatin particularly localized to the nucleus periphery in trophozoites and schizonts (Flueck et al., 2009; Pérez-Toledo et al., 2009). Similarly, PfHP1 was predominantly found at the nucleus periphery of immature and activated gametocytes, while in mature gametocytes PfHP1 was often found in concentrated foci within the nuclei (Figure S6). Immunolabeling with NMS served as negative control and did not result in any labeling (Figure S7).

The ChIP-qPCR analysis on precipitated acetylated histones using anti-H3K9ac antibody demonstrated a higher recovery of the five genes transcriptionally up-regulated in TSA-treated mature gametocytes (**Figure 5B**). The increased recovery rates

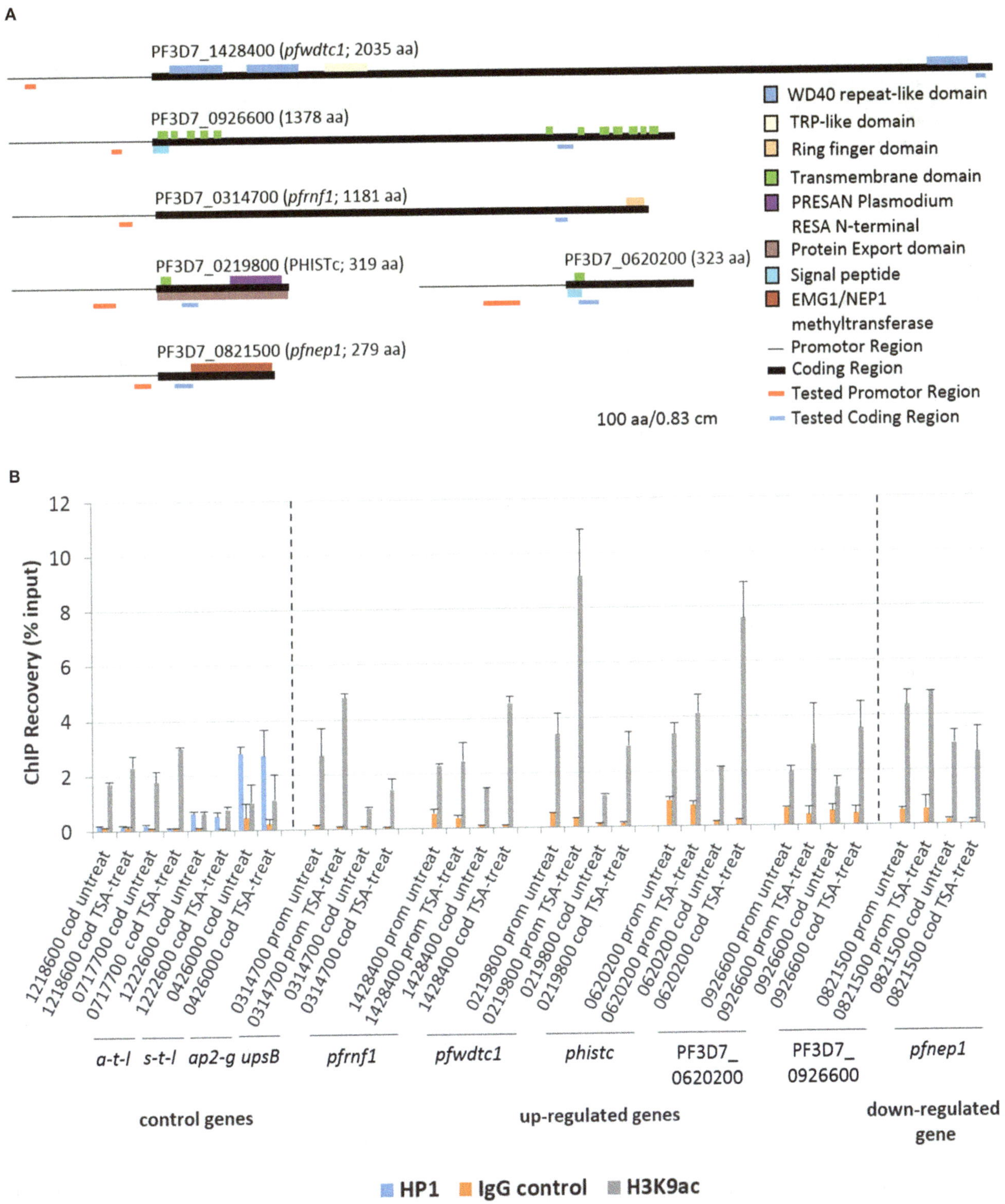

FIGURE 5 | Association of genes affected by TSA-treatment with acetylated histone H3. **(A)** Predicted domain structures of the six genes deregulated in mature gametocytes by TSA-treatment. Promotor (thin black line) and coding (black box) regions as well as location of the primers specific to the promotor (red line) and to the coding region (blue line) are indicated. **(B)** ChIP-qPCR analysis of five up-regulated genes and one down-regulated gene as identified by microarray using rabbit anti-H3K9ac antibody to demonstrate potential association between the genes and acetylated histone H3. Crosslinked chromatin from mature gametocytes treated with TSA at IC_{90} concentrations or with 0.5% vol. ethanol (untreated control) for 6 h was precipitated with rabbit anti-H3K9ac antibody or with rabbit

(Continued)

FIGURE 5 | Continued
anti-PfHP1antibody and IgG as controls. The immunoprecipitated material was analyzed by qPCR to confirm specific enrichment of selected genes including *pfrnf1* (PF3D7_0314700), *pfwdtc1* (PF3D7_1428400), *phistc* (PF3D7_0219800), PF3D7_0620200, and PF3D7_0926600. As a down-regulated gene *pfnep1* (PF3D7_0821500) was analyzed. The genes encoding arginine tRNA-ligase a-t-l (PF3D7_1218600) and seryl tRNA-ligase s-t-l (PF3D7_0717700) as well as *ap2-g* (PF3D7_1222600) and the *var* gene *upsB* (PF3D7_0426000) were used as controls. Primers targeting either the coding regions (cod.) or promoter regions (prom.) were used for qPCR. The values represent the proportion of chromatin recovered from the input samples. Results shown are representative for two to three independent experiments.

were detected both when primers corresponding to the promotor regions or the coding regions were used. A slightly higher recovery was also seen for the two control tRNA-ligase-encoding control genes, when the gametocytes were treated with TSA. No increased recovery rate, on the other hand, was detected, when primers corresponding to the promotor and coding regions of *pfnep1* were used in the qPCR analyses. Furthermore, the genes *ap2-g* and *var upsB* were precipitated with the anti-HP1 antibody (**Figure 5B**). The recovery rates for the *var* gene *upsB* were higher than the ones for *ap2-g* and neither of the recovery rates changed upon TSA-treatment of the gametocytes. Generally, similar higher recovery rates were observed for the TSA-dependent transcriptionally up-regulated genes, when the anti-H4Kac4 antibody was used for precipitation. No higher recoveries of *pfrnf1* and *pfwdtc1* were achieved, though, when the promotor regions were amplified, indicating that these promotors might associate particularly with acetylated H3 (Figure S8). Furthermore, no higher recovery for PF3D7_0620200 was detected. The overall high recovery rates observed when using anti-H4Kac4 antibody for precipitation might be due to the fact that this antibody also reacts with acetylated H2B (compare with **Figures 2C,D**). The combined data demonstrate an association of acetylated histones with the five selected genes that were transcriptionally up-regulated in TSA-treated gametocytes.

Treatment of Mature Gametocytes with TSA Results in Increased PfRNF1 Synthesis

In a final set of experiments, we aimed to determine, if up-regulation of transcript expression following TSA-treatment also corroborates with increased protein synthesis. We selected one gene, *pfrnf1*, whose transcript level was up-regulated in mature gametocytes following TSA-treatment, for further investigations. *In-silico* analyses disclose the ring finger-domain protein PfRNF1 as a putative E3-ligase (Ponts et al., 2008). A recombinant protein corresponding to the N-terminal region of PfRNF1 was bacterially expressed and used to generate antisera against PfRNF1 in mice. IFA were performed in the different asexual and sexual blood stages of *P. falciparum*. Asexual blood stage parasites were highlighted by MSP-1 labeling; gametocytes and activated gametocytes were highlighted by Pfs230 immunolabeling. The IFA revealed a prominent expression of PfRNF1 in immature gametocytes with peak expression in stage II gametocytes. Here, the protein localized to the gametocyte cytoplasm and nucleus (**Figure 6A**). PfRNF1 was also detected at low levels in mature gametocytes and in gametocytes 30 min post-activation as well as in schizonts.

Expression of PfRNF1, which has a calculated molecular weight of 135 kDa, was then investigated in immature and mature gametocytes via WB analysis. A predominant protein band was detected in both, immature and mature gametocyte lysates, when immunoblotted with anti-PfRNF1 antisera, which was migrating at a molecular weight of roughly 200 kDa. An additional protein band at ~140 kDa was also observed (**Figure 6B**). No protein bands were present in lysates of the non-infected RBC control. For loading control, immunoblotting with anti-Pf39 antisera, directed against the endoplasmic reticulum-specific protein Pf39 (Templeton et al., 1997), was performed, and Pf39 was detected in all parasite lysates. We also investigated the sub-cellular localization of PfRNF1 in gametocytes via WB, using cytosolic and nuclear fractions of mixed gametocyte cultures. WB revealed the presence of PfRNF1 as a 200-kDa protein in both fractions (**Figure 6C**). Antibodies against PfActin1, which is predominantly present in the cytoplasm and to a minor level in the nuclei were used as a fraction control. The purity of the fractions was further confirmed by immunoblotting with anti-H4Kac4 antibody, which labeled histones in the nuclear fraction, but which did not result in any protein band in the cytoplasmic fraction (**Figure 6C**).

To validate the protein expression data, we generated a *P. falciparum* transfectant line, which expresses PfRNF1 C-terminally tagged with HA-Strep (Figure S1B). Successful integration was confirmed by diagnostic PCR (Figure S1C). Subsequent WB analyses, using rabbit anti-HA antibody, detected a protein band with an approximate molecular weight of 200 kDa in lysates of immature gametocytes from the transfectant line, but not from wild-type parasites used as a negative control (**Figure 6D**). Further, no protein band was detected in lysates of non-infected RBCs. The combined WB data indicate that PfRNF1 migrates at a higher molecular weight than expected, which might be caused by PTMs. When the PfRNF1-HA-Strep-expressing parasite line was used in IFA and immunolabeled with anti-HA antibody, a similar protein expression pattern was observed as has been described above (Figure S9).

Finally, we assessed whether treatment of mature gametocytes with TSA results in up-regulation of PfRNF1 on the protein level. In this regard, mature gametocytes, both of the wild-type strain and the PfRNF1-HA-Strep-expressing transfectant line, were treated with TSA at IC_{90} concentration or 0.5% vol. ethanol (untreated control) for 24 h, lysates were generated and PfRNF1 was detected by WB analysis using the anti-PfRNF1 antisera. Immunoblotting revealed increased PfRNF1 levels in lysates of TSA-treated gametocytes compared to the untreated control for both wild-type and transfectant (**Figure 7A**, Figure S10A). Quantitative WB analysis showed a significant up-regulation of

PfRNF1 following TSA-treatment as compared to the untreated control (**Figure 7B**, Figure S10B).

DISCUSSION

Histone PTMs are emerging as major regulatory mechanisms thought to modulate gene expression in eukaryotes. While these mechanisms have been extensively studied during the erythrocytic replication of *P. falciparum*, little is known about this process during parasite human-to-mosquito transmission. In this study, we aimed to determine the role of histone acetylation and deacetylation in the control of gene expression in *P. falciparum* gametocytes during their development and transmission to the mosquito. To achieve our goal, we used the chemical loss-of-function approach using the HDAC inhibitor TSA (inhibitor of HDACs I and II) on the *P. falciparum* gametocyte-producing NF54 strain. Treatment with TSA results in a mean IC_{50} value of 29 nM. The killing of the *P. falciparum* asexual blood stages by TSA with IC_{50} values in nM ranges have already been reported before for the chloroquine-sensitive 3D7 (8 nM) and chloroquine resistant strain DD2 (11 nM) (Andrews et al., 2008).

In order to determine the effect of TSA on gametocyte development and transmission to the mosquito, we treated stage II gametocytes with the HDAC inhibitor and followed gametocyte development. We show that gametocyte development was strongly affected, and here stage II and III gametocytes appeared to be more vulnerable to TSA treatment then stage IV and V gametocytes. On the other hand, TSA only moderately effected macrogamete and zygote development. In a previous study, it was also reported that microgametes were only moderately affected following treatment with a variety of HDAC inhibitors (Trenholme et al., 2014). The fact that TSA has strong gametocytocidal activities, but only exerts minor effects on gametes and zygotes indicates that histone acetylation-mediated gene regulation is important during gametocytogenesis, but not during the early phase of midgut-stage development. This is in accord with findings in *P. falciparum* and *P. berghei* that transcript required for the midgut stage formation is synthesized and stored in female gametocytes, where it is translationally repressed by binding to regulatory ribonucleoprotein complexes, like the RNA helicase DOZI (development of zygote inhibited) and the Sm-like factor CITH (homolog of worm CAR-I and fly Trailer Hitch), as identified in *P. berghei*, or the Pumilio/FBF (Puf) family RNA-binding protein Puf2, as was shown for *P. falciparum* (Mair et al., 2006, 2010; Miao et al., 2013; Guerreiro et al., 2014). A recent analysis integrating transcriptome and proteome data revealed 512 highly expressed transcripts in *P. falciparum* female gametocytes without corresponding protein expression, indicating large scale translational repression (Lasonder et al., 2016). Repression of the stored transcript is released and translation is initiated, once the gametocytes become activated in the mosquito midgut.

To confirm histone acetylation in gametocytes, we used two commercially available histone acetylation antibodies (anti-H3K9ac and anti-H4Kac4) to detect the acetylated histones in the nuclei of different gametocyte stages. By means of these

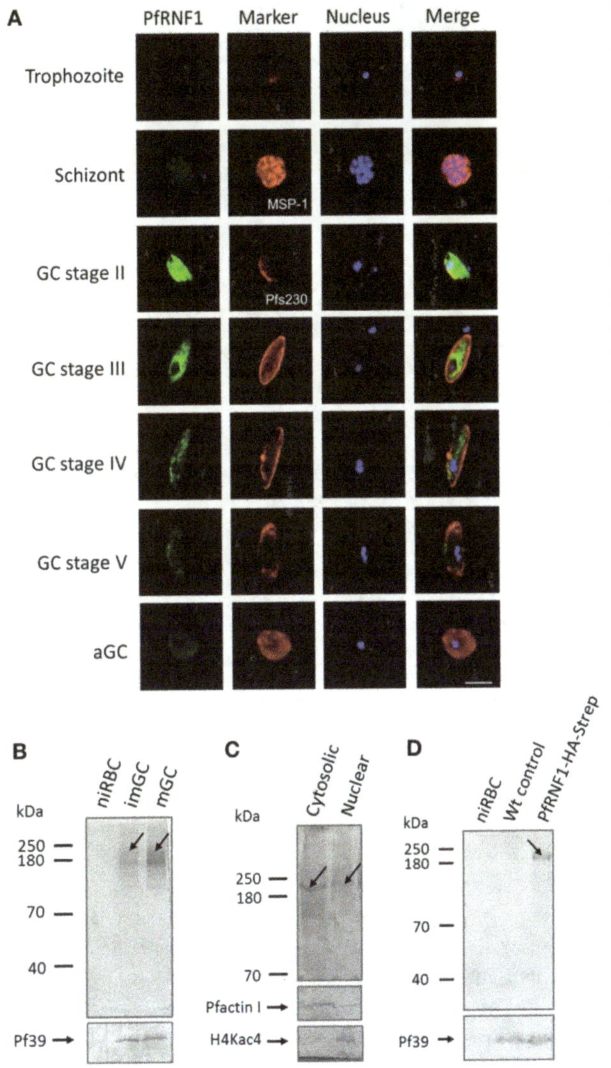

FIGURE 6 | Characterization of PfRNF1. **(A)** Localization of PfRNF1 in the *P. falciparum* asexual blood and gametocyte stages. Mouse anti-PfRNF1 antisera was used to immunolabel fixed samples of trophozoites, schizonts and mature gametocytes (GC) of stages II to V as well as of activated gametocytes (aGC) at 30 min post-activation (green). Schizonts were visualized by labeling with rabbit anti-MSP-1 antibody and gametocytes were visualized by rabbit anti-Pfs230 antisera (red); nuclei were highlighted by Hoechst nuclear stain 33342 (blue). Bar, 5 μm. Results shown are representative for four independent experiments. **(B)** Expression of PfRNF1 in gametocyte lysates of immature (imGC) and mature (mGC) gametocytes were immunoblotted with anti-PfRNF1 antibody and detected two protein bands of approximate molecular weights of 200 kDa (arrow) and 140 kDa. Lysates of non-infected red blood cells (niRBCs) were used for negative control. Immunoblotting with mouse anti-Pf39 antisera served as loading control. **(C)** Sub-cellular localization of PfRNF1. Cytosolic and nuclear fractions of enriched immature gametocytes were subjected to WB using anti-PfRNF1 antisera and detected a 200-kDa band (arrow) in both fractions. Mouse antibodies against PfActinI (41 kDa) and rabbit antibodies against H4Kac4 detecting acetylated histone H4 (~11 kDa) were used as fraction controls. **(D)** Detection of PfRNF1-HA-Strep in gametocytes of parasite line PfRNF1-HA-Strep. Lysates of PfRNF1-HA-Strep immature gametocytes were immunoblotted with rabbit anti-HA antibody and detected a protein band of 200 kDa (arrow). Lysates of non-infected red blood cells (niRBCs) as well as wild-type (Wt) gametocytes were used as negative control. Results shown (for **A–D**) are representative for three to four independent experiments.

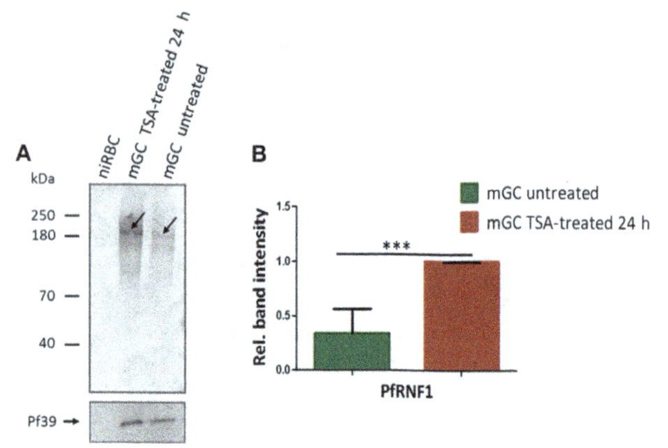

FIGURE 7 | Up-regulation of PfRNF1 levels in mature gametocytes following TSA-treatment. **(A)** Lysates from mature gametocytes (mGC) following treatment with TSA at IC_{90} concentrations or 0.5% vol. ethanol (untreated control) for 24 h were subjected to WB using mouse anti-PfRNF1 antisera and detected a 200 kDa band (arrow). Immunoblotting of lysates of non-infected red blood cells (niRBC) was used for negative control; immunoblotting with mouse anti-Pf39 antisera served as loading control. **(B)** Quantification of PfRNF1 protein expression following TSA-treatment of mature gametocytes. Lysates of mature gametocytes were subjected to immunoblotting as described above and PfRNF1 levels were quantified between TSA-treated and untreated samples by measuring the band intensities via Image J for six different experiments; the values were normalized with the band intensities of Pf39 used as loading control (set to 1). Results shown (for **A,B**) are representative for six independent experiments. $^{***}P < 0.001$, Student's *t*-test.

antibodies, we demonstrated that gametocyte treatment with TSA results in histone hyper-acetylation thereby leading to transcriptional activation. Histone hyper-acetylation following treatment of the malaria parasite with HDAC inhibitors have been earlier reported for *P. falciparum* blood stages (Andrews et al., 2008; Trenholme et al., 2014) and the asexual blood stages of *P. knowlesi* (Chua et al., 2017).

As a next step we aimed to investigate any deregulation of gene expression in immature, mature and activated gametocytes caused by TSA-treatment via microarray- and real-time RT-PCR-based analyses. Comparative transcriptomics between untreated and inhibitor-treated gametocytes identified 453 genes, which were more than 2-fold deregulated after 1 or 6 h following TSA-treatment. Among these 303 were more than 2-fold up-regulated, while 150 genes were down-regulated. Up-regulation of gene expression can be explained by increased euchromatin formation due to the loose contact between the negatively charged DNA and the acetylated histones, which hence counteracts gene silencing. Down-regulation of gene expression following TSA-treatment, on the other hand, which occurs in less than half of the identified genes, might be due to indirect effects. As mentioned earlier, PfHP1 was reported to bind to H3K9me3 to maintain the heterochromatin state, resulting in *ap2-g* repression (Brancucci et al., 2014), a process also involving PfHda2. It is postulated that the removal of acetyl groups by PfHda2 promotes histone methylation leading to PfHP1 binding (Coleman et al., 2014). Other studies have also reported the down-regulation of gene expression following treatment with HDAC inhibitors (Glaser et al., 2003; Chaal et al., 2010; Andrews et al., 2012b). Subsequent ChIP-qPCR analyses confirmed the general association of genes up-regulated in gametocytes following TSA-treatment with acetylated histones, particularly acetylated H3 and H4. The observed higher recovery rates achieved, when anti-H4Kac4 was used in the ChIP assays may be due to the facts that the antibody recognizes several lysine acetylation sites in H4 and that it additionally exhibits a minor binding to acetylated H2B.

An interesting finding in this study is the fact that the impairment of gene silencing during gametocytogenesis re-activates genes known to be crucial for blood stage replication. This was particularly observed for genes assigned to antigenic variation and cytoadherence and to RBC invasion by merozoites, or genes encoding exported proteins, which are particularly characteristic for the intraerythrocytic trophozoites. Interestingly, genes involved in antigenic variation and cytoadherence included ones coding for RIFINs and SURFINs, while only one out of 60 known *var* genes was identified. This might be explained by the fact that *var* gene activation and silencing is mostly accredited to the NAD-dependent histone deacetylases PfSir2A and PfSir2B (Duraisingh et al., 2005; Freitas-Junior et al., 2005; Tonkin et al., 2009) which are not affected following TSA-treatment. *Var* gene regulation is also linked to histone methylation, like H3K4me3-mediated *var* gene activation and H3K9me3-mediated *var* gene silencing (Chookajorn et al., 2007; Lopez-Rubio et al., 2007, 2009; Salcedo-Amaya et al., 2009), which further substantiate the reason why *var* genes were hardly identified. RIFINs are encoded by about 135 *rif* genes and comprise the largest family of antigenically variable molecules in *P. falciparum* (reviewed in Kirkman and Deitsch, 2014). H3K9 acetylation has been shown to control the expression of *rif* genes, which probably accounts for the reason why RIFINs were affected (Cabral et al., 2012). SURFINs are encoded by 10 surface-associated interspersed (*surf*) genes, which are located close or within the subtelomeric region of chromosomes. Little is known whether they are epigenetically regulated, but it is likely that they are regulated by histone PTMs (Mphande et al., 2008). Not identified by the microarray analyses were any of the genes coding for the 15 variant antigen-encoding *mc-2tm* genes. Furthermore, only one out of 35 STEVOR-encoding genes was up-regulated in gametocytes following TSA-treatment, suggesting that these gene families are not primarily affected in their expression levels by histone acetylation.

The majority of exported proteins regulated in their synthesis by histone acetylation include members of the PHIST (*Plasmodium* helical interspersed subtelomeric) family. The PHIST family comprises 89 proteins, the most of which have yet unknown functions. The PHIST protein family is characterized by a conserved domain of ~150 amino acids predicted to form four consecutive alpha helices and have been shown to be differentially expressed during the *Plasmodium* life-cycle (Warncke et al., 2016). The differential expression of these proteins may suggest an epigenetic mechanism. Invasion-related genes regulated in their expression by histone acetylation include previously identified surface proteins of merozoites, e.g., members of the MSP (merozoite surface protein) and the RON

(Rhoptry neck) families (Proellocks et al., 2010; Beeson et al., 2016; Lin et al., 2016). Noteworthy, all of these identified gene families, i.e., *rif* and *stevor* and the ones encoding the PHIST family as well as the merozoite invasion-related families were reported to associate with heterochromatin markers (Flueck et al., 2009; Lopez-Rubio et al., 2009; Salcedo-Amaya et al., 2009) thereby maintaining default silencing of the majority of redundant members of multi-gene families (reviewed in Duffy et al., 2012).

While the above mentioned genes appear to be silenced by deacetylations of the associated histones after the parasites have entered the sexual pathways, other genes were apparently waiting to be activated by histone acetylation, once the parasite has been transmitted to the mosquito vector. Among others, these genes encode proteins important for midgut extravasation by the ookinete, like the secreted ookinete protein 25 (PSOP25), the secreted ookinete adhesive protein (SOAP), the von Willebrand factor A-domain related protein (WARP), the circumsporozoite and thrombospondin-related adhesion protein-related protein (CTRP), the cell traversal protein for ookinetes and sporozoites (CelTOS), or chitinase (CHT1) (reviewed in Pradel, 2007; Bennink et al., 2016).

To further justify our data, we selected one gene, *pfrnf1* (PF3D7_0314700), whose transcript was up-regulated following TSA-treatment of mature gametocytes, for further characterization. PfRNF1 possesses a C-terminal RING finger domain, which shows a high homology with the human E3 ubiquitin-protein ligase Praja-1. PfRNF1 has been annotated as a potential E3 ligase in *P. falciparum* as a component of the ubiquitin-mediated pathway (Ponts et al., 2008). TSA-treatment caused increased transcript and protein levels of PfRNF1 in mature gametocytes. Based on our data we postulate that under normal conditions deacetylation of histones H3 and H4 down-regulates PfRNF1 expression in mature gametocytes. The regulation of expression by histone deacetylases was recently also reported for the human RING finger domain protein RNF148 (Liu et al., 2013). We therefore suspect that PfRNF1 is a potential HDAC-regulated E3 ligase involved in ubiquitin-mediated pathways during gametocyte development, which might be important for regulatory processes during human-to-mosquito transmission of *Plasmodium*.

Our combined data highlight the role of histone acetylation in the control of gene expression during gametocyte development and transmission from the human to the mosquito, which may be exploited in malaria transmission-blocking strategies.

AUTHOR CONTRIBUTIONS

Conceived and designed the experiments: CN, MK, ML, TV, and GP. Performed the experiments: CN, MK, OP, LO, and MF. Analyzed the data: CN, MK, OP, LO, AR, and GP. Wrote the manuscript: CN, MK, and GP. All authors read and approved the manuscript.

FUNDING

We thank Alex Maier (ANU Canberra) for kindly providing vector pHAST. The work was funded by grant PR905/7-1 of the Deutsche Forschungsgemeinschaft (to GP) and further supported by grant 01DR14019 of the German Ministry for Education and Research (to GP) and an ERS Start-Up grant of RWTH Aachen University (to CN). MK received a short-term fellowship by the Deutscher Akademischer Austauschdienst; CN received a Theodore von Kármán fellowship from the RWTH Aachen University. GP is recipient of a Heisenberg professorship of the Deutsche Forschungsgemeinschaft.

REFERENCES

Alves Avelar, L. A., Held, J., Engel, J. A., Sureechatchaiyan, P., Hansen, F. K., Hamacher, A., et al. (2017). Design and synthesis of novel anti-plasmodial histone deacetylase inhibitors containing an alkoxyamide connecting unit. *Arch. Pharm.* 350:1600347. doi: 10.1002/ardp.2016 00347

Aminake, M. N., Arndt, H.-D., and Pradel, G. (2012). The proteasome of malaria parasites: a multi-stage drug target for chemotherapeutic intervention? *Int. J. Parasitol. Drugs Drug Resist.* 2, 1–10. doi: 10.1016/j.ijpddr.2011. 12.001

Aminake, M. N., Schoof, S., Sologub, L., Leubner, M., Kirschner, M., Arndt, H.-D., et al. (2011). Thiostrepton and derivatives exhibit antimalarial and gametocytocidal activity by dually targeting parasite proteasome and apicoplast. *Antimicrob. Agents Chemother.* 55, 1338–1348. doi: 10.1128/AAC.01096-10

Andrews, K. T., Gupta, A. P., Tran, T. N., Fairlie, D. P., Gobert, G. N., and Bozdech, Z. (2012b). Comparative gene expression profiling of *P. falciparum* malaria parasites exposed to three different histone deacetylase inhibitors. *PLoS ONE* 7:e31847. doi: 10.1371/journal.pone.0031847

Andrews, K. T., Tran, T. N., and Fairlie, D. P. (2012a). Towards histone deacetylase inhibitors as new antimalarial drugs. *Curr. Pharm. Des.* 18, 3467–3479. doi: 10.2174/138161212801327257

Andrews, K. T., Tran, T. N., Lucke, A. J., Kahnberg, P., Le, G. T., Boyle, G. M., et al. (2008). Potent antimalarial activity of histone deacetylase inhibitor analogues. *Antimicrob. Agents Chemother.* 52, 1454–1461. doi: 10.1128/AAC.00757-07

Andrews, K. T., Tran, T. N., Wheatley, N. C., and Fairlie, D. P. (2009). Targeting histone deacetylase inhibitors for anti-malarial therapy. *Curr. Top. Med. Chem.* 9, 292–308. doi: 10.2174/156802609788085313

Aurrecoechea, C., Brestelli, J., Brunk, B. P., Dommer, J., Fischer, S., Gajria, B., et al. (2009). PlasmoDB: a functional genomic database for malaria parasites. *Nucleic Acids Res.* 37, 539–543. doi: 10.1093/nar/gkn814

Balaji, S., Babu, M. M., Iyer, L. M., and Aravind, L. (2005). Discovery of the principal specific transcription factors of Apicomplexa and their implication for the evolution of the AP2-integrase DNA binding domains. *Nucleic Acids Res.* 33, 3994–4006. doi: 10.1093/nar/gki709

Beeson, J. G., Drew, D. R., Boyle, M. J., Feng, G., Fowkes, F. J. I., and Richards, J. S. (2016). Merozoite surface proteins in red blood cell invasion, immunity and vaccines against malaria. *FEMS Microbiol. Rev.* 40, 343–372. doi: 10.1093/femsre/fuw001

Bennink, S., Kiesow, M. J., and Pradel, G. (2016). The development of malaria parasites in the mosquito midgut. *Cell. Microbiol.* 18, 905–918. doi: 10.1111/cmi.12604

Bozdech, Z., Llinás, M., Pulliam, B. L., Wong, E. D., Zhu, J., and DeRisi, J. L. (2003). The transcriptome of the intraerythrocytic developmental cycle of *Plasmodium falciparum*. *PLoS Biol.* 1:e5. doi: 10.1371/journal.pbio.0000005

Brancucci, N. M. B., Bertschi, N. L., Zhu, L., Niederwieser, I., Chin, W. H., Wampfler, R., et al. (2014). Heterochromatin protein 1 secures survival and transmission of malaria parasites. *Cell Host Microbe* 16, 165–176. doi: 10.1016/j.chom.2014.07.004

Cabral, F. J., Fotoran, W. L., and Wunderlich, G. (2012). Dynamic activation and repression of the *Plasmodium falciparum* rif gene family and their relation to chromatin modification. *PLoS ONE* 7:e29881. doi: 10.1371/journal.pone.0029881

Chaal, B. K., Gupta, A. P., Wastuwidyaningtyas, B. D., Luah, Y. H., and Bozdech, Z. (2010). Histone deacetylases play a major role in the transcriptional regulation of the *Plasmodium falciparum* life cycle. *PLoS Pathog.* 6:e1000737. doi: 10.1371/journal.ppat.1000737

Chookajorn, T., Dzikowski, R., Frank, M., Li, F., Jiwani, A. Z., Hartl, D. L., et al. (2007). Epigenetic memory at malaria virulence genes. *Proc. Natl. Acad. Sci. U.S.A.* 104, 899–902. doi: 10.1073/pnas.0609084103

Chua, M. J., Arnold, M. S. J., Xu, W., Lancelot, J., Lamotte, S., Späth, G., et al. (2017). Effect of clinically approved HDAC inhibitors on plasmodium, Leishmania and Schistosoma parasite growth. *Int. J. Parasitol. Drugs Drug Resist.* 7, 42–50. doi: 10.1016/j.ijpddr.2016.12.005

Coleman, B. I., Skillman, K. M., Jiang, R. H. Y., Childs, L. M., Altenhofen, L. M., Ganter, M., et al. (2014). A *Plasmodium falciparum* histone deacetylase regulates antigenic variation and gametocyte conversion. *Cell Host Microbe* 16, 177–186. doi: 10.1016/j.chom.2014.06.014

Crowley, V. M., Rovira-Graells, N., de Pouplana, L. R., and Cortés, A. (2011). Heterochromatin formation in bistable chromatin domains controls the epigenetic repression of clonally variant *plasmodium falciparum* genes linked to erythrocyte invasion. *Mol. Microbiol.* 80, 391–406. doi: 10.1111/j.1365-2958.2011.07574.x

Cui, L., and Miao, J. (2010). Chromatin-Mediated epigenetic regulation in the malaria parasite *Plasmodium falciparum*. *Eukaryot. Cell* 9, 1138–1149. doi: 10.1128/EC.00036-10

Cui, L., Fan, Q., Cui, L., and Miao, J. (2008). Histone lysine methyltransferases and demethylases in *Plasmodium falciparum*. *Int. J. Parasitol.* 38, 1083–1097. doi: 10.1016/j.ijpara.2008.01.002

Cui, L., Miao, J., and Cui, L. (2007b). Cytotoxic effect of curcumin on malaria parasite *Plasmodium falciparum*: inhibition of histone acetylation and generation of reactive oxygen species. *Antimicrob. Agents Chemother.* 51, 488–494. doi: 10.1128/AAC.01238-06

Cui, L., Miao, J., Furuya, T., Li, X., Su, X. Z., and Cui, L. (2007a). PfGCN5-mediated histone H3 acetylation plays a key role in gene expression in *Plasmodium falciparum*. *Eukaryot. Cell* 6, 1219–1227. doi: 10.1128/EC.00062-07

Dinko, B., and Pradel, G. (2016). Immune evasion by *Plasmodium falciparum* Parasites: converting a host protection mechanism for the parasite's benefit. *Adv. Infect. Dis.* 6, 82–95. doi: 10.4236/aid.2016.62011

Duffy, M. F., Selvarajah, S. A., Josling, G. A., and Petter, M. (2012). The role of chromatin in Plasmodium gene expression. *Cell. Microbiol.* 14, 819–828. doi: 10.1111/j.1462-5822.2012.01777.x

Duffy, M. F., Selvarajah, S. A., Josling, G. A., and Petter, M. (2014). Epigenetic regulation of the *Plasmodium falciparum* genome. *Brief. Funct. Genomics* 13, 203–216. doi: 10.1093/bfgp/elt047

Duraisingh, M. T., and Horn, D. (2016). Epigenetic regulation of virulence gene expression in parasitic protozoa. *Cell Host Microbe* 19, 629–640. doi: 10.1016/j.chom.2016.04.020

Duraisingh, M. T., Voss, T. S., Marty, A. J., Duffy, M. F., Good, R. T., Thompson, J. K., et al. (2005). Heterochromatin silencing and locus repositioning linked to regulation of virulence genes in *Plasmodium falciparum*. *Cell* 121, 13–24. doi: 10.1016/j.cell.2005.01.036

Engel, J. A., Jones, A. J., Avery, V. M., Sumanadasa, S. D. M., Ng, S. S., Fairlie, D. P., et al. (2015). Profiling the anti-protozoal activity of anti-cancer HDAC inhibitors against Plasmodium and Trypanosoma parasites. *Int. J. Parasitol. Drugs Drug Resist.* 5, 117–126. doi: 10.1016/j.ijpddr.2015.05.004

Fivelman, Q. L., McRobert, L., Sharp, S., Taylor, C. J., Saeed, M., Swales, C. A., et al. (2007). Improved synchronous production of *Plasmodium falciparum* gametocytes *in vitro*. *Mol. Biochem. Parasitol.* 154, 119–123. doi: 10.1016/j.molbiopara.2007.04.008

Florens, L., Washburn, M. P., Raine, J. D., Anthony, R. M., Grainger, M., Haynes, J. D., et al. (2002). A proteomic view of the *Plasmodium falciparum* life cycle. *Nature* 419, 520–526. doi: 10.1038/nature01107

Flueck, C., Bartfai, R., Volz, J., Niederwieser, I., Salcedo-Amaya, A. M., Alako, B. T. F., et al. (2009). *Plasmodium falciparum* heterochromatin protein 1 marks genomic loci linked to phenotypic variation of exported virulence factors. *PLoS Pathog.* 5:e1000569. doi: 10.1371/journal.ppat.1000569

Freitas-Junior, L. H., Hernandez-Rivas, R., Ralph, S. A., Montiel-Condado, D., Ruvalcaba-Salazar, O. K., Rojas-Meza, A. P., et al. (2005). Telomeric heterochromatin propagation and histone acetylation control mutually exclusive expression of antigenic variation genes in malaria parasites. *Cell* 121, 25–36. doi: 10.1016/j.cell.2005.01.037

Gardner, M. J., Hall, N., Fung, E., White, O., Berriman, M., Hyman, R. W., et al. (2002). Genome sequence of the human malaria parasite *Plasmodium falciparum*. *Nature* 419, 498–511. doi: 10.1038/nature01097

Glaser, K. B., Staver, M. J., Waring, J. F., Stender, J., Ulrich, R. G., and Davidsen, S. K. (2003). Gene expression profiling of multiple Histone Deacetylase (HDAC) inhibitors: defining a common gene set produced by HDAC inhibition in T24 and MDA carcinoma cell lines. *Mol. Cancer Ther.* 2, 151–163.

Gómez-Díaz, E., Yerbanga, R. S., Lefèvre, T., Cohuet, A., Rowley, M. J., Ouedraogo, J. B., et al. (2017). Epigenetic regulation of *Plasmodium falciparum* clonally variant gene expression during development in *Anopheles gambiae*. *Sci. Rep.* 7:40655. doi: 10.1038/srep40655

Guerreiro, A., Deligianni, E., Santos, J. M., Silva, P. A. G. C., Louis, C., Pain, A., et al. (2014). Genome-wide RIP-Chip analysis of translational repressor-bound mRNAs in the Plasmodium gametocyte. *Genome Biol.* 15:493. doi: 10.1186/s13059-014-0493-0

Hansen, F. K., Sumanadasa, S. D. M., Stenzel, K., Duffy, S., Meister, S., Marek, L., et al. (2014). Discovery of HDAC inhibitors with potent activity against multiple malaria parasite life cycle stages. *Eur. J. Med. Chem.* 82, 204–213. doi: 10.1016/j.ejmech.2014.05.050

Hu, G., Cabrera, A., Kono, M., Mok, S., Chaal, B. K., Haase, S., et al. (2010). Transcriptional profiling of growth perturbations of the human malaria parasite *Plasmodium falciparum*. *Nat. Biotechnol.* 28, 91–98. doi: 10.1038/nbt.1597

Ifediba, T., and Vanderberg, J. P. (1981). Complete *in vitro* maturation of *Plasmodium falciparum* gametocytes. *Nature* 294, 364–366.

Joshi, M. B., Lin, D. T., Chiang, P. H., Goldman, N. D., Fujioka, H., Aikawa, M., et al. (1999). Molecular cloning and nuclear localization of a histone deacetylase homologue in *Plasmodium falciparum*. *Mol. Biochem. Parasitol.* 99, 11–19. doi: 10.1016/S0166-6851(98)00177-7

Josling, G. A., and Llinás, M. (2015). Sexual development in Plasmodium parasites: knowing when it's time to commit. *Nat. Rev. Microbiol.* 13, 573–587. doi: 10.1038/nrmicro3519

Kafsack, B. F. C., Painter, H. J., and Llinás, M. (2012). New Agilent platform DNA microarrays for transcriptome analysis of *Plasmodium falciparum* and *Plasmodium berghei* for the malaria research community. *Malar. J.* 11:187. doi: 10.1186/1475-2875-11-187

Kafsack, B. F. C., Rovira-Graells, N., Clark, T. G., Bancells, C., Crowley, V. M., Campino, S. G., et al. (2014). A transcriptional switch underlies commitment to sexual development in malaria parasites. *Nature* 507, 248–252. doi: 10.1038/nature12920

Kariuki, M. M., Kiaira, J. K., Mulaa, F. K., Mwangi, J. K., Wasunna, M. K., and Martin, S. K. (1998). *Plasmodium falciparum*: purification of the various gametocyte developmental stages from *in vitro*-cultivated parasites. *Am. J. Trop. Med. Hyg.* 59, 505–508.

Kirkman, L. A., and Deitsch, K. W. (2014). Recombination and diversification of the variant antigen encoding genes in the malaria parasite *Plasmodium falciparum*. *Microbiol. Spectr.* 2, 1–12. doi: 10.1128/microbiolspec.MDNA3-0022-2014

Kuehn, A., and Pradel, G. (2010). The coming-out of malaria gametocytes. *J. Biomed. Biotechnol.* 2010:976827. doi: 10.1155/2010/976827

Lambros, C., and Vanderberg, J. P. (1979). Synchronization of *Plasmodium falciparum* erythrocytic stages in culture. *J. Parasitol.* 65, 418–420.

Lasonder, E., Ishihama, Y., Andersen, J. S., Vermunt, A. M. W., Pain, A., Sauerwein, R. W., et al. (2002). Analysis of the *Plasmodium falciparum* proteome by high-accuracy mass spectrometry. *Nature* 419, 537–542. doi: 10.1038/nature01111

Lasonder, E., Rijpma, S. R., Van Schaijk, B. C. L., Hoeijmakers, W. A. M., Kensche, P. R., Gresnigt, M. S., et al. (2016). Integrated transcriptomic and proteomic analyses of *P. falciparum* gametocytes: molecular insight into sex-specific processes and translational repression. *Nucleic Acids Res.* 44, 6087–6101. doi: 10.1093/nar/gkw536

Le Roch, K. G., Zhou, Y., Blair, P. L., Grainger, M., Moch, J. K., Haynes, J. D., et al. (2003). Discovery of gene function by expression profiling of the malaria parasite life cycle. *Science* 301, 1503–1508. doi: 10.1126/science.1087025

Lin, C. S., Uboldi, A. D., Epp, C., Bujard, H., Tsuboi, T., Czabotar, P. E., et al. (2016). Multiple *Plasmodium falciparum* merozoite surface protein 1 complexes mediate merozoite binding to human erythrocytes. *J. Biol. Chem.* 291, 7703–7715. doi: 10.1074/jbc.M115.698282

Liu, Y. Q., Tao, D. C., Liao, S. Y., Yang, Y., Ma, Y. X., and Zhang, S. Z. (2013). Identification of a novel human testicular interstitial gene, RNF148, and its expression regulated by histone deacetylases. *Genet. Mol. Res.* 12, 4060–4069. doi: 10.4238/2013.September.27.7

Livak, K. J., and Schmittgen, T. D. (2001). Analysis of relative gene expression data using real-time quantitative PCR and the $2^{-\Delta\Delta C_T}$ method. *Methods* 25, 402–408. doi: 10.1006/meth.2001.1262

Llinás, M., Deitsch, K. W., and Voss, T. S. (2008). Plasmodium gene regulation: far more to factor in. *Trends Parasitol.* 24, 551–556. doi: 10.1016/j.pt.2008.08.010

Lopez-Rubio, J. J., Riviere, L., and Scherf, A. (2007). Shared epigenetic mechanisms control virulence factors in protozoan parasites. *Curr. Opin. Microbiol.* 10, 560–568. doi: 10.1016/j.mib.2007.10.003

Lopez-Rubio, J.-J., Mancio-Silva, L., and Scherf, A. (2009). Genome-wide analysis of heterochromatin associates clonally variant gene regulation with perinuclear repressive centers in malaria parasites. *Cell Host Microbe* 5, 179–190. doi: 10.1016/j.chom.2008.12.012

Mair, G. R., Braks, J. A. M., Garver, L. S., Wiegant, J. C. A. G., Hall, N., Dirks, R. W., et al. (2006). Regulation of sexual development of Plasmodium by translational repression. *Science* 313, 667–669. doi: 10.1126/science.1125129

Mair, G. R., Lasonder, E., Garver, L. S., Franke-Fayard, B. M. D., Carret, C. K., Wiegant, J. C. A. G., et al. (2010). Universal features of post-transcriptional gene regulation are critical for Plasmodium zygote development. *PLoS Pathog.* 6:e1000767. doi: 10.1371/journal.ppat.1000767

Miao, J., Fan, Q., Cui, L., Li, X., Wang, H., Ning, G., et al. (2010). The MYST family histone acetyltransferase regulates gene expression and cell cycle in malaria parasite *Plasmodium falciparum*. *Mol. Microbiol.* 78, 883–902. doi: 10.1111/j.1365-2958.2010.07371.x

Miao, J., Fan, Q., Parker, D., Li, X., Li, J., and Cui, L. (2013). Puf Mediates translation repression of transmission-blocking vaccine candidates in malaria parasites. *PLoS Pathog.* 9:e1003268. doi: 10.1371/journal.ppat.1003268

Mphande, F. A., Ribacke, U., Kaneko, O., Kironde, F., Winter, G., and Wahlgren, M. (2008). SURFIN4.1, a schizont-merozoite associated protein in the SURFIN family of *Plasmodium falciparum*. *Malar. J.* 7:116. doi: 10.1186/1475-2875-7-116

Narum, D. L., and Thomas, A. W. (1994). Differential localization of full-length and processed forms of PF83/AMA-1 an apical membrane antigen of *Plasmodium falciparum* merozoites. *Mol. Biochem. Parasitol.* 67, 59–68.

Ngwa, C. J., Scheuermayer, M., Mair, G. R., Kern, S., Brügl, T., Wirth, C. C., et al. (2013). Changes in the transcriptome of the malaria parasite *Plasmodium falciparum* during the initial phase of transmission from the human to the mosquito. *BMC Genomics* 14:256. doi: 10.1186/1471-2164-14-256

Pérez-Toledo, K., Rojas-Meza, A. P., Mancio-Silva, L., Hernández-Cuevas, N. A., Delgadillo, D. M., Vargas, M., et al. (2009). *Plasmodium falciparum* heterochromatin protein 1 binds to tri-methylated histone 3 lysine 9 and is linked to mutually exclusive expression of var genes. *Nucleic Acids Res.* 37, 2596–2606. doi: 10.1093/nar/gkp115

Peterson, M. G., Marshall, V. M., Smythe, J. A., Crewther, P. E., Lew, A., Silva, A., et al. (1989). Integral membrane protein located in the apical complex of *Plasmodium falciparum*. *Mol. Cell. Biol.* 9, 3151–3154.

Petter, M., Lee, C. C., Byrne, T. J., Boysen, K. E., Volz, J., Ralph, S. A., et al. (2011). Expression of *P. falciparum* var genes involves exchange of the histone variant H2A.Z at the promoter. *PLoS Pathog.* 7:e1001292. doi: 10.1371/journal.ppat.1001292

Ponts, N., Yang, J., Chung, D. W. D., Prudhomme, J., Girke, T., Horrocks, P., et al. (2008). Deciphering the ubiquitin-mediated pathway in apicomplexan parasites: a potential strategy to interfere with parasite virulence. *PLoS ONE* 3:e2386. doi: 10.1371/journal.pone.0002386

Pradel, G. (2007). Proteins of the malaria parasite sexual stages: expression, function and potential for transmission blocking strategies. *Parasitology* 134, 1911–1929. doi: 10.1017/S0031182007003381

Pradel, G., Hayton, K., Aravind, L., Iyer, L. M., Abrahamsen, M. S., Bonawitz, A., et al. (2004). A multidomain adhesion protein family expressed in *Plasmodium falciparum* is essential for transmission to the mosquito. *J. Exp. Med.* 199, 1533–1544. doi: 10.1084/jem.20031274

Proellocks, N. I., Coppel, R. L., and Waller, K. L. (2010). Dissecting the apicomplexan rhoptry neck proteins. *Trends Parasitol.* 26, 297–304. doi: 10.1016/j.pt.2010.02.012

Recker, M., Buckee, C. O., Serazin, A., Kyes, S., Pinches, R., Christodoulou, Z., et al. (2011). Antigenic variation in *Plasmodium falciparum* malaria involves a highly structured switching pattern. *PLoS Pathog.* 7:e1001306. doi: 10.1371/journal.ppat.1001306

Rug, M., and Maier, A. G. (2013). Transfection of *Plasmodium falciparum*. *Methods Mol Biol.* 923, 75–98. doi: 10.1007/978-1-62703-026-7_6

Salanti, A., Staalsoe, T., Lavstsen, T., Jensen, A. T. R., Sowa, M. P. K., Arnot, D. E., et al. (2003). Selective upregulation of a single distinctly structured var gene in chondroitin sulphate A-adhering *Plasmodium falciparum* involved in pregnancy-associated malaria. *Mol. Microbiol.* 49, 179–191. doi: 10.1046/j.1365-2958.2003.03570.x

Salcedo-Amaya, A. M., van Driel, M. A., Alako, B. T., Trelle, M. B., van den Elzen, A. M. G., Cohen, A. M., et al. (2009). Dynamic histone H3 epigenome marking during the intraerythrocytic cycle of *Plasmodium falciparum*. *Proc. Natl. Acad. Sci. U.S.A.* 106, 9655–9660. doi: 10.1073/pnas.0902515106

Sautel, C. F., Cannella, D., Bastien, O., Kieffer, S., Aldebert, D., Garin, J., et al. (2007). SET8-mediated methylations of histone H4 lysine 20 mark silent heterochromatic domains in apicomplexan genomes. *Mol. Cell. Biol.* 27, 5711–5724. doi: 10.1128/MCB.00482-07

Scherf, A., Lopez-Rubio, J. J., and Riviere, L. (2008). Antigenic Variation in *Plasmodium falciparum*. *Annu. Rev. Microbiol.* 62, 445–470. doi: 10.1146/annurev.micro.61.080706.093134

Schmidt, I., Pradel, G., Sologub, L., Golzmann, A., Ngwa, C. J., Kucharski, A., et al. (2016). Bistacrine derivatives as new potent antimalarials. *Bioorg. Med. Chem.* 24, 3636–3642. doi: 10.1016/j.bmc.2016.06.003

Schobert, R., and Biersack, B. (2017). Multimodal HDAC inhibitors with improved anticancer activity. *Curr. Cancer Drug Targets.* doi: 10.2174/1568009617666170206102613. [Epub ahead of print].

Scholz, S. M., Simon, N., Lavazec, C., Dude, M.-A., Templeton, T. J., and Pradel, G. (2008). PfCCp proteins of *Plasmodium falciparum*: gametocyte-specific expression and role in complement-mediated inhibition of exflagellation. *Int. J. Parasitol.* 38, 327–340. doi: 10.1016/j.ijpara.2007.08.009

Simon, N., Kuehn, A., Williamson, K. C., and Pradel, G. (2016). Adhesion protein complexes of malaria gametocytes assemble following parasite transmission to the mosquito. *Parasitol. Int.* 65, 27–30. doi: 10.1016/j.parint.2015.09.007

Sinha, A., Hughes, K. R., Modrzynska, K. K., Otto, T. D., Pfander, C., Dickens, N. J., et al. (2014). A cascade of DNA-binding proteins for sexual commitment and development in Plasmodium. *Nature* 507, 253–257. doi: 10.1038/nature 12970

Sumanadasa, S. D. M., Goodman, C. D., Lucke, A. J., Skinner-Adams, T., Saham, I., Haque, A., et al. (2012). Antimalarial activity of the anticancer histone deacetylase inhibitor SB939. *Antimicrob. Agents Chemother.* 56, 3849–3856. doi: 10.1128/AAC.00030-12

Sun, W., Tanaka, T. Q., Magle, C. T., Huang, W., Southall, N., Huang, R., et al. (2014). Chemical signatures and new drug targets for gametocytocidal drug development. *Sci. Rep.* 4, 1–11. doi: 10.1038/srep03743

Templeton, T. J., Fujioka, H., Aikawa, M., Parker, K. C., and Kaslow, D. C. (1997). *Plasmodium falciparum* Pfs40, renamed Pf39, is localized to an intracellular membrane-bound compartment and is not sexual stage-specific. *Mol. Biochem. Parasitol.* 90, 359–365. doi: 10.1016/S0166-6851(97)00164-3

Tonkin, C. J., Carret, C. K., Duraisingh, M. T., Voss, T. S., Ralph, S. A., Hommel, M., et al. (2009). Sir2 paralogues cooperate to regulate virulence genes and antigenic variation in *Plasmodium falciparum*. *PLoS Biol.* 7:e1000084. doi: 10.1371/journal.pbio.1000084

Trenholme, K., Marek, L., Duffy, S., Pradel, G., Fisher, G., Hansen, F. K., et al. (2014). Lysine acetylation in sexual stage malaria parasites is a target for antimalarial small molecules. *Antimicrob. Agents Chemother.* 58, 3666–3678. doi: 10.1128/AAC.02721-13

Volz, J., Carvalho, T. G., Ralph, S. A., Gilson, P., Thompson, J., Tonkin, C. J., et al. (2010). Potential epigenetic regulatory proteins localise to distinct nuclear sub-compartments in *Plasmodium falciparum*. *Int. J. Parasitol.* 40, 109–121. doi: 10.1016/j.ijpara.2009.09.002

Voss, T. S., Bozdech, Z., and Bártfai, R. (2014). Epigenetic memory takes center stage in the survival strategy of malaria parasites. *Curr. Opin. Microbiol.* 20, 88–95. doi: 10.1016/j.mib.2014.05.007

Voss, T. S., Mini, T., Jenoe, P., and Beck, H.-P. (2002). *Plasmodium falciparum* possesses a cell cycle-regulated short type replication protein a large subunit encoded by an unusual transcript. *J. Biol. Chem.* 277, 17493–17501. doi: 10.1074/jbc.M200100200

Warncke, J. D., Vakonakis, I., and Beck, H.-P. (2016). Plasmodium Helical Interspersed Subtelomeric (PHIST) proteins, at the center of host cell remodeling. *Microbiol. Mol. Biol. Rev.* 80, 905–927. doi: 10.1128/MMBR.00014-16

Wheatley, N. C., Andrews, K. T., Tran, T. L., Lucke, A. J., Reid, R. C., and Fairlie, D. P. (2010). Antimalarial histone deacetylase inhibitors containing cinnamate or NSAID components. *Bioorg. Med. Chem. Lett.* 20, 7080–7084. doi: 10.1016/j.bmcl.2010.09.096

Wirth, C. C., Glushakova, S., Scheuermayer, M., Repnik, U., Garg, S., Schaack, D., et al. (2014). Perforin-like protein PPLP2 permeabilizes the red blood cell membrane during egress of *Plasmodium falciparum* gametocytes. *Cell. Microbiol.* 16, 709–733. doi: 10.1111/cmi.12288

World Malaria Report, WHO (2016). Available online at: http://www.who.int/malaria/publications/world-malaria-report-2016/report/en/

Zagni, C., Floresta, G., Monciino, G., and Rescifina, A. (2017). The search for potent, small-molecule HDACIs in cancer treatment: a decade after vorinostat. *Med. Res. Rev.* doi: 10.1002/med.21437. [Epub ahead of print].

4

Nematode Species Identification: Current Status, Challenges and Future Perspectives for Cyathostomins

Christina M. Bredtmann[1], *Jürgen Krücken*[1], *Jayaseelan Murugaiyan*[2], *Tetiana Kuzmina*[3] *and Georg von Samson-Himmelstjerna*[1*]

[1] Department of Veterinary Medicine, Institute for Parasitology and Tropical Veterinary Medicine, Freie Universität Berlin, Berlin, Germany, [2] Department of Veterinary Medicine, Institute for Animal Hygiene and Environmental Health, Freie Universität Berlin, Berlin, Germany, [3] Department of Parasitology, I.I. Schmalhausen Institute of Zoology, Kyiv, Ukraine

Edited by:
Lilach Sheiner,
Wellcome Trust Centre for Molecular Parasitology, United Kingdom

Reviewed by:
Elias Papadopoulos,
Aristotle University of Thessaloniki, Greece
Martin Krarup Nielsen,
University of Kentucky, United States

***Correspondence:**
Georg von Samson-Himmelstjerna
gvsamson@fu-berlin.de

Human and animal health is globally affected by a variety of parasitic helminths. The impact of co-infections and development of anthelmintic resistance requires improved diagnostic tools, especially for parasitic nematodes e.g., to identify resistant species or attribute pathological effects to individual species or particular species combinations. In horses, co-infection with cyathostomins is rather a rule than an exception with typically 5 to 15 species (out of more than 40 described) per individual host. In cyathostomins, reliable morphological species differentiation is currently limited to adults and requires highly specialized expertize while precise morphological identification of eggs and early stage larvae is impossible. The situation is further complicated by a questionable validity of some cyathostomins while others might actually represent cryptic species complexes. Several molecular methods using different target sequences were established to overcome these limitations. For adult worms, PCR followed by sequencing of mitochondrial genes or external or internal ribosomal RNA spacers is suitable to genetically confirm morphological identifications. The most commonly used method to differentiate eggs or larvae is the reverse-line-blot hybridization assay. However, both methods suffer from the fact that target sequences are not available for many species or even that GenBank® entries are unreliable regarding the cyathostomin species. Recent advances in proteomic tools for identification of metazoans including insects and nematodes of the genus *Trichinella* will be evaluated for suitability to diagnose cyathostomins. Future research should focus on the comparative analysis of morphological, molecular and proteomic data from the same cyathostomin specimen to optimize tools for species-specific identification.

Keywords: cyathostomins, nematodes, diagnostic, PCR, MALDI-TOF MS

INTRODUCTION

Parasitic helminths globally affect human and animal health and can be of zoonotic relevance (e.g., *Ascaris* spp.). In equines, the most important intestinal nematodes belong to the family Strongylidae and are comprised of two subfamilies: The Strongylinae encompassing 14 species in 5 genera (*Strongylus*, *Oesophagodontus*, *Triodontophorus*, *Bidentostomum*, and *Craterostomum*), and the Cyathostominae encompassing currently 50 valid species in 14 genera (*Caballonema*,

Coronocyclus, *Cyathostomum*, *Cylicocyclus*, *Cylicodontophorus*, *Cylicostephanus*, *Cylindropharynx*, *Gyalocephalus*, *Hsiungia*, *Parapoteriostomum*, *Petrovinema*, *Poteriostomum*, *Scrjabinodentus*, *Tridentoinfundibulum*) (Lichtenfels et al., 2008), in contrast to previous publications listing 51 or 52 species in 13 genera (Lichtenfels, 1975; Lichtenfels et al., 2002). In the literature, the term "small strongyles" has either been coined to include only the Cyathostominae or all equine strongylidae except the genus *Strongylus*, which were designated "large strongyles" (Lyons et al., 1999). Although, still widely used, it is now recommended to avoid the terms small and large strongyles (Lichtenfels et al., 2002).

Since prevalence of the highly pathogenic *Strongylus* species declined after introduction of the macrocyclic lactones (Herd, 1990), the cyathostomins are currently recognized as the most important equine parasites because of (i) their up to 100% prevalence in equids (Lyons et al., 1999), (ii) numerous reports of anthelmintic resistance and (iii) their pathogenicity which becomes particularly manifest in cases of sometimes fatal larval cyathostominosis (Love et al., 1999). Anthelmintic resistance against benzimidazoles is highly prevalent worldwide and pyrantel resistance is also frequently observed whereas reduced efficacy of macrocylic lactones has rarely been reported (Kaplan, 2002; Kuzmina and Kharchenko, 2008; Von Samson-Himmelstjerna, 2012; Matthews, 2014; Nielsen et al., 2014).

Cyathostomins have a direct life-cycle with adults located in the lumen of caecum and colon, shedding eggs with the feces. First larvae (L1) hatch in the feces, molt twice to infectious third larvae (L3) which are ingested by equids. In the large intestine, L3 encyst inside the intestinal wall and may also undergo hypobiosis for months, before molting to fourth larvae (L4) (Corning, 2009). Synchronous excystation of large numbers of hypobiotic larvae potentially causes larval cyathostominosis characterized by severe inflammation leading to weight-loss, diarrhea, colic, or even death (Love et al., 1999).

Although, Cyathostomins are a threat to equine welfare and scientific efforts to address this problem are frequently undertaken, research is impaired by the lack of sufficient identification methods (Lichtenfels, 2008). This perspective addresses the different methods, their advantages and limitations and gives an outlook on possible future methods for nematode identification using the cyathostomins as paradigm.

SAMPLES AND SAMPLING

The first challenge for species identification is the availability of suitable specimens. While strongylid eggs can be easily collected from feces, they have virtually no diagnostically useful morphological features. Strongylid L3 can be obtained from eggs using different fecal cultures methods (Smyth, 1990). However, only some L3 can be identified to the genus level, and this requires a high experience level. Only for a few species *in vitro* culture to the L4 (Chapman et al., 1994; Brianti et al., 2009) has been described. Therefore, adult parasites must be collected from naturally infected hosts. In horses, only a few adult strongyles are occasionally shed with the feces but collection of adult nematodes from feces after anthelmintic treatment is possible (Osterman Lind et al., 2003; Kuzmina et al., 2005; Kuzmina and Kharchenko, 2008). However, the complete worm burden representing all species in the living horse will only be documented by examination of all feces over several days, which may be associated with degradation of worms leading to distorted results. A more exact and meaningful method is the collection of adult nematodes from the content of the horse intestine (Drudge and Lyons, 1977). The critical test method, which is described in detail by Drudge et al. (1963), is a combination of both, the fecal collection over a week and collection during necropsy. This method is widely used to study the effectiveness of anthelmintic compounds (e.g., Lyons et al., 2007, 2010). Due to the need of sacrificed or slaughtered horses, these methods are restricted to research. Thus, there is a great need to develop alternatives for precise nematode diagnosis for living horses. The immediate research aim is therefore the development of effective and specific non-invasive cyathostomin identification methods.

MORPHOLOGICAL IDENTIFICATION

For more than 100 years (Molin, 1861; Loos, 1900), a large number of cyathostomin species has been morphologically described using 93 different names. In the meantime, several previously described species are considered synonyms (Lichtenfels et al., 1998) and currently 50 species are recognized as valid. Comprehensive identification keys summing up the descriptions were published (Lichtenfels, 1975; Tolliver, 2000; Lichtenfels et al., 2008).

Morphological identification of adult strongyles relies on careful examination of faint characters at the anterior end of the adult nematodes or of the reproductive system. These traits include the size and shape of buccal capsules, internal and external leaf crowns and its extra-chitinous support as illustrated in **Figure 1** to point out that differences are very faint. Fine morphological structures of posterior end such as size and shape of the bursa, genital cone, gubernaculum, and spicules in males and shape of the tail, size and proportion of different parts of the reproductive system in females are also valuable for species differentiation (Lichtenfels, 1975; Dvojnos and Kharchenko, 1994; Lichtenfels et al., 2008). However, reliable morphological identification of adult cyathostomins can only be achieved following several years of intensive training and currently only few experts are available worldwide (Lichtenfels et al., 2008).

Whereas, adult cyathostomins can be discriminated, eggs, L1 and L2 cannot be differentiated from other nematodes of the family Strongylidae. Identification of L3 is possible for some genera such as *Strongylus*, *Triodontophorus*, *Gyalocephalus*, or *Poteriostomum* while most others can only be assigned to several cyathostomin larval types (Bevilaqua et al., 1993; Santos et al., 2016). The morphological features include qualitative and quantitative traits such as the number, arrangement and shape of intestinal/midgut cells, the length of the intestine and the length of the sheath tail.

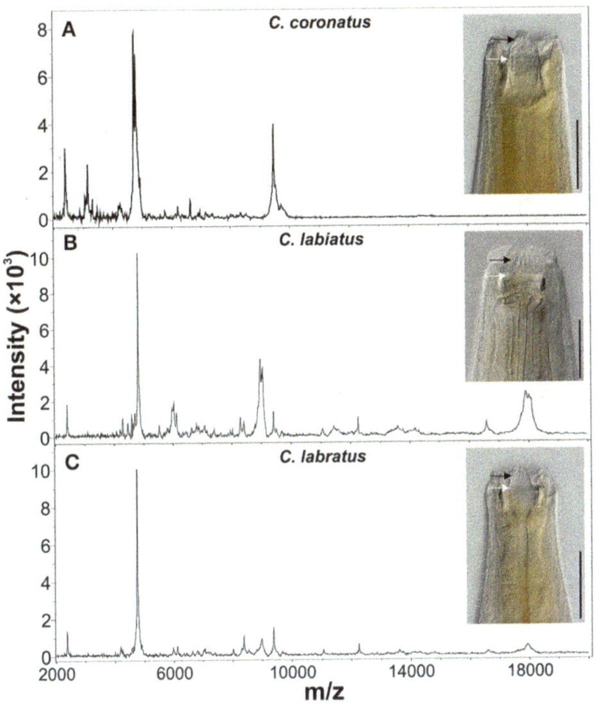

FIGURE 1 | Comparison of morphological and proteomic species identification methods. Anterior ends and representative MALDI-TOF MS spectra of three cyathostomin species from the closely related species **(A)** *Coronocyclus coronatus*, **(B)** *Coronocyclus labiatus*, and **(C)** *Coronocyclus labratus* are shown. Scale bars represent 100 μm. The x-axes show mass charge ratios while y-axes represent arbitrary intensity units. Spectra were baseline subtracted and smoothed using default parameters in the flexAnalysis software (Bruker Daltonics). Specimen were cleared with lactophenol to improve visibility of structural features of the cuticle. External and internal leaf crown are indicated by black and white arrows, respectively.

MOLECULAR METHODS

To overcome the limitations of morphological identification, research has focused on molecular cyathostomin identification. These methods, once target-sequences are implemented correctly, can be applied independently of the nematode life-stage.

A target locus which proved to be useful in developing genetic markers for diagnostic and phylogenetic purposes is the ribosomal DNA (rDNA) (reviewed by Gasser and Newton, 2000; Chilton, 2004). Eukaryotic nuclear rDNA is organized in clusters of sometimes several hundred repeats. Coding sequences for 18S, 5.8S, and 28S rRNAs are interrupted by the first and second internal-transcribed spacers (ITS-1 and ITS-2) (Long and Dawid, 1980). The similarity of ITS sequences is higher within than among different species (Elder and Turner, 1995). This was also shown for strongyles, where the extent of intraspecific variation was low (0–0.3%) in comparison to interspecific differences (0.6–23.7% for the ITS-1 region, 1.3–56.3% for the ITS-2 region) (Hung et al., 1999b).

An early approach for molecular species identification based on the ITS-2 locus is the PCR-linked restriction fragment length polymorphism (PCR-RFLP) analysis, which was first used for differentiation of single eggs of the Strongylinae (Campbell et al., 1995) and was then applied to show that the morphologically very similar *Cylicocyclus ashworthi* and *Cylicocyclus nassatus* actually represent separate species (Hung et al., 1997). Another method is the PCR-linked single-strand-conformation-polymorphism technique (SSCP-PCR; Gasser and Monti, 1997), which allows the delineation of 14 strongyle species, including 9 cyathostomins, based on ITS-2 PCR products (Hung et al., 1999a). These methods rely on the DNA from individual worms or eggs and are thus associated with time-consuming procedures if it is desired to screen a representative subset of a strongyle community.

Species identification from mixed parasite DNA from fecal samples and/or copro-cultures was demonstrated after ITS-2 sequences for 28 strongyle species (including 22 cyathostomin species) were determined and species specific primers evaluated for four common species (Hung et al., 1999b). Although, this method theoretically allows species-specific research on pooled samples, it is limited to the identification of only few species.

The variability of the 26S-18S rDNA intergenic-spacer (IGS) was used for species differentiation of 16 cyathostomin species with a range of interspecies variation of 31–56% (Kaye et al., 1998). The obtained sequences were used to develop a PCR-ELISA for the identification of six common cyathostomin species (Hodgkinson et al., 2003) and a Reverse-Line-Blot-Assay (RLB) to simultaneously identify 13 strongyle species (Traversa et al., 2007). Both methods have been used to monitor the species composition before and after anthelmintic treatment (Hodgkinson et al., 2005; Čerňanská et al., 2009; Ionita et al., 2010; Traversa et al., 2010). Re-evaluation and validation of existing and new oligo-probes increased the number of species that can be identified with RLB to 18 (Cwiklinski et al., 2012). PCR-ELISA and RLB are qualitative methods detecting the presence or absence of the different species. A semi-quantitative approach applying replicates of pooled larvae was positively evaluated to enable screening of many cyathostomin populations in parallel (Kooyman et al., 2016).

Despite being recognized as "a less suitable target than ITS for quick diagnostic tests," due to its high substitution rates and high possibility of intraspecific polymorphisms, the mitochondrial Cytochrome oxidase c subunit I (COI) is used for species differentiation and could indicate cryptic species (Blouin, 2002). Twenty two COI sequence haplotypes (overall 10.8% rate of intraspecific nucleotide difference) were found within *C. nassatus* using specimen from different hosts and geographic origins, while only little variation (0.0–0.6% differences) was seen in the ITS-2 sequences suggesting cryptic species within *C. nassatus* (Traversa et al., 2008) and maybe other cyathostomin morpho-species as well. Analysis of ITS-1 and ITS-2 sequences of *Cylicostephanus minutus* individuals showed 3.0 and 7.4% differences also indicating the presence of a cryptic species complex (Hung et al., 1999a). The combination of markers on questionable species appears useful to investigate the occurrence of cryptic species complexes.

Whereas the objective of research on cyathostomin species identification is on the one hand to improve the available diagnostic tools, it aims on the other hand to contribute to the understanding of the phylogenetic relationships between the different taxa. Therefore, three gene loci, the ITS-2, COI and 28S rRNA were compared for their phylogenetic usefulness in strongyles. It was encountered that the high level of substitution saturation renders COI unsuitable for phylogenetic analysis. The remaining loci, ITS-2 and 28S rRNA, both showed similar groupings of cyathostomins. Combining both loci resulted in a tree with improved bootstrapping support for the internal nodes (McDonnell et al., 2000) pointing towards the importance of the simultaneous application of different molecular markers. This can also be seen in a study analyzing ITS-1 and ITS-2 sequences of 30 strongyle nematode species, including 23 cyathostomin species that questions the widely accepted separation of Strongylinae and Cyathostominae and proposes a framework to systematically analyze future datasets of strongyle nematodes (Hung et al., 2000). Findings consistent with the latter phylogenetic analysis were shown in a study focusing on the genus *Cylicocyclus* which proposed a separation of *Cylicocyclus* in two clades but statistical support for this hypothesis was relatively weak (Bu et al., 2013).

SEROLOGICAL METHODS

Larval cyathostominosis is caused by the simultaneous re-activation and emergence of high numbers of hypobiotic larvae (Love et al., 1999) causing severe pathology. Usually, no eggs are expelled due to absence of adults making coproscopic diagnosis unfeasible (Murphy and Love, 1997). This leads to the aim of pre-patent detection of cyathostomin infections using serology to be able to assess the risk of larval cyathostominosis based on the estimation of the mucosal cyathostomin worm burden.

One promising approach identified anti-larval IgG(T) serum antibody responses to two antigen complexes, only elicited by larvae, as potential markers for prepatent cyathostomin infections (Dowdall et al., 2002). Subsequent purification of native antigenic complexes from larvae resulted in higher IgG(T) signals in an ELISA and reduced the number of false positive responses (Dowdall et al., 2003). Further evidence for an immunodiagnostic potential of these markers is given by a study where the mucosal worm burden of naïve and infected horses was assessed and found to significantly correlate with the IgG(T) serum levels. Additionally, sera from horses with clinical suspicion of larval cyathostominosis had significantly increased antigen-specific IgG(T) levels (Dowdall et al., 2004). One antigenic complex could be identified as cyathostomin gut-associated larval antigen-1 (Cy-GALA-1) and allocated to the species *Cyathostomum pateratum* (McWilliam et al., 2010), followed by the characterization of the orthologous antigens of four additional common cyathostomin species. An ELISA was developed based on recombinant Cy-GALA proteins, which allows the detection of the immune response to cyatostomin larvae. Cross-reactivity to other parasites was not observed and is unlikely, because of the diversity of orthologous GALA sequences of non-cyathostomin species (Mitchell et al., 2016). In the absence of experimental single species infections, cross-reactivity between cyathostomin species is hard to evaluate and diagnostic tests should therefore include a panel of different Cy-GALA proteins to detect most larval cyathostomin infections.

If in future available for routine diagnosis this approach could be of clinical relevance and help ruling out or confirming a larval cyathostominosis in horses with unspecific symptoms of wasting or colic. However, due to the lack of species-specificity serological methods will not help gaining detailed knowledge on the role of individual species in larval cyathostominosis.

PROTEOMICS METHOD

The proteome based matrix-assisted laser desorption/ionization time-of-flight mass spectrometry (MALDI-TOF MS profiling) species identification of microorganisms has already revolutionized diagnostic microbiology. Species identification is based on the molecular masses of proteins such as ribosomal and other abundant proteins. A small amount of microorganisms or crude extracted intact proteins is transferred to specially designed target plates and allowed to co-crystallize with an inert, UV absorbing matrix such as α-Cyano-4-hydroxycinnamic acid. A pulsed 337 nm laser beam irradiates the samples to form a dense ion plume. The resultant ions are accelerated through a vacuum tube to reach the detector and separated according to their charge/mass (*m/z*) ratio and the time of flight (TOF) for each is measured. The mass range *m/z* 2,000–20,000 is generally applied for species identification through pattern matching of the spectra peaks with that of a reference spectra database. The method is popular due to its cost-effectiveness, reliability and availability of specially designed linear MALDI machines equipped with software tools and reference databases. This method has been evaluated for a variety of microorganisms such as bacterial, fungal, and viral pathogens (Wieser et al., 2012; Clark et al., 2013). In the past two decades, this technique was established for rapid characterization of eukaryotic cell lines and for species differentiation of protozoan parasites (e.g., *Leishmania, Giardia*) and arthropods (e.g., mosquitoes, ticks, tsetse flies) (Hoppenheit et al., 2013; Singhal et al., 2016; Yssouf et al., 2016). Regarding nematodes, first diagnostic use of MALDI-TOF has been described to identify different races of *Ditylensus dipsaci* (Perera et al., 2009) and closely related species of root-knot and seed-gall nematodes (Perera et al., 2005; Ahmad et al., 2012). Despite these developments, extensive studies on the application of MALDI-TOF MS for rapid species identification for helminth have not been reported. Recently, MALDI-TOF MS was applied for rapid species identification of *Trichinella* spp. after adopting a simple formic-acid/acetonitrile extraction from pooled larvae and compilation of a reference database (Mayer-Scholl et al., 2016). This approach could also be extended to cyathostomin species identification. Preliminary data to evaluate the potential for MALDI-TOF MS for cyathostomins revealed distinct patterns for adult individuals of different species (**Figure 1**).

Of course, master-spectra libraries can only be generated with validated, correctly identified material. This requires that proteomic data are obtained from morphologically and molecularly identified individual specimen. For arthropods, this

TABLE 1 | Comparison of methods for cyathostomin species identification.

Identification method		Life stage	Usefulness and limitations	References
MORPHOLOGICAL IDENTIFICATION				
		Eggs	No species differentiation possible	Lichtenfels, 1975, 2008; Dvojnos and Kharchenko, 1994; Tolliver, 2000; Lichtenfels et al., 2008; Kharchenko et al., 2009; Kornaś et al., 2009; Santos et al., 2016
		Larvae	L3 can be allocated to different larvae types, but not to individual species	
		Adults	Identification keys published but species identification is difficult for inexperienced workers	
MOLECULAR METHODS				
Marker	**Method**			
ITS-1 and ITS-2	PCR and sequencing	All	Species identification and phylogenetic analysis, identification of cryptic species Sometimes only small differences between closely related species Not applicable for mixed samples, isolation of DNA from individual specimen necessary	Campbell et al., 1995; Chilton et al., 1997; Hung et al., 1999a, 2000; Bu et al., 2013
	SSCP-PCR	All	Delineation of 14 Strongylida species (9 Cyathostomin species), Isolation of DNA from individual specimen necessary	Gasser and Monti, 1997
	PCR-RFLP	All	Distinction of Strongylinae eggs, Distinction of two Cyathstomin species (*C.ashworthi, C.nassatus*). Isolation of DNA from individual specimen necessary, established for larvae	Campbell et al., 1995; Hung et al., 1997
IGS	PCR-ELISA	All	Screening for 6 cyathostomin species in mixed samples possible. Established for eggs and larvae	Hodgkinson et al., 2003, 2005
	RLB	All	Differentiation of up to 18 common species, less time consuming and costly than other molecular methods, screening of strongyle population before and after anthelmintic treatment possible, mixed samples possible, but more viable for individual worms; semi-quantitative approach possible	Traversa et al., 2007; Ionita et al., 2010; Cwiklinski et al., 2012; Kooyman et al., 2016
COI	PCR and sequencing	All	Investigation of intraspecies genetic variability, identification of cryptic species, not applicable for mixed samples, isolation of DNA from individual specimen necessary	Hung et al., 1999a; Traversa et al., 2008
SEROLOGICAL METHODS				
Protein-based ELISA		Larvae	Pre-patent detection of four common cyathostomin species possible from serum, no cyathostomin species differentiation possible	Mitchell et al., 2016
PROTEMICS METHOD				
		Potentially all	Method is established for bacteria, fungi, several species of arthropods; only one study on nematodes (*Trichinella* spp.), protocols and reference spectra data base have to be established	Karger et al., 2012; Yssouf et al., 2013, 2016; Mayer-Scholl et al., 2016; Singhal et al., 2016;

issue can be solved by using always e.g., a wing or leg for proteomic and any other body part for molecular analysis. For nematodes, which are not segmented, this is not trivial since no defined body parts can be reproducibly cut off at exactly the same position without altering the protein spectrum. Therefore, methods need to be developed that reliably allow to conduct both methods using exactly the same starting material, despite the fact that the protein extraction usually involves conditions that damage DNA. Nevertheless, it was possible to extract DNA of sufficient quality from the acetonitrile/formic acid insoluble material to successfully amplify and sequence the ITS-2 region for the three specimen shown in **Figure 1**. These were 100, 99, and 97% identical to Genbank accession numbers JN786951.2, JN786947.2, JN786949 respectively, which confirmed the morphological identification in each case.

Possible limitations could be the different spectra elicited by different development stages, as seen in tick species identification. However, despite changes of the overall MS protein profiles, the ticks could be classified correctly according to certain specific peaks (Karger et al., 2012). Characterization of species-specific peak patterns, independent of development stages, therefore needs to be part of future research to implement MALDI-TOF MS as a possible diagnostic tool.

CONCLUSION

Different approaches have been used over the past decades to improve cyathostomin species delineation. All methods have their advantages and limitations (**Table 1**) and none is already fully satisfying for the research questions to be answered and all are far away from applicability in routine laboratory diagnosis. Comprehensive research on different aspects improving the discrimination of individual cyathostomin species, such as inclusion of several molecular markers and additional proteomic profiles could be of great help in the future. This should include the morphological identification together with the description of the genotype (molecular) and phenotype (proteomic) data in association with the currently accepted taxonomic classification. Ideally, morphological, molecular and proteomic data from the same individual should be used to take advantage of all three approaches to identify the complete species spectrum in the Cyathostominae and delineate their phylogenetic relationship.

AUTHOR CONTRIBUTIONS

CB performed MALDI-TOF experiments and literature surveys. CB and JK drafted and edited the manuscript. TK contributed microphotographs. TK, JM, and GS contributed to writing of the manuscript. CB, JK, JM, and GS designed the general outline.

FUNDING

The work received financial support from the Deutsche Forschungsgemeinschaft (DFG GRK2046).

REFERENCES

Ahmad, F., Gopal, J., and Wu, H. (2012). Rapid and highly sensitive detection of single nematode via direct MALDI Mass Spectrometry. *Talanta* 93, 182–185. doi: 10.1016/j.talanta.2012.02.009

Bevilaqua, C. M. L., Rodrigues, M., de, L., and Concordet, D. (1993). Identification of infective larvae of some common nematode strongylids of horses. *Rev. Med. Vet.* 144, 989–995.

Blouin, M. S. (2002). Molecular prospecting for cryptic species of nematodes: mitochondrial DNA versus internal transcribed spacer. *Int. J. Parasitol.* 32, 527–531. doi: 10.1016/S0020-7519(01)00357-5

Brianti, E., Giannetto, S., Traversa, D., Chirgwin, S. R., Shakya, K., and Klei, T. R. (2009). *In vitro* development of cyathostomin larvae from the third stage larvae to the fourth stage: morphologic characterization, effects of refrigeration, and species-specific patterns. *Vet. Parasitol.* 163, 348–356. doi: 10.1016/j.vetpar.2009.04.029

Bu, Y., Niu, H., and Zhang, L. (2013). Phylogenetic analysis of the genus Cylicocyclus (Nematoda: Strongylidae) based on nuclear ribosomal sequence data. *Acta Parasitol.* 58, 167–173. doi: 10.2478/s11686-013-0124-z

Campbell, A. J. D., Gasser, R. B., and Chilton, N. B. (1995). Differences in a Ribosomal DNA sequence of strongylus species allows identification of single eggs. *Int. J. Parasitol.* 25, 359–365. doi: 10.1016/0020-7519(94)00116-6

Chapman, M. R., Hutchinson, G. W., Cenac, M. J., and Klei, T. R. (1994). *In vitro* culture of equine strongylidae to the fourth larval stage in a cell-free medium. *J. Parasitol.* 80, 225–231. doi: 10.2307/3283751

Chilton, N. B. (2004). The use of nuclear ribosomal DNA markers for the identification of bursate nematodes (order Strongylida) and for the diagnosis of infections. *Anim. Heal. Res. Rev.* 5, 173–187. doi: 10.1079/AHR200497

Chilton, N. B., Gasser, R. B., and Beveridge, I. (1997). Phylogenetic relationships of australian strongyloid nematodes inferred from ribosomal DNA sequence data. *Int. J. Parasitol.* 27, 1481–1494. doi: 10.1016/S0020-7519(97)00134-3

Clark, A. E., Kaleta, E. J., Arora, A., and Wolk, D. M. (2013). Matrix-Assisted laser desorption ionization-time of flight mass spectrometry: a fundamental shift in the routine practice of clinical microbiology. *Clin. Microbiol. Rev.* 26, 547–603. doi: 10.1128/CMR.00072-12

Corning, S. (2009). Equine cyathostomins: a review of biology, clinical significance and therapy. *Parasit. Vectors* 2(Suppl. 2):S1. doi: 10.1186/1756-3305-2-s2-s1

Cwiklinski, K., Kooyman, F. N. J., Van Doorn, D. C. K., Matthews, J. B., and Hodgkinson, J. E. (2012). New insights into sequence variation in the IGS region of 21 cyathostomin species and the implication for molecular identification. *Parasitology* 139, 1063–1073. doi: 10.1017/S0031182012000467

Dowdall, S. M. J., Matthews, J. B., Mair, T., Murphy, D., Love, S., and Proudman, C. J. (2002). Antigen-specific IgG (T) responses in natural and experimental cyathostominae infection in horses. *Vet. Parasitol.* 106, 225–242. doi: 10.1016/S0304-4017(02)00085-7

Dowdall, S. M. J., Proudman, C. J., Klei, T. R., Mair, T., and Matthews, J. B. (2004). Characterisation of IgG(T) serum antibody responses to two larval antigen complexes in horses naturally- or experimentally-infected with cyathostomins. *Int. J. Parasitol.* 34, 101–108. doi: 10.1016/j.ijpara.2003.09.008

Dowdall, S. M. J., Proudman, C. J., Love, S., Klei, T. R., and Matthews, J. B. (2003). Purification and analyses of the specificity of two putative diagnostic antigens for larval cyathostomin infection in horses. *Res. Vet. Sci.* 75, 223–229. doi: 10.1016/S0034-5288(03)00116-4

Čerňanská, D., Paoletti, B., Král'ová-Hromadová, I., and Iorio, R., Čudeková, P., Milillo, P., et al. (2009). Application of a Reverse Line Blot hybridisation assay for the species-specific identification of cyathostomins (Nematoda, Strongylida) from benzimidazole-treated horses in the Slovak Republic. *Vet. Parasitol.* 160, 171–174. doi: 10.1016/j.vetpar.2008.10.078

Drudge, J. H., and Lyons, E. T. (1977). Methods in the evaluation of antiparasitic drugs in the horse. *Am. J. Vet. Res.* 38, 1581–1586.

Drudge, J. H., Szanto, J., Wyant, Z. N., and Elam, G. (1963). Critical tests of thiabendazole as an anthelmintic in the horse. *Am. J. Vet. Res.* 24, 1217–1222.

Dvojnos, G. M., and Kharchenko, V. O. (1994). *Strongylids of Wild and Domestic Horses (in Russian)*. Kiev: Naukova Dumka.

Elder, J. F. J., and Turner, B. J. (1995). Concerted evolution of repetitive DNA sequences in eukaryotes. *Q. Rev. Biol.* 70, 297–320. doi: 10.1086/419073

Gasser, R. B., and Monti, J. R. (1997). Identification of parasitic nematodes by PCR-SSCP of ITS-2 rDNA. *Mol. Cell. Probes* 11, 201–209. doi: 10.1006/mcpr.1997.0106

Gasser, R. B., and Newton, S. E. (2000). Genomic and genetic research on bursate nematodes: significance, implications and prospects. *Int. J. Parasitol.* 30, 509–534. doi: 10.1016/S0020-7519(00)00021-7

Herd, R. P. (1990). The changing world of worms: the rise of the cyathostomes and the decline of strongylus vulgaris. *Compend. Contin. Educ. Pract. Vet.* 12, 732–736.

Hodgkinson, J. E., Freeman, K. L., Lichtenfels, J. R., Palfreman, S., Love, S., and Matthews, J. B. (2005). Identification of strongyle eggs from anthelmintic-treated horses using a PCR-ELISA based on intergenic DNA sequences. *Parasitol. Res.* 95, 287–292. doi: 10.1007/s00436-004-1289-z

Hodgkinson, J. E., Lichtenfels, J. R., Mair, T. S., Cripps, P., Freeman, K. L., Ramsey, Y. H., et al. (2003). A PCR-ELISA for the identification of cyathostomin fourth-stage larvae from clinical cases of larval cyathostominosis. *Int. J. Parasitol.* 33, 1427–1435. doi: 10.1016/S0020-7519(03)00140-1

Hoppenheit, A., Murugaiyan, J., Bauer, B., Steuber, S., Clausen, P. H., and Roesler, U. (2013). Identification of Tsetse (*Glossina* spp.) using matrix-assisted laser desorption/ionisation time of flight mass spectrometry. *PLoS Negl. Trop. Dis.* 7:e2305. doi: 10.1371/journal.pntd.0002305

Hung, G. C., Chilton, N. B., Beveridge, I., and Gasser, R. B. (2000). A molecular systematic framework for equine strongyles based on ribosomal DNA sequence data. *Int. J. Parasitol.* 30, 95–103. doi: 10.1016/S0020-7519(99)00166-6

Hung, G. C., Chilton, N. B., Beveridge, I., McDonnell, A., Lichtenfels, J. R., and Gasser, R. B. (1997). Molecular delineation of *Cylicocyclus nassatus* and *C. ashworthi* (Nematoda: *Strongylidae). Int. J. Parasitol.* 27, 601–605. doi: 10.1016/S0020-7519(96)00192-0

Hung, G. C., Chilton, N. B., Beveridge, I., Zhu, X. Q., Lichtenfels, J. R., and Gasser, R. B. (1999a). Molecular evidence for cryptic species within *Cylicostephanus minutus* (Nematoda: Strongylidae). *Int. J. Parasitol.* 29, 285–291. doi: 10.1016/S0020-7519(98)00203-3

Hung, G. C., Gasser, R. B., Beveridge, I., and Chilton, N. B. (1999b). Species-specific amplification by PCR of ribosomal DNA from some equine strongyles. *Parasitol.* 119(Pt 1), 69–80.

Ionita, M., Howe, D. K., Lyons, E. T., Tolliver, S. C., Kaplan, R. M., Mitrea, I. L., et al. (2010). Use of a reverse line blot assay to survey small strongyle (Strongylida: Cyathostominae) populations in horses before and after treatment with ivermectin. *Vet. Parasitol.* 168, 332–337. doi: 10.1016/j.vetpar.2009.11.021

Kaplan, R. M. (2002). Anthelmintic resistance in nematodes of horses. *Vet. Res.* 33, 491–507. doi: 10.1051/vetres:2002035

Karger, A., Kampen, H., Bettin, B., Dautel, H., Ziller, M., Hoffmann, B., et al. (2012). Species determination and characterization of developmental stages of ticks by whole-animal matrix-assisted laser desorption/ionization mass spectrometry. *Ticks Tick Borne Dis.* 3, 78–89. doi: 10.1016/j.ttbdis.2011.11.002

Kaye, J. N., Love, S., Lichtenfels, J. R., and McKeand, J. B. (1998). Comparative sequence analysis of the intergenic spacer region of cyathostome species. *Int. J. Parasitol.* 28, 831–836. doi: 10.1016/S0020-7519(98)00031-9

Kharchenko, V., Kuzmina, T., Trawford, A., Getachew, M., and Feseha, G. (2009). Morphology and diagnosis of some fourth-stage larvae of cyathostomines (Nematoda: Strongyloidea) in donkeys *Equus asinus* L. from Ethiopia. *Syst. Parasitol.* 72, 1–13. doi: 10.1007/s11230-008-9152-8

Kooyman, F. N. J., van Doorn, D. C. K., Geurden, T., and Wagenaar, J. A. (2016). Semi-quantitative differentiation of cyathostomin larval cultures by reverse line blot. *Vet. Parasitol.* 216, 59–65. doi: 10.1016/j.vetpar.2015.12.009

Kornaś, S., Gawor, J., Cabaret, J., Molenda, K., Skalska, M., and Nowosad, B. (2009). Morphometric identification of equid cyathostome (Nematoda: Cyathostominae) infective larvae. *Vet. Parasitol.* 162, 290–294. doi: 10.1016/j.vetpar.2009.03.018

Kuzmina, T. A., Kharchenko, V. A., Starovir, A. I., and Dvojnos, G. M. (2005). Analysis of the strongylid nematodes (Nematoda: Strongylidae) community after deworming of brood horses in Ukraine. *Vet. Parasitol.* 131, 283–290. doi: 10.1016/j.vetpar.2005.05.010

Kuzmina, T. A., and Kharchenko, V. O. (2008). Anthelmintic resistance in cyathostomins of brood horses in Ukraine and influence of anthelmintic treatments on strongylid community structure. *Vet. Parasitol.* 154, 277–288. doi: 10.1016/j.vetpar.2008.03.024

Lichtenfels, J. R. (1975). Helminths of Domestic Equids. Illustrated keys to genera and species with emphasis on North American forms. *Proc. Helminthol. Soc. Wash.* 42, 1–83.

Lichtenfels, J. R. (2008). Preface. *Vet. Parasitol.* 156, 1–3. doi: 10.1016/j.vetpar.2008.06.026

Lichtenfels, J. R., Gibbons, L. M., and Krecek, R. C. (2002). Recommended terminology and advances in the systematics of the Cyathostominea (Nematoda: Strongyloidea) of horses. *Vet. Parasitol.* 107, 337–342. doi: 10.1016/S0304-4017(02)00167-X

Lichtenfels, J. R., Kharchenko, V. A., and Dvojnos, G. M. (2008). Illustrated identification keys to strongylid parasites (Strongylidae: Nematoda) of horses, zebras and asses (Equidae). *Vet. Parasitol.* 156, 4–161. doi: 10.1016/j.vetpar.2008.04.026

Lichtenfels, J. R., Kharchenko, V. A., Krecek, R. C., and Gibbons, L. M. (1998). An annotated checklist by genus and species of 93 species level names for 51 recognized species of small strongyles (Nematoda: Strongyloidea: Cyathostominea) of horses, asses and zebras of the world. *Vet. Parasitol.* 79, 65–79. doi: 10.1016/S0304-4017(98)00149-6

Long, E. O., and Dawid, I. B. (1980). Repeated genes in eukaryotes. *Annu. Rev. Biochem.* 49, 727–764. doi: 10.1146/annurev.bi.49.070180.003455

Loos, A. (1900). Notizen zur Helminthologie Egyptens. III. Die Sclerostomen der Pferde und Esel in Egypten. *Cent. Bakteriol.* 1, 150–160–192.

Love, S., Murphy, D., and Mellor, D. (1999). Pathogenicity of cyathostome infection. *Vet. Parasitol.* 85, 113–122. doi: 10.1016/S0304-4017(99)00092-8

Lyons, E. T., Tolliver, S. C., and Collins, S. S. (2007). Study (1991 to 2001) of drug-resistant Population B small strongyles in critical tests in horses in Kentucky at the termination of a 40-year investigation. *Parasitol. Res.* 101, 689–701. doi: 10.1007/s00436-007-0535-6

Lyons, E. T., Tolliver, S. C., and Drudge, J. (1999). Historical perspective of cyathostomes: prevalence, treatment and control programs. *Vet. Parasitol.* 85, 97–112. doi: 10.1016/S0304-4017(99)00091-6

Lyons, E. T., Tolliver, S. C., Kuzmina, T. A., and Collins, S. S. (2010). Critical tests evaluating efficacy of moxidectin against small strongyles in horses from a herd for which reduced activity had been found in field tests in Central Kentucky. *Parasitol. Res.* 107, 1495–1498. doi: 10.1007/s00436-010-2025-5

Matthews, J. B. (2014). Anthelmintic resistance in equine nematodes. *Int. J. Parasitol. Drugs Drug Resis.* 4, 310–315. doi: 10.1016/j.ijpddr.2014.10.003

Mayer-Scholl, A., Murugaiyan, J., Neumann, J., Bahn, P., Reckinger, S., and Nöckler, K. (2016). Rapid identification of the foodborne pathogen Trichinella spp. by matrix-assisted laser desorption/ionization mass spectrometry. *PLoS ONE* 11:e0152062. doi: 10.1371/journal.pone.0152062

McDonnell, A., Love, S., Tait, A., Lichtenfels, J. R., and Matthews, J. B. (2000). Phylogenetic analysis of partial mitochondrial cytochrome oxidase c subunit I and large ribosomal RNA sequences and nuclear internal transcribed spacer I sequences from species of Cyathostominae and Strongylinae (Nematoda, Order Strongylida), parasites of the horse. *Parasitology* 121, 649–659. doi: 10.1017/s003118200000696x

McWilliam, H. E. G., Nisbet, A. J., Dowdall, S. M. J., Hodgkinson, J. E., and Matthews, J. B. (2010). Identification and characterisation of an immunodiagnostic marker for cyathostomin developing stage larvae. *Int. J. Parasitol.* 40, 265–275. doi: 10.1016/j.ijpara.2009.08.004

Mitchell, M. C., Tzelos, T., Handel, I., McWilliam, H. E. G., Hodgkinson, J. E., Nisbet, A. J., et al. (2016). Development of a recombinant protein-based ELISA for diagnosis of larval cyathostomin infection. *Parasitology* 143, 1055–1066. doi: 10.1017/S0031182016000627

Molin, R. (1861). Il sottordine degli acrofalli ordinato scientificamente secondo i risultamenti delle indagini anatomiche ed embrigeniche. *Mem. R. Ist. Veneto Sc. Lett Arti* 9, 427–633.

Murphy, D., and Love, S. (1997). The pathogenic effects of experimental cyathostome infections in ponies. *Vet. Parasitol.* 70, 99–110. doi: 10.1016/S0304-4017(96)01153-3

Nielsen, M. K., Reinemeyer, C. R., Donecker, J. M., Leathwick, D. M., Marchiondo, A. A., and Kaplan, R. M. (2014). Anthelmintic resistance in equine parasites-Current evidence and knowledge gaps. *Vet. Parasitol.* 204, 55–63. doi: 10.1016/j.vetpar.2013.11.030

Osterman Lind, E., Eysker, M., Nilsson, O., Uggla, A., and Höglund, J. (2003). Expulsion of small strongyle nematodes (cyathostomin spp) following deworming of horses on a stud farm in Sweden. *Vet. Parasitol.* 115, 289–299. doi: 10.1016/S0304-4017(03)00200-0

Perera, M. R., Vanstone, V. A., and Jones, M. G. (2005). A novel approach to identify plant parasitic nematodes using matrix-assisted laser desorption/ionization time-of-flight mass spectrometry. *Rapid Commun. Mass Spectrom.* 19, 1454–1460. doi: 10.1002/rcm.1943

Perera, M., Taylor, S., Jones, M., and Vanstone, V. (2009). Protein biomarkers to distinguish oat and lucerne races of the stem nematode, Ditylenchus dipsaci, with quarantine significance for Western Australia. *Nematology* 11, 555–563.doi: 10.1163/138855409X12465362560557

Santos, D. W., Dias de Castro, L. L., Giese, E. G., and Molento, M. B. (2016). Morphometric study of infective larvae of cyathostomins of horses and their distribution. *J. Equine Vet. Sci.* 44, 49–53. doi: 10.1016/j.jevs.2016.02.237

Singhal, N., Kumar, M., and Virdi, J. S. (2016). MALDI-TOF MS in clinical parasitology: applications, constraints and prospects. *Parasitology* 143, 1491–1500. doi: 10.1017/S0031182016001189

Smyth, J. D. (1990). *In Vitro Cultivation of Parasitic Helminths.* Boca Raton, FL: CRC Press Inc.

Tolliver, S. C. (2000). *A Practical Method of Identification of the North American Cyathostomes (Small Strongyles) in Equid in Kentucky.* Lexington: University of Kentucky, Department of Veterinary Science.

Traversa, D., Iorio, R., Klei, T. R., Kharchenko, V. A., Gawor, J., Otranto, D., et al. (2007). New method for simultaneous species-specific identification of equine strongyles (nematoda, strongylida) by reverse line blot hybridization. *J. Clin. Microbiol.* 45, 2937–2942. doi: 10.1128/JCM.00714-07

Traversa, D., Kuzmina, T., Kharchenko, V. A., Iorio, R., Klei, T. R., and Otranto, D. (2008). Haplotypic variability within the mitochondrial gene encoding for the cytochrome c oxidase 1 (cox1) of *Cylicocyclus nassatus* (Nematoda, Strongylida): evidence for an affiliation between parasitic populations and domestic and wild equid hosts. *Vet. Parasitol.* 156, 241–247. doi: 10.1016/j.vetpar.2008.05.031

Traversa, D., Milillo, P., Barnes, H., von Samson-Himmelstjerna, G., Schurmann, S., Demeler, J., et al. (2010). Distribution and species-specific occurrence of cyathostomins (Nematoda, Strongylida) in naturally infected horses from Italy, United Kingdom and Germany. *Vet. Parasitol.* 168, 84–92. doi: 10.1016/j.vetpar.2009.10.006

Von Samson-Himmelstjerna, G. (2012). Anthelmintic resistance in equine parasites - detection, potential clinical relevance and implications for control. *Vet. Parasitol.* 185, 2–8. doi: 10.1016/j.vetpar.2011.10.010

Wieser, A., Schneider, L., Jung, J., and Schubert, S. (2012). MALDI-TOF MS in microbiological diagnostics-identification of microorganisms and beyond (mini review). *Appl. Microbiol. Biotechnol.* 93, 965–974. doi: 10.1007/s00253-011-3783-4

Yssouf, A., Almeras, L., Raoult, D., and Parola, P. (2016). Emerging tools for identification of arthropod vectors. *Future Microbiol.* 11, 549–566. doi: 10.2217/fmb.16.5

Yssouf, A., Socolovschi, C., Flaudrops, C., Ndiath, M. O., Sougoufara, S., Dehecq, J. S., et al. (2013). Matrix-assisted laser desorption ionization - time of flight mass spectrometry: an emerging tool for the rapid identification of mosquito vectors. *PLoS ONE* 8:e72380. doi: 10.1371/journal.pone.0072380

5

Chronic *Toxoplasma gondii* Infection Exacerbates Secondary Polymicrobial Sepsis

*Maria C. Souza [1], Denise M. Fonseca [1], Alexandre Kanashiro [2], Luciana Benevides [1], Tiago S. Medina [1], Murilo S. Dias [1], Warrison A. Andrade [3], Giuliano Bonfá [1], Marcondes A. B. Silva [2], Aline Gozzi [4], Marcos C. Borges [4], Ricardo T. Gazzinelli [3], José C. Alves-Filho [2], Fernando Q. Cunha [2] and João S. Silva [1]**

[1] Department of Biochemistry and Immunology, Ribeirão Preto Medical School, University of São Paulo, São Paulo, Brazil, [2] Department of Pharmacology, Ribeirão Preto Medical School, University of São Paulo, São Paulo, Brazil, [3] Department of Medicine, University of Massachusetts Medical School, Worcester, MA, USA, [4] Department of Internal Medicine, Ribeirão Preto Medical School, University of São Paulo, São Paulo, Brazil

Edited by:
Kai Matuschewski,
Humboldt University of Berlin,
Germany

Reviewed by:
Frank C. Gibson, III,
University of Florida, USA
Serge Ankri,
Technion, Israel

***Correspondence:**
João S. Silva
jsdsilva@fmrp.usp.br

Sepsis is a severe syndrome that arises when the host response to an insult is exacerbated, leading to organ failure and frequently to death. How a chronic infection that causes a prolonged Th1 expansion affects the course of sepsis is unknown. In this study, we showed that mice chronically infected with *Toxoplasma gondii* were more susceptible to sepsis induced by cecal ligation and puncture (CLP). Although *T. gondii*-infected mice exhibited efficient control of the bacterial burden, they showed increased mortality compared to the control groups. Mechanistically, chronic *T. gondii* infection induces the suppression of Th2 lymphocytes via *Gata3*-repressive methylation and simultaneously induces long-lived IFN-γ-producing $CD4^+$ T lymphocytes, which promotes systemic inflammation that is harmful during CLP. Chronic *T. gondii* infection intensifies local and systemic Th1 cytokines as well as nitric oxide production, which reduces systolic and diastolic arterial blood pressures after sepsis induction, thus predisposing the host to septic shock. Blockade of IFN-γ prevented arterial hypotension and prolonged the host lifespan by reducing the cytokine storm. Interestingly, these data mirrored our observation in septic patients, in which sepsis severity was positively correlated to increased levels of IFN-γ in patients who were serologically positive for *T. gondii*. Collectively, these data demonstrated that chronic infection with *T. gondii* is a critical factor for sepsis severity that needs to be considered when designing strategies to prevent and control the outcome of this devastating disease.

Keywords: sepsis, septic shock, *Toxoplasma gondii*, coinfection, chronic disease

INTRODUCTION

The majority of studies regarding host-pathogen relationships have focused on the interaction of a single pathogen with its host. However, humans are commonly exposed recurrently or simultaneously to multiple pathogens (Jamieson et al., 2010; Telfer et al., 2010). Understanding how previous/simultaneous infections can modify the host immune response and consequently affect the outcome of a secondary infection is crucial to designing new therapeutic strategies to control coinfections.

Sepsis, a life-threatening disease associated with high morbidity and mortality worldwide, is caused by a dysregulation of the immune system to different infectious agents (Schmid et al., 2004). An uncontrolled infection induces a systemic inflammatory reaction that culminates in a cytokine storm. Such inflammatory mediators deregulate the cardiovascular system, cause vascular permeability, and lead to severe sepsis and septic shock characterized by severe hypotension, multi-organ failure, and death (Bone et al., 1997; Hotchkiss et al., 2009).

Toxoplasmosis is a highly prevalent protozoan infection, affecting approximately one-third of the world population (Robert-Gangneux and Darde, 2012). The oral route of infection favors the disruption of the intestinal epithelium caused by inflammatory stressors induced against the parasite and facilitates the spread of the parasite toward different target organs (Dubey et al., 1998; Montoya and Liesenfeld, 2004). Locally, innate cells express sensors such as Toll-like receptors (TLRs) that are indispensable to parasite recognition (Debierre-Grockiego et al., 2007; Andrade et al., 2013). *T. gondii* infection induces a scenario of intense inflammation, characterized by IFN-γ-producing long-lived $CD4^+$ and $CD8^+$ T lymphocytes (Gazzinelli et al., 1994; Mashayekhi et al., 2011; Hand et al., 2012). Although the parasite growth is controlled efficiently, it triggers intense tissue damage that is commonly harmful to the host (Mashayekhi et al., 2011). After the acute phase of infection, the parasite is maintained latently in the brain and skeletal muscle, leading to a chronic state (Munoz et al., 2011). This evidence suggests that long-lived *T. gondii*-induced lymphocytes have an intrinsic molecular programme that is promptly activated to release excessive amounts of IFN-γ after a secondary pathogenic exposure. Although clear evidence exists that sepsis modulates secondary infections (Nascimento et al., 2010), it is currently unknown whether previous infections can interfere with the sepsis outcome.

In this study, we showed that IFN-γ-producing lymphocytes induced by *T. gondii* parasites persist after the acute phase of infection and are deleterious during polymicrobial sepsis. Mechanistically, *T. gondii* infection is followed by *Gata3* methylation and increased transcription of IFN-γ-related genes in $CD4^+$ T cells, thus inducing long-lived memory T cells. The partial blockage of IFN-γ prevented massive cytokine production, arterial hypotension, and prolonged host lifespan. Notably, these data mirrored our observation in patients because elevated serum levels of IFN-γ correlate with sepsis severity. Additionally, patients serologically positive for *T. gondii* had increased serum levels of IFN-γ compared to patients who were serologically negative. These observations demonstrate that chronic infection with *T. gondii* aggravates the course of sepsis and opens new avenues to design strategies to control the severity of *T. gondii*-sepsis coinfection.

MATERIALS AND METHODS

Ethics Statement

The research was approved by the Ethics Committee on Animal Experiments of Ribeirão Preto Medical School (CETEA-107-2009) and the Institutional Animal Care and Use Committee of the University of Massachusetts Medical School (IACUC-2371-12). The study on human samples was approved by the Human Research Ethics Committee at Hospital das Clínicas of Faculdade de Medicina da Universidade de São Paulo (research protocol n°. 536/2008). After obtaining written informed consent from all of the patient's relatives, venous blood samples were collected.

Mice and Parasites

Female C57BL/6 mice were used. The low-virulent ME-49 strain of *T. gondii* was harvested from the brains of infected mice (Benevides et al., 2008). Since our major aim was to address sepsis susceptibility in chronically infected mice, we only used the ME-49 strain that allows mice to progress to chronic phase of infection.

Polymicrobial Sepsis Model

Sepsis was induced using a cecal ligation and puncture (CLP) model. Two punctures with sterile 21-G needles were used to standardize the sub-lethal sepsis (Benjamim et al., 2003; Nascimento et al., 2010).

Bacteria Count Determination and Leukocyte Migration to the Peritoneum

The quantification of the bacterial load in the blood and peritoneal exudates was performed at 6, 12, and 24 h after CLP. For these analyses, the animals were anesthetized, and blood was collected via cardiac puncture, following which the animals were euthanized in a CO_2 chamber. The peritoneal exudates were collected via an injection of 1.5 mL of PBS/EDTA into the peritoneal cavity. After the sample collection, 10 μL of blood or peritoneal wash without dilutions were plated on Mueller-Hinton agar (Difco Laboratories, Detroit, MI, US) and incubated at 37°C under aerobic conditions for 24 h. Colony-forming units (CFUs) were expressed as Log2 of CFU/10 μL of blood or peritoneal wash. All procedures were performed under sterile conditions (Nascimento et al., 2010). Leukocyte migration and differential count were assessed 6, 12, and 24 h after the induction of CLP. The cells present in the peritoneal cavity were harvested via washing of the peritoneal cavity using 1.5 ml of phosphate buffered saline (PBS) containing EDTA (1 mM). The total leukocyte counts were obtained with a cell counter (Coulter AC T series analyser, Coulter, Miami, FL), and the differential count was performed using flow cytometry (BD Immunocytometry System, Franklin Lakes, NJ, USA). The results were expressed as the number of total leukocytes, neutrophils or lymphocytes in the peritoneal cavity (Alves-Filho et al., 2006).

Histopathological Analyses

For pathological analyses, the gut was washed to remove the intestinal contents, and the ileum fragment was individually wrapped in a "Swiss roll," fixed in 10% formalin, embedded in paraffin and processed routinely for haematoxylin and eosin staining. Slides were imaged using light microscopy. The images were acquired with a digital camera (Leica DC300F, Switzerland) coupled to a microscope for histological analysis.

Flow Cytometry

All antibodies used for flow cytometry were purchased from BD Biosciences or eBiosciences and used according to the manufacturer's instructions. For neutrophil staining, Ly6G (FITC, 1A8), CD11c (APC-Cy7, N418), CD11b (PE Cy7, M170) and F4/80 (Percp Cy5, BM8) were used. For intracellular cytokine staining, CD3 (FITC, 145-2C11), CD4 (PercP, RM4-5), CD8 (PE Cy7, 53-6.7), IFN-γ (APC, XMG1.2) and TNF-α (PE, MP6X722) were used. For transcription factors, CD3 (FITC, 145-2C11), CD4 (APC Cy7, RM4-5), CD44 (PercP, IM7) and Tbet (Alexa 647, 4B10) or CD3 (PE, 145-2C11), CD4 (APC Cy7, RM4-5), CD44 (PercP, IM7), RorγT (APC, Q31-378) and Gata3 (Alexa 488, L50-823) were used. For memory cells, CD3 (PE, 145-2C11), CD4 (APC Cy7, RM4-5), CCR7 (Alexa 647, 3D12) and CD62L (FITC, MEL-14) were used. Briefly, tissue-isolated cells were incubated with monoclonal antibodies in buffer containing blocking antibody. For intracellular staining, the cells were harvested and plated with PMA-ionomycin and Brefeldin A (Golgi plug BD bioscience), and stained for flow cytometry analysis. After incubation, cells were fixed and permeabilized with the BD Cytofix/Cytoperm kit (BD Biosciences and eBiosciences, CA, USA). Cell acquisition was performed on the BD CANTO II cell analyser (BD Biosciences) using FACSDiva software (BD Biosciences), and data were analyzed using FlowJo software (Tree Star, Ashland, OR).

Measurement of Cytokine and Chemokine Levels

The levels of mouse TNF-α, IFN-γ, IL-6, and KC were measured using DuoSet ELISA kits (R&D Systems).

Induction of Colitis

Chronic dextran sodium sulfate (DSS) colitis was induced by administering 3% (w/v−1) DSS (molecular mass, 36–50 kDa; MP Biomedicals, OH) for 14 days, followed by 26 days of normal drinking water.

Antibody Treatment

The cytokine IFN-γ was neutralized by intraperitoneal (i.p.) injection of 10 μg of purified mAb 24 h before CLP. The mouse anti-IFN-γ mAb was purified from the ascites of mice injected with an anti-IFN-γ hybridoma (XMG1.2). Controls received 500 μg of normal rat IgG diluted in PBS. The IgG was isolated from naïve rats using protein G column purification.

Antibiotic Treatment

The broad-spectrum antibiotic treatment regimen was followed as described by Hand et al. (2012) with modifications. Briefly, each animal received a daily combination of 5 mg neomycin trisulfate (Sigma), 2.5 mg vancomycin (Sigma), 5 mg metronidazole (sigma) and 5 mg ampicillin sodium (sigma) diluted in 200 μL water via oral gavage for 2 weeks before and 2 weeks post-infection with *T. gondii*.

Epigenetics Analysis

For cell isolation, $CD4^+$ T cells were negatively selected using the EasySep kit (StemCell Technologies, Canada), and DNA extraction was subsequently performed. The epigenetic analysis was performed using the PCR kit EpiTect Methyl II PCR Arrays (Qiagen Sciences, USA) to determine the methylated CpG islands and indicate the percentage of methylated DNA. The DNA in each individual enzymatic reaction was quantified using real-time PCR with primers that flanked the promoter region of interest as follows: *tbx21* - Chr11, CpG-start 96975880, CpG-end 96976654; *eomes* - Chr9, CpG-start 1183859814, CpG-end 118386331; *gata3* - Chr2, CpG-start 9802719, CpG-end 9803061 and *rora* - Chr9, CpG-start 68501352, CpG-end 68502769.

Blood Pressure Analysis

Arterial blood pressure was non-invasively measured by determining the tail blood volume with a pressure recording sensor and an occlusion tail cuff (CODA System, Kent Scientific, CT) 24 h after CLP. The results were expressed in millimeters of mercury (mmHg).

Patient Samples and Experiments

The patients' blood was collected in the first 24 h after admission. The samples were processed and analyzed for cytokine production and *Toxoplasma gondii* serology. The levels of the cytokine IFN-γ were measured using DuoSet ELISA as indicated by the manufacturer's instructions (R&D Systems). The *Toxoplasma gondii* serology was performed by indirect immunofluorescence assay as indicated by the manufacturer's instructions (FLUOCON IgG/IgM WAMA, Belgium).

Statistics

The animal survival was expressed as the percentage of surviving animals analyzed using the Mantel-Cox log-rank test (X_2, chi-squared). For comparison of multiple parametric data, the variance (ANOVA) tests were used followed by the *post-hoc* Tukey-Kramer test. Data are expressed as the means ± standard error of the mean (SEM). Statistical analysis and graphics were performed using the GraphPad Prism version 5.0 (GraphPad Software, San Diego, CA, USA).

RESULTS

Chronic *T. gondii* Infection Increases the Susceptibility to Polymicrobial Sepsis

Mice chronically infected with *T. gondii* for 40 days were subjected to sublethal sepsis induced by CLP surgery (coinfected mice). Herein, we observed increased mortality of coinfected mice compared to sublethal CLP-subjected mice (**Figure 1A**). These data indicate that chronic *T. gondii* infection aggravated polymicrobial sepsis, which was not due to toxoplasmosis reactivation (Figures S1A,B).

To investigate whether coinfected mice were able to control bacterial proliferation, the bacterial burden was quantified in the blood and peritoneum. We found that 24 h after CLP, coinfected mice were more efficient in controlling bacterial replication both systemically (**Figure 1B**) and locally (**Figure 1C**) compared to septic mice. Moreover, we counted the number of leukocytes recovered from the peritoneal cavity after CLP. The total leukocyte count strikingly decreased in the blood

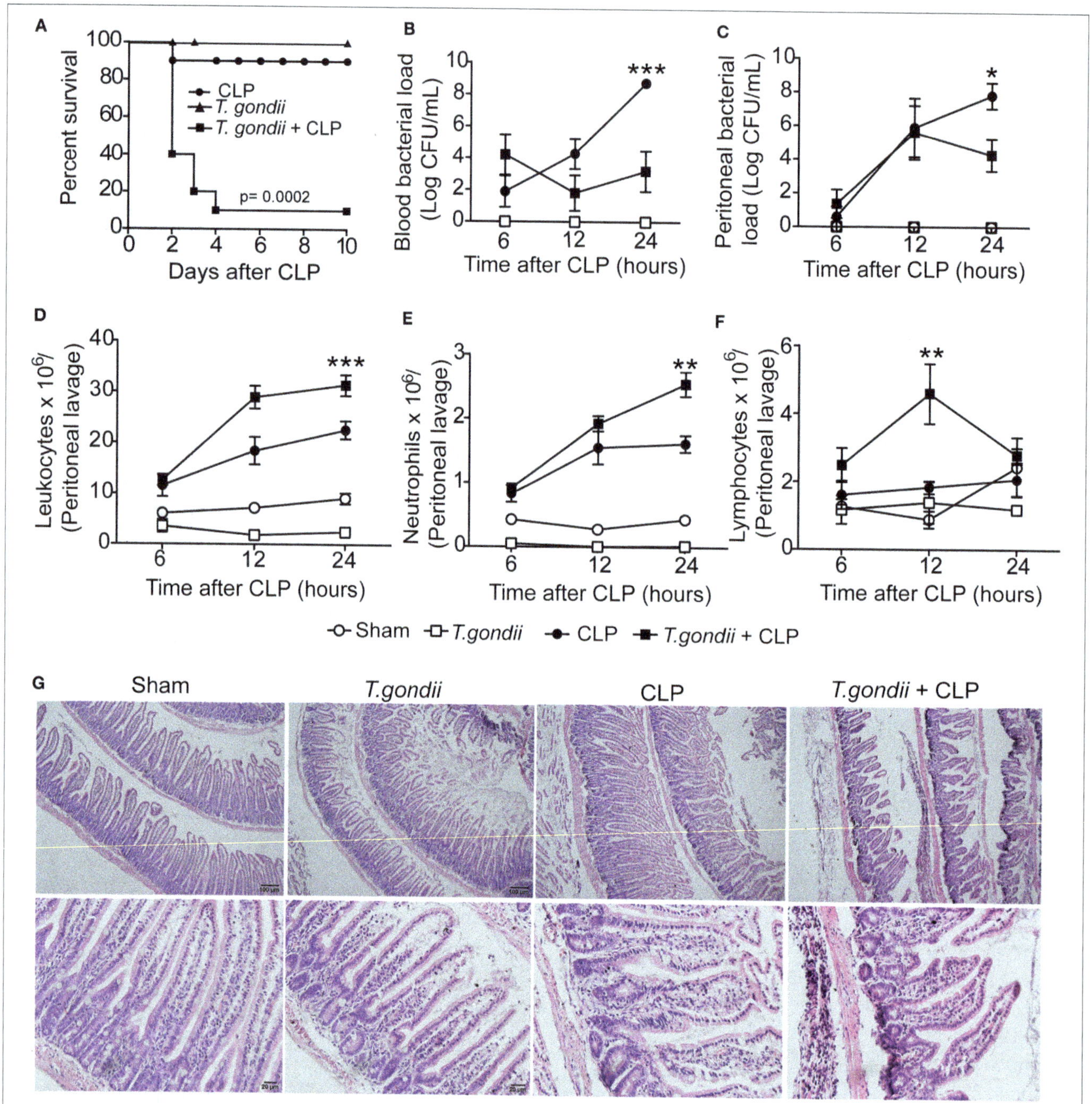

FIGURE 1 | Chronic *T. gondii* infection aggravates polymicrobial sepsis. Forty days after *T. gondii* infection, C57BL/6 mice were subjected to CLP for different analyses. The survival rate was evaluated until the 10th day post-CLP induction **(A)**. These data are representative of three independent experiments ($n = 10$), and the statistical analysis was determined using the Mantel-Cox log-rank test. The bacterial load was analyzed in the blood **(B)** and peritoneal lavage **(C)** at 6, 12, or 24 h post-CLP induction. The results are expressed as the log of the colony-forming units (CFU) per microliter. The leukocytes from the peritoneum **(D)** were stained with May-Grünwald Giemsa, and the number of neutrophils **(E)** and lymphocytes **(F)** were determined using a cell counter. Data are presented as the means ± SEM for 4 animals per group in four independent experiments (ANOVA, followed by Tukey's test; $^{*}p < 0.05$; $^{**}p < 0.01$; $^{***}p < 0.001$). At 24 h post-CLP, histopathological features of the ileum were analyzed after staining with haematoxylin and eosin (H&E). The results are representative of three independent experiments using 4 mice per group **(G)**.

of coinfected mice (data not shown); however, the leukocytes increased in the peritoneum of coinfected mice compared to septic mice (**Figure 1D**). The neutrophil recruitment to the peritoneal cavity was increased in coinfected mice compared to CLP-subjected mice (**Figure 1E**), which paralleled the bacterial clearance. We also observed increased migration of lymphocytes in mice 12 h after CLP (**Figure 1F**). To investigate whether intense cellular recruitment to the peritoneal cavity reflects intestinal inflammation and tissue damage, we evaluated the histological features in the intestine 24 h after sepsis induction. We found extensive neutrophil infiltrate mainly in the ileum of coinfected mice along with decreased mRNA expression of occludin, a tight junction protein (Figures S2A,B), and massive intestinal tissue damage (**Figure 1G**). These data suggest that chronic *T. gondii* infection promotes a microenvironment in the intestine that favors the inflammatory response during CLP. Notably, we did not find evidence of vital organ failure in coinfected mice, which was evaluated by either histopathological analysis or biochemical biomarkers for renal, hepatic, cardiac, and muscular dysfunctions.

Chronic *T. gondii* Infection Intensifies Proinflammatory Cytokine Production during Sepsis

The major factor leading to host susceptibility during sepsis is the increased production of inflammatory cytokines, which can promote septic shock (Ebong et al., 1999). To evaluate whether the high mortality of coinfected mice mirrored the production of inflammatory mediators, we quantified the cytokines in the serum and peritoneal lavage 24 h after CLP. Notably, coinfected mice showed increased levels of IFN-γ (**Figures 2A,E**), TNF-α (**Figures 2B,F**), IL-6 (**Figures 2C,G**), and KC (**Figures 2D,H**) in both the serum and peritoneal lavage compared to the control groups. For the immuneregulatory cytokines, IL-4 was not detected and the levels of IL-10 in the peritoneal lavage were similar in all groups studied. Splenic $CD4^+$ and $CD8^+$ T cells of *T. gondii*-infected mice produced elevated levels of IFN-γ and TNF-α even in the absence of a secondary stimulus (**Figures 3A–D**). Although the size of the spleen from *T. gondii*-infected mice was similar to naïve mice, after the induction of sepsis, *T. gondii*-infected mice experienced a notable reduction in spleen size along with a striking emergence of IFN-γ- and TNF-α-producing $CD4^+$ (**Figures 3E–G**) and $CD8^+$ (**Figures 3H–J**) T cells into the peritoneum. These data suggest that inflammatory cells were leaving the spleen/bloodstream and reaching the peritoneal cavity. Thus, *T. gondii*-programmed $CD4^+$ and $CD8^+$ T cells may be recruited to the site of sepsis and are the primary source of inflammatory mediators during sepsis in infected mice.

Long-Lived $CD4^+$ *T. gondii*-Primed T Cells Release IFN-γ and TNF-α during Sepsis

To further gain insights into the mechanisms by which chronic *T. gondii* infection aggravates sepsis, we assessed whether chronic infection maintained a pool of long-lived lymphocytes that act as first responders in polymicrobial sepsis. As expected, chronic *T. gondii* infection maintained a pool of $CD4^+$ and $CD8^+$ T cells ($CD4^+CD44^+$ and $CD8^+CD44^+$ T cells, respectively) independent of sepsis (Figures S3A,B), thus confirming that such cells were activated by *T. gondii*. Indeed, chronic infection deeply induced the transcription of IFN-γ-related genes, which

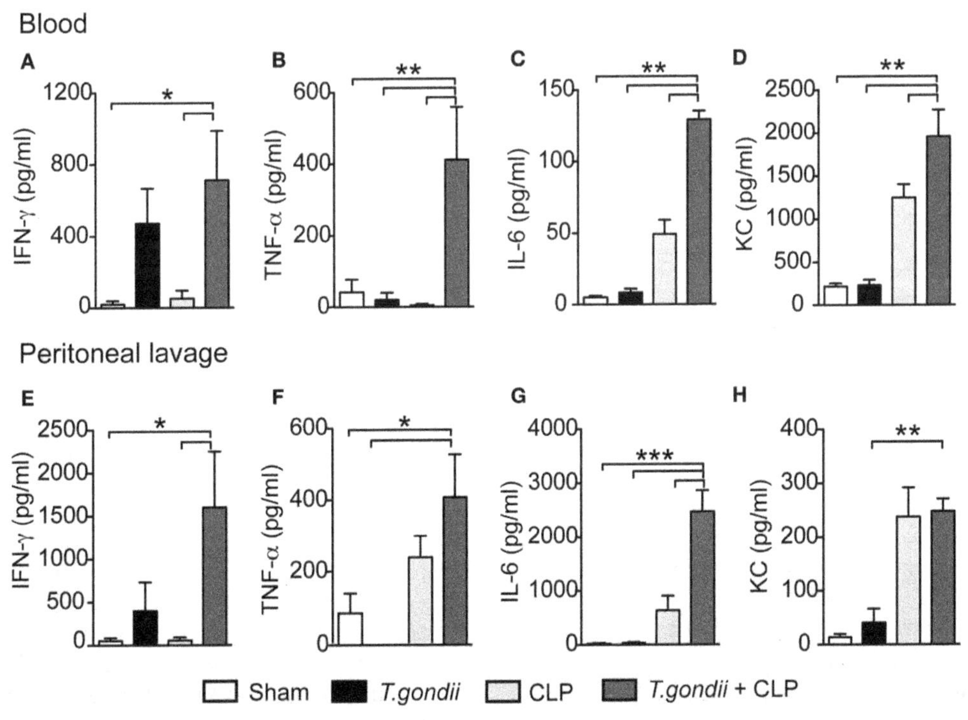

FIGURE 2 | The *T. gondii*-primed immune response promotes a storm of cytokines associated with CLP. C57BL/6 mice were infected with 5 cysts of *T. gondii*, and 40 days after infection, the mice were subjected to CLP. Twenty-four hours after CLP, the serum and peritoneal lavage were collected for cytokine analysis. The levels of pro-inflammatory cytokines IFN-γ **(A,E)**, TNF-α **(B,F)**, IL-6 **(C,G)**, and the chemokine KC **(D,H)** were determined using ELISA. Data are presented as the means ± SEM for 4 animals per group in three different experiments (ANOVA followed by Tukey's test; $^*p < 0.05$; $^{**}p < 0.01$; $^{***}p < 0.001$).

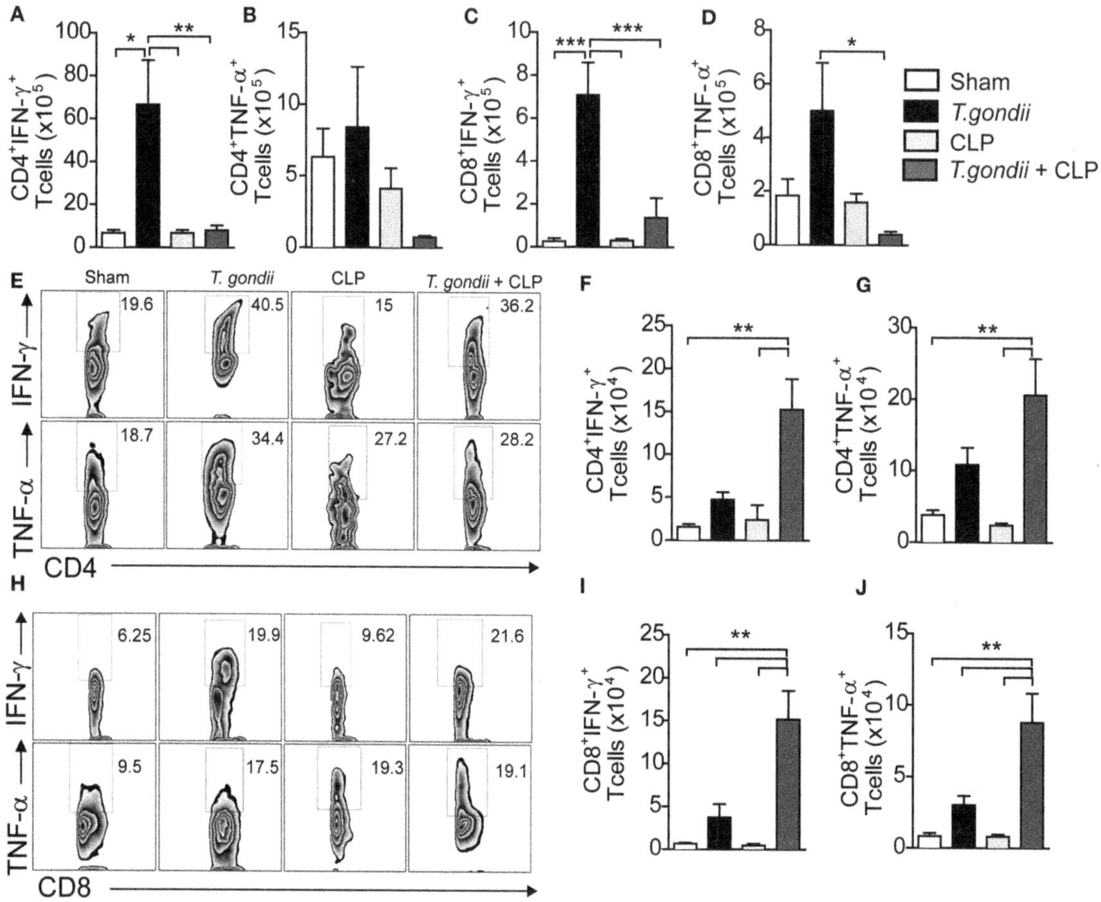

FIGURE 3 | The *T. gondii*-experienced CD4+ and CD8+ T cells are programmed to produce inflammatory mediators during sepsis. Naïve or chronically *T. gondii*-infected mice were subjected to CLP to evaluate the frequencies of IFN-γ- or TNF-α-producing $CD4^+$ and $CD8^+$ T cells in the spleen **(A–D)**. Peritoneal leukocytes were recovered from the peritoneal lavage 24 h after CLP, then stimulated with PMA-ionomycin, and stained for flow cytometry analysis **(E–J)**. Data are presented as the means ± SEM for 4 animals in three different experiments. Statistical analysis was performed using ANOVA followed by Tukey's test; $^*p < 0.05$; $^{**}p < 0.01$; $^{***}p < 0.001$.

were intensified during sepsis development (Figure S3C). As long-lived T cells comprise a pool of central and effector memory cells (Wherry et al., 2003), we explored whether *T. gondii* exposure maintained a pool of memory T cells during its chronic phase. Chronic *T. gondii* infection induced an increased number of $CD4^+CD44^{high}CD62L^+CCR7^+$ T lymphocytes, named here as central memory-like T lymphocytes (**Figures 4A,B**) that were converted to effector memory-like ($CD4^+CD44^{high}CD62L^-CCR7^-$) T lymphocytes after CLP surgery (**Figures 4C,D**). Herein, sepsis induction reactivated long-lived *T. gondii*-experienced T cells to produce IFN-γ and TNF-α in both the mesenteric lymph nodes (**Figures 4E,G**) and peritoneum (**Figures 4F,H**). To evaluate the involvement of microbiota in promoting long-lived T cells, we induced colitis with a classical intestinal stressor dextran sodium sulfate (DSS) to promote bacterial translocation followed by CLP. Surprisingly, DSS-induced bacterial translocation was unable to induce central and effector memory-like T lymphocytes (**Figures 4A–D**) and IFN-γ and TNF-α production after sepsis induction (**Figures 4E–H**). These results rule out a potential role of the microbiota in generating deleterious long-lived T cells that cross-react against released bacteria via CLP.

Chronically *T. gondii*-Infected Mice Develop Hypotension during Sepsis

T. gondii-primed $CD4^+$ T lymphocytes are polarized toward a Th1 profile (Gazzinelli et al., 1994), and recently, it was demonstrated that IFN-γ suppresses permissive chromatin remodeling in the regulatory region of the *Il4* gene (Nishida et al., 2013). To test whether the microenvironment elicited by chronic toxoplasmosis could promote epigenetic reprogramming of lymphocytes, we purified splenic $CD4^+$ T cells and investigated the repressive methylation status of their transcription factors. During the chronic phase of *T. gondii* infection, *Gata3* was found significantly methylated compared to the naïve $CD4^+$ T splenic cells (**Figure 5A**). Additionally, repressive methylation of Th17- (*Rora*) and Th1-associated transcription factors (*Tbx21* and *Eomes*) were undetectable in chronically infected mice (**Figure 5A**). The epigenetic changes observed indicate that Th1-induced expression can be due to *Gata3* repression. This provides

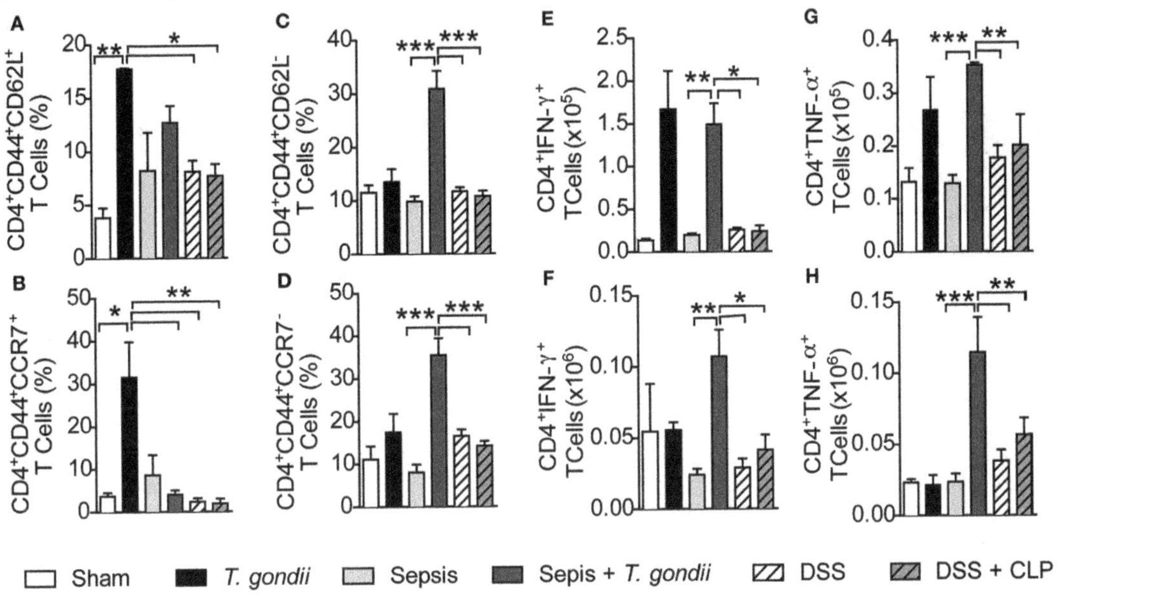

FIGURE 4 | *T. gondii*-infected mice induce long-lived CD4$^+$ T cells that are reactivated during sepsis. C57BL/6 mice were infected with 5 cysts of *T. gondii* or treated with 3% dextran sodium sulfate (DSS) to induce colitis. After 40 days of *T. gondii* infection or DSS treatment, the animals were subjected to CLP. The frequency of central memory-like (CD4$^+$CD44$^+$CD62L$^+$ or CCR7$^+$) **(A,B)** and effector memory-like (CD4$^+$CD44$^+$CD62L$^-$ or CCR7$^-$) **(C,D)** T cells was quantified in the mesenteric lymph nodes of control, coinfected, and colitis-induced mice. IFN-γ- or TNF-α-producing CD4$^+$ T cells were recovered from the mesenteric lymph nodes **(E,G)** or peritoneal lavage and quantified **(F,H)**. Data are presented as the means ± SEM for 4 animals in three different experiments. The lymphocytes were analyzed using flow cytometry, and statistical analysis was performed using ANOVA followed by Tukey's test; $^*p < 0.05$; $^{**}p < 0.01$; $^{***}p < 0.001$.

further evidence for our hypothesis that *Gata3* repression during *T. gondii* infection drives the immune response toward a Th1 pattern. To characterize whether CD4$^+$ T lymphocytes are driven to long-lived Th1 lymphocytes during the chronic infection, we analyzed the transcription factors expressed by the Th1 lymphocytes (*Tbet*). We observed that the *T. gondii*-induced inflammatory milieu reprogrammed naïve CD4$^+$ T lymphocytes into long-lived Th1 lymphocytes independent of CLP (**Figure 5B**). In contrast, *T. gondii*-primed T cells did not express significant amounts of the transcription factors *Rorγt* and *Gata3* with or without a secondary infection, which excludes the role of long-lived Th17 and Th2 cells in our model.

Nitric oxide (NO) production and the subsequent cytokine storm induced during sepsis are major inductors of hypotension and septic shock (Bone et al., 1997). Indeed, we detected increased NO production in coinfected mice compared to CLP-subjected mice (Figure S4). Since coinfected mice also had increased inflammatory cytokines, mainly IFN-γ, we explored whether chronic *T. gondii* infection could aggravate sepsis by reducing systolic and diastolic arterial blood pressures. Only coinfected mice developed hypotension through the reduction of systolic and diastolic blood pressures (**Figure 5C**). Moreover, the partial blockage of IFN-γ prevented hypotension in these mice (**Figure 5C**).

Recent data have revealed that *T. gondii* infection promotes long-lived IFN-γ-producing microbiota-specific CD4$^+$ T cells (Hand et al., 2012). To verify a possible role of the microbiota in controlling arterial blood pressure of coinfected mice, we treated them with broad-spectrum antibiotics to prevent bacterial translocation during the acute phase of *T. gondii* infection. We found that depletion of the microbiota did not prevent cytokine production and arterial hypotension (**Figure 5C**). These observations reveal that chronic *T. gondii* infection intensifies the plethora of cytokines during sepsis and predisposes the host to septic shock. Since the blockade of IFN-γ prevented host hypotension, we evaluated whether treatment with monoclonal anti-IFN-γ antibody could prevent the susceptibility of coinfected mice. The pretreatment with 10 μg/kg of anti-IFN-γ significantly improved the survival of these mice (**Figure 5D**).

Positive Serology for Toxoplasmosis Increases IFN-γ during Sepsis

To determine whether the IFN-γ-mediated mechanism described in coinfected mice is also observed in coinfected humans, we collected the blood of patients with sepsis to test the serology for toxoplasmosis and to measure IFN-γ production. Our data showed that patients with more severe clinical forms of sepsis had increased IFN-γ serum levels (**Figures 6A,B**), which strongly supports that IFN-γ production contributes to sepsis severity. In addition, patients serologically positive for toxoplasmosis had increased levels of IFN-γ during sepsis compared to serologically negative patients or healthy controls (**Figure 6C**). Similarly, previous exposure to *T. gondii* was deleterious to the host because mortality was increased in coinfected patients compared to patients who were serologically negative for toxoplasmosis (**Figure 6D**). Collectively, our data supports the hypothesis that

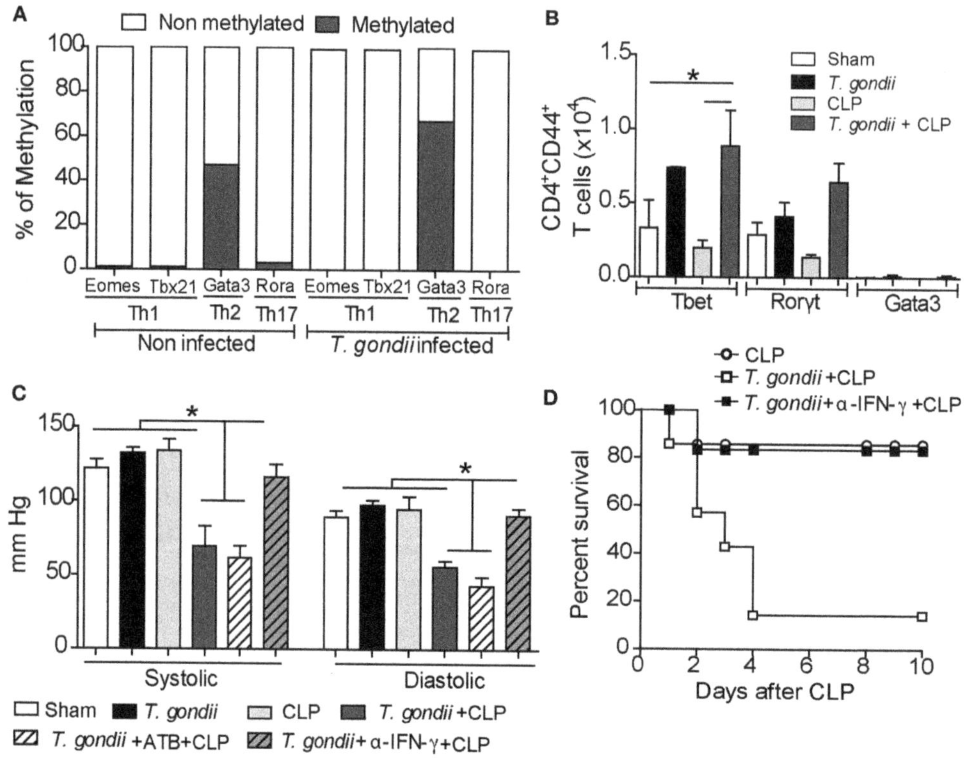

FIGURE 5 | Treatment with anti-IFN-γ prevents hypotension and ameliorates host survival. For the methylation analysis, $CD4^+$ T cells were separated from spleen cells by negative selection for DNA extraction. The pattern of DNA methylation was determined using the EpiTect Methyl II PCR Arrays kit. This analysis was performed in two independent trials, and the variation rate ≥ 10% was considered significant **(A)**. The expression of the transcription factors *T-bet*, *Gata-3* and *RorγT* was determined in $CD44^{high}CD4^+$ T cells using flow cytometry **(B)**. For blood pressure analysis, a group of coinfected mice was pretreated with broad-spectrum antibiotics (ATB) 2 weeks before and after *T. gondii* infection, and another group was treated with anti-IFN-γ antibodies 24 h before CLP induction. After 40 days of *T. gondii* infection, the mice were subjected to CLP, and at 24 h post-CLP, the blood pressure (mmHg) was evaluated in the animal tail using a sphygmomanometer **(C)**. The bars represent the means ± SEM for 4 animals per group ($^*p < 0.05$). The survival assay was monitored for 10 days after treatment with a 10 μg/kg dose of anti-IFN-γ antibodies **(D)**. The results are expressed as a percentage of survival, and the *p*-value was considered when comparing chronic *T. gondii* infected/CLP mice who received antibody treatment vs. animals that were not treated.

patients with positive serology for toxoplasmosis are at risk for the development of severe sepsis.

DISCUSSION

Several studies demonstrated that a variety of outcomes is possible during a secondary infection, depending on the route of infection, the type of pathogen, or even the temporal proximity (Gardner, 1981; Navarini et al., 2006; Barton et al., 2007; Gumenscheimer et al., 2007; Humphreys et al., 2008; Miller et al., 2009; Jamieson et al., 2010; Fenoy et al., 2012). In this context, the involvement of a chronic infection followed by acute infections has been poorly explored. *T. gondii* creates a scenario of intense intestinal inflammation featured by the high prevalence of Th1 lymphocytes. Similarly, sepsis is a multifactorial disease characterized by systemic inflammatory response syndrome (SIRS). In the present study, considering their worldwide prevalence and their inflammatory condition, we conjectured that patients serologically positive for toxoplasmosis could aggravate the outcome of sepsis by intensifying the inflammatory response. Surprisingly, the majority of patients who died of septic shock were serologically positive for toxoplasmosis, which led us to investigate the cellular and humoral mechanisms involved in the immune response in mice that were chronically infected with *T. gondii* during sepsis development.

Leukocytes are required to control bacterial replication during a microorganism's invasion (Reddy and Standiford, 2010; Kovach and Standiford, 2012). Interestingly, although mice chronically infected with *T. gondii* were more susceptible to sepsis, they had better control of bacterial proliferation by enhancing leukocyte recruitment to the site of infection, suggesting that the infection provides intrinsic factors for modulating the host immune response that can interfere with the outcome of sepsis. This phenomenon can be possible because the inflammation developed during *T. gondii* infection is maintained during its chronic phase and interferes with the outcome of the secondary infection caused by CLP. Interestingly, this phenomenon is specific of *T. gondii*, since other protozoa as *Trypanosoma cruzi*, *Plasmodium chabaudi*, or even a fungus, *Paracoccidiodes brasiliensis*, do not induce an increased susceptibility to sepsis in mice.

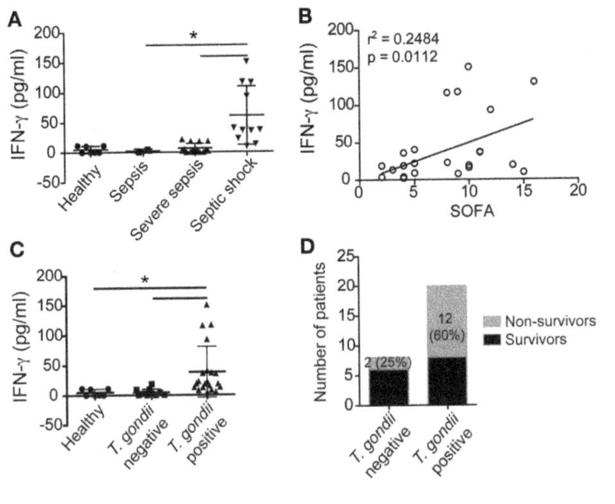

FIGURE 6 | Patients exposed to *T. gondii* have increased INF-γ during sepsis. The serum concentrations of IFN-γ in septic patients or healthy individuals (healthy = 7, sepsis = 2, severe sepsis = 15, and septic shock = 11) were determined using ELISA **(A–C)**. The data shown are the mean values of individual subjects from triplicate experiments **(A–C)**. The statistical analysis was performed using ANOVA followed by Tukey's test; $^*p < 0.05$. Linear regression analysis of the means of IFN-γ from septic patients in relationship to changes in the Sepsis-related Organ Failure Assessment (SOFA) scores are shown ($r^2 = 0.2484$; $p < 0.0112$) **(B)**. The number of non-survivors is presented as a percentage **(D)**.

It is well known that $CD4^+$ and $CD8^+$ memory T cells are essential for the control of *T. gondii* proliferation, preventing the de-encystation and reactivation of the disease (Gazzinelli et al., 1992). Our findings revealed that *T. gondii* infection robustly induces long-lived IFN-γ- and TNF-α-producing $CD4^+$ and $CD8^+$ T cells that are maintained, reprogrammed and amplified to act against a secondary challenge of sepsis. Our data suggests that central memory-like T cells are induced and maintained in the secondary lymphoid organs during chronic *T. gondii* infection by expressing the surface receptors CCR7 and CD62L. After sepsis induction, such cells are reprogrammed and quickly converted to effector memory-like cells by reducing their expression of both CCR7 and CD62L, which facilitates their migration to peripheral organs where they produce robust amounts of NO, IFN-γ and TNF-α to control the bacterial burden.

There are several factors that must be considered when analyzing *T. gondii* oral infection. During its acute phase, intestinal injury is responsible for the transient release of bacterial microbiota in the mesenteric lymph nodes, spleen, and liver, thereby triggering the activation and differentiation of memory cells that are specific not only for the parasite but also for antigens of the microbiota (Benson et al., 2009; Hand et al., 2012). Nevertheless, we showed that bacterial translocation did not influence the outcome of sepsis severity because intestinal damage induced by DSS did not induce memory cells or interfere with the host survival after CLP. Thus, the presence of long-lived *T. gondii*-experienced $CD4^+$ and $CD8^+$ T cells was more influential in aggravating sepsis than bacterial translocation.

Oral *T. gondii* infection induces highly inflammatory responses that dysregulate the intestinal epithelium and cause ileitis (Craven et al., 2012). Our findings support that inflammation due to chronic *T. gondii* infection aggravated the intestinal tissue damage after CLP. Such characteristic features promote a synergistic cytokine effect that can lead to septic shock (Fong et al., 1989; Calandra and Glauser, 1990; Dofferhoff et al., 1991; Dinarello, 1997). Chronic *T. gondii* infection promoted the overexpression of IFN-γ-related genes, which were exacerbated by CLP. Indeed, the blockade of IFN-γ prevented hypotension and improved the host survival upon sepsis induction.

Recent studies have shown that epigenetic changes, such as methylation, can induce gene silencing and heterochromatin remodeling that inhibits the access of transcription factors to DNA (Jaenisch and Bird, 2003; Esteller, 2007; Gómez-Díaz et al., 2012; Fernández-Sánchez et al., 2013). Here, *T. gondii* infection promoted the methylation of the *gata3* gene, which inhibited access to this gene and impaired the Th2 immune response, what could explain the absence of IL-4 in the peritoneum. IL-10 apparently does not take part of the immunoregulation, since it is produced equally in not infected or infected groups. In contrast, the *Tbx21* and *Eomes* genes were not inhibited by the methylation process, which facilitated the induction of the Th1 immune response and its maintenance during sepsis. Interestingly, naïve C57BL/6 mice exhibited 47% *gata3* methylation, which explains in part why such mice strains have an intrinsic susceptibility to pathogens that promote the Th1 immune response.

Since the overproduction of inflammatory cytokines is the primary cause of mortality in septic patients (Puneet et al., 2010), we reduced the robust inflammatory response using an IFN-γ monoclonal antibody. When subjects were treated with low doses of anti-IFN-γ, we observed a significant improvement in the survival rate of septic mice that were previously infected by *T. gondii*. These results support that although this cytokine is necessary to control chronic *T. gondii* infection (Gazzinelli et al., 1994), the overproduction of it may contribute to sepsis severity.

Robustness of systemic inflammation is the main factor that aggravates sepsis and predisposes patients to septic shock (Tumes et al., 2013). Our findings showed that previous exposure to *T. gondii* was a factor that intensified IFN-γ production and aggravated sepsis severity. Patients previously exposed to *T. gondii* had an increased mortality rate during sepsis compared to non-exposed patients. In this study, we proposed that serology for toxoplasmosis should be monitored in septic patients to predict sepsis severity. Because serology for toxoplasmosis is not time-consuming and laborious, it could be used to optimize the screening of sepsis severity.

In conclusion, we described that toxoplasmosis imprints intracellular signals that activate $CD4^+$ and $CD8^+$ T cells to produce IFN-γ. During infection, such cells are converted to memory-like T cells to maintain a pool of central memory-like $CD4^+$ T cells in secondary lymphoid organs. Our data suggest that during sepsis induction, central memory-like T cells specific to *T. gondii* are properly converted to effector memory-like T cells. Although their specificity against *T. gondii* is not impaired, such cells can cross-react against bacteria to control secondary bacterial infections. Nevertheless, the exacerbated systemic inflammatory response is deleterious to the host because it aggravates SIRS, leading to hypotension with consequent septic shock. Collectively, these data demonstrate that environmental features, such as previous chronic and non-lethal infections, may explain why sepsis has a broad spectrum of clinical forms.

AUTHOR CONTRIBUTIONS

MCS, DF, AK, LB, JA, FC, RG, and JS designed the study. MCS, DF, AK, LB, GB, MD, WA, and MABS performed the mouse experiments. MCS, AG, and MB provided the samples and performed the patient's experiments. MCS, AK, and TM wrote the manuscript. MCS, LB, AK, RG, and JS edited the manuscript.

FUNDING

This work was supported by the Coordination for the Improvement of Higher Education Personnel (CAPES) and the National Counsel of Technological and Scientific Development (CNPq). "The research leading to these results received funding from the Sao Paulo Research Foundation (FAPESP) under grant agreement n 2013/08216-2 (Center for Research in Inflammatory Disease), from the University of Sao Paulo NAP-DIN under grant agreement no. 11.1.21625.01.0."

ACKNOWLEDGMENTS

The authors would like to thank Cristiane Milanezi for technical support, as well as Vanessa Carregaro for providing anti-IFN-γ antibody.

REFERENCES

Alves-Filho, J. C., Freitas, A, Russo, M., and Cunha, F. Q. (2006). Toll-like receptor 4 signaling leads to neutrophil migration impairment in polymicrobial sepsis. *Crit. Care Med.* 34, 461–470. doi: 10.1097/01.CCM.0000198527.71819.E1

Andrade, W. A., Souza, M. C., Ramos-Martinez, E., Nagpal, K., Dutra, M. S., Melo, M. B., et al. (2013). Combined action of nucleic acid-sensing Toll-like receptors and TLR11/TLR12 heterodimers imparts resistance to *Toxoplasma gondii* in mice. *Cell Host Microbe* 13, 42–53. doi: 10.1016/j.chom.2012.12.003

Barton, E. S., White, D. W., Cathelyn, J. S., Brett-McClellan, K. A., Engle, M., Diamond, M. S., et al. (2007). Herpesvirus latency confers symbiotic protection from bacterial infection. *Nature* 447, 326–329. doi: 10.1038/nature05762

Benevides, L., Milanezi, C. M., Yamauchi, L. M., Benjamim, C. F., Silva, J. S., and Silva, N. M. (2008). CCR2 receptor is essential to activate microbicidal mechanisms to control *Toxoplasma gondii* infection in the central nervous system. *Am. J. Pathol.* 173, 741–751. doi: 10.2353/ajpath.2008.080129

Benjamim, C. F., Hogaboam, C. M., Lukacs, N. W., and Kunkel, S. L. (2003). Septic mice are susceptible to pulmonary aspergillosis. *Am. J. Pathol.* 163, 2605–2617. doi: 10.1016/S0002-9440(10)63615-2

Benson, A., Pifer, R., Behrendt, C. L., Hooper, L. V., and Yarovinsky, F. (2009). Gut commensal bacteria direct a protective immune response against *Toxoplasma gondii. Cell Host Microbe* 6, 187–196. doi: 10.1016/j.chom.2009.06.005

Bone, R. C., Grodzin, C. J., and Balk, R. A. (1997). Sepsis: a new hypothesis for pathogenesis of the disease process. *Chest* 112, 235–243. doi: 10.1378/chest.112.1.235

Calandra, T., and Glauser, M. P. (1990). Cytokines and septic shock. *Diagn. Microbiol. Infect. Dis.* 13, 377–381. doi: 10.1016/0732-8893(90)90006-H

Craven, M., Egan, C. E., Dowd, S. E., McDonough, S. P., Dogan, B., Denkers, E., et al. (2012). Inflammation drives dysbiosis and bacterial invasion in murine models of ileal Crohn's disease. *PLoS ONE* 7:e41594. doi: 10.1371/journal.pone.0041594

Debierre-Grockiego, F., Campos, M. A., Azzouz, N., Schmidt, J., Bieker, U., Resende, M. G., et al. (2007). Activation of TLR2 and TLR4 by glycosylphosphatidylinositols derived from *Toxoplasma gondii. J. Immunol.* 179, 1129–1137. doi: 10.4049/jimmunol.179.2.1129

Dinarello, C. A. (1997). Proinflammatory and anti-inflammatory cytokines as mediators in the pathogenesis of septic shock. *Chest* 112, 321S–329S. doi: 10.1378/chest.112.6_Supplement.321S

Dofferhoff, A. S., Vellenga, E., Limburg, P. C., van Zanten, A., Mulder, P. O., and Weits, J. (1991). Tumour necrosis factor (cachectin) and other cytokines in septic shock: a review of the literature. *Neth. J. Med.* 39, 45–62.

Dubey, J. P., Lindsay, D. S., and Speer, C. A. (1998). Structures of *Toxoplasma gondii* tachyzoites, bradyzoites, and sporozoites and biology and development of tissue cysts. *Clin. Microbiol. Rev.* 11, 267–299.

Ebong, S. J., Call, D. R., Bolgos, G., Newcomb, D. E., Granger, J. I., O'Reilly, M., et al. (1999). Immunopathologic responses to non-lethal sepsis. *Shock* 12, 118–126. doi: 10.1097/00024382-199908000-00005

Esteller, M. (2007). Epigenetic gene silencing in cancer: the DNA hypermethylome. *Hum. Mol. Genet.* 16, 50–59. doi: 10.1093/hmg/ddm018

Fenoy, I. M., Chiurazzi, R., Sánchez, V. R., Argenziano, M. A., Soto, A., Picchio, M. S., et al. (2012). *Toxoplasma gondii* infection induces suppression in a mouse model of allergic airway inflammation. *PLoS ONE* 7:e43420. doi: 10.1371/journal.pone.0043420

Fernández-Sánchez, A., Baragaño Raneros, A., Carvajal Palao, R., Sanz, A. B., Ortiz, A., Ortega, F., et al. (2013). DNA demethylation and histone H3K9 acetylation determine the active transcription of the NKG2D gene in human $CD8^+$ T and NK cells. *Epigenetics* 8, 66–78. doi: 10.4161/epi.23115

Fong, Y., Tracey, K. J., Moldawer, L. L., Hesse, D. G., Manogue, K. B., Kenney, J. S., et al. (1989). Antibodies to cachectin/tumor necrosis factor reduce interleukin 1 beta and interleukin 6 appearance during lethal bacteremia. *J. Exp. Med.* 170, 1627–1633. doi: 10.1084/jem.170.5.1627

Gardner, I. D. (1981). Suppression of antibacterial immunity by infection with influenza virus. *J. Infect. Dis.* 144, 225–231. doi: 10.1093/infdis/144.3.225

Gazzinelli, R. T., Wysocka, M., Hayashi, S., Denkers, E. Y., Hieny, S., Caspar, P., et al. (1994). Parasite-induced IL-12 stimulates early IFN-gamma synthesis and resistance during acute infection with *Toxoplasma gondii. J. Immunol.* 153, 2533–2543.

Gazzinelli, R., Xu, Y., Hieny, S., Cheever, A., and Sher, A. (1992). Simultaneous depletion of $CD4^+$ and $CD8^+$ T lymphocytes is required to reactivate chronic infection with *Toxoplasma gondii. J. Immunol.* 149, 175–180.

Gómez-Díaz, E., Jordá, M., Peinado, M. A., and Rivero, A. (2012). Epigenetics of host-pathogen interactions: the road ahead and the road behind. *PLoS Pathog.* 8:e1003007. doi: 10.1371/journal.ppat.1003007

Gumenscheimer, M., Balkow, S., Simon, M. M., Jirillo, E., Galanos, C., and Freudenberg, M. A. (2007). Stage of primary infection with lymphocytic choriomeningitis virus determines predisposition or resistance of mice to secondary bacterial infections. *Med. Microbiol. Immunol.* 196, 79–88. doi: 10.1007/s00430-006-0030-1

Hand, T. W., Dos Santos, L. M., Bouladoux, N., Molloy, M. J., Págan, A. J., Pepper, M., et al. (2012). Acute gastrointestinal infection induces long-lived microbiota-specific T cell responses. *Science* 337, 1553–1556. doi: 10.1126/science.1220961

Hotchkiss, R. S., Coopersmith, C. M., McDunn, J. E., and Ferguson, T. A. (2009). The sepsis seesaw: tilting toward immunosuppression. *Nat. Med.* 15, 496–497. doi: 10.1038/nm0509-496

Humphreys, T. D., Khanolkar, A., Badovinac, V. P., and Harty, J. T. (2008). Generation and maintenance of Listeria-specific $CD8^+$ T cell responses in perforin-deficient mice chronically infected with LCMV. *Virology* 370, 310–322. doi: 10.1016/j.virol.2007.08.038

Jaenisch, R., and Bird, A. (2003). Epigenetic regulation of gene expression: how the genome integrates intrinsic and environmental signals. *Nat. Genet.* 33, 245–254. doi: 10.1038/ng1089

Jamieson, A. M., Yu, S., Annicelli, C. H., and Medzhitov, R. (2010). Influenza virus-induced glucocorticoids compromise innate host defense against a secondary bacterial infection. *Cell Host Microbe* 7, 103–114. doi: 10.1016/j.chom.2010.01.010

Kovach, M. A., and Standiford, T. J. (2012). The function of neutrophils in sepsis. *Curr. Opin. Infect. Dis.* 25, 321–327. doi: 10.1097/QCO.0b013e32835 28c9b

Mashayekhi, M., Sandau, M. M., Dunay, I. R., Frickel, E. M., Khan, A., Goldszmid, R. S., et al. (2011). CD8a$^+$ dendritic cells are the critical source of interleukin-12 that controls acute infection by *Toxoplasma gondii* tachyzoites. *Immunity* 35, 249–259. doi: 10.1016/j.immuni.2011.08.008

Miller, C. M. D., Smith, N. C., Ikin, R. J., Boulter, N. R., Dalton, J. P., and Donnelly, S. (2009). Immunological interactions between 2 common pathogens, Th1-inducing protozoan *Toxoplasma gondii* and the Th2-inducing helminth *Fasciola hepatica*. *PLoS ONE* 4:e5692. doi: 10.1371/journal.pone.00 05692

Montoya, J. G., and Liesenfeld, O. (2004). Toxoplasmosis. *Lancet* 363, 1965–1976. doi: 10.1016/S0140-6736(04)16412-X

Munoz, M., Liesenfeld, O., and Heimesaat, M. M. (2011). Immunology of *Toxoplasma gondii*. *Immunol. Rev.* 240, 269–285. doi: 10.1111/j.1600-065X. 2010.00992.x

Nascimento, D. C., Alves-Filho, J. C., Sônego, F., Fukada, S. Y., Pereira, M. S., Benjamim, C., et al. (2010). Role of regulatory T cells in long-term immune dysfunction associated with severe sepsis. *Crit. Care Med.* 38, 1718–1725. doi: 10.1097/CCM.0b013e3181e78ad0

Navarini, A. A., Recher, M., Lang, K. S., Georgiev, P., Meury, S., Bergthaler, A., et al. (2006). Increased susceptibility to bacterial superinfection as a consequence of innate antiviral responses. *Proc. Natl. Acad. Sci. U.S.A.* 103, 15535–15539. doi: 10.1073/pnas.0607325103

Nishida, J., Li, Y., Zhuang, Y., Huang, Z., and Huang, H. (2013). IFN-gamma suppresses permissive chromatin remodeling in the regulatory region of the Il4 gene. *Cytokine* 62, 91–95. doi: 10.1016/j.cyto.2013.02.010

Puneet, P., Yap, C. T., Wong, L., Lam, Y., Koh, D. R., Moochhala, S., et al. (2010). SphK1 regulates proinflammatory responses associated with endotoxin and polymicrobial sepsis. *Science* 328, 1290–1294. doi: 10.1126/science.1188635

Reddy, R. C., and Standiford, T. J. (2010). Effects of sepsis on neutrophil chemotaxis. *Curr. Opin. Hematol.* 17, 18–24. doi: 10.1097/MOH.0b013e32833 338f3

Robert-Gangneux, F., and Dardé, M. L. (2012). Epidemiology of and diagnostic strategies for toxoplasmosis. *Clin. Microbiol. Rev.* 25, 264–296. doi: 10.1128/CMR.05013-11

Schmid, A., Pugin, J., Chevrolet, J. C., Marsch, S., Ludwig, S., Stocker, R., et al. (2004). Burden of illness imposed by severe sepsis in Switzerland. *Swiss Med. Wkly.* 134, 97–102.

Telfer, S., Lambin, X., Birtles, R., Beldomenico, P., Burthe, S., Paterson, S., et al. (2010). Species interactions in a parasite community drive infection risk in a wildlife population. *Science* 330, 243–246. doi: 10.1126/science.1190333

Tumes, D. J., Onodera, A., Suzuki, A., Shinoda, K., Endo, Y., Iwamura, C., et al. (2013). The polycomb protein Ezh2 regulates differentiation and plasticity of CD4$^+$ T helper type 1 and type 2 cells. *Immunity* 39, 819–832. doi: 10.1016/j.immuni.2013.09.012

Wherry, E. J., Teichgräber, V., Becker, T. C., Masopust, D., Kaech, S. M., Antia, R., et al. (2003). Lineage relationship and protective immunity of memory CD8 T cell subsets. *Nat. Immunol.* 4, 225–234. doi: 10.1038/ni889

6

Giardia's Epithelial Cell Interaction *In Vitro*: Mimicking Asymptomatic Infection?

Martin R. Kraft[1,2], Christian Klotz[1], Roland Bücker[2], Jörg-Dieter Schulzke[2] and Toni Aebischer[1]**

[1] Unit 16 Mycotic and Parasitic Agents and Mycobacteria, Robert Koch-Institute, Berlin, Germany, [2] Institute of Clinical Physiology, Charité Campus Benjamin Franklin, Berlin, Germany

Edited by:
Mario Alberto Rodriguez, Center for Research and Advanced Studies of the National Polytechnic Institute (CINVESTAV), Mexico

Reviewed by:
Maria Del Consuelo Gomez, Instituto Politécnico Nacional, Mexico
James H. McKerrow, University of California, San Diego, United States
Elisa Azuara-Liceaga, Universidad Autónoma de la Ciudad de México, Mexico

***Correspondence:**
Martin R. Kraft
kraftm@rki.de
Toni Aebischer
aebischera@rki.de

The protozoan parasite *Giardia duodenalis* is responsible for more than 280 million cases of gastrointestinal complaints ("giardiasis") every year, worldwide. Infections are acquired orally, mostly via uptake of cysts in contaminated drinking water. After transformation into the trophozoite stage, parasites start to colonize the duodenum and upper jejunum where they attach to the intestinal epithelium and replicate vegetatively. Outcome of *Giardia* infections vary between individuals, from self-limiting to chronic, and asymptomatic to severely symptomatic infection, with unspecific gastrointestinal complaints. One proposed mechanism for pathogenesis is the breakdown of intestinal barrier function. This has been studied by analyzing trans-epithelial electric resistances (TEER) or by indicators of epithelial permeability using labeled sugar compounds in *in vitro* cell culture systems, mouse models or human biopsies and epidemiological studies. Here, we discuss the results obtained mainly with epithelial cell models to highlight contradictory findings. We relate published studies to our own findings that suggest a lack of barrier compromising activities of recent *G. duodenalis* isolates of assemblage A, B, and E in a Caco-2 model system. We propose that this epithelial cell model be viewed as mimicking asymptomatic infection. This view will likely lead to a more informative use of the model if emphasis is shifted from aiming to identify *Giardia* virulence factors to defining non-parasite factors that arguably appear to be more decisive for disease.

Keywords: Giardia, giardiasis, TEER, barrier function, Caco-2, transwell, permeability

INTRODUCTION

Giardia duodenalis (also *Giardia lamblia* or *Giardia intestinalis*) is an ubiquitous protozoan parasite of the order diplomonadida and forms a species complex of eight different phylogenetic groups (assemblages) characterized by different host specificities. Assemblages A and B are infectious to humans and other mammals (Thompson and Monis, 2012). It is responsible for more than 280 million symptomatic cases of infection, i.e., cases of giardiasis associated with gastrointestinal malfunctions (see below), every year, worldwide. Infections are acquired by uptake of dormant cyst forms of the parasite mostly via contaminated drinking water, and highest prevalences are reported for countries with poor access to higher sanitation standards, though it is one of the most common reported parasitic infections in other countries as well. Since 2004, more attention is paid to this pathogen due to WHO's "Neglected Diseases Initiative" (Adam, 2001; Savioli et al., 2006; Ankarklev et al., 2010). *Giardia* sp. cysts transform into their trophozoite stage after passing the host's stomach and the latter forms colonize the duodenum and upper jejunum where they replicate, attach to the intestinal epithelium using their adhesive disc and feed on luminal nutrients.

THE CHALLENGE: SYMPTOMATIC VS. ASYMPTOMATIC INFECTIONS

In the context of this article, we define a symptomatic infection, i.e., giardiasis disease, as being characterized by acute gastrointestinal complaints, like diarrhea, abdominal pain, nausea, and vomiting (Adam, 2001; Ankarklev et al., 2010) and we like to distinguish it from asymptomatic infections defined by the absence of such acute symptoms. Asymptomatic infections according to this definition would include infections that—particularly if recurring—result in malabsorption/malnutrition phenotypes or may represent pure colonization without any pathology, which was recently shown by Garzon et al. (2017) on asymptomatic children, who found no correlation between *Giardia*-infection and barrier dysfunction, but only of barrier dysfunction and wasting and stunting. However, infections may also trigger post-infectious syndromes such as irritable bowel disease (D'Anchino et al., 2002; Wensaas et al., 2012; Hanevik et al., 2014; Litleskare et al., 2015; Halliez et al., 2016; Nakao et al., 2017).

The reasons for these fundamental differences of the outcomes of infections remain unclear (Adam, 2001; Troeger et al., 2007; Klotz and Aebischer, 2015; Tysnes and Robertson, 2015). A mechanism that was proposed to link to acute symptoms was the breakdown of the intestinal barrier function of the epithelium, leading to increased permeability with bacterial invasion as a possible result (Buret, 2007; Ankarklev et al., 2010). This was probably inspired by the impressive *in vitro* phenotypes obtained with certain bacterial, gastrointestinal pathogens and their products/toxins/proteases (Malago et al., 2003; Fajdiga et al., 2006; Rees et al., 2008; Liu et al., 2012; Anderson et al., 2013; Fiorentino et al., 2013) as well as other parasitic protozoans like *Entamoeba histolytica*, *Cryptosporidium parvum*, or *Blastocystis* sp. (Li et al., 1994; Leroy et al., 2000; Buret et al., 2003; Betanzos et al., 2014; Wu et al., 2014). It is fair to say that this has motivated numerous studies with the implicit goal of identifying a similar functional correlate of acutely symptomatic giardiasis in *in vitro* models. Here, we review *in vitro* investigations that aimed at finding such a robust correlate for acute clinical symptoms and conclude that, frustratingly, this goal was largely missed. We hypothesize that this is because these models reproduce the prevailing inconspicuous course of *G. duodenalis* infection, rather than one that is associated with acute symptoms. We propose, as others did (Bartelt and Sartor, 2015), that non-parasite factors in combination with *G. duodenalis* infection are most likely causing acute symptoms and adapting *in vitro* models to search for such factors should be attempted. We also propose that a number of epithelial functions that may give insight into non-acute but probably more relevant symptoms linked to malabsorption/malnutrition phenotypes have not yet been investigated *in vitro* but should become a focus of future work.

Two studies can serve to illustrate the dilemma that we face when trying to define pathological correlates of *Giardia* infection at the histological/cellular level. One study performed by Oberhuber et al. (1997) analyzed 567 *Giardia*-positive cases identified in a retrospective study of gastrointestinal biopsy samples collected consecutively over an eight-year period in the frame of a gastrointestinal pathology service in Germany. This number of *Giardia* positive cases represented ~0.3% of all samples analyzed in that period. Reasons for soliciting histopathological analyses were described as follows: "most of the patients experienced unspecific gastrointestinal complaints that prompted an upper endoscopy" (Oberhuber et al., 1997). The authors conclude that "the histology of the small-bowel mucosa is inconspicuous in most subjects with giardiasis." It is reasonable to assume that such a consecutive study on biopsies sampled a random cross-sectional collection of mostly adult patients and therefore, it is justified to conclude that most *Giardia*-infections do not lead to acute symptoms. In contrast, a study focusing on acutely symptomatic cases reported epithelial barrier dysfunction, altered *tight junction* composition, and increased signs of apoptosis (Troeger et al., 2007).

Epidemiological Findings on Epithelial Dysfunction

There have been several epidemiological studies investigating functional correlates of disease such as gut permeability in different patient collectives suffering from *G. duodenalis* infection. Very recently Rogawski et al. (2017) and Kosek (2017), through a multisite birth-cohort study, showed that persisting infection within the first 6 months of life was correlated with reduced weight and height for age Z scores at 2 years of age. However, this was not dependent on diarrhea, i.e., independent of acutely symptomatic infection. More likely, stunting was the result of changes to gut permeability, assessed by Lactulose (L) and mannitol (M) excretion assays according to which permeability was positively correlated with parasite detection, which agrees with some earlier findings (Dagci et al., 2002; Goto et al., 2002) but contradicts others (Serrander et al., 1984; Campbell et al., 2004; Goto et al., 2009). Even studies using the same method vary in their results. For example, Goto et al. (2002) assessed in a cross-sectional study intestinal parasite infection and permeability of 210 Nepali children aged 0–60 months who were living in poor conditions. Fourteen percent of 173 were acutely infected with *Giardia*. L:M ratios suggested increased permeability in *Giardia*-infected (0.43; $n = 8$) compared to uninfected children (0.25; $n = 45$; $p = 0{,}014$). However, standard deviations were very high and the stepwise multiple and logistic regression analyses used is known to be prone to type I errors (Burnham and Anderson, 2004). On the other hand, in a later longitudinal study by Goto et al. (2009) the examination of 298 children from Bangladesh until their second year of age and with comparable living conditions did not find a correlation of L:M ratios and *Giardia*-infection. Similar results were found in Gambian children (2–15 months of age) by another longitudinal L:M study by Campbell et al. (2004). In other studies, even a negative correlation of *Giardia*-infection to severe diarrhea could be observed (Bilenko et al., 2004; Kotloff et al., 2013; Muhsen et al., 2014).

Overall, epidemiological evidence for altered permeability as a consequence of frequent *G. duodenalis* infection exists. Effects are weak and appear to be inconsistent probably because data are confounded by non-acute, asymptomatic cases included in studied patient collectives. However, the evidence is rather against *G. duodenalis* infection alone as being a clear cause of acute symptoms such as diarrhea. In view of this data, the quest is open for improved *in vitro* models and respective readout parameters that may link to distinct symptoms, such as changes of permeability, molecular transport, and absorption mechanisms.

Investigations of Epithelial Barrier Functions *in Vitro*

Thinking of giardiasis disease as being linked to different syndromes of altered gut barrier function, acute and non-acute, should allow derivation of distinct readout parameters as proxies for the diverse symptoms when interrogating *in vitro* cell culture models with *Giardia* parasites. Current readouts include probing electrophysiological properties of epithelial cell monolayers such as trans-epithelial electric resistance (TEER), assessing transport and permeability changes using tracer molecules, or inferring monolayer integrity from changes of abundance and localization of proteins that make up *tight junctions* (**Figure 1**). In addition, epithelial tissues also function as communication layers relaying signals to other organs such as the immune system, and cyto- and chemokine responses were also used as readout parameters to characterize the effect of infection.

TEER as a Surrogate of Acute Effects on Tissue Integrity

The measurement of TEER as an indicator for paracellular permeability is a well-accepted method to estimate acute pathophysiological effects on cell barrier function of intestinal epithelial cells (Srinivasan et al., 2015). An important prerequisite for a robust readout is the presence of an electro-physiologically intact monolayer. TEER measurements to investigate the effect of *Giardia* trophozoites on epithelial function have been used by several groups in diverse setups but were implemented with possibly relevant experimental differences (Supplementary Table 1). Our own data (**Figure 2**) suggest that exposure of Caco-2 cells *in vitro* to diverse *G. duodenalis* isolates derived from samples of symptomatic patients does not affect epithelial monolayer integrity. This is in good agreement with some previous studies (Chavez et al., 1986, 1995; Tysnes and Robertson, 2015) but is in contrast to others (Teoh et al., 2000; Humen et al., 2011; Maia-Brigagao et al., 2012), who described a TEER decrease of up to 45%. If one assumes, as also proposed by others (Bartelt and Sartor, 2015), that *G. duodenalis* infection alone is insufficient to cause acute disease and, therefore, that infections are mostly asymptomatic, then one would not expect an effect on TEER. Since several studies have reported the contrary, however, it seems justified to analyze possible reasons for the discrepancies as they may point toward the currently elusive additional factors that are postulated here and elsewhere (Bartelt and Sartor, 2015) to precipitate acute symptoms.

As listed in Supplementary Table 1, studies differ in experimental detail and it is of interest to analyze whether these could have affected the overall outcome of the respective TEER measurements. For example, one variable of the popular Caco-2 model is that several clonal Caco-2 populations exist and their response can vary according to a particular readout (Katelaris et al., 1995; Sambuy et al., 2005; Liévin-Le Moal, 2013; Srinivasan et al., 2015). Therefore, we tested the parental cell-line and the clonal cell line Caco-2 bbe in a similar setting—with the same result (Supplementary Figures 1A,B). Of note, different subpopulations—also unintentionally established by ongoing passaging of those heterogeneous cells—may explain highly different basic TEER values between setups, which range from ~160 Ωcm^2 (Teoh et al., 2000) to >1,200 Ωcm^2 (Scott et al., 2002). In our experiments, Caco-2 (parental) had a basic TEER of ~300 Ωcm^2, whereas Caco-2 bbe offered initially ~200 Ωcm^2 (Supplementary Figure 2) but increased this value in a linear manner after 37 passages to 350 Ωcm^2 at passage #53 (Supplementary Figure 3), which is a known phenomenon (Sambuy et al., 2005; Srinivasan et al., 2015).

Parasite number is another factor that varies between studies, where MOIs of 0.5–8 have been described (Humen et al., 2011). In our experiments, we used MOIs of similar range (1 and 10; Supplementary Figure 1C) as well as very high parasite doses up to MOIs of 100 (**Figure 2B** or Supplementary Figures 1A,B). Thus, it seems unlikely that parasite:enterocyte ratios can explain conflicting results between studies. Specific characteristics of chosen parasite isolates cannot be excluded, but several identical isolates were tested in more than one study—including our own experiments—with different outcome (Supplementary Table 1). Thus, other differences in experimental setups must be considered.

It has been discussed that trophozoites' physical attachment alone may increase TEER and therefore obscure possible barrier defects (Chavez et al., 1995; Teoh et al., 2000; Chin et al., 2002; Tysnes and Robertson, 2015). However, exposure to the potent *Giardia* detachment reagent formononetin, known to remove trophozoites almost instantly without affecting their viability (Fisher et al., 2013), also did not led to normal TEERs of infected conditions (Supplementary Figure 4A). Though, formononetin-treatment right after infection seem to reduce its magnitude (Supplementary Figure 4B), this contrasts to data by Humen et al. (2011), who noted a TEER decrease which was dependent on trophozoite attachment that could not be triggered by spent medium. However, spent medium and sonicates led to a decline in TEER in other studies (Teoh et al., 2000).

In many studies, infected monolayers were washed intensively with ice cold PBS to remove parasites and subsequently measured TEER (Supplementary Table 1). Our experiences with such washing procedures led to erroneously high TEERs and highly increased variances of measurements, an effect that required several hours of re-incubation to normalize (Supplementary Figure 5). In experiments that do not rely on washing, such as the use of sonicated lysates or trophozoite-conditioned DMEM, Caco-2 monolayers were shown to reduce their TEERs when

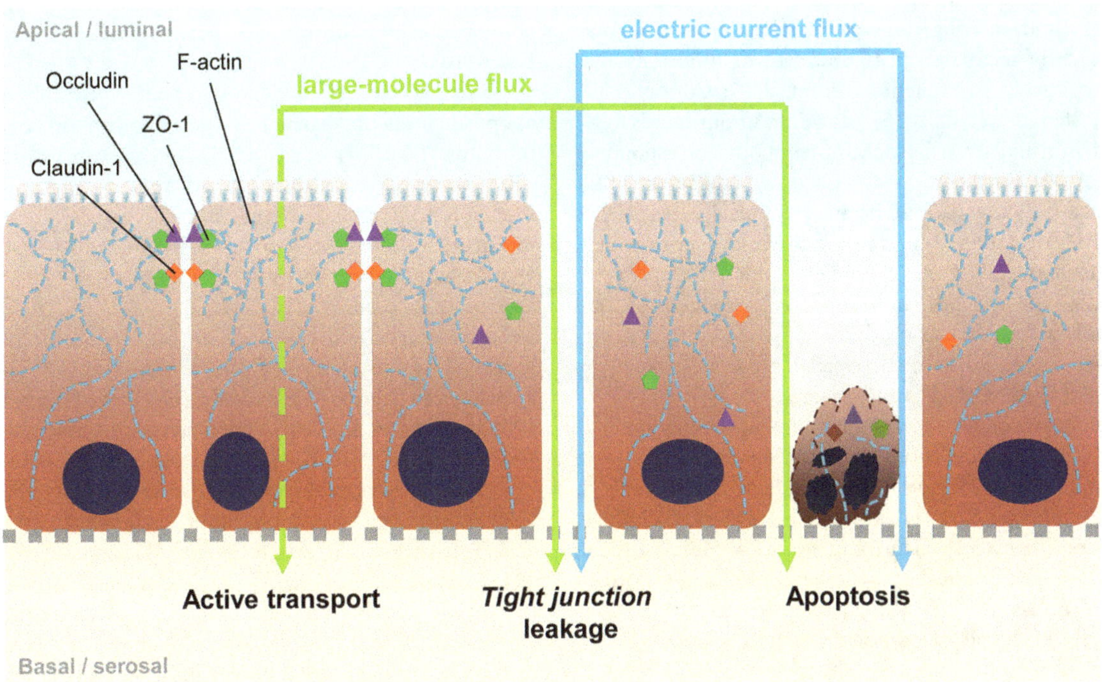

FIGURE 1 | Epithelial barrier. Scheme depicts the epithelia barrier and possible ways of its impairment. *Tight junctions* are located at the lateral sides in apical proximity and consist of membrane-spanning proteins like occludin and different claudins, as well as scaffold proteins like ZO-1 which connect the cytosolic ends of *tight junction* proteins to the actin cytoskeleton. Exchange of those proteins, leading to different *tight junction* compositions, affect specific permeability. Degradation of *tight junctions* is followed by an increase of unspecific permeability. Loss of cellular contacts lead to apoptosis and vice versa, apoptosis induces *tight junction* degradation. With measuring TEER, open breaches in the epithelium can be detected directly. The use of labeled molecules can also detect such leaks, however molecules can also be actively transported transcellularly e.g., via pinocytosis.

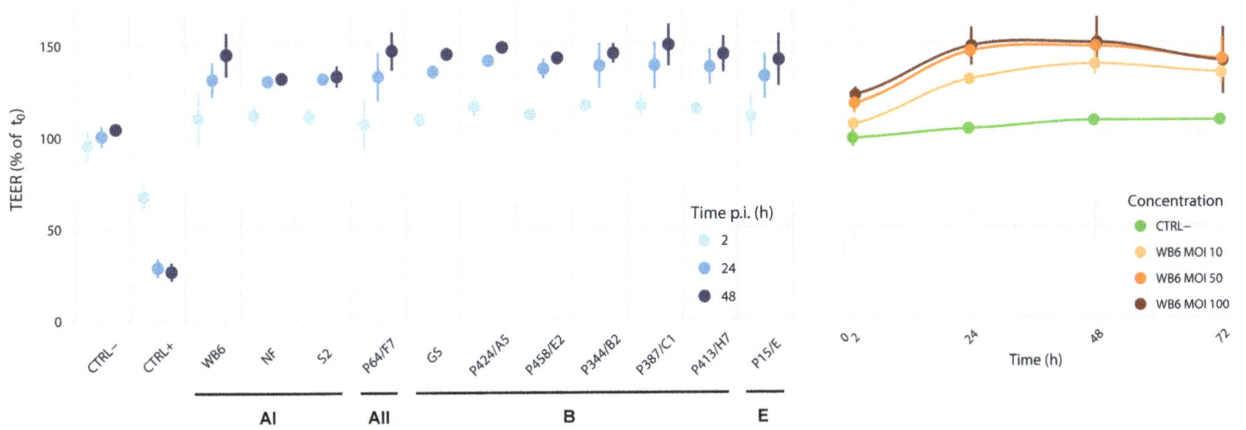

FIGURE 2 | Isolate comparison and dose dependency. We analyzed the effects of *Giardia* colonization of epithelial monolayers on TEER using the Caco-2 clone bbe, since it is reportedly more homogeneous than other clones or its parental line (Sambuy et al., 2005; Liévin-Le Moal, 2013; Srinivasan et al., 2015). Although, Caco-2 cells have been derived from a human colon cancer patient, a 21-day phase of confluent incubation ensures their differentiation toward a polarized small intestinal enterocyte-like cell type, considered as a model for the small intestinal epithelial barrier (ibid.). In this setup, we tested 11 different *G. duodenalis* isolates at MOIs of 20, including 5 reference strains WB6, NF, S2 (assemblage AI), GS (assemblage B), P15 (assemblage E) and 6 newly established clinical isolates (1 assemblage AII and 5 assemblage B). Data is relative to measurements before infection. Uninfected controls (CTRL-) were sham treated, monolayers with induced apoptosis using 1 μM staurosporine served as positive (leaky) controls (CTRL+). Each point represents the mean of 3 independent experiments with 3 monolayers per condition per experiment. Error bars indicate standard deviation. No evidence for parasite-induced decreases in TEER was found. In contrast, all tested isolates led consistently to a dose-dependent TEER-increase, without significant differences between isolates or assemblages.

exposed to, for example, NF or S2 lysates already after 24 h (Teoh et al., 2000). By destroying compartmentalization, lysates may lead to release of factors such as proteases or other enzymes that affect epithelial cell function (Buret, 2007; Cotton et al., 2011, 2014; Bhargava et al., 2015). However, in our hands WB6 lysates and heat-inactivated trophozoites, both corresponding to a MOI of 20, did not influence Caco-2 monolayers' TEER (Supplementary Figure 6A), while filtered apical supernatants from a WB6-MOI-100-72-h condition weakly recapitulated the TEER increase noted in experiments with intact parasites (Supplementary Figure 6B), indicating that products of vital *Giardia* trophozoites, such as products of secreted microvesicles (Evans-Osses et al., 2017) or stressed Caco-2 cells, may be responsible for the observed TEER increase.

Another variation in experimental design is the time of culture and differentiation before infection (Supplementary Table 1). Since monolayers change TEER properties over time of cultivation (Supplementary Figure 2) and less differentiated cells may be more sensitive to disturbing stimuli, findings can be confounded which can explain the disparate results in seemingly similar studies (Teoh et al., 2000; Humen et al., 2011; Maia-Brigagao et al., 2012, and for own data see Supplementary Figure 7).

The medium composition is another important parameter in *Giardia* co-culture experiments. Complete substitution of apical DMEM volume with *Giardia* growth-medium TYI-S-33 can lead to a steep initial TEER increase of monolayers, that can be further accentuated if monolayers are infected with WB6 trophozoites. However, the presence of TYI-S-33 will eventually lead to the collapse of infected and non-infected monolayers (Chavez et al., 1986; Supplementary Figure 8). Thus, takeover of TYI-S-33 components can clearly be a confounder.

Although, presence of O_2 for a microaerophilic pathogen is of relevance, this parameter does not seem to be decisive either. When aerobic and anaerobic conditions were compared using Caco-2 with WB6 trophozoites, anaerobic conditions showed no TEER decrease within 77 h, but indicated a higher TEER increase in both infected and uninfected Caco-2 monolayers. Prolonged incubation led to barrier failure within 139 h in all anaerobically cultivated Caco-2 monolayers, whereas TEER of aerobic cultivated monolayers remained stable and—for infected conditions—elevated (Supplementary Figure 9). Of note, viability of WB6 in our setups remained high with 57–75% of trophozoites still alive after 48 h and 32–48% after 72 h in unmodified culture conditions (data not shown).

The sodium-dependent glucose cotransporter (SGLT)-1 has been shown to inhibit enterocyte apoptosis in Caco-2 cells under high glucose conditions (Yu et al., 2005, 2008). Therefore, it is possible that depending on the cell culture media applied apoptotic effects of *Giardia* are masked by high glucose concentrations, e.g., in the often-used standard DMEM. However, such an effect is unlikely to have occurred in studies that used the parental Caco-2 since they do not express SGLT-1 in relevant amounts (Turner et al., 1996; Yu et al., 2008). In studies that used the Caco-2 bbe line which express this transporter (Turner et al., 1996) this is difficult to rule out, but in our experiments with the Caco-2 bbe line and low glucose conditions, comparable to Yu et al. did not affect TEER values when compared with cultures using normal DMEM (Supplementary Figure 10).

Serum is another possible component, capable of masking apoptosis induction, since it is known to contain corresponding inhibitors (Zoellner et al., 1996). In our experiments without FBS, however, no significant differences regarding *Giardia*-infection were found (Supplementary Figure 7). In contrast, the magnitude of effects of staurosporine which was used as a apoptosis-inducing control on TEER was clearly affected by FBS as predicted (Zoellner et al., 1996).

Another interesting confounder may be the *Giardia lamblia* virus (GLV). It is described as a double-stranded RNA virus of 7 kb size and belongs to the family *Totiviridae* (Wang and Wang, 1986; Janssen et al., 2015). GLV can infect several but not all *Giardia* isolates (Miller et al., 1988), depending on the expression of a specific surface receptor (Sepp et al., 1994). The related *Leishmania*-specific endosymbiont "*Leishmania* RNA virus-1" (LRV1) is known to affect the severity of leishmaniasis (Ives et al., 2011). Likewise, GLV could also influence *Giardia*'s virulence, though no correlation regarding GLV infestation of *Giardia* isolates to symptomatic or asymptomatic patients were found in the past (Jonckheere and Gordts, 1987). Our experiments—at least regarding TEER—also suggest no detectable differences between GLV-infected or uninfected WB6 and GS trophozoites on Caco-2 monolayers (Supplementary Figure 11).

In summary, variations in experimental design due to the lack of standardization confound the search for robust effects on TEER induced by *G. duodenalis*. The current data in particular of the Caco-2 *in vitro* co-culture model rather suggests that *Giardia* alone does not induce acute barrier-defects.

Alteration in *Tight Junction* Composition

Intestinal epithelial barrier function is highly dependent on cytoskeleton architecture and *tight junction* composition (Hidalgo et al., 1989; Troeger et al., 2007). *Giardia*-induced changes in the F-actin cytoskeleton were observed after incubation with sonicates (Scott et al., 2002), with living trophozoites, sonicates and spent medium (Teoh et al., 2000) or only with attached trophozoites (Humen et al., 2011). All these studies found also alterations to respective TEER values (Supplementary Table 1). *Tight junction* proteins, ZO-1 and claudin-1 showed in some studies altered localization, that could be prevented by various treatments, e.g., by EGF- (Buret et al., 2002) or caspase-3 inhibitor treatment (Chin et al., 2002), or MLCK-inhibitor addition (Scott et al., 2002; see summary in Supplementary Table 1). *Ex vivo*-analysis of epithelial tissue from symptomatic patients, showed 30% reduced claudin-1 abundance (Troeger et al., 2007), which was not evident in any *in vitro* study. On a technical note, all *in vitro* studies which showed alterations of the *tight junction* complex, experiments were conducted on plastic (chamber slides) or glass (coverslips) support which alter Caco-2 monolayer morphologies (Supplementary Figure 12).

In contrast, but in agreement with the TEER measurements, no significant differences between infected or uninfected monolayers with respect to F-actin and *tight junction* proteins were observed on electrophysiologically tight filter-supported

Caco-2 layers (**Figures 3, 4**). Occasionally, effects as described in other studies, were detectable but lacked any correlation with infection (**Figure 5**). Due to heterogeneity of Caco-2 monolayers leading to a mosaic of microvilli formation (Katelaris et al., 1995; Sambuy et al., 2005; Liévin-Le Moal, 2013), the reported *G. duodenalis* induced microvilli depletion (Chavez et al., 1986, 1995; Buret et al., 1990, 1991) that should manifest as apical cytoskeletal changes could have been missed since changes reported were not drastic.

In conclusion, integrity of the *tight junction* protein complex also suggests an asymptomatic interaction of *Giardia* alone with the Caco-2 model. Alterations described by others may be related to growth in non-transwell systems. Of note, described disruptive effects on ZO-1 have been described as secondary to apoptosis and not directly induced by the parasite (Chin et al., 2002; Buret et al., 2003; Bojarski et al., 2004; Zehendner et al., 2011).

Epithelial Barrier Dysfunction Due To Apoptosis

Apoptosis is a tightly regulated process in the gut epithelium. For giardiasis, reported rates vary greatly between studies from no changes to controls (Chavez et al., 1986, 1995; Katelaris et al., 1995; Maia-Brigagao et al., 2012; Tysnes and Robertson, 2015, and own findings), to minor increases from 1 to 1.5% in symptomatic patients' mucosa (Troeger et al., 2007), to isolate specific effects of sonicates (Chin et al., 2002), to significant increases up to 41% with a rather low MOI of 3 after just 16 h using HCT-8 cells (Panaro et al., 2007) or only significant after long term co-culture (Fisher et al., 2013). HCT-8 cells were also shown to undergo increased apoptosis in mixed isolate infections (Koh et al., 2013); a finding that we could not reproduce with Caco-2 cells using NF and S2 (data not shown). Thus, effects on apoptosis also seem to be highly dependent on experimental setup and lack the robustness to allow a clear conclusion.

Tissue Permeability as a Surrogate of Altered Molecular Fluxes

Absorption and trans-epithelial transport of biomolecules are key functions of the gut epithelia (Kiela and Ghishan, 2016) and permeation assays can be used to probe these functions.

Labeled Compounds as Marker for Paracellular Permeability

A number of *in vitro* studies assessed paracellular permeability using fluorescein isothiocyanate (FITC)-conjugated dextran. Buret et al. (2002) noted a more than 40-fold increase of the trans-epithelial FITC-dextran flux in co-cultures with *Giardia* trophozoites. This effect was associated with alterations on *tight junction* protein distributions (Buret et al., 2002) and could be abolished when monolayers were pretreated with epidermal growth factor (EGF). Since bovine EGF can act on human cells, and since serum used in co-culture experiments provides several growth factors with overlapping effects, differences between serum batches must be considered as potential confounders. Similar results in a comparable setting were also reported using sonicates of various *Giardia* isolates (WB, PB, NF, and S2; all assemblage A; Chin et al., 2002) and on SCBN monolayers (Scott et al., 2002). Interestingly, large molecule permeability could be abolished using Myosin light-chain kinase (MLCK)-Inhibitor ML-9 (Scott et al., 2002). The mechanism proposed implicates phosphorylation of Myosin light-chain (MLC) by MLCK activity that leads to alterations in the F-actin and ZO-1 composition and eventually to increased permeability. An *ex vivo* study using FITC-dextran in *Giardia* GS infected mice compared effects on FITC-dextran permeability on day 7 (colonization phase) and 35 (post-clearance phase) after infection and found a slight increase in permeability at both time points of ~30% that was correlated with cleavage of occludin and also increased endocytosis of bacteria (Chen et al., 2013). Our findings using FITC-dextran correlate with our respective TEER measurements (Supplementary Figure 13), showing no increased permeability of *Giardia*-infected monolayers, but of apoptosis-induced controls. Thus, like before the *in vitro* findings are as contradictory—also with respect to this parameter—as the *in vivo* studies mentioned before.

Combined Assessment of Para- and Transcellular Flux

It is known, at least for *in vivo* studies, that individual sugars alone are not a reliable indicator of intestinal permeability and therefore disaccharide/monosaccharide ratios should be used instead (Johnston et al., 2000). Lactulose and mannitol for example are not transported via active monosaccharide transport systems but due to their difference in size can serve as a marker for transcellular permeability through channels (mannitol) and paracellular permeability, or *tight junction* leakage (lactulose; Andre et al., 1988). However, L:M ratios are not used very often *in vitro*, but other compounds had been used instead to assess and distinguish paracellular and transcellular flux. Using horse radish peroxidase (HRP) and creatinine as trans- and paracellular markers, respectively, infection with both a lab adapted and a field isolate, led to increased mucosal to serosal transcellular flux. Also paracellular permeability was increased by the field isolate (R-2), which is contradictory to the observed TEER increase in the same study (Tysnes and Robertson, 2015). Another study by Hardin et al. (1997) on *Giardia* S2-infected Mongolian gerbils could not find increased permeability to [^{51}Cr]EDTA (permeability similar to lactulose), but macromolecular transport of BSA was induced. A study on rats also suggest *Giardia*'s interference with active transport, but the other way around: Glucose and glycine absorption was decreased, whereas potassium which diffuses passively through the epithelium was unaffected (Anand et al., 1980). However, one should keep in mind that malabsorption could be either a result of impaired uptake due to dissipated osmotic and ion gradients originated from leaky *tight junctions* and apoptotic cells, or due to a reduction in the absorptive area because of villus shortening and microvilli depletion. The latter, a reduction in absorptive area, has been shown to be one of the more consistently found pathological features of *Giardia* (Chavez et al., 1986, 1995; Buret et al., 1990, 1991; Troeger et al., 2007) and could explain some study discrepancies.

Results with Caco-2 cells in permeability assays have to be interpreted with caution as these cells are known to actively and passively transport contents and are extensively used in

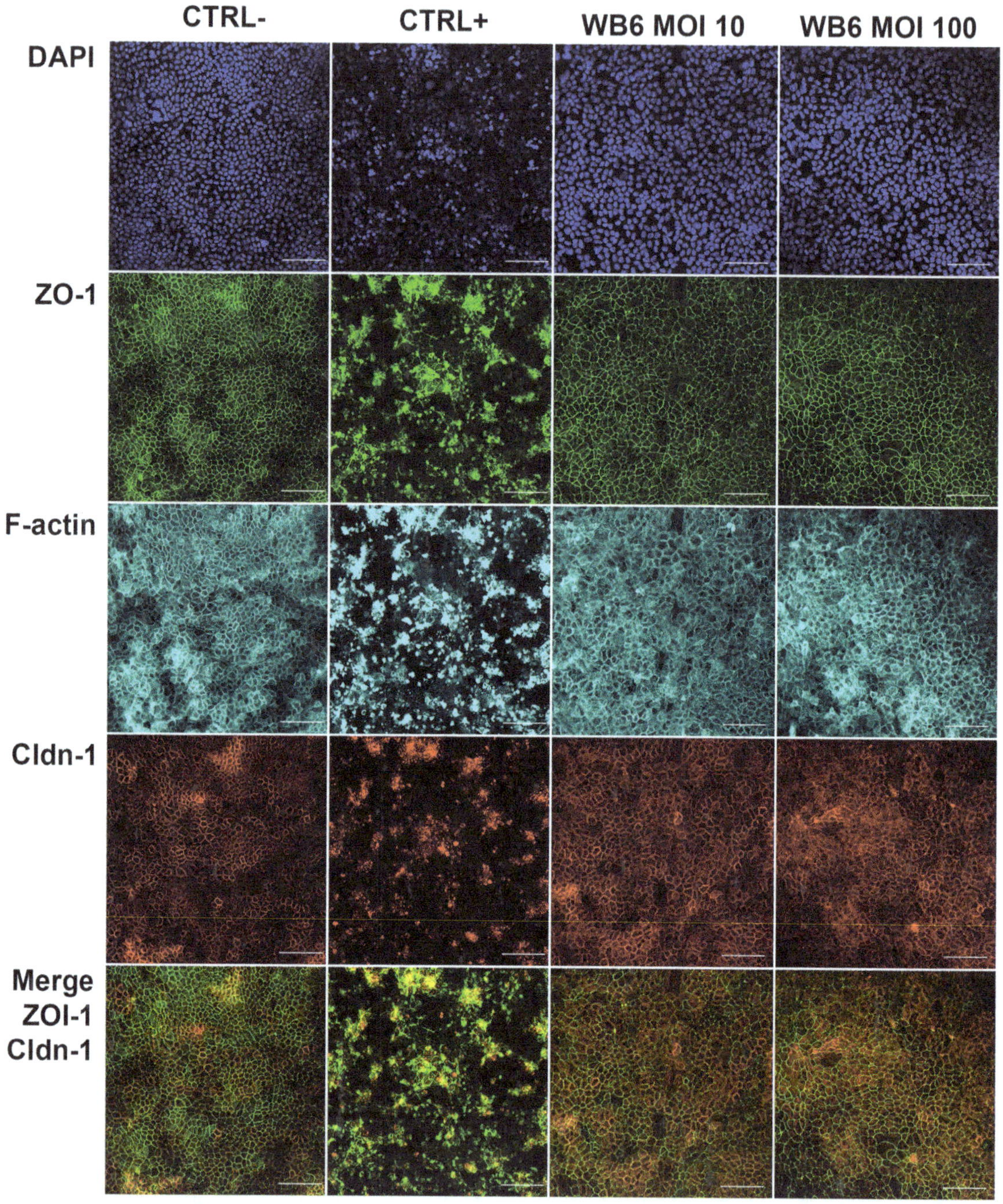

FIGURE 3 | *Tight junction* integrity. Micrographs depict *tight junction* proteins ZO-1 (green), claudin-1 (red), and F-actin cytoskeleton (cyan) after 72 h, comparing uninfected control (CTRL−), 1 μM staurosporine control (CTRL+), and *G. duodenalis* isolate WB6 of MOI 10 and 100. Scale bars indicate 100 μm. Nuclear staining with DAPI is shown in blue. No significant changes in any of the observed proteins due to *Giardia*-infection are detectable.

pharmaceutical drug absorption assays (Hidalgo et al., 1989; Artursson et al., 2001; Sambuy et al., 2005; Sun et al., 2008). When cultivated on plastic surfaces and not on transwell-filters, these cells tend to form large liquid-filled vacuole-like structures (Supplementary Figure 12) probably because they are not able to route those volumes through to a basally located compartment. Also, osmotically active marker substances, like sugars, can confound results by interfering with osmotic gradients. Enhanced active transport by *Giardia*, however, is understudied, but, should become more of a focus also because antigens or whole microbes of the intestinal lumen can be transported and be of pathological relevance. Indeed, Chen et al. (2013) found evidence for enhanced endocytosis of bacteria, rendering such a scenario possible.

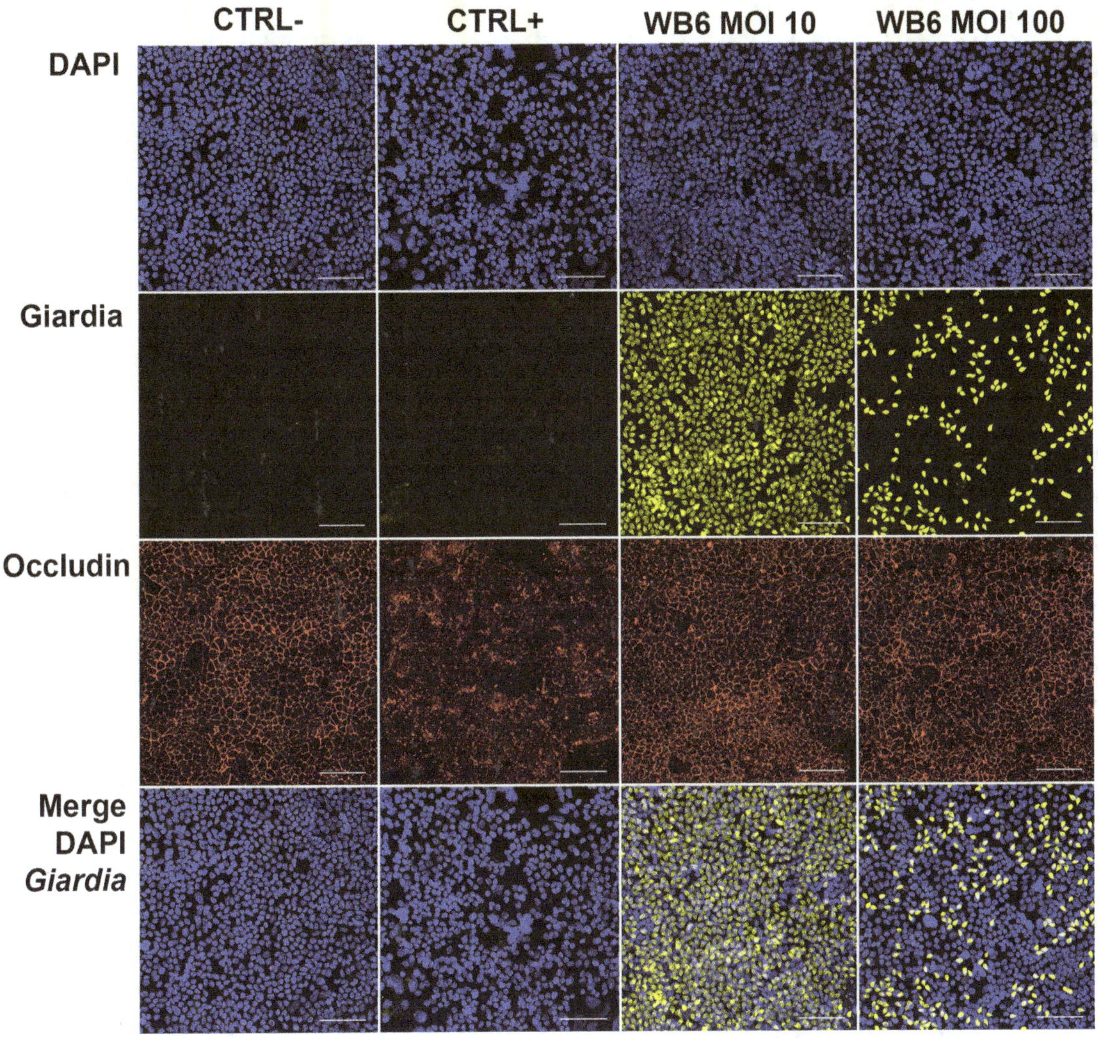

FIGURE 4 | *Tight junction* integrity and trophozoites. Micrographs depict *tight junction* protein occludin (red) and trophozoites (yellow) in Caco-2 bbe monolayer after 24 h, comparing uninfected control (CTRL-), 1 μM staurosporine control (CTRL+) and *G. duodenalis* isolate WB6 of MOI 10 and 100. Scale bars indicate 100 μm. Nuclear staining with DAPI is shown in blue. No significant changes concerning occludin due to *Giardia*-infection are detectable. A MOI of 10 is sufficient to completely cover the Caco-2 monolayer. Of note, MOI 100 show artificially less trophozoites attached than MOI 10 condition, possibly due to rapid nutrient consumption followed by starvation and subsequent detachment of the trophozoites.

Analysis of Chemokine/Cytokine Profiles in *Giardia* Epithelial Cell Co-cultures

In order to validate the asymptomatic outcome of our Caco-2 setup further, several chemokines/cytokines potentially or claimed to be upregulated during giardiasis were investigated. Most of the cytokine analyses that have been published were performed using cell monolayers grown on cell culture plastic. A seminal study used micro-array analysis of *Giardia*-infected Caco-2 cells during the first 18 h and showed an increase in CCL20, CCL2, and CXCL1/2 mRNA abundance among others (Roxström-Lindquist et al., 2005). However, increased IL-8 and TNFα mRNAs were not detected. Another study indicated no changes to IL-8, CCL2, GM-CSF, and TNFα (Jung et al., 1995). Hence, it appears that responses to *Giardia* infections differ from the generalized response by enterocytes of colonic origin to bacterial infections (Jung et al., 1995). This was corroborated by Fisher et al. (2013) for CCL2, GRO-isoforms (CXCL1/2), or IL-8 in the Caco-2 co-culture system. Interestingly, Caco-2 co-cultured with macrophages alone elicited GRO-isoform and IL-8 expression but this was abolished again when *Giardia* trophozoites were added, indicating immune-modulatory capabilities of the parasite (Fisher et al., 2013). *Giardia*'s ability to alter immune responses has been described by others, too (Kamda and Singer, 2009; Cotton et al., 2014, 2015). Our data using the Caco-2 transwell culture system also suggest no triggering of basolateral release of CCL2/20, CXCL1/2, IL-8, TNFα, or GM-CSF by different isolates or MOIs tested (**Figure 6**). Overall, our cytokine data also suggest an asymptomatic *Giardia*-infection. Whether this may be due to parasites' immune-modulatory features (Kamda

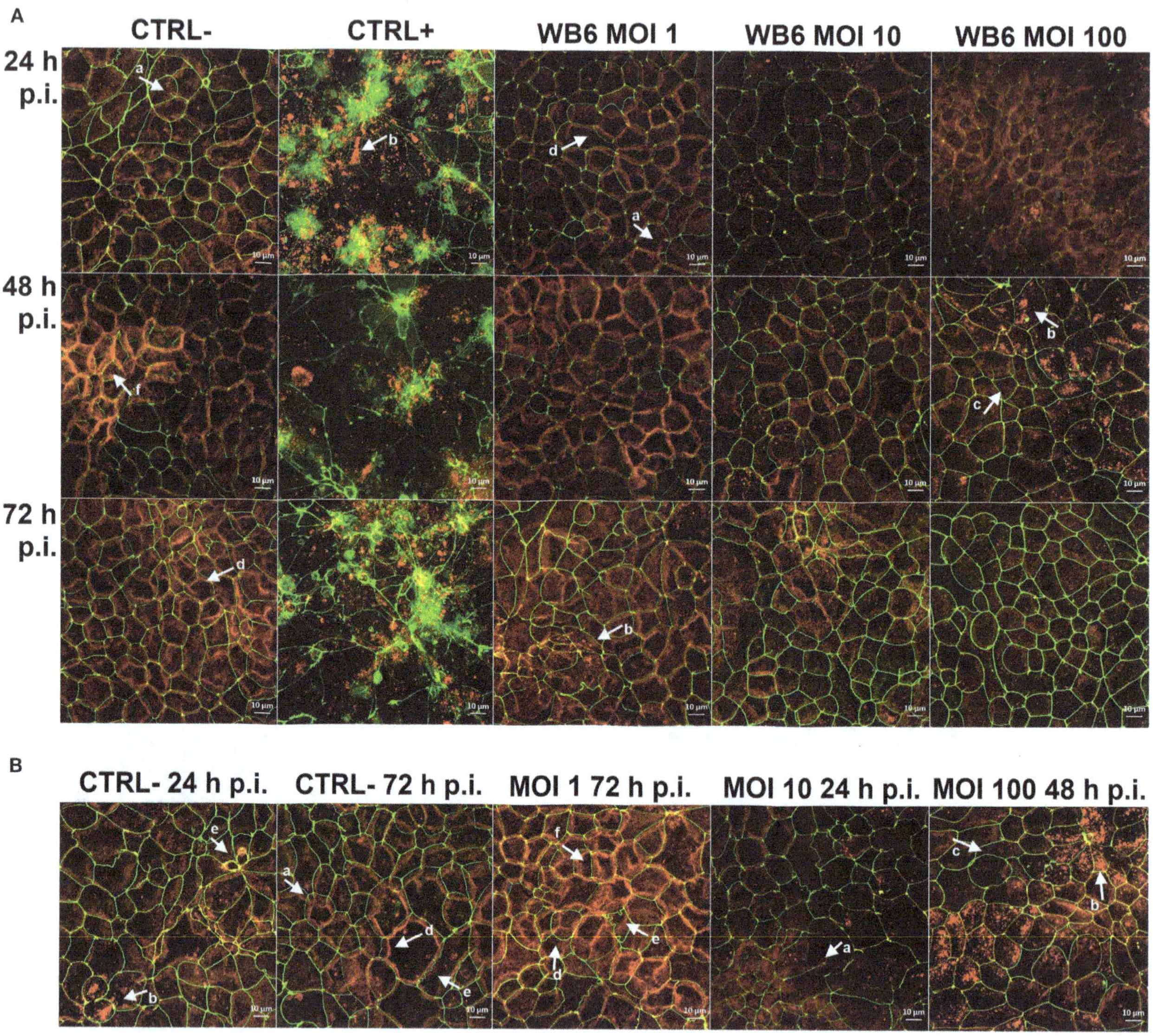

FIGURE 5 | Effects on *tight junction* proteins. Micrographs are derived from z-stacks, spanning whole cells, by using maximum intensity projection and depict *tight junction* proteins ZO-1 (green) and claudin-1 (red) in Caco-2 bbe monolayer, comparing uninfected control (CTRL−), 1 μM staurosporine control (CTRL+) and *G. duodenalis* isolate WB6 of MOI 1, 10 and 100 after 24, 48, and 72 h **(A)**. An additional selection of micrographs of same samples is shown in **(B)**, illustrating Caco-2 peculiarities. Arrows in **(A,B)** indicate observed random phenotypes like ZO-1 "branching" (a), claudin-1 flocculation and delocalization (b) or its absence directly next to it (c), mismatch of ZO-1 and claudin-1 localization (d), odd cellular contacts (e), and areas of increased claudin-1 presence (f).

and Singer, 2009; Cotton et al., 2014, 2015) requires further studies.

CONCLUSION

As mentioned in the introduction, one of the major enigmas in giardiasis is what distinguishes acutely symptomatic from asymptomatic outcomes of *Giardia*-infections. In this work, we reviewed and discussed current *in vitro* epithelial cell culture systems that we propose do reproduce asymptomatic host-parasite interaction rather than acutely symptomatic giardiasis. We propose for further development of these systems a structured approach that aims at identifying appropriate *in vitro* correlates for distinct clinical symptoms: The search for correlates of acute manifestations such as diarrhea could focus on readouts such as TEER, *tight junction* function, and ion secretion, but should focus on testing combinations of parasite and non-parasite factors. Food factors, or the lack of certain nutrients, could determine trophozoite virulence as well as bile or pancreatic secretions. Especially bile is a requirement for axenic trophozoite cultivation (Keister, 1983; Halliday et al., 1988) and it could stimulate the parasite not only to grow, but also to increase its virulence. It is also imaginable that certain host proteases could cleave *Giardia* proteins in a way that an inactive virulence function is activated, similar to what has been shown as a necessity for host cell

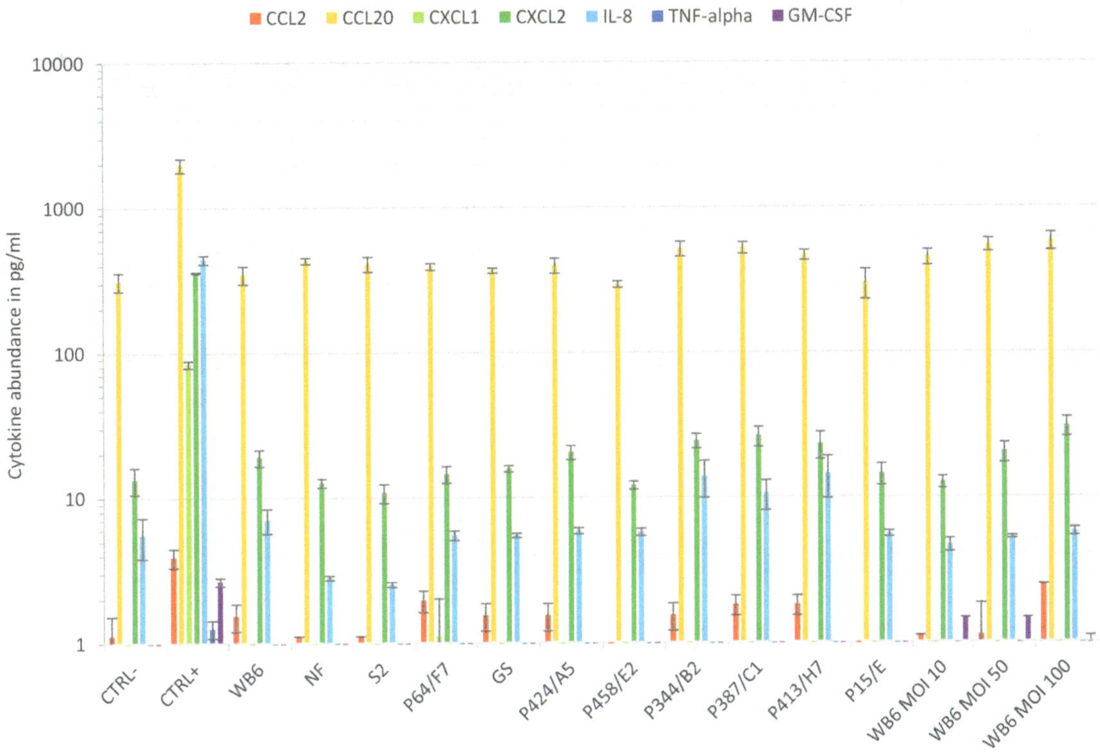

FIGURE 6 | Cytokine response. Cytokine levels of CCL2, CCL20, CXCL1, CXCL2, IL-8, TNFα, and GM-CSF were compared using basal supernatants of the conducted 48–72 h TEER experiments and the Luminex® technology. Data show means and standard deviation of cytokine levels of supernatants, gathered from at least two independent TEER experiments. Except for CCL20, cytokines were barely detected in this compartment independent of infection. In contrast, monolayers insulted with staurosporine (CTRL+) increased amounts of CCL20, CXCL1/2, and IL-8, whereas CCL2, TNFα, and GM-CSF remained below the lower quantification limit.

entry of influenza virus particles (Kido et al., 2012). Of note, *Giardia* specifically decreases the activity of pancreatic trypsin, but not of chymotrypsin (Seow et al., 1993), which suggests that certain proteases can be hazardous for *Giardia* and may disturb a finely balanced silent infection to provoke pathogenic reactions. Additionally, a host's genetic background linked to hypogammaglobulinemia, IgA deficiency or cystic fibrosis or a host's phenotype comprising reduced gastric acidity, stress, co-infections, or other concomitant diseases, could contribute to the pathogenesis (DuPont, 2013). Furthermore, since the mechanisms of trans-epithelial transport are as diverse as the respective substrates (Kiela and Ghishan, 2016) and our lack of knowledge if and how *Giardia* affects those transport systems, the search for correlates and explanations for more protracted effects such as stunted growth that may be linked to altered fluxes of particular biomolecules, should focus on a systematic assessment of epithelial cell functions related to those transcellular transport and absorption mechanisms. Another important factor relevant for the symptomatic outcome may be the host's microbiome, as suggested by others (Singer and Nash, 2000; Chen et al., 2013; Slapeta et al., 2015). The fact that young children after the lactation period are generally more affected by *Giardia* infestation than older children or adults may be an epidemiological correlate of a not-yet-settled microbiome that is more susceptible to interference by the parasite. Moreover, differences in food resources and cultural habits, resulting in distinct intestinal bacterial colonization may underlay the variances noted between studies that cover different geographic regions. Additionally, very recent publications reporting experimental findings also point toward an increasing role of the intestinal microbiota during *Giardia* infections (Allain et al., 2017; Barash et al, 2017; Beatty et al., 2017). Finally, since giardiasis resembles symptoms of food allergies, hypersensitivity or intolerance like coeliac disease, pathogenesis could be more related to the host's individual immune reaction (Scott et al., 2004). This might explain why *Giardia*-infections are less severe or even protective in developing countries, where allergic diseases are usually not as prevalent. However, due to the parasite's ability to enhance sensitization toward food antigens (Di Prisco et al., 1998), the causal relationship will be difficult to investigate. Moreover, the general *in vitro* methodology of *Giardia*-host interaction studies requires better standardization with the goal to offer robust, inter-laboratory evaluated models.

AUTHOR CONTRIBUTIONS

All authors contributed equally to design and conception of this work. MK conducted research on literature and collected experimental data. CK, RB, JS, and TA contributed to experimental design and intellectual input. RB and JS helped interpreting data and MK, CK, and TA contributed to the manuscript.

FUNDING

This work was financially supported by grant GRK 2046 from the German Research Foundation (DFG). The funding bodies had no role in the design of the study, collection, analysis, and interpretation of data or in writing the manuscript.

ACKNOWLEDGMENTS

We thank Ms. Wibke Krüger and Ms. Petra Gosten-Heinrich for technical assistance, as well as Prof. Staffan Svärd and Prof. Andre Buret for intellectual input. Furthermore, we thank Prof. Andre Buret (Department of Biological Sciences, University of Calgary, Canada) for sending us NF and S2 *Giardia* isolates and Dr. Marco Lalle (Istituto Superiore di Sanità, Rome, Italy) for sending us "*Giardia lamblia* virus"-infected isolates. Finally, we thank Mr. Jonnel Jaurigue for proof-reading the manuscript.

REFERENCES

Adam, R. D. (2001). Biology of *Giardia lamblia*. *Clin. Microbiol. Rev.* 14, 447–475. doi: 10.1128/CMR.14.3.447-475.2001

Allain, T., Amat, C. B., Motta, J.-P., Manko, A., and Buret, A. G. (2017). Interactions of *Giardia* sp. with the intestinal barrier: epithelium, mucus, and microbiota. *Tissue Barriers* 5:e1274354. doi: 10.1080/21688370.2016.1274354

Anand, B. S., Kumar, M., Chakravarti, R. N., Sehgal, A. K., and Chhuttani, P. N. (1980). Pathogenesis of malabsorption in Giardia infection: an experimental study in rats. *Trans. R. Soc. Trop. Med. Hyg.* 74, 565–569. doi: 10.1016/0035-9203(80)90139-X

Anderson, R. C., Young, W., Clerens, S., Cookson, A. L., McCann, M. J., Armstrong, K. M., et al. (2013). Human oral isolate *Lactobacillus* fermentum AGR1487 reduces intestinal barrier integrity by increasing the turnover of microtubules in Caco-2 cells. *PLoS ONE* 8:e78774. doi: 10.1371/journal.pone.0078774

Andre, F., Andre, C., Emery, Y., Forichon, J., Descos, L., and Minaire, Y. (1988). Assessment of the lactulose-mannitol test in Crohn's disease. *Gut* 29, 511–515. doi: 10.1136/gut.29.4.511

Ankarklev, J., Jerlström-Hultqvist, J., Ringqvist, E., Troell, K., and Svärd, S. G. (2010). Behind the smile: cell biology and disease mechanisms of Giardia species. *Nat. Rev. Microbiol.* 8, 413–422. doi: 10.1038/nrmicro2317

Artursson, P., Palm, K., and Luthman, K. (2001). Caco-2 monolayers in experimental and theoretical predictions of drug transport. *Adv. Drug Deliv. Rev.* 46, 27–43. doi: 10.1016/S0169-409X(96)00415-2

Barash, N. R., Maloney, J. G., Singer, S. M., and Dawson, S. C. (2017). *Giardia* alters commensal microbial diversity throughout the murine gut. *Infect. Immun.* 85:e00948-16. doi: 10.1128/IAI.00948-16

Bartelt, L. A., and Sartor, R. B. (2015). Advances in understanding Giardia: determinants and mechanisms of chronic sequelae. *F1000Prime Rep.* 7:62. doi: 10.12703/P7-62

Beatty, J. K., Akierman, S. V., Motta, J.-P., Muise, S., Workentine, M. L., Harrison, J. J., et al. (2017). *Giardia duodenalis* induces pathogenic dysbiosis of human intestinal microbiota biofilms. *Int. J. Parasitol.* 47, 311–326. doi: 10.1016/j.ijpara.2016.11.010

Betanzos, A., Schnoor, M., Javier-Reyna, R., García-Rivera, G., Bañuelos, C., Pais-Morales, J., et al. (2014). Analysis of the epithelial damage produced by *Entamoeba histolytica* infection. *J. Vis. Exp.* e51668. doi: 10.3791/51668

Bhargava, A., Cotton, J. A., Dixon, B. R., Gedamu, L., Yates, R. M., and Buret, A. G. (2015). *Giardia duodenalis* surface cysteine proteases induce cleavage of the intestinal epithelial cytoskeletal protein villin via myosin light chain kinase. *PLoS ONE* 10:e0136102. doi: 10.1371/journal.pone.0136102

Bilenko, N., Levy, A., Dagan, R., Deckelbaum, R. J., El-On, Y., and Fraser, D. (2004). Does co-infection with *Giardia lamblia* modulate the clinical characteristics of enteric infections in young children? *Eur. J. Epidemiol.* 19, 877–883. doi: 10.1023/B:EJEP.0000040533.75646.9c

Bojarski, C., Weiske, J., Schoneberg, T., Schroder, W., Mankertz, J., Schulzke, J.-D., et al. (2004). The specific fates of tight junction proteins in apoptotic epithelial cells. *J. Cell Sci.* 117, 2097–2107. doi: 10.1242/jcs.01071

Buret, A. G. (2007). Mechanisms of epithelial dysfunction in giardiasis. *Gut* 56, 316–317. doi: 10.1136/gut.2006.107771

Buret, A. G., Chin, A. C., and Scott, K. G. (2003). Infection of human and bovine epithelial cells with *Cryptosporidium* andersoni induces apoptosis and disrupts tight junctional ZO-1: effects of epidermal growth factor. *Int. J. Parasitol.* 33, 1363–1371. doi: 10.1016/S0020-7519(03)00138-3

Buret, A. G., Mitchell, K., Muench, D. G., and Scott, K. G. (2002). *Giardia lamblia* disrupts tight junctional ZO-1 and increases permeability in non-transformed human small intestinal epithelial monolayers: effects of epidermal growth factor. *Parasitology* 125, 11–19. doi: 10.1017/S0031182002001853

Buret, A., Gall, D. G., and Olson, M. E. (1990). Effects of murine giardiasis on growth, intestinal morphology, and disaccharidase activity. *J. Parasitol.* 76, 403–409. doi: 10.2307/3282675

Buret, A., Gall, D. G., and Olson, M. E. (1991). Growth, activities of enzymes in the small intestine, and ultrastructure of microvillous border in gerbils infected with *Giardia duodenalis*. *Parasitol. Res.* 77, 109–114. doi: 10.1007/BF00935423

Burnham, K. P., and Anderson, D. R. (2004). *Model Selection and Multimodel Inference: A Practical Information-Theoretic Approach, 2nd Edn.* New York, NY: Springer. doi: 10.1007/b97636

Campbell, D. I., McPhail, G., Lunn, P. G., Elia, M., and Jeffries, D. J. (2004). Intestinal inflammation measured by fecal neopterin in Gambian children with enteropathy: association with growth failure, *Giardia lamblia*, and intestinal permeability. *J. Pediatr. Gastroenterol. Nutr.* 39, 153–157. doi: 10.1097/00005176-200408000-00005

Chavez, B., Gonzalez-Mariscal, L., Cedillo-Rivera, R., and Martinez-Palomo, A. (1995). *Giardia lamblia*: *in vitro* cytopathic effect of human isolates. *Exp. Parasitol.* 80, 133–138. doi: 10.1006/expr.1995.1015

Chavez, B., Knaippe, F., Gonzalez-Mariscal, L., and Martinez-Palomo, A. (1986). *Giardia lamblia*: electrophysiology and ultrastructure of cytopathology in cultured epithelial cells. *Exp. Parasitol.* 61, 379–389. doi: 10.1016/0014-4894(86)90194-3

Chen, T.-L., Chen, S., Wu, H.-W., Lee, T.-C., Lu, Y.-Z., Wu, L.-L., et al. (2013). Persistent gut barrier damage and commensal bacterial influx following eradication of Giardia infection in mice. *Gut. Pathog.* 5:26. doi: 10.1186/1757-4749-5-26

Chin, A. C., Teoh, D. A., Scott, K. G.-E., Meddings, J. B., MacNaughton, W. K., and Buret, A. G. (2002). Strain-dependent induction of enterocyte apoptosis by *Giardia lamblia* disrupts epithelial barrier function in a caspase-3-dependent manner. *Infect. Immun.* 70, 3673–3680. doi: 10.1128/IAI.70.7.3673-3680.2002

Cotton, J. A., Amat, C. B., and Buret, A. G. (2015). Disruptions of host immunity and inflammation by *Giardia duodenalis*: potential consequences for co-infections in the Gastro-intestinal tract. *Pathogens* 4, 764–792. doi: 10.3390/pathogens4040764

Cotton, J. A., Beatty, J. K., and Buret, A. G. (2011). Host parasite interactions and pathophysiology in Giardia infections. *Int. J. Parasitol.* 41, 925–933. doi: 10.1016/j.ijpara.2011.05.002

Cotton, J. A., Motta, J.-P., Schenck, L. P., Hirota, S. A., Beck, P. L., and Buret, A. G. (2014). *Giardia duodenalis* infection reduces granulocyte infiltration in an *in vivo* model of bacterial toxin-induced colitis and attenuates inflammation in human intestinal tissue. *PLoS ONE* 9:e109087. doi: 10.1371/journal.pone.0109087

Dagci, H., Ustun, S., Taner, M. S., Ersoz, G., Karacasu, F., and Budak, S. (2002). Protozoon infections and intestinal permeability. *Acta Trop.* 81, 1–5. doi: 10.1016/S0001-706X(01)00191-7

D'Anchino, M., Orlando, D., and Feudis, L., de (2002). *Giardia lamblia* infections become clinically evident by eliciting symptoms of irritable bowel syndrome. *J. Infect.* 45, 169–172. doi: 10.1053/jinf.2002.1038

Di Prisco, M. C., Hagel, I., Lynch, N. R., Jimenez, J. C., Rojas, R., Gil, M., et al. (1998). Association between giardiasis and allergy. *Ann. Aller. Asthma Immunol.* 81, 261–265. doi: 10.1016/S1081-1206(10)62823-2

DuPont, H. L. (2013). Giardia: both a harmless commensal and a devastating pathogen. *J. Clin. Invest.* 123, 2352–2354. doi: 10.1172/JCI69932

Evans-Osses, I., Mojoli, A., Monguio-Tortajada, M., Marcilla, A., Aran, V., Amorim, M., et al. (2017). Microvesicles released from *Giardia intestinalis* disturb host-pathogen response *in vitro*. *Eur. J. Cell Biol.* 96, 131–142. doi: 10.1016/j.ejcb.2017.01.005

Fajdiga, S., Koninkx, J. F. J. G., Tooten, P. C. J., and Marinsek-Logar, R. (2006). Interference of *Salmonella* enteritidis and *Lactobacillus* spp. with IL-8 levels and transepithelial electrical resistance of enterocyte-like Caco-2 cells. *Folia Microbiol.* 51, 268–272. doi: 10.1007/BF02931810

Fiorentino, M., Ding, H., Blanchard, T. G., Czinn, S. J., Sztein, M. B., and Fasano, A. (2013). Helicobacter pylori-induced disruption of monolayer permeability and proinflammatory cytokine secretion in polarized human gastric epithelial cells. *Infect. Immun.* 81, 876–883. doi: 10.1128/IAI.01406-12

Fisher, B. S., Estrano, C. E., and Cole, J. A. (2013). Modeling long-term host cell-*Giardia lamblia* interactions in an *in vitro* co-culture system. *PLoS ONE* 8:e81104. doi: 10.1371/journal.pone.0081104

Garzon, M., Pereira-da-Silva, L., Seixas, J., Papoila, A. L., Alves, M., Ferreira, F., et al. (2017). Association of enteric parasitic infections with intestinal inflammation and permeability in asymptomatic infants of Sao Tome Island. *Pathog. Glob. Heal.* 111, 116–127. doi: 10.1080/20477724.2017.1299831

Goto, R., Mascie-Taylor, C. G., and Lunn, P. G. (2009). Impact of intestinal permeability, inflammation status and parasitic infections on infant growth faltering in rural Bangladesh. *Br. J. Nutr.* 101, 1509–1516. doi: 10.1017/S0007114508083554

Goto, R., Panter-Brick, C., Northrop-Clewes, C. A., Manahdhar, R., and Tuladhar, N. R. (2002). Poor intestinal permeability in mildly stunted Nepali children: associations with weaning practices and *Giardia lamblia* infection. *Br. J. Nutr.* 88, 141–149. doi: 10.1079/BJN2002599

Halliday, C. E., Clark, C., and Farthing, M. J. (1988). Giardia-bile salt interactions *in vitro* and *in vivo*. *Trans. R. Soc. Trop. Med. Hyg.* 82, 428–432. doi: 10.1016/0035-9203(88)90153-8

Halliez, M. C. M., Motta, J.-P., Feener, T. D., Guerin, G., LeGoff, L., Francois, A., et al. (2016). *Giardia duodenalis* induces para-cellular bacterial translocation and causes post-infectious visceral hypersensitivity. *Am. J. Physiol. Gastrointest. Liver Physiol.* 310, G574–G585. doi: 10.1152/ajpgi.00 144.2015

Hanevik, K., Wensaas, K.-A., Rortveit, G., Eide, G. E., Morch, K., and Langeland, N. (2014). Irritable bowel syndrome and chronic fatigue 6 years after giardia infection: a controlled prospective cohort study. *Clin. Infect. Dis.* 59, 1394–1400. doi: 10.1093/cid/ciu629

Hardin, J. A., Buret, A. G., Olson, M. E., Kimm, M. H., and Gall, D. G. (1997). Mast cell hyperplasia and increased macromolecular uptake in an animal model of giardiasis. *J. Parasitol.* 83, 908–912. doi: 10.2307/3284287

Hidalgo, I. J., Raub, T. J., and Borchardt, R. T. (1989). Characterization of the human colon carcinoma cell line (Caco-2) as a model system for intestinal epithelial permeability. *Gastroenterology* 96, 736–749. doi: 10.1016/S0016-5085(89)80072-1

Humen, M. A., Pérez, P. F., and Liévin-Le Moal, V. (2011). Lipid raft-dependent adhesion of *Giardia intestinalis* trophozoites to a cultured human enterocyte-like Caco-2/TC7 cell monolayer leads to cytoskeleton-dependent functional injuries. *Cell. Microbiol.* 13, 1683–1702. doi: 10.1111/j.1462-5822.2011.0 1647.x

Ives, A., Ronet, C., Prevel, F., Ruzzante, G., Fuertes-Marraco, S., Schutz, F., et al. (2011). Leishmania RNA virus controls the severity of mucocutaneous leishmaniasis. *Science* 331, 775–778. doi: 10.1126/science.1199326

Janssen, M. E. W., Takagi, Y., Parent, K. N., Cardone, G., Nibert, M. L., and Baker, T. S. (2015). Three-dimensional structure of a protozoal double-stranded RNA virus that infects the enteric pathogen *Giardia lamblia*. *J. Virol.* 89, 1182–1194. doi: 10.1128/JVI.02745-14

Johnston, S. D., Smye, M., Watson, R. G., McMillan, S. A., Trimble, E. R., and Love, A. H. (2000). Lactulose-mannitol intestinal permeability test: a useful screening test for adult coeliac disease. *Ann. Clin. Biochem.* 37, 512–519. doi: 10.1177/ 000456320003700413

Jonckheere, J. F., de, and Gordts, B. (1987). Occurrence and transfection of a Giardia virus. *Mol. Biochem. Parasitol.* 23, 85–89. doi: 10.1016/0166-6851(87)90190-3

Jung, H. C., Eckmann, L., Yang, S. K., Panja, A., Fierer, J., Morzycka-Wroblewska, E., et al. (1995). A distinct array of proinflammatory cytokines is expressed in human colon epithelial cells in response to bacterial invasion. *J. Clin. Invest.* 95, 55–65. doi: 10.1172/JCI117676

Kamda, J. D., and Singer, S. M. (2009). Phosphoinositide 3-kinase-dependent inhibition of dendritic cell interleukin-12 production by *Giardia lamblia*. *Infect. Immun.* 77, 1–9. doi: 10.1128/IAI.00718-08

Katelaris, P. H., Naeem, A., and Farthing, M. J. (1995). Attachment of *Giardia lamblia* trophozoites to a cultured human intestinal cell line. *Gut* 37, 512–518. doi: 10.1136/gut.37.4.512

Keister, D. B. (1983). Axenic culture of *Giardia lamblia* in TYI-S-33 medium supplemented with bile. *Trans. R. Soc. Trop. Med. Hyg.* 77, 487–488. doi: 10.1016/0035-9203(83)90120-7

Kido, H., Okumura, Y., Takahashi, E., Pan, H.-Y., Wang, S., Yao, D., et al. (2012). Role of host cellular proteases in the pathogenesis of influenza and influenza-induced multiple organ failure. *Biochim. Biophys. Acta* 1824, 186–194. doi: 10.1016/j.bbapap.2011.07.001

Kiela, P. R., and Ghishan, F. K. (2016). Physiology of intestinal absorption and secretion. *Best Pract. Res. Clin. Gastroenterol.* 30, 145–159. doi: 10.1016/j.bpg.2016.02.007

Klotz, C., and Aebischer, T. (2015). The immunological enigma of human Giardiasis. *Curr. Trop. Med. Rep.* 2, 119–127. doi: 10.1007/s40475-015-0050-2

Koh, W. H., Geurden, T., Paget, T., O'Handley, R., Steuart, R. F., Thompson, R. C. A., et al. (2013). *Giardia duodenalis* assemblage-specific induction of apoptosis and tight junction disruption in human intestinal epithelial cells: effects of mixed infections. *J. Parasitol.* 99, 353–358. doi: 10.1645/GE-3021.1

Kosek, M. N. (2017). Causal pathways from enteropathogens to environmental enteropathy: findings from the MAL-ED birth cohort study. *EBioMedicine* 18, 109–117. doi: 10.1016/j.ebiom.2017.02.024

Kotloff, K. L., Nataro, J. P., Blackwelder, W. C., Nasrin, D., Farag, T. H., Panchalingam, S., et al. (2013). Burden and aetiology of diarrhoeal disease in infants and young children in developing countries (the Global Enteric Multicenter Study, GEMS): a prospective, case-control study. *Lancet* 382, 209–222. doi: 10.1016/S0140-6736(13)60844-2

Leroy, A., Lauwaet, T., Bruyne, G., de, Cornelissen, M., and Mareel, M. (2000). *Entamoeba histolytica* disturbs the tight junction complex in human enteric T84 cell layers. *FASEB J.* 14, 1139–1146.

Li, E., Stenson, W. F., Kunz-Jenkins, C., Swanson, P. E., Duncan, R., and Stanley, S. L. (1994). *Entamoeba histolytica* interactions with polarized human intestinal Caco-2 epithelial cells. *Infect. Immun.* 62, 5112–5119.

Liévin-Le Moal, V. (2013). Dysfunctions at human intestinal barrier by water-borne protozoan parasites: lessons from cultured human fully differentiated colon cancer cell lines. *Cell. Microbiol.* 15, 860–869. doi: 10.1111/cmi.12126

Litleskare, S., Wensaas, K.-A., Eide, G. E., Hanevik, K., Kahrs, G. E., Langeland, N., et al. (2015). Perceived food intolerance and irritable bowel syndrome in a population 3 years after a giardiasis-outbreak: a historical cohort study. *BMC Gastroenterol.* 15:164. doi: 10.1186/s12876-015-0393-0

Liu, Q., Mittal, R., Emami, C. N., Iversen, C., Ford, H. R., and Prasadarao, N. V. (2012). Human isolates of *Cronobacter sakazakii* bind efficiently to intestinal epithelial cells *in vitro* to induce monolayer permeability and apoptosis. *J. Surg. Res.* 176, 437–447. doi: 10.1016/j.jss.2011.10.030

Maia-Brigagao, C., Morgado-Diaz, J. A., and de Souza, W. (2012). Giardia disrupts the arrangement of tight, adherens and desmosomal junction proteins of intestinal cells. *Parasitol. Int.* 61, 280–287. doi: 10.1016/j.parint.2011.11.002

Malago, J. J., Koninkx, J. F. J. G., Ovelgonne, H. H., van Asten, F. J. A. M., Swennenhuis, J. F., and van Dijk, J. E. (2003). Expression levels of heat shock proteins in enterocyte-like Caco-2 cells after exposure to *Salmonella enteritidis*. *Cell Stress Chaperones* 8, 194–203. doi: 10.1379/1466-1268(2003)008<0194:ELOHSP>2.0.CO;2

Miller, R. L., Wang, A. L., and Wang, C. C. (1988). Identification of *Giardia lamblia* isolates susceptible and resistant to infection by the double-stranded RNA virus. *Exp. Parasitol.* 66, 118–123. doi: 10.1016/0014-4894(88)90056-2

Muhsen, K., Cohen, D., and Levine, M. M. (2014). Can *Giardia lamblia* infection lower the risk of acute diarrhea among preschool children? *J. Trop. Pediatr.* 60, 99–103. doi: 10.1093/tropej/fmt085

Nakao, J. H., Collier, S. A., and Gargano, J. W. (2017). Giardiasis and subsequent irritable bowel syndrome: a longitudinal cohort study using health insurance data. *J. Infect. Dis.* 215, 798–805. doi: 10.1093/infdis/jiw621

Oberhuber, G., Kastner, N., and Stolte, M. (1997). Giardiasis: a histologic analysis of 567 cases. *Scand. J. Gastroenterol.* 32, 48–51. doi: 10.3109/00365529709025062

Panaro, M. A., Cianciulli, A., Mitolo, V., Mitolo, C. I., Acquafredda, A., Brandonisio, O., et al. (2007). Caspase-dependent apoptosis of the HCT-8 epithelial cell line induced by the parasite *Giardia intestinalis*. *FEMS Immunol. Med. Microbiol.* 51, 302–309. doi: 10.1111/j.1574-695X.2007.00304.x

Rees, L. E. N., Cogan, T. A., Dodson, A. L., Birchall, M. A., Bailey, M., and Humphrey, T. J. (2008). Campylobacter and IFNgamma interact to cause a rapid loss of epithelial barrier integrity. *Inflamm. Bowel Dis.* 14, 303–309. doi: 10.1002/ibd.20325

Rogawski, E. T., Bartelt, L. A., Platts-Mills, J. A., Seidman, J. C., Samie, A., Havt, A., et al. (2017). Determinants and impact of giardia infection in the first 2 years of life in the MAL-ED birth cohort. *J. Pediatr. Infect. Dis. Soc.* 6, 153–160. doi: 10.1093/jpids/piw082

Roxström-Lindquist, K., Ringqvist, E., Palm, D., and Svärd, S. (2005). *Giardia lamblia*-induced changes in gene expression in differentiated Caco-2 human intestinal epithelial cells. *Infect. Immun.* 73, 8204–8208. doi: 10.1128/IAI.73.12.8204-8208.2005

Sambuy, Y., Angelis, I., de, Ranaldi, G., Scarino, M. L., Stammati, A., and Zucco, F. (2005). The Caco-2 cell line as a model of the intestinal barrier: influence of cell and culture-related factors on Caco-2 cell functional characteristics. *Cell Biol. Toxicol.* 21, 1–26. doi: 10.1007/s10565-005-0085-6

Savioli, L., Smith, H., and Thompson, A. (2006). Giardia and Cryptosporidium join the 'Neglected diseases initiative'. *Trends Parasitol.* 22, 203–208. doi: 10.1016/j.pt.2006.02.015

Scott, K. G., Meddings, J. B., Kirk, Lees-Miller, S. P., and Buret, A. G. (2002). Intestinal infection with *Giardia* spp. reduces epithelial barrier function in a myosin light chain kinase-dependent fashion. *Gastroenterology* 123, 1179–1190. doi: 10.1053/gast.2002.36002

Scott, K. G.-E., Yu, L. C. H., and Buret, A. G. (2004). Role of CD8+ and CD4+ T lymphocytes in jejunal mucosal injury during murine giardiasis. *Infect. Immun.* 72, 3536–3542. doi: 10.1128/IAI.72.6.3536-3542.2004

Seow, F., Katelaris, P., and Ngu, M. (1993). The effect of *Giardia lamblia* trophozoites on trypsin, chymotrypsin and amylase *in vitro*. *Parasitology* 106, 233. doi: 10.1017/S0031182000075053

Sepp, T., Wang, A. L., and Wang, C. C. (1994). Giardiavirus-resistant *Giardia lamblia* lacks a virus receptor on the cell membrane surface. *J. Virol.* 68, 1426–1431.

Serrander, R., Magnusson, K. E., and Sundqvist, T. (1984). Acute infections with *Giardia lamblia* and rotavirus decrease intestinal permeability to low-molecular weight polyethylene glycols (PEG 400). *Scand. J. Infect. Dis.* 16, 339–344. doi: 10.3109/00365548409073958

Singer, S. M., and Nash, T. E. (2000). The role of normal flora in *Giardia lamblia* infections in mice. *J. Infect. Dis.* 181, 1510–1512. doi: 10.1086/315409

Slapeta, J., Dowd, S. E., Alanazi, A. D., Westman, M. E., and Brown, G. K. (2015). Differences in the faecal microbiome of non-diarrhoeic clinically healthy dogs and cats associated with *Giardia duodenalis* infection: impact of hookworms and coccidia. *Int. J. Parasitol.* 45, 585–594. doi: 10.1016/j.ijpara.2015.04.001

Srinivasan, B., Kolli, A. R., Esch, M. B., Abaci, H. E., Shuler, M. L., and Hickman, J. J. (2015). TEER measurement techniques for *in vitro* barrier model systems. *J. Lab. Autom.* 20, 107–126. doi: 10.1177/2211068214561025

Sun, H., Chow, E. C., Liu, S., Du, Y., and Pang, K. S. (2008). The Caco-2 cell monolayer: usefulness and limitations. *Expert Opin. Drug Metab. Toxicol.* 4, 395–411. doi: 10.1517/17425255.4.4.395

Teoh, D. A., Kamieniecki, D., Pang, G., and Buret, A. G. (2000). *Giardia lamblia* rearranges F-actin and alpha-actinin in human colonic and duodenal monolayers and reduces transepithelial electrical resistance. *J. Parasitol.* 86, 800–806. doi: 10.1645/0022-3395(2000)086[0800:GLRFAA]2.0.CO;2

Thompson, R. A., and Monis, P. (2012). Giardia—from genome to proteome. *Adv. Parasitol.* 78, 57–95. doi: 10.1016/B978-0-12-394303-3.00003-7

Troeger, H., Epple, H.-J., Schneider, T., Wahnschaffe, U., Ullrich, R., Burchard, G.-D., et al. (2007). Effect of chronic *Giardia lamblia* infection on epithelial transport and barrier function in human duodenum. *Gut* 56, 328–335. doi: 10.1136/gut.2006.100198

Turner, J. R., Lencer, W. I., Carlson, S., and Madara, J. L. (1996). Carboxy-terminal vesicular stomatitis virus G protein-tagged intestinal Na+-dependent glucose cotransporter (SGLT1): maintenance of surface expression and global transport function with selective perturbation of transport kinetics and polarized expression. *J. Biol. Chem.* 271, 7738–7744. doi: 10.1074/jbc.271.13.7738

Tysnes, K. R., and Robertson, L. J. (2015). Investigation of effects of *Giardia duodenalis* on transcellular and paracellular transport in enterocytes using *in vitro* Ussing chamber experiments. *Parasitology* 142, 691–697. doi: 10.1017/S0031182014001772

Wang, A. L., and Wang, C. C. (1986). Discovery of a specific double-stranded RNA virus in *Giardia lamblia*. *Mol. Biochem. Parasitol.* 21, 269–276. doi: 10.1016/0166-6851(86)90132-5

Wensaas, K.-A., Langeland, N., Hanevik, K., Morch, K., Eide, G. E., and Rortveit, G. (2012). Irritable bowel syndrome and chronic fatigue 3 years after acute giardiasis: historic cohort study. *Gut* 61, 214–219. doi: 10.1136/gutjnl-2011-300220

Wu, Z., Mirza, H., Teo, J. D. W., and Tan, K. S. W. (2014). Strain-dependent induction of human enterocyte apoptosis by blastocystis disrupts epithelial barrier and ZO-1 organization in a caspase 3- and 9-dependent manner. *Biomed. Res. Int.* 2014:209163. doi: 10.1155/2014/209163

Yu, L. C. H., Flynn, A. N., Turner, J. R., and Buret, A. G. (2005). SGLT-1-mediated glucose uptake protects intestinal epithelial cells against LPS-induced apoptosis and barrier defects: a novel cellular rescue mechanism? *FASEB J.* 19, 1822–1835. doi: 10.1096/fj.05-4226com

Yu, L. C., Huang, C. Y., Kuo, W. T., Sayer, H., Turner, J. R., and Buret, A. G. (2008). SGLT-1-mediated glucose uptake protects human intestinal epithelial cells against *Giardia duodenalis*-induced apoptosis. *Int. J. Parasitol.* 38, 923–934. doi: 10.1016/j.ijpara.2007.12.004

Zehendner, C. M., Librizzi, L., Curtis, M., de, Kuhlmann, C. R. W., and Luhmann, H. J. (2011). Caspase-3 contributes to ZO-1 and Cl-5 tight-junction disruption in rapid anoxic neurovascular unit damage. *PLoS ONE* 6:e16760. doi: 10.1371/journal.pone.0016760

Zoellner, H., Hofler, M., Beckmann, R., Hufnagl, P., Vanyek, E., Bielek, E., et al. (1996). Serum albumin is a specific inhibitor of apoptosis in human endothelial cells. *J. Cell Sci.* *109*, 2571–2580.

7

Behavior of Neutrophil Granulocytes during *Toxoplasma gondii* Infection in the Central Nervous System

Aindrila Biswas[1], Timothy French[1], Henning P. Düsedau[1], Nancy Mueller[1], Monika Riek-Burchardt[2], Anne Dudeck[2], Ute Bank[2], Thomas Schüler[2†] and Ildiko Rita Dunay[1†]*

[1] Institute of Inflammation and Neurodegeneration, Otto-von-Guericke University Magdeburg, Magdeburg, Germany,
[2] Institute for Molecular and Clinical Immunology, Otto-von-Guericke University Magdeburg, Magdeburg, Germany

Edited by:
Anton Aebischer,
Robert Koch-Institute, Germany

Reviewed by:
Emma Harriet Wilson,
University of California, Riverside,
United States
Michal Adam Olszewski,
University of Michigan, United States

***Correspondence:**
Ildiko Rita Dunay
ildikodunay@gmail.com

† These authors have contributed equally to this work.

Cerebral toxoplasmosis is characterized by activation of brain resident cells and recruitment of specific immune cell subsets from the periphery to the central nervous system (CNS). Our studies revealed that the rapidly invaded Ly6G$^+$ neutrophil granulocytes are an early non-lymphoid source of interferon-gamma (IFN-γ), the cytokine known to be the major mediator of host resistance to *Toxoplasma gondii* (*T. gondii*). Upon selective depletion of Ly6G$^+$ neutrophils, we detected reduced IFN-γ production and increased parasite burden in the CNS. Ablation of Ly6G$^+$ cells resulted in diminished recruitment of Ly6C^{hi} monocytes into the CNS, indicating a pronounced interplay. Additionally, we identified infiltrated Ly6G$^+$ neutrophils to be a heterogeneous population. The Ly6G$^+$CD62-L^{hi}CXCR4$^+$ subset released cathelicidin-related antimicrobial peptide (CRAMP), which can promote monocyte dynamics. On the other hand, the Ly6G$^+$CD62-L^{lo}CXCR4$^+$ subset produced IFN-γ to establish early inflammatory response. Collectively, our findings revealed that the recruited Ly6G$^+$CXCR4$^+$ neutrophil granulocytes display a heterogeneity in the CNS with a repertoire of effector functions crucial in parasite control and immune regulation upon experimental cerebral toxoplasmosis.

Keywords: *Toxoplasma gondii*, neutrophil granulocytes, cerebral toxoplasmosis, neuroinflammation, neutrophil Infiltration

INTRODUCTION

T. gondii is a highly successful parasite capable of crossing most biological barriers of the body (Barragan, 2002; Harker et al., 2015). The parasite can infect migratory immune cells such as dendritic cells (DCs), macrophages and neutrophil granulocytes to enter immunoprivileged sites (Barragan, 2002; Da Gama et al., 2004; Courret et al., 2006; Lambert et al., 2006). During the acute phase of infection, enterocytes secrete chemokines including monocyte chemotactic protein-1 (MCP-1) and macrophage inflammatory protein-2 (MIP-2), which recruit neutrophil granulocytes, inflammatory monocytes and DCs to the site of infection (Robben et al., 2005; Courret et al., 2006; Pittman and Knoll, 2015). We have previously detected that the CD8α^+ DC subset is the crucial source of interleukin-12 (IL-12), the cytokine that stimulates natural killer (NK) cells and T cells to produce the cytokine IFN-γ (Mashayekhi et al., 2011). IFN-γ is a major mediator of host resistance to *T. gondii*, regulating a plethora of intracellular mechanisms to eliminate the parasite (Gazzinelli et al., 1993; Hunter et al., 1994; Kang and Suzuki, 2001; Kim and Weiss, 2004; Gazzinelli and Sher, 2014). Recent studies revealed that neutrophil granulocytes, besides innate lymphoid cells, NK cells and T cells, are able to produce IFN-γ (Sturge et al., 2013). They also produce IFN-γ independently from toll-like receptor (TLR)11-induced IL-12 during acute toxoplasmosis in the periphery (Sturge et al., 2013, 2015). Our previous experiments provided evidence that unlike inflammatory monocytes, neutrophil granulocytes worsened ileal pathology upon specific depletion in the acute phase of toxoplasmosis (Dunay et al., 2010). These studies were carried out in mice, which had an intact TLR-recognition system responsible for IL-12 dependent IFN-γ production by NK and T cells. However, the relative contribution of neutrophil granulocytes to IFN-γ production was not elucidated.

The parasites can enter the CNS within immune cells, initially infecting endothelial cells of the blood-brain barrier, where they egress, and invade brain resident cells (Konradt et al., 2016). Cyst formation within neurons undergoing a stress-mediated response is followed by ongoing basal inflammation, establishing a chronic persistent infection (Parlog et al., 2014; Blanchard et al., 2015). Chronic cerebral toxoplasmosis is characterized by the activation of resident cells such as microglia and astrocytes, which carry out distinct antiparasitic functions (Strack et al., 2002; Schluter et al., 2003; Drögemüller et al., 2008; Kamerkar and Davis, 2012; Cabral et al., 2016). In addition, peripheral immune cell subsets of myeloid and lymphoid origin are recruited to the inflamed CNS (John et al., 2011). Recently, we characterized the behavior of infiltrating $CD11b^{+}Ly6C^{hi}$ myeloid derived cells, which carry out a pivotal role upon cerebral toxoplasmosis (Möhle et al., 2014, 2016; Biswas et al., 2015). Several studies have highlighted the role of brain-resident cells, lymphocytes, DCs, and macrophages (Strack et al., 2002; John et al., 2011), however, the function of neutrophil granulocytes in host defense in the CNS is still uncertain.

Neutrophil granulocytes differentiating from the common myeloid progenitor in the bone marrow (BM) form the first line of defense during infection and inflammation (Soehnlein et al., 2008b). Upon reaching the site of infection, neutrophils can execute many immune functions including production of reactive oxygen species (ROS) or proinflammatory modulators (Denkers et al., 2012; Bardoel et al., 2014; Perez-de-Puig et al., 2015). The surface marker Ly6G, exclusively expressed on neutrophil granulocytes, facilitates distinction from monocytes, enabling specific functional studies. The role of neutrophil granulocytes in the periphery and the CNS has been investigated in multiple neurodegenerative diseases and infections, however, their impact on cerebral toxoplasmosis remains to be elucidated (Zhou et al., 2003; Zehntner et al., 2005; Mildner et al., 2008; Ransohoff and Engelhardt, 2012; Sturge et al., 2013; Wantha et al., 2013; Marais et al., 2014).

Here we characterized the phenotype and behavior of $Ly6G^{+}$ neutrophil granulocytes in chronic *T. gondii* infection. We detected their influx into the CNS during the acute stage of cerebral toxoplasmosis, which was associated with the upregulation of expression of certain activation markers and co-stimulatory molecules. Importantly, intracellular cytokine analysis revealed that neutrophil granulocytes form a non-lymphoid source of the pro-inflammatory cytokine IFN-γ at the acute stage of infection. Upon using a specific anti-granulocyte monoclonal antibody (mAb) 1A8, we measured a significant increase in the parasite burden. We also detected a reduction in monocyte recruitment and IFN-γ production confirming the specific contribution of neutrophil granulocytes. Neutrophils exhibited heterogeneity based on specific expression of the adhesion molecule CD62-L and the chemokine receptor CXCR4, respectively. This implies that multiple signals at the site of the inflammation can influence the functional characteristics and phenotype of neutrophils.

MATERIALS AND METHODS

Animals

Age and sex matched C57BL/6 wild-type (WT) mice, obtained from Janvier (Cedex, France) were used. All animal care was in accordance with institutional guidelines. Food and water were available *ad libitum*. Experiments were performed in accordance to German and European legislation.

Infection

T. gondii cysts of type II strain ME 49 were harvested from the brains of female NMRI mice infected intra-peritoneally (i.p.) with *T. gondii* cysts 8–10 months earlier. Brains obtained from infected mice were mechanically homogenized in 1 ml sterile phosphate-buffered saline (PBS). Cyst numbers were counted in a 10 μl brain suspension using a light microscope. Two cysts were administered i.p. in a total volume of 200 μl per mouse as described before (Möhle et al., 2016). Control mice were mock-infected with sterile PBS. The mice were perfused intracardially with 60 ml sterile ice-cold PBS. The brains were removed for further analysis. The acute stage of infection was defined between day 10 and day 14 whereas the chronic stage of infection was starting at day 21. Therefore, to investigate the recruited neutrophil granulocytes in chronic cerebral toxoplasmosis, mice were sacrificed 4 weeks post-infection for further analysis.

1A8 mAb Treatment

Depletion of neutrophils was performed by i.p. administration of anti-Ly6G mAb (clone 1A8, BioXCell). Mice were injected with 500 μg (as described before by Daley et al., 2008; Dunay et al., 2010) of the antibody i.p. on alternate days from days 10 to 23 post-infection. Mice were sacrificed 24 h after the last antibody treatment. Rat IgG2a (BioXCell) was used as a control to mAb.

Cell Isolation

Brains were homogenized in a buffer containing 1M HEPES (pH 7.3) and 45% glucose and then sieved through a 70 μm strainer. The cell suspension was washed and fractionated on 25–75% Percoll gradient (GE Healthcare). Isolated cells were washed with PBS and used immediately for further experiments. Peripheral blood was obtained from posterior vena cava and lysed with erythrocyte (RBC) lysis buffer (eBioscience). Subsequently, these cells were stained with the desired fluorescent conjugated antibodies (Biswas et al., 2015).

Flow Cytometry

Isolated mononuclear cells were incubated with Zombie NIR™ or Violet™ fixable dye (Biolegend) for live/dead discrimination. Unspecific antibody binding was blocked by incubation with anti-FcγIII/II receptor antibody (clone 93). Thereafter, cells were stained with fluorochrome-conjugated antibodies against cell surface markers: CD45 (30-F11), CD11b (M1/70), Ly6C (HK1.4), MHC I H-2D^b (28-14-8), MHC II I-A/I-E (M5/114.15.2), CD80 (16-10A1), and CD86 (GL1), all purchased from eBioscience, CXCR2 (SA04E1), CXCR4 (L27GF12), and CD64 (X54-5/7.1) from Biolegend, Ly6G (1A8), CD62-L (MEL-14) from BD Bioscience, then washed and fixed in 4% paraformaldehyde. Matched isotype controls were used to assess the level of unspecific binding.

For intracellular cytokine staining, single-cell suspensions (5×10^5 cells/well) were stimulated in 96-well plates in the presence of *Toxoplasma* lysate antigen (5 μg/ml) and Brefeldin A (10 μg/ml, GolgiPlug, BD Biosciences). After 6 h, cells were incubated with Zombie NIR™ or Violet™ fixable dye and anti-FcγIII/II receptor antibody (clone 93) and surface stained for CD45 (30-F11), CD11b (M1/70), Ly6G (1A8), Ly6C (HK1.4), CRAMP (R-170), washed in FACS buffer [PBS with 1% of fetal calf serum (FCS)] and fixed in 4% paraformaldehyde. Cells were permeabilized using Permeabilization Buffer (Biolegend). To measure the cytokine expression, the staining was performed with the following antibodies: IL-1α (ALF-161), TNF (MP6-XT22), NOS2 (CXNFT), IFN-γ (XMG1.2), IL-1β (NJTEN3), and IL-10 (JES5-16E3) from eBioscience in Permeabilization Buffer (Biolegend) (Biswas et al., 2015).

A total of 100,000 cells was acquired using a flow cytometer (BD FACS Canto II). Data were analyzed using FlowJo software (Version 10 Tree Star). Matched isotype controls were used to assess the level of unspecific binding.

Detection of Reactive Oxygen Species

Isolated cells were stained for CD45 (30-F11), CD11b (M1/70), Ly6G (1A8), Ly6C (HK1.4), CXCR4 (L27GF12), and CD62-L (MEL-14) in FACS buffer for 30 min after blocking FcγRs. ROS production was measured by Total ROS Detection Kit (ENZO, 51011), according to the manufacturer's instructions.

q- and qRT-PCR

RNA and DNA was isolated from the right hemisphere of the infected mice as previously described (Möhle et al., 2016). Following the isolation of the nucleic acids, semi-quantitative PCR was performed to measure the parasite burden and the cytokine gene expression levels in the brain.

Immunofluorescence

Mice were anesthetized with isoflurane and perfused intracardially with saline followed by paraformaldehyde (PFA, 4%) in phosphate buffer (pH 7.4). The brain was removed, post-fixed with PFA overnight, cryoprotected in 30% sucrose, frozen, and 20-μm-thick sections were prepared in a cryostat. The sections were fixed with ethanol, blocked with normal serum and incubated overnight at 4°C with the primary antibody SAG-1 (D61S clone; 1:20, Invitrogen) or PECAM-1/CD31 (MEC13.3 clone; 1:500) and Ly6G (1A8 clone; 1:200). Following the primary antibody staining, lectin staining was performed (Fluorescein labeled Dolichos Biflorus Agglutinin (DBA); 1:500, Vector Laboratories) according to the manufacturer's guidelines. Then, sections were incubated for 2 h at room temperature with secondary antibodies (Alexa Fluor-488, Thermo Fischer Scientific). Controls were carried out by omission of the primary antibodies. Sections were counterstained with Sytox Red Dead Cell Stain (1:20,000, Thermo Fischer Scientific) to visualize the cell nuclei and slides were observed under a confocal laser microscope (LSM510, Carl Zeiss).

Statistical Analysis

Data were analyzed by Mann-Whitney test for two groups or one-way ANOVA for several groups followed by Tukey's post-test with GraphPad Prism 6 (San Diego, CA). In all cases, results were presented as mean ± standard deviation (SD) and were considered significant, with $p < 0.05$.

RESULTS

Rapid Influx of Neutrophil Granulocytes into the Brain upon Cerebral Toxoplasmosis

Infection of mice with *T. gondii* induces egress of Ly6C^{hi} monocytes and Ly6G$^+$ neutrophil granulocytes from the BM to the blood. Following our previous characterization of BM derived monocytes in the CNS in 4 weeks *T. gondii*-infected mice, we analyzed neutrophil dynamics using the same experimental model. CD11b and Ly6C expression were used to identify the inflammatory monocytes (Ly6C^{hi}), neutrophils (Ly6C^{int}) and resident monocytes (Ly6C^{lo}) in the blood (**Figures 1A,C**). The CD11b$^+$ cells were further differentiated based on their Ly6C and Ly6G expression (**Figures 1B,D**). The neutrophil specific Ab Ly6G (1A8) was applied to distinguish neutrophil granulocytes (Ly6G$^+$) from monocytes (Ly6G$^-$) (**Figures 1B,D**). We observed increased percentages of circulating neutrophil granulocytes in peripheral blood of infected mice (30 ± 3.06%) as compared to non-infected controls (15.7 ± 1%; **Figures 1B,D**).

Alongside the enhanced egress of immune cells in the periphery, cerebral toxoplasmosis leads to the activation of brain resident cells and infiltration of circulating immune cells to the CNS (Möhle et al., 2014; Biswas et al., 2015). Peripheral immune cell influx into the infected brain is characterized by initial invasion of neutrophils, followed by the recruitment of BM-derived monocytes and the lymphocytes. While in non-infected controls the main immune cell population was resting resident microglia (CD45^{lo}CD11b$^+$; **Figures 1E,F**), we observed the entry of CD45^{hi} myeloid derived population in the brains of *T. gondii*-infected mice (**Figure 1G**). The recruited cells included two populations, CD45^{hi}CD11b$^-$ cells (ungated; **Figure 1G**) and CD45^{hi}CD11b$^+$ cells (upper gate; 10.0 ± 2.1% of the parent population). The CD45^{hi}CD11b$^+$ cells comprised of BM-derived myeloid cells, namely monocytes, neutrophil granulocytes, macrophages and DCs. Upon infection,

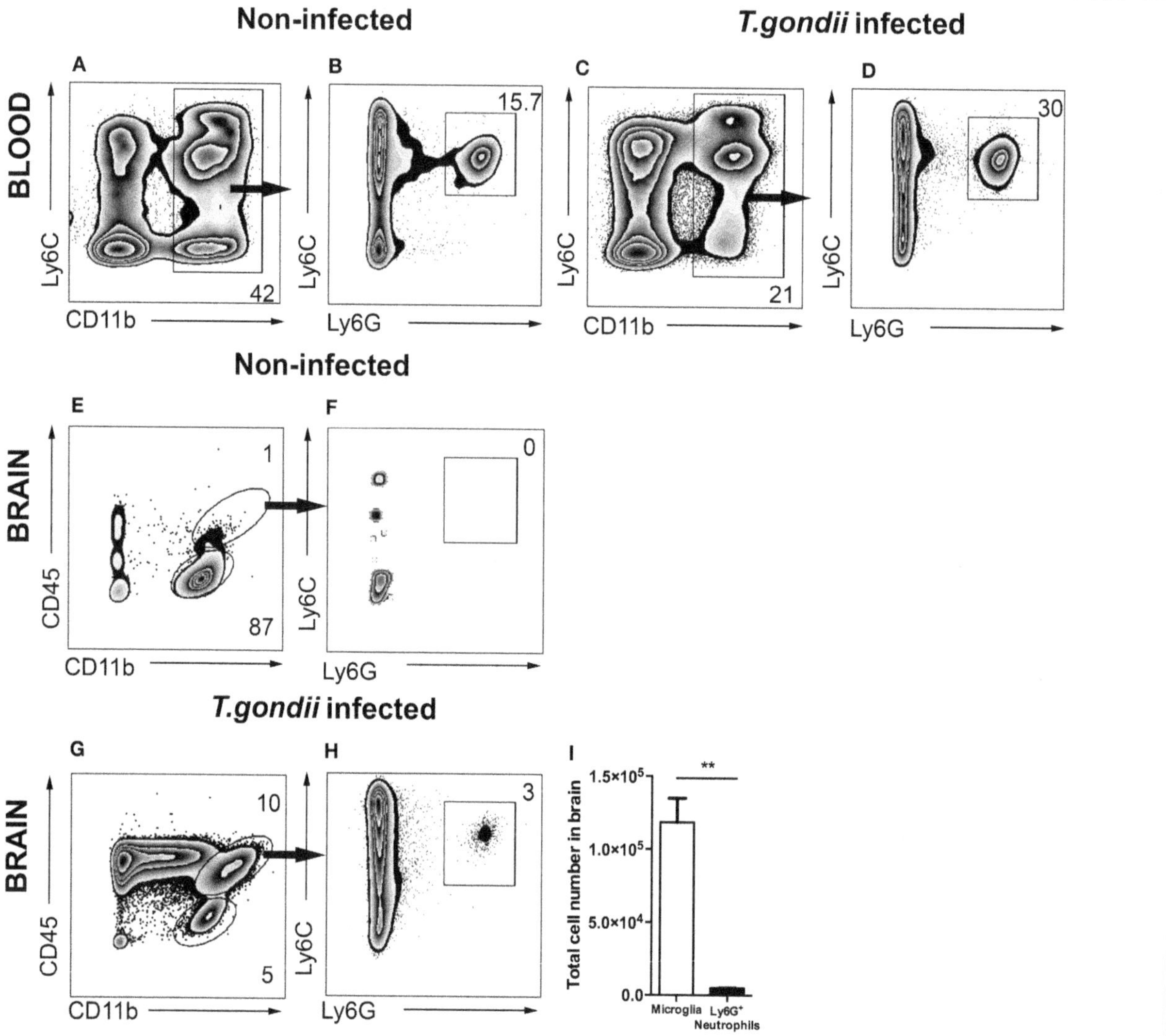

FIGURE 1 | Gating strategy of neutrophil granulocytes in blood and in brain. Cells were isolated from the blood and brain of non-infected mice **(A,B,E,F)** and the blood and brain of 4 weeks *T. gondii*-infected mice **(C,D,G,H)** and analyzed by flow cytometry. Following FSC-SSC, singlet gating and exclusion of dead cells (not shown), live cells were used for further analysis. **(A,C)** Show gating of CD11b$^+$ cells in the blood which are further characterized into Ly6C$^+$Ly6G$^+$ neutrophil granulocytes **(B,D)**. **(E)** Shows the resident microglia (CD11b$^+$CD45^{lo}, lower gate), and **(F)** shows the percentage of neutrophil granulocytes (Ly6C$^+$Ly6G$^+$) from myeloid populations in the brains of non-infected animals (CD11b$^+$CD45^{hi}, upper gate). **(G,H)** Shows the exact same gating strategy in the infected brains. **(I)** The bar graphs represent total number of cells (activated microglia - white bar and neutrophil granulocytes - black bar) in the infected brains. Numbers represent % of parent population. The data shown is representative for 3 independent experiments with 5 mice per group for each experiment. Mann-Whitney test was performed for comparisons (**$p < 0.01$).

brain resident activated microglia cells expressed elevated CD45 levels (CD45^{int}CD11b$^+$; 5.0 ± 1.06% of the parent population). The anti-Ly6G (1A8) antibody was applied to distinguish Ly6G$^+$ neutrophil granulocytes (**Figure 1H**; 3.0 ± 1.02% of the CD45^{hi}CD11b$^+$) from monocytes. Next, the total number of mononuclear cells was quantified in the brain during chronic cerebral toxoplasmosis (**Figure 1I**). Thus, CD45^{hi}CD11b$^+$Ly6G$^+$ neutrophil granulocytes ($6 \times 10^3 \pm 50$) formed a small yet defined population, when compared to the absolute numbers of CD45^{int}CD11b$^+$ microglia ($1 \times 10^5 \pm 2{,}000$). These data demonstrate that cerebral toxoplasmosis leads to the activation of resident microglia and the recruitment of lymphoid and myeloid immune cells including neutrophil granulocytes.

Localization of Neutrophil Granulocytes in the CNS during the Course of Cerebral Toxoplasmosis

Neutrophil granulocytes, the earliest immune cells to arrive at the site of infection, can deploy a plethora of mechanisms to attack invading pathogens (Denkers et al., 2012; Bardoel et al., 2014; Perez-de-Puig et al., 2015). To study their localization around *T. gondii* in the CNS, we performed immunofluorescence analysis of mice brain slices at the acute stage and chronic stage of the infection. We observed that neutrophil granulocytes were not only in the blood vessels, marked by PECAM1, but entered the brain parenchyma (**Figure 2A**). The recruited neutrophils were in close proximity to the *T. gondii* tachyzoites in the cerebral cortex during the acute stage infection (**Figure 2B**). Upon encystation of the *T. gondii* parasites in the chronic phase, we observed the absence of neutrophils in the vicinity of bradyzoite containing cysts (**Figure 2C**). These immunofluorescence results indicate the affinity of the neutrophil granulocytes to the infective stage of *T. gondii* in contrast to the dormant stage during the course of the cerebral toxoplasmosis.

Phenotypic Analysis of Infiltrating Neutrophils Upon Cerebral *T. gondii* Infection

To further characterize neutrophil granulocytes in inflamed brains upon 4 weeks of *T. gondii* infection, the expression profiles of various cell surface markers were determined by flow cytometry. As control, microglia were selected, because under homeostatic condition neutrophils are not present in the CNS, and immune cells from the same isolate chosen for the comparison. A large percentage of infiltrating neutrophils expressed enhanced levels of MHC I and MHC II (83 ± 1% MHC I; 95 ± 0.5% MHC II) (**Figures 3M–P**) unlike in the periphery (25 ± 4% MHC I; 3 ± 0.5% MHC II) (**Figures 3A–D**). According to their function as antigen presenting cells (APCs) of the brain, activated microglia also expressed significant levels of MHC I and MHC II (100% MHC I; 100% MHC II) (**Figures 3M–P**). We further compared the expression of the co-stimulatory molecules CD80 and CD86 and detected these on small parts of the neutrophil population (15 ± 0.5% CD80; 17 ± 0.5% CD86) and activated microglia (18 ± 1% CD80; 52 ± 1% CD86) (**Figures 3Q–T**). The phagocytosis mediating receptor CD64 (FcgR1), which was present on a large proportion of activated microglia (89 ± 1% CD64), was only detectable on a small percentage of neutrophils (11 ± 0.5%) (**Figures 3U,V**). The chemokine receptor CXCR2 was detected on more than half of the neutrophils (65 ± 0.5%). However, only a small percentage of activated microglia expressed CXCR2 (5 ± 0.5%) (**Figures 3W,X**). The neutrophil granulocytes in the periphery did not express any significant levels of CD80, CD86 and CD64 (**Figures 3E–J**). However, the entire neutrophil population expressed CXCR2 (**Figures 3K,L**). Hence, activated microglia and neutrophils express immune modulatory molecules in infected brains indicating their contribution to the establishment of local immunity in response to *T. gondii* infection.

Cytokine Production of Infiltrating Neutrophils upon Cerebral *T. gondii* Infection

Several studies have demonstrated that neutrophil granulocytes secrete plenty of immune modulatory molecules including cytokines upon infection (Sturge et al., 2013; Bardoel et al., 2014). To determine their cytokine expression profile, in experimental cerebral toxoplasmosis (4 weeks *T. gondii* infection), myeloid cells from the infected brain were analyzed by intracellular flow cytometry. We observed that neutrophil granulocytes hardly produced pro-inflammatory cytokines such as IL-1α and TNF (3 ± 1% and 5 ± 0.5%, respectively). On the contrary, microglia served as a considerable source of both cytokines (50 ± 3% and 80 ± 1%, respectively) (**Figures 4A,B,E,F**). Importantly, 65 ± 0.5% of neutrophil granulocytes synthesized IL-1β (**Figures 4C,D**). Interestingly, IFN-γ was also produced by the neutrophils (85 ± 0.5%) contrary to activated microglia (**Figures 4I,J**). IL-10 and iNOS were synthesized by negligible numbers of neutrophil granulocytes (0 ± 0.5% IL-10; 2 ± 0.5% iNOS) and microglial cells (0 ± 0.5% IL-10; 8 ± 1% iNOS) (**Figures 4G,H,K,L**). Besides, all neutrophils synthesized ROS unlike activated microglia (95 ± 0.5%) (**Figures 4M,N**). In summary, these data demonstrate that neutrophil granulocytes produce multiple immune modulatory molecules including IFN-γ.

IFN-γ Production by Neutrophil Granulocytes over the Course of Cerebral Toxoplasmosis

IFN-γ plays a critical role in the host response to cerebral toxoplasmosis. Previous studies defined NK cells, T cells and microglia as sources of IFN-γ during cerebral toxoplasmosis

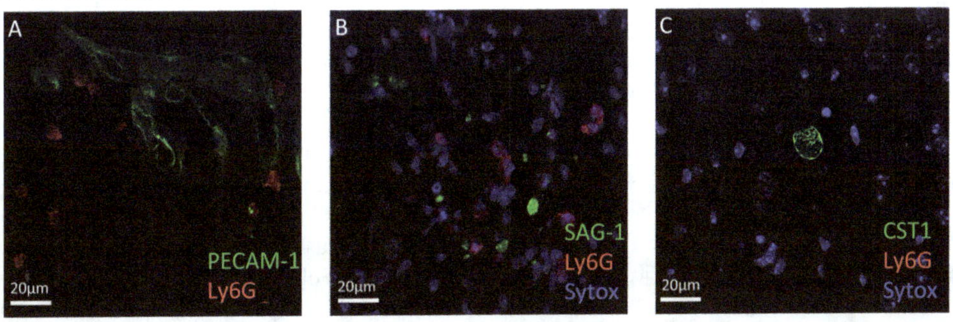

FIGURE 2 | Immunofluorescence staining of Ly6G$^+$ neutrophil granulocytes and *T. gondii* in brain slices. Immunostaining of PECAM-1 or SAG1 or CST1 (green), Ly6G (red), and Sytox Dead Cell stain (blue) in the cortex of *T. gondii*-infected C57BL/6 mice **(A–C)**. **(A)** In acute cerebral toxoplasmosis, recruitment of Ly6G$^+$ neutrophil granulocytes into the brain from the circulation is shown. **(B)** Further, massive infiltration of Ly6G$^+$ neutrophil granulocytes around *T. gondii* tachyzoites (green) is shown. **(C)** In chronic cerebral toxoplasmosis, no localization of Ly6G$^+$ neutrophil granulocytes is shown. Eight coronal slides per mouse were analyzed with a maginification of 63x; $n = 4$ mice. This experiment was repeated two times. Scale bars, 20 μm in **(A–C)**.

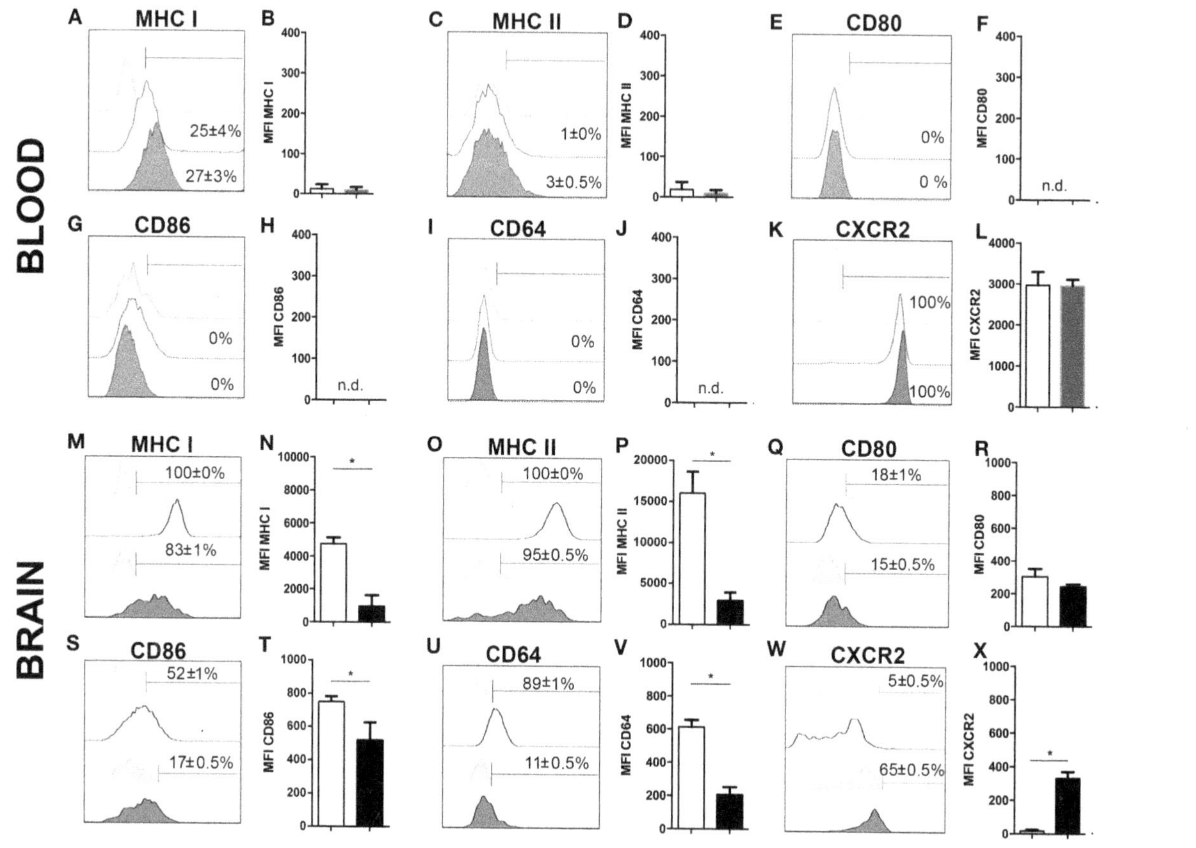

FIGURE 3 | Phenotypic analysis of neutrophil granulocytes and activated microglia **(A–X)**. Expression of activation markers and chemokine receptors in mice blood and brains after 4 weeks of *T. gondii* infection, were analyzed by flow cytometry, respectively. The cells were gated as described and shown in the representative plots of **Figure 1**. Neutrophils from the infected and non-infected blood ($CD11b^+CD45^{hi}Ly6G^+Ly6C^+$), activated microglia ($CD11b^+CD45^{int}$), and neutrophil granulocytes from the infected brain ($CD11b^+CD45^{hi}Ly6G^+Ly6C^+$), were assessed for their relative expression of the indicated molecules. **(A,C,E,G,I,K,M,O,Q,S,U,W)** Histograms show the representative expression level of the surface maker by the cell population in comparison to the corresponding isotype control (light gray without tint or light gray tinted). Bars mark cells positively expressing particular surface markers and numbers above bars represent the percentage of cells in the respective population: neutrophils in non-infected blood ($CD11b^+Ly6G^+$) (without any tint, dotted line), neutrophils in infected blood ($CD11b^+Ly6G^+$) (tinted, dotted line), activated microglia ($CD11b^+CD45^{int}$) (without any tint), neutrophil granulocytes ($CD11b^+Ly6G^+$) (tinted). **(B,D,F,H,J,L,N,P,R,T,V,X)** Bar graphs represent the median fluorescence intensity (MFI) for the specific marker MFI ± SD ($n = 4$) (neutrophils in non-infected blood: white bars; neutrophils in infected blood: gray bars; activated microglia: white bars; and neutrophils: black bars). Data represent 2 independent experiments with 5 mice per experiment. Mann-Whitney test was performed for comparisons ($^*p < 0.05$).

(Gazzinelli et al., 1993; Hunter et al., 1994; Gavrilescu et al., 2004; Kim et al., 2012; Gazzinelli and Sher, 2014). However, the contribution of neutrophil granulocytes to IFN-γ production in the brain has not been elucidated (Suzuki, 2002; Sa et al., 2015).Therefore, we performed flow cytometry from the brains of mice during the acute (2 weeks) as well as the chronic stage (4 weeks) of *T. gondii* infection. In the acute phase, 83.5 ± 0.5% of neutrophil granulocytes produced IFN-γ (1.5 * 10 ^ 3 ± 200 cells). This was the case for only 47 ± 0.5% of activated microglia. At this time-point, only negligible numbers of $CD11b^-$ lymphocytes (247 ± 50 cells) were detectable in the brain to make a significant contribution (6 ± 0.5%) (**Figures 5A,B**). However, during the chronic phase of infection enhanced number of lymphocytes infiltrated the brain, which then became the major IFN-γ producers (88 ± 0.5%) (1.5 * 10 ^ 6 ± 550 cells) (**Figures 5C–F**). Neutrophils were secondary producers of IFN-γ at the chronic stage of infection (85 ± 4%) (1.4 * 10 ^ 3 ± 60 cells) (**Figures 5C–F**). Thus, our results demonstrate that $Ly6G^+$ neutrophil granulocytes are representing an important early source of early IFN-γ in the acute phase of cerebral toxoplasmosis.

Depletion of Neutrophil Granulocytes in Experimental Cerebral Toxoplasmosis

It is still unclear whether neutrophils contribute to control of cerebral toxoplasmosis. To investigate this, we took advantage of the previously described specific depleting anti-Ly6G mAb (clone 1A8). Following our observation that $Ly6G^+$ neutrophils are early IFN-γ producers in the acute phase of cerebral toxoplasmosis, we started the ablation at day 10 post-infection when neutrophil granulocytes began entering the brain. We continued the ablation, injecting Ly6G mAb or control IgG2 mAb every alternate day, as the infection progressed from the acute to chronic stage. Twenty-four hours after the last Ab treatment,

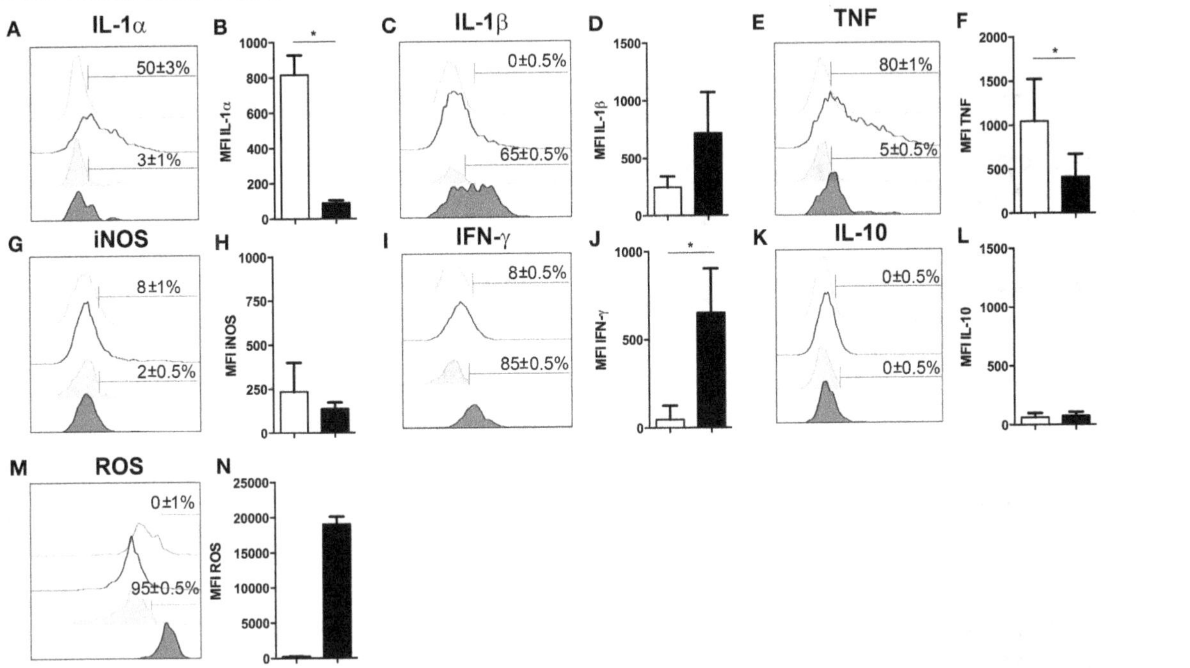

FIGURE 4 | Functional properties of neutrophil granulocytes and activated microglia in the infected brain. **(A–N)** Cells isolated from brains of mice infected with 4 weeks of *T. gondii*, were re-stimulated with *Toxoplasma* lysate antigen *in vitro* and analyzed by flow cytometry. The cells were gated as described in the **Figure 1 (E–H)**. **(A,C,E,G,I,K,M)** Histograms show the representative expression levels of the indicated molecules in comparison to the corresponding isotype control (light gray without tint or light gray tinted). Bars mark cells positive for the particular cytokine. Numbers above bars represent the percentage of cells positive for the cytokine of the respective population: activated microglia ($CD11b^+CD45^{int}$) (without any tint), neutrophil granulocytes ($CD11b^+Ly6G^+$) (tinted). **(B,D,F,H,J,L,N)** Bar graphs represent the MFI of the respective fluorochrome for a particular cytokine, MFI ± SD (activated microglia: white bars; and neutrophils: black bars). Data are representative of 2 independent experiments with 5 mice per experiment. Mann-Whitney test was performed for comparisons ($^*p < 0.05$). White bars and black bars represent activated microglia and neutrophil granulocytes respectively.

mice were sacrificed and the successful depletion of $CD11b^+$ $Ly6G^+$ monocytes in the blood was confirmed (7.0 ± 0.13 to 0%; **Figures 6A,B**).

In agreement with this, anti-Ly6G treatment of infected mice also resulted in a significant reduction of neutrophils in the brain. Further characterization revealed a reduction of recruited myeloid cells (24.0 ± 1.5 to 19.0 ± 0.28%) in the brains of anti-Ly6G treated infected mice (**Figure 6C**, upper panel). This observation was further confirmed with a significant decrease of $Ly6G^+$ neutrophils (**Figure 6C**, middle panel; 3.0 ± 0.5% to 0.6 ± 0.3%). Further investigation revealed reduced recruitment of $CD11b^+Ly6C^{hi}$ inflammatory monocytes (**Figure 6C**, lower panel; 48.0 ± 3.0% to 32.0 ± 1.3%) in the brains of anti-Ly6G treated mice. Moreover, absolute cell numbers of $CD45^{hi}$ $CD11b^+$ myeloid cells ($p < 0.05$), $Ly6G^+$ neutrophils ($p < 0.001$) and $Ly6C^{hi}$ monocytes ($p < 0.01$) were significantly reduced. On the contrary, numbers of T lymphocytes ($CD45^{hi}CD11b^-CD4^+$ and $CD45^{hi}CD11b^-CD8^+$) and microglia ($CD45^{int}CD11b^+$) remained unaltered (**Figures 6D,E**).

Using q and qRT-PCR we investigated whether the ablation of $Ly6G^+$ neutrophil granulocytes affected parasite burden and cytokine gene expression levels in brains of anti-Ly6G treated mice. We found that anti-Ly6G treatment was associated with elevated parasite burden (**Figure 7A**). Correspondingly, we observed a 40 and 60% reduction of pro-inflammatory TNF and IFN-γ, respectively, as compared to IgG treated controls (**Figures 7C,E**). Furthermore, IL-10 and IL-1β mRNA levels were reduced in anti-Ly6G treated mice (**Figure 7B,D**). Together, these results demonstrate that increased parasite burden correlates inversely with the reduced levels of TNF, IFN-γ, IL-1 β, and IL-10 in brains of neutrophil-depleted mice with cerebral toxoplasmosis. Hence, the recruitment of neutrophil granulocytes and their early cytokine production appear to promote inflammatory immune responses restricting pathogen load in brains of *T. gondii*-infected mice.

Heterogeneity of Neutrophil Granulocyte Subsets in Cerebral Toxoplasmosis

Depending on the infection model, different subsets of neutrophil granulocytes can be discriminated based on their phenotypic and functional properties (Tsuda et al., 2004; Pillay et al., 2010; Beyrau et al., 2012). However, in the case of cerebral toxoplasmosis, it was largely unclear whether recruited neutrophils represent a heterogeneous or rather homogeneous population in the brain. Therefore, $CD45^+CD11b^+Ly6C^+Ly6G^+$ neutrophil granulocytes from 4 weeks *T. gondii*-infected mice were analyzed by flow cytometry (**Figures 8A,B**). We found that this population contained cells expressing different levels of CD62-L (**Figure 8C**). Contrary to CD62-L^{lo} neutrophils (20 ± 0.5%), a high percentage of CD62-L^{hi} neutrophils (50 ± 0.5%) expressed

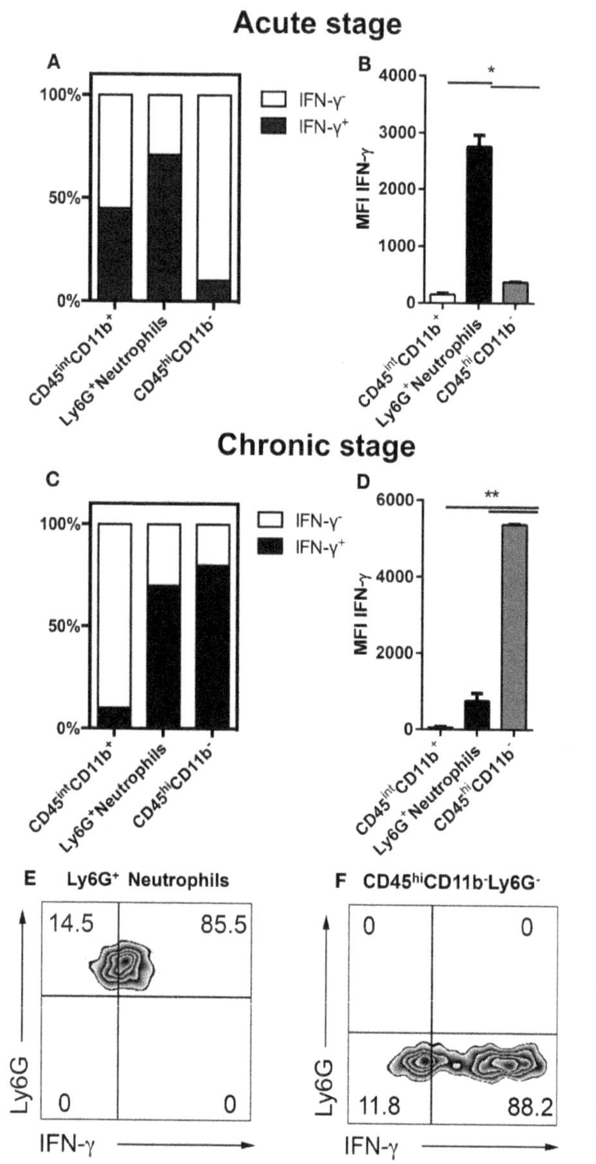

FIGURE 5 | IFN-γ production over the course of cerebral toxoplasmosis **(A–F)**. Cells isolated from brains of mice infected with 2 and 4 weeks of *T. gondii*, were re-stimulated with *Toxoplasma* lysate antigen *in vitro* and analyzed by flow cytometry. The cells were gated as shown in **Figures 1E,F**. **(A,C)** The fraction of the total cell population expressing IFN-γ was plotted in stacked bar graphs. **(B,D)** Bar graphs represent the MFI of the respective fluorochrome for a particular cytokine, MFI ± SD ($n = 4$). **(E,F)** The representative plots show the gating strategy of Ly6G$^+$ neutrophils and CD11b$^-$CD45^{hi}Ly6G$^-$ cells producing IFN-γ. The quadrant was set on isotype control. Data are representative of 2 independent experiments with 5 mice per experiment. Significant differences (*$p < 0.05$, **$p < 0.01$) were determined using the Mann-Whitney test. White bars, black bars and gray bars represent CD45^{int}CD11b$^+$ activated microglia, Ly6G$^+$ neutrophils and CD45^{hi}CD11b$^-$ lymphocytes, respectively.

CRAMP (**Figures 8D,E**). On the contrary, only 25 ± 0.5% of CD62-L^{hi} neutrophils secreted IFN-γ while this was the case for 45 ± 0.5% of CD62-L^{lo} neutrophils (**Figures 8F,G**). However, CD62-L^{hi} and CD62-L^{lo} neutrophil granulocytes produced similar levels of ROS (90 ± 0.5% vs. 95 ± 0.5%) (**Figures 8H,I**). These data suggest the phenotypic heterogeneity of brain-derived neutrophil granulocytes further defining CD62-L^{lo} neutrophils as a source of protective IFN-γ.

DISCUSSION

Neutrophil granulocytes are the first immune cells recruited from the periphery to secrete initial effector molecules upon injury and infection. They play a critical role in infection to eliminate pathogens via multiple mechanisms (Zhou et al., 2003; Nathan, 2006; Kolaczkowska and Kubes, 2013). The response of neutrophil granulocytes to parasitic infection is well described in the periphery, but their role within the CNS in chronic infections is not thoroughly defined. One previous study concluded that neutrophil granulocytes are the limiting factor against uncontrolled tachyzoite replication in cerebral toxoplasmosis (Bliss et al., 2001), but this conclusion was based on depletion of Gr1$^+$ cells. However, later it turned out that Gr1 expression is not restricted to neutrophil granulocytes but also expressed by monocytes (Daley et al., 2008).

We defined the phenotype and function of Ly6G$^+$ neutrophil granulocytes in the course of chronic toxoplasmosis in the CNS. Initially, we observed increased percentages of Ly6G$^+$ neutrophils in the blood of *T. gondii*-infected mice. In the chronic stage of the infection, brain resident microglia cells displayed an activated phenotype, and peripheral immune cells including CD11b$^-$ lymphoid and CD11b$^+$ myeloid cells infiltrated the brain. In line with previous reports, characterization of brain immune cells revealed that recruited CD11b$^+$ myeloid cells contained Ly6G$^-$ inflammatory monocytes and Ly6G$^+$ neutrophil granulocytes (Möhle et al., 2014; Biswas et al., 2015). Despite low absolute numbers of neutrophils in the chronic stage, they form a substantial portion of the myeloid cell compartment in the CNS in the acute stage of the infection. Confocal microscopic analysis identified neutrophil granulocytes adjacent to *T. gondii* tachyzoites in the acute infection, albeit they were distant from cysts in the chronic stage. This observation suggests that the active infective form of the parasite could potentially trigger the host defense and effector functions of neutrophil granulocytes such as generation of ROS or even phagocytosis as it has been shown in acute toxoplasma infection in the periphery (Abdallah et al., 2011).

We measured MHC I and MHC II expression on both microglia and neutrophil granulocytes. This indicates that neutrophils can acquire an APC phenotype in cerebral toxoplasmosis. Neutrophil granulocytes are generally regarded as professional phagocytes responding early to tissue infection and injury. In line with our observations, increasing evidence suggests that neutrophils can also modulate adaptive immune responses by activating CD4$^+$ T cells *in vitro* via upregulation of MHC class molecules (Wagner and Hug, 2005; Abdallah et al., 2011). On the contrary, the co-stimulatory molecule CD86 and the phagocytosis-related receptor CD64 (FcγR1) were detected primarily on activated microglia as opposed to neutrophils. The chemokine receptor CXCR2, typically expressed by neutrophil

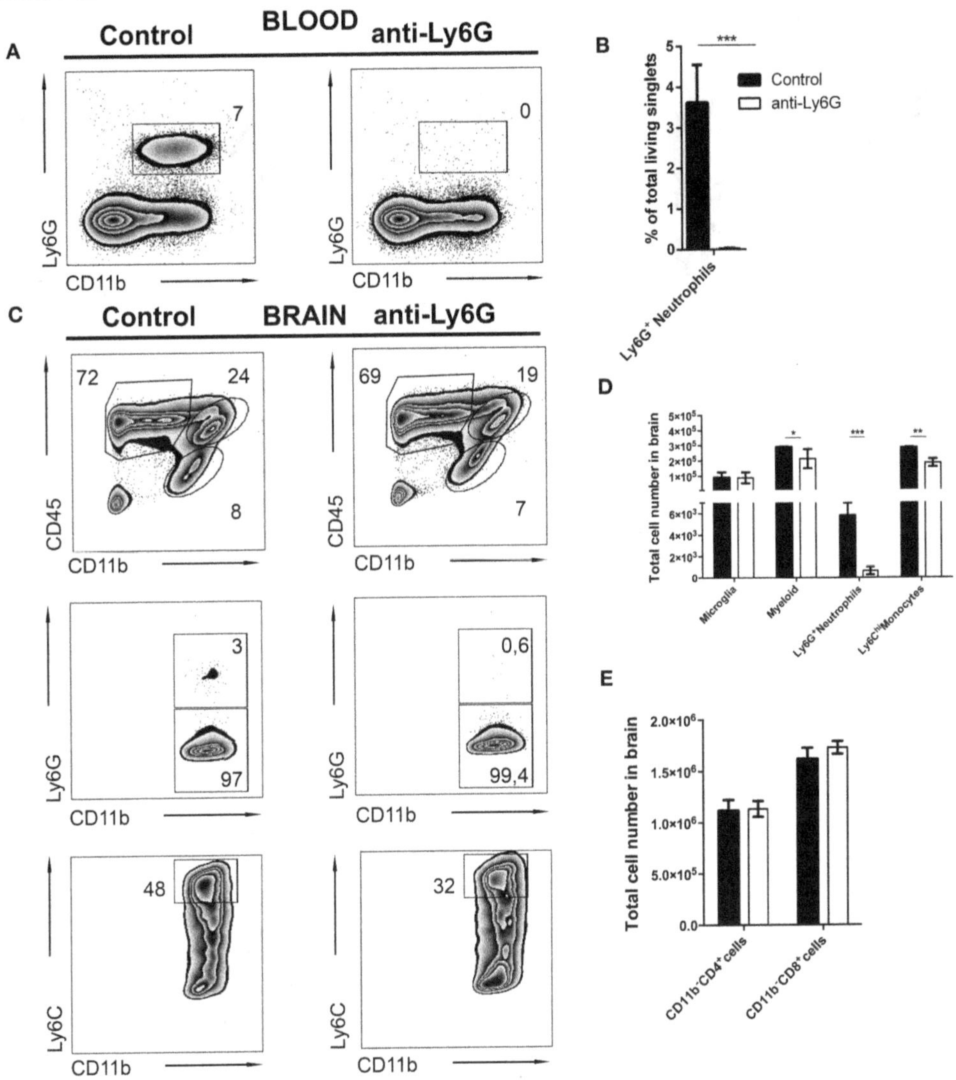

FIGURE 6 | Selective depletion of Ly6G$^+$ neutrophil granulocytes. C57BL/6 mice were infected with *T. gondii*. From day 10 to day 23 post-infection mice were alternatively treated with either IgG mAb (control, left), or anti-Ly6G (Anti-Ly6G, right) to deplete neutrophil granulocytes. The cells were gated as shown in **Figures 1E–H**. Panel **(A)** displays representative plots to define CD11b$^+$Ly6G$^+$ circulating neutrophil granulocytes (upper gate) in the blood. **(B)** The bar graph represents the percentage of Ly6G$^+$ cells in the blood. **(C)** The upper plots show the gating of lymphocytes (CD11b$^-$CD45^{hi}), activated microglia (CD11b$^+$CD45^{int}) and the myeloid population (CD11b$^+$CD45^{hi}) in infected brains. Middle plots display the myeloid subsets: Ly6G$^+$(neutrophil granulocytes) and Ly6G$^-$ (monocytes) in the brain. Lower plots display the inflammatory monocyte subset (from the Ly6G$^-$ gate): Ly6C^{hi}. **(D)** The bar graphs represent the total cell number of the respective subsets in the brain (black bars: control; white bars: anti-Ly6G). **(E)** The bar graphs represent the total cell number of the respective CD4$^+$ and CD8$^+$ lymphoid cell population. Data shown here is the representative of 2 individual experiments with 4 mice per group for each experiment. The numbers in the representative contour plots are % of the parent population. Significant differences ($^*p < 0.05$, $^{**}p < 0.01$, $^{***}p < 0.001$) were determined using the Mann-Whitney test.

granulocytes, was down-regulated upon entering the brain (Liu et al., 2010). Despite being also expressed on oligodendrocytes and neurons (Liu et al., 2010), where it mediates a wide range of functions, CXCR2 is not present on the activated microglia. Similarly, activated microglia do not express CD62-L which is crucial for leukocyte rolling, transmigration and accumulation at sites of inflammation (Rainer, 2002; Biswas et al., 2015). We identify the existence of two subsets of neutrophils in the infected brain, which can be discriminated based on their differential CD62-L expression (Zenaro et al., 2015). CXCL12, the ligand of CXCR4 is constitutively expressed on endothelial cells in the CNS (McCandless et al., 2006; Wilson et al., 2010). We showed that cerebral toxoplasmosis leads to increased expression of CXCR4 on neutrophil granulocytes. In conclusion, we demonstrate that CNS infiltrating neutrophils display distinct phenotypes in cerebral *T. gondii* infection.

Following surface characterization, we studied the secretion of certain inflammatory mediators by Ly6G$^+$ neutrophil granulocytes and activated microglia. The proinflammatory molecules IL-1β and ROS were primarily produced by

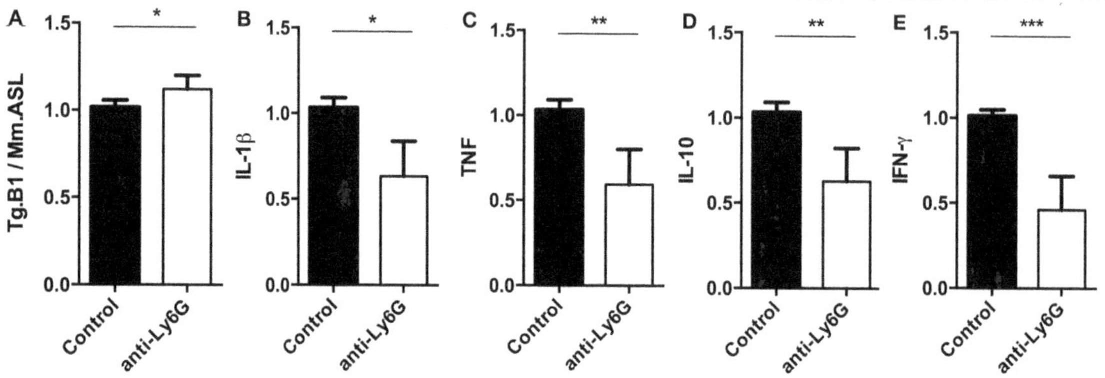

FIGURE 7 | Semi-quantitative RT-PCR analysis of Ly6G$^+$ neutrophil granulocytes-depleted mice. Quantitative and Semi-quantitative RT-PCR analyses of pathogen load and cytokine gene expression in brains of *T. gondii*-infected C57BL/6 mice (for 23 days) after treatment with IgG mAb (black bars) or anti-Ly6G (white bars). **(A–E)** Relative expression was calculated by normalization to the expression of the housekeeping genes mouse argininosuccinate lyase and hypoxanthine phosphoribosyltransferase. Resulting data were further normalized on mean values of control groups. Data shown is the representative of 2 individual experiments with 4 mice per group for each experiment. Significant differences ($^*p < 0.05$, $^{**}p < 0.01$, $^{***}p < 0.001$) were determined using the Mann-Whitney test.

neutrophils in line with previous studies (Bardoel et al., 2014). Most importantly, we detected that the cytokine IFN-γ, which is the main driving factor of the host immune response against *T. gondii*, was secreted by neutrophil granulocytes. Neutrophils can produce IFN-γ in *Nocardia asteroides*-infected lungs (Ellis and Beaman, 2002) and *Salmonella typhimurium*-infected intestines (Kirby et al., 2002; Sturge et al., 2013). Our observation are in contrast to Sa et al. (2015) who reported that microglia are the main source of myeloid cell-derived IFN-γ in a reactivation model of cerebral toxoplasmosis in RAG$^{-/-}$and IFN-γ$^{-/-}$ mice with a Balb/c background. However, it is important to stress that our results were obtained in WT C57BL/6 mice, which may explain the disparity. Interestingly, our observation is in line with Sturge et al. (2015) who reported that the neutrophils store IFN-γ at the promyelocyte stage in the absence of inflammation. Additionally, they showed that during acute toxoplasmosis neutrophils form an important non-lymphoid source of IFN-production (Sturge et al., 2013). Importantly, we reveal that infiltrating neutrophil granulocytes are an important source of myeloid cell-derived IFN-γ particularly in the early phase of cerebral toxoplasmosis.

The ablation of Ly6G$^+$ neutrophils in the periphery resulted in a reduced infiltration to the CNS. The depletion was also associated with a significant reduction of IFN-γ mRNA levels in infected brains. IFN-γ is crucial for survival during *T. gondii* infection (Gazzinelli et al., 1993; Hunter et al., 1994; Gavrilescu et al., 2004; Kim et al., 2012; Gazzinelli and Sher, 2014). Increased parasite loads after anti-Ly6G treatment may have been a direct consequence of the antibody-mediated elimination of IFN-γ-producing neutrophils. Nonetheless, we cannot exclude indirect effects such as those resulting from impaired recruitment of other immune cells. It is important to mention that the neutrophil granulocytes ablation had no effect on the recruitment of CD4$^+$ and CD8$^+$ T lymphocytes to the brain. This suggests non-significant interaction with the T lymphocytes in terms of recruitment, however T cell activation may have been affected as it not part of the investigation. One study reported that ablation of neutrophils resulted in impaired maturation of resident microglia and brain macrophages into professional APCs, altering the T cell function (Steinbach et al., 2013). In contrary, we did not detect impaired differentiation or activation status of microglia into MHC II expressing professional CD11c$^+$ APCs (data not shown).

We previously showed that Ly6C^{hi} monocytes express TNF and IL-10 in the CNS during cerebral toxoplasmosis (Biswas et al., 2015). Thus, the reduction of TNF and IL-10 levels after neutrophil depletion may be due to the reduced recruitment of Ly6C^{hi} monocytes. However, the reduced IFN-γ and IL-1β levels were most likely caused by the complete ablation of Ly6G$^+$ neutrophil granulocytes as there was no change in the lymphocyte compartment.

In the current study, based on CXCR4 expression, neutrophil granulocytes displayed certain heterogeneity. Ly6G$^+$ neutrophils comprised of CD62-L^{hi}CXCR4$^+$ and CD62-L^{lo}CXCR4$^+$ subsets. On one hand the Ly6G$^+$CD62-L^{hi}CXCR4$^+$ subset expressed higher levels of CRAMP and produced lower levels of IFN-γ, but on the other hand Ly6G$^+$CD62-L^{lo}CXCR4$^+$ neutrophil granulocytes expressed lower levels of CRAMP and produced higher levels of IFN-γ. Differential expression of CRAMP and IFN-γ suggest functional heterogeneity of Ly6G$^+$ neutrophil granulocytes. One subset Ly6G$^+$CD62-L^{hi}CXCR4$^+$ with high CRAMP expression may promote monocyte recruitment. The Ly6G$^+$ neutrophil granulocytes have been described to influence the recruitment of monocytes in injury models (Zhou et al., 2003; Soehnlein et al., 2008a,b). The other subset Ly6G$^+$CD62-L^{lo}CXCR4$^+$ with higher IFN-γ production may establish the inflammatory response against cerebral toxoplasmosis.

Here we report that cerebral toxoplasmosis leads to infiltration of Ly6G$^+$ neutrophil granulocytes to the CNS. These neutrophils contribute to IFN-γ production during the early stages of the developing neuroinflammation. Importantly, we

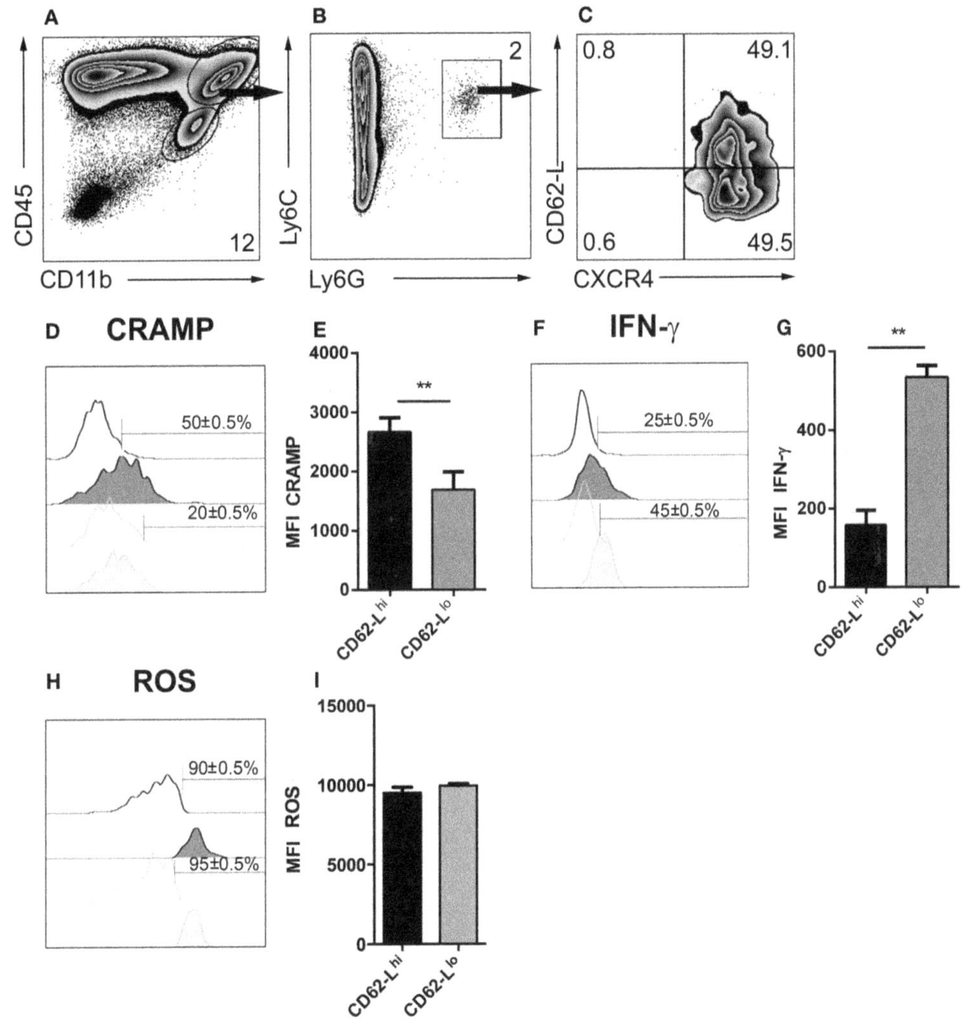

FIGURE 8 | Emergence of neutrophil subsets in the CNS. **(A,B)** Cells isolated from 4 week *T. gondii*-infected mice were gated on $CD45^+CD11b^+Ly6C^+Ly6G^+$ neutrophils **(C)**, and their CXCR4 and CD62-L expression was determined. The neutrophil granulocyte subsets $CXCR4^+CD62\text{-}L^{lo}$ and $CXCR4^+CD62\text{-}L^{hi}$ were studied for their CRAMP, IFN-γ and ROS expression. **(D,F,H)** Representative histograms show CRAMP, IFN-γ, and ROS expression of $CXCR4^+CD62\text{-}L^{hi}$ (black filled) and $CXCR4^+CD62\text{-}L^{lo}$ (gray filled) neutrophils as compared to the corresponding isotype control (black or gray, not filled). Bars mark the cells positive for the particular markers. Numbers above the bars represent percentage of cells positive for the marker of the respective population: $CXCR4^+CD62\text{-}L^{hi}$ (black) and $CXCR4^+CD62\text{-}L^{lo}$ (gray). **(E,G,I)** Bar graphs represent the MFI of the respective fluorochrome for a particular marker, MFI ± SD ($n = 4$) ($CXCR4^+CD62\text{-}L^{hi}$ (black) and $CXCR4^+CD62\text{-}L^{lo}$ (gray)). The numbers in the representative contour plots are % of the parent population. Data are representative of 2 independent experiments with $n = 4$ mice per experiment. Significant differences ($^{**}p < 0.01$) in the bar graphs were determined using the Mann-Whitney test.

identified two distinct $Ly6G^+CXCR4^+$ neutrophil granulocyte subsets based on their CD62-L and CRAMP expression. Moreover, we detected a neutrophil-dependent recruitment of $Ly6C^{hi}$ monocytes to the CNS in chronic *T. gondii* infection. In summary, our findings suggest that neutrophil granulocytes perform important functions to promote host defense and exhibit heterogeneity in experimental cerebral toxoplasmosis.

AUTHOR CONTRIBUTIONS

ID designed the experiments and supervised the project. AB, TF, HD, NM, MR, AD, UB, performed the experiments. AB, AD, UB, ID, and TS interpreted the data. AB, ID, and TS contributed to manuscript preparation. ID funded the project.

FUNDING

This study was supported by the Deutsche Forschungsgemeinschaft (SFB 854, TP25, DU1112-5-1) to ID. The funders had no role in study design, data collection and analysis, decision to publish, or preparation of the manuscript.

ACKNOWLEDGMENTS

We thank Dana Zabler and Dr. Sarah Abidat Schneider for excellent technical assistance.

REFERENCES

Abdallah, D. S. A., Egan, C. E., Butcher, B. A., and Denkers, E. Y. (2011). Mouse Neutrophils are professional antigen- presenting cells programmed to instruct T_h1 and T_h17 T-cell differentiation. *Int. Immunol.* 23, 317–326. doi: 10.1093/intimm/dxr007

Bardoel, B. W., Kenny, E. F., Sollberger, G., and Zychlinsky, A. (2014). The balancing act of neutrophils. *Cell Host Microbe* 15, 526–536. doi: 10.1016/j.chom.2014.04.011

Barragan, A. (2002). Transepithelial migration of *Toxoplasma gondii* is linked to parasite motility and virulence. *J. Exp. Med.* 195, 1625–1633. doi: 10.1084/jem.20020258

Beyrau, M., Bodkin, J. V., and Nourshargh, S. (2012). Neutrophil heterogeneity in health and disease: a revitalized avenue in inflammation and immunity. *Open. Biol.* 2:120134. doi: 10.1098/rsob.120134

Biswas, A., Bruder, D., Wolf, S. A., Mack, M., Heimesaat, M. M., and Dunay, I. R. (2015). Ly6C (high) monocytes control cerebral Toxoplasmosis. *J. Immunol.* 194, 3223–3235. doi: 10.4049/jimmunol.1402037

Blanchard, N., Dunay, I. R., and Schlüter, D. (2015). Persistence of *Toxoplasma gondii* in the central nervous system: a fine-tuned balance between the parasite, the brain and the immune system. *Parasite Immunol.* 37, 150–158. doi: 10.1111/pim.12173

Bliss, S. K., Gavrilescu, L. C., Alcaraz, A., and Denkers, E. Y. (2001). Neutrophil depletion during *Toxoplasma gondii* infection leads to impaired immunity and lethal systemic pathology. *Infect. Immun.* 69, 4898–4905. doi: 10.1128/IAI.69.8.4898-4905.2001

Cabral, C. M., Tuladhar, S., Dietrich, H. K., and Nguyen, E. (2016). Neurons are the primary target cell for the brain-tropic intracellular parasite *Toxoplasma gondii*. *PLoS Pathog.* 12:e1005447. doi: 10.1371/journal.ppat.1005447

Konradt, C., Ueno, N., Christian, D. A., Delong, J. H., Pritchard, G. H., Herz, J., et al. (2016). Endothelial cells are a replicative niche for entry of *Toxoplasma gondii* to the central nervous system. *Nat. Microbiol.* 1:16001. doi: 10.1038/nmicrobiol.2016.1

Courret, N., Darche, S., Sonigo, P., Milon, G., Buzoni-Gâtel, D., and Tardieux, I. (2006). CD11c- and CD11b-expressing mouse leukocytes transport single *Toxoplasma gondii* tachyzoites to the brain. *Blood* 107, 309–316. doi: 10.1182/blood-2005-02-0666

Da Gama, L. M., Gomes, F. L. R., Guimarães, U., and Arnholdt, A. C. V. (2004). Reduction in adhesiveness to extracellular matrix components, modulation of adhesion molecules and *in vivo* migration of murine macrophages infected with *Toxoplasma gondii*. *Microbes Infect.* 6, 1287–1296. doi: 10.1016/j.micinf.2004.07.008

Daley, J. M., Thomay, A. A., Connolly, M. D., Reichner, J. S., and Albina, J. E. (2008). Use of Ly6G-specific monoclonal antibody to deplete neutrophils in mice. *J. Leukoc. Biol.* 83, 64–70. doi: 10.1189/jlb.0407247

Denkers, E. Y., Schneider, A. G., Cohen, S. B., and Butcher, B. A. (2012). Phagocyte responses to protozoan infection and how *Toxoplasma gondii* Meets the Challenge. *PLoS Pathog.* 8:1002794. doi: 10.1371/journal.ppat.1002794

Drögemüller, K., Helmuth, U., Brunn, A., Sakowicz-Burkiewicz, M., Gutmann, D. H., Mueller, W., et al. (2008). Astrocyte gp130 expression is critical for the control of *Toxoplasma* encephalitis. *J. Immunol.* 181, 2683–2693. doi: 10.4049/jimmunol.181.4.2683

Dunay, I. R., Fuchs, A., and Sibley, L. D. (2010). Inflammatory monocytes but not neutrophils are necessary to control infection with *Toxoplasma gondii* in Mice. *Infect. Immun.* 78, 1564–1570. doi: 10.1128/IAI.00472-09

Ellis, T. N., and Beaman, B. L. (2002). Murine polymorphonuclear neutrophils produce interferon-gamma in response to pulmonary infection with *Nocardia asteroides*. *J. Leukoc. Biol.* 72, 373–381.

Gavrilescu, L. C., Butcher, B. A., Rio, L. D., Taylor, G. A., and Denkers, E. Y. (2004). STAT1 is essential for antimicrobial effector function but dispensable for gamma interferon production during *Toxoplasma gondii* infection. *Infect. Immun.* 72, 1257–1264. doi: 10.1128/IAI.72.3.1257

Gazzinelli, R. T., Thomas, A., and Sher, A. (1993). Acute cerebral toxoplasmosis is induced by *in vivo* neutralization of TNF-alpha and correlates with the down-regulated expression of inducible nitric oxide synthase and other markers of macrophage activation. *J. Immunol.* 151, 3672–36781.

Gazzinelli, R., and Sher, A. (2014). Innate resistance against *Toxoplasma gondii*: an evolutionary tale of mice, cats, and men. *Cell Host Microbe* 15, 132–138. doi: 10.1016/j.chom.2014.01.004

Harker, K. S., Ueno, N., and Lodoen, M. B. (2015). *Toxoplasma gondii* dissemination: a parasite's journey through the infected host. *Parasite Immunol.* 37, 141–149. doi: 10.1111/pim.12163

Hunter, C. A., Subauste, C. S., Cleave, V. H. V., and Remington, J. S. (1994). Production of gamma interferon by natural killer cells from *Toxoplasma gondii*-infected SCID mice: regulation by interleukin-10, interleukin- 12, and tumor necrosis factor alpha. *Infect. Immun.* 62, 2818–2824.

John, B., Ricart, B., Tait Wojno, E. D., Harris, T. H., Randall, L. M., Christian, D. A., et al. (2011). Analysis of behavior and trafficking of dendritic cells within the brain during Toxoplasmic encephalitis. *PLoS Pathog.* 7:e1002246. doi: 10.1371/journal.ppat.1002246

Kamerkar, S., and Davis, P. H. (2012). *Toxoplasma* on the brain: understanding host-pathogen interactions in chronic CNS infection. *J. Parasitol. Res.* 2012:589295. doi: 10.1155/2012/589295

Kang, H., and Suzuki, Y. (2001). Requirement of non-T cells that produce gamma interferon for prevention of reactivation of *Toxoplasma gondii* infection in the brain. *Infect. Immun.* 69, 2920–2927. doi: 10.1128/IAI.69.5.2920-2927.2001

Kim, B. H., Shenoy, A. R., Kumar, P., Bradfield, C. J., and MacMicking, J. D. (2012). IFN-Inducible GTPases in host defense. *Cell Host Microbe* 12, 432–444. doi: 10.1016/j.chom.2012.09.007

Kim, K. and Weiss, L. M. (2004). *Toxoplasma gondii*: the model apicomplexan. *Int. J. Parasitol.* 34, 423–432. doi: 10.1016/j.ijpara.2003.12.009

Kirby, A. C., Yrlid, U., and Wick, M. J. (2002). The innate immuneresponse differs in primary and secondary *Salmonella* infection. *J. Immunol.* 169, 4450–4459. doi: 10.4049/jimmunol.169.8.4450

Klose, C. S. N., Flach, M., Möhle, L., Rogell, L., Hoyler, T., Ebert, K., et al. (2014). Differentiation of type 1 ILCs from a common progenitor to all helper-like innate lymphoid cell lineages. *Cell* 157, 340–356. doi: 10.1016/j.cell.2014.03.030

Kolaczkowska, E., and Kubes, P. (2013). Neutrophil recruitment and function. *Nat. Rev. Immun.* 13, 159–175. doi: 10.1038/nri3399

Lambert, H., Hitziger, N., Dellacasa, I., Svensson, M., and Barragan, A. (2006). Induction of dendritic cell migration upon *Toxoplasma gondii* infection potentiates parasite dissemination. *Cell. Microbiol.* 8, 1611–1623. doi: 10.1111/j.1462-5822.2006.00735.x

Liu, L. P., Belkadi, A., Darnall, L., Hu, T., Drescher, C., Cotleur, A. C., et al. (2010). CXCR2-positive neutrophils are essential for cuprizone-induced demyelination: relevance to multiple sclerosis. *Nat. Neurosci.* 13, 319–326. doi: 10.1038/nn.2491

Marais, S., Wilkinson, K. A., Lesosky, M., Coussens, A. K., Deffur, A., Pepper, D., et al. J. (2014). Neutrophil-associated central nervous system inflammation in *Tuberculous meningitis* immune reconstitution Inflammatory syndrome. *Clin. Infect. Dis.* 59, 1638–1647. doi: 10.1093/cid/ciu641

Mashayekhi, M., Sandau, M. M., Dunay, I. R., Frickel, E. M., Khan, A., Goldszmid, R. S., et al. (2011). $CD8\alpha^+$ dendritic cells are the critical source of interleukin-12 that controls acute infection by *Toxoplasma gondii* tachyzoites. *Immunity* 35, 249–259. doi: 10.1016/j.immuni.2011.08.008

McCandless, E. E., Wang, Q., Woerner, B. M., Harper, J. M., and Klein, R. S. (2006). CXCL12 limits inflammation by localizing mononuclear infiltrates to the perivascular space during experimental autoimmune encephalomyelitis. *J. Immunol.* 177, 8053–8064. doi: 10.4049/jimmunol.177.11.8053

Mildner, A., Djukic, M., Garbe, D., Wellmer, A., Kuziel, W. A., Mack, M., et al. (2008). Ly-$6G^+CCR2^-$ myeloid cells rather than Ly-$6C^{high}CCR2^+$ monocytes are required for the control of bacterial infection in the central nervous system. *Nat. Rev. Immunol.* 181, 2713–2722. doi: 10.4049/jimmunol.181.4.2713

Möhle, L., Israel, N., Paarmann, K., Krohn, M., Pietkiewicz, S., Müller, A., et al. (2016). Chronic *Toxoplasma gondii* infection enhances β-amyloid phagocytosis and clearance by recruited monocytes. *Acta Neuropathol. Commun.* 4:25. doi: 10.1186/s40478-016-0293-8

Möhle, L., Parlog, A., Pahnke, J., and Dunay, I. R. (2014). Spinal cord pathology in chronic experimental *Toxoplasma gondii* infection. *Eur. J. Microbiol. Immunol.* 4, 65–75. doi: 10.1556/EuJMI.4.2014.1.6

Nathan, C. (2006). Neutrophils and immunity: challenges and opportunities. *Nat. Rev. Immunol.* 6, 173–182. doi: 10.1038/nri1785

Parlog, A., Harsan, L.-A., Zagrebelsky, M., Weller, M., von Elverfeldt, D., Mawrin, C., et al. (2014). Chronic murine Toxoplasmosis is defined by subtle changes in neuronal connectivity. *Dis. Model. Mech.* 7, 459–469. doi: 10.1242/dmm.014183

Perez-de-Puig, I., Miró-Mur, F., Ferrer-Ferrer, M., Gelpi, E., Pedragosa, J., Justicia, C., et al. (2015). Neutrophil recruitment to the brain in mouse and human ischemic stroke. *Acta Neuropathol.* 129, 239–257. doi: 10.1007/s00401-014-1381-0

Pillay, J., Ramakers, B. P., Kamp, V. M., Loi, A. L. T., Lam, S. W., Hietbrink, F., et al. (2010). Functional heterogeneity and differential priming of circulating neutrophils in human experimental endotoxemia. *J. Leukoc. Biol.* 88, 211–220. doi: 10.1189/jlb.1209793

Pittman, K. J., and Knoll, L. J. (2015). Long-term relationships: the complicated interplay between the host and the developmental stages of *Toxoplasma gondii* during acute and chronic infections. *Microbiol. Mol. Biol. Rev.* 79, 387–401. doi: 10.1128/MMBR.00027-15

Rainer, T. H. (2002). L-Selectin in health and sisease. *Resuscitation* 52, 127–141. doi: 10.1016/S0300-9572(01)00444-0

Ransohoff, R. M., and Engelhardt, B. (2012). The anatomical and cellular basis of immune surveillance in the central nervous system. *Nat. Rev. Immunol.* 12, 623–635. doi: 10.1038/nri3265

Robben, P. M., Regina, M. L., Kuziel, W. A., and Sibley, L. D. (2005). Recruitment of Gr-1+ monocytes is essential for control of acute Toxoplasmosis. *J. Exp. Med.* 201, 1761–1769. doi: 10.1084/jem.20050054

Sa, Q., Ochiai, E., Tiwari, A., Perkins, S., Mullins, J., Gehman, M., et al. (2015). Cutting Edge: IFN-γ produced by brain-resident cells is crucial to control cerebral infection with *Toxoplasma gondii*. *J. Immunol.* 195, 796–800. doi: 10.4049/jimmunol.1500814

Schluter, D., Kwok, L.-Y., Lütjen, S., Soltek, S., Hoffmann, S., Körner, H., et al. (2003). Both lymphotoxin- and TNF are crucial for control of *Toxoplasma gondii* in the central nervous system. *J. Immunol.* 170, 6172–6182. doi: 10.4049/jimmunol.170.12.6172

Soehnlein, O., Kai-Larsen, Y., Frithiof, R., Sorensen, O. E., Kenne, E., Scharffetter-Kochanek, K., et al. (2008a). Neutrophil primary granule proteins HBP and HNP1-3 boost bacterial phagocytosis by human and murine macrophages. *J. Clin. Invest.* 118, 3491–3502. doi: 10.1172/JCI35740

Soehnlein, O., Zernecke, A., Eriksson, E. E., Rothfuchs, A. G., Pham, C. T., Herwald, H., et al. (2008b). Neutrophil secretion products pave the way for inflammatory monocytes. *Blood* 112, 1461–1471. doi: 10.1182/blood-2008-02-139634

Steinbach, K., Piedavent, M., Bauer, S., Neumann, J. T., and Friese, M. A., (2013). Neutrophils amplify autoimmune central nervous system infiltrates by maturing local APCs. *J. Immunol.* 91, 4531–4539 doi: 10.4049/jimmunol.1202613

Strack, A., Asensio, V. C., Campbell, I. L., Schlüter, D., and Deckert, M. (2002). Chemokines are differentially expressed by astrocytes, microglia and inflammatory leukocytes in *Toxoplasma* encephalitis and critically regulated by interferon-gamma. *Acta Neuropathol.* 103, 458–468. doi: 10.1007/s00401-001-0491-7

Sturge, C. R., Benson, A., Raetz, M., Wilhelm, C. L., Mirpuri, J., Vitetta, E. S., et al. (2013). TLR-independent neutrophil-derived IFN-γ is important for host resistance to intracellular pathogens. *Proc. Natl. Acad. Sci. U.S.A.* 110, 10711–10716. doi: 10.1073/pnas.1307868110

Sturge, C. R., Burger, E., Raetz, M., Hooper, L. V., and Yarovinsky, F. (2015). Cutting edge: developmental regulation of IFN-γ production by mouse neutrophil precursor cells. *J. Immunol.* 195, 36–40. doi: 10.4049/jimmunol.1500366

Suzuki, Y. (2002). Immunopathogenesis of cerebral toxoplasmosis. *J. Infect. Dis.* 186(Suppl.), S234–S240. doi: 10.1086/344276

Tsuda, Y., Takahashi, H., Kobayashi, M., Hanafusa, T., Herndon, D. N., and Suzuki, F. (2004). Three different neutrophil subsets exhibited in mice with different susceptibilities to infection by Methicillin-resistant *Staphylococcus aureus*. *Immunity* 21, 215–226. doi: 10.1016/j.immuni.2004.07.006

Wagner, C., and Hug, F. (2005). Cellular inflammatory response to persistent localized *Staphylococcus aureus* infection: phenotypical and functional characterization of polymorphonuclear neutrophils (PMN). *Clin. Exp. Immunol.* 143, 70–77. doi: 10.1111/j.1365-2249.2005.02963.x

Wantha, S., Alard, J. E., Megens, R. T., van der Does, A. M., Döring, Y., Drechsler, M., et al. (2013). Neutrophil-derived cathelicidin promotes adhesion of classical monocytes. *J. Immunol.* 190, 3570–3578. doi: 10.1161/CIRCRESAHA.112.300666

Wilson, E. H., Weninger, W., and Hunter, C. A. (2010). Trafficking of immune cells in the central nervous system. *J. Clin. Invest.* 120, 1368–1379. doi: 10.1172/JCI41911.1368

Zehntner, S. P., Brickman, C., Bourbonnière, L., Remington, L., Caruso, M., and Owens, T. (2005). Neutrophils that infiltrate the central nervous system regulate T cell responses. *J. Immunol.* 174, 5124–51231. doi: 10.4049/jimmunol.174.8.5124

Zenaro, E., Pietronigro, E., Bianca, V. D., Piacentino, G., Marongiu, L., Budui, S., et al. (2015). Neutrophils promote Alzheimer's disease - like pathology and cognitive decline via LFA-1 integrin. *Nat. Med.* 21, 880–886. doi: 10.1038/nm.3913

Zhou, J., Stohlman, S. A., Hinton, D. R., and Marten, N. W. (2003). Neutrophils promote mononuclear cell infiltration during Viral-induced encephalitis. *J. Immunol.* 170, 3331–3336. doi: 10.4049/jimmunol.170.6.3331

8

Modeling Immune Response to *Leishmania* Species Indicates Adenosine as an Important Inhibitor of Th-Cell Activation

Henrique A. L. Ribeiro[1,2]*, *Tatiani U. Maioli*[2], *Leandro M. de Freitas*[3], *Paolo Tieri*[1] *and Filippo Castiglione*[1]

[1] Consiglio Nazionale delle Ricerche, Istituto per le Applicazioni del Calcolo, Rome, Italy, [2] Departamento de Nutrição, Universidade Federal de Minas Gerais, Belo Horizonte, Brazil, [3] Núcleo de Biointegração, Universidade Federal da Bahia, Vitória da Conquista, Brazil

Edited by:
Anton Aebischer,
Robert Koch-Insitute, Germany

Reviewed by:
Weihuan Fang,
Zhejiang University, China
Antonio M. Mendes,
Instituto de Medicina Molecular (IMM),
Portugal

***Correspondence:**
Henrique A. L. Ribeiro
h.deassis@iac.cnr.it

Infection by *Leishmania* protozoan parasites can cause a variety of disease outcomes in humans and other mammals, from single self-healing cutaneous lesions to a visceral dissemination of the parasite. The correlation between chronic lesions and ecto-nucleotidase enzymes activity on the surface of the parasite is addressed here using damage caused in epithelial cells by nitric oxide. In order to explore the role of purinergic metabolism in lesion formation and the outcome of the infection, we implemented a cellular automata/lattice gas model involving major immune characters (Th1 and Th2 cells, IFN-γ, IL-4, IL-12, adenosine –Ado–, NO) and parasite players for the dynamic analysis of the disease progress. The model were analyzed using partial ranking correlation coefficient (PRCC) to indicate the components that most influence the disease progression. Results show that low Ado inhibition rate over Th-cells is shared by *L. major* and *L. braziliensis,* while in *L. amazonensis* infection the Ado inhibition rate over Th-cells reaches 30%. IL-4 inhibition rate over Th-cell priming to Th1 independent of IL-12 are exclusive of *L. major*. The lesion size and progression showed agreement with published biological data and the model was able to simulate cutaneous leishmaniasis outcomes. The sensitivity analysis suggested that Ado inhibition rate over Th-cells followed by Leishmania survival probability were the most important characteristics of the process, with PRCC of 0.89 and 0.77 respectively. The simulations also showed a non-linear relationship between Ado inhibition rate over Th-cells and lesion size measured as number of dead epithelial cells. In conclusion, this model can be a useful tool for the quantitative understanding of the immune response in leishmaniasis.

Keywords: leishmaniasis, cutaneous, adenosine (Ado), model, lattice-gas, inflammation

INTRODUCTION

Leishmaniasis is an infectious disease caused by parasites from *Leishmania* species. It is considered a neglected tropical disease, affecting 96 countries worldwide (Alvar et al., 2012). More than 700.000 new cases are reported by WHO every year (WHO, 2017). The disease presents in two main different clinical forms, visceral and cutaneous leishmaniasis, and their outcome ranges from self-healing cutaneous lesions to disseminated lesions or to visceral dissemination of the parasite, possibly leading to death if not properly treated (Carvalho et al., 1985; Alvar et al., 2012). The clinical form and severity of leishmaniasis depend on the parasite species/strain involved and on the host immune response mounted (Sacks and Noben-Trauth, 2002; Hurdayal and Brombacher, 2014).

The immune response involved in leishmaniasis has mainly been studied in mice. The animal models most frequently used are BALB/c and C57BL/6 mice infected with *L. major*, which represent typical models for susceptibility and resistance respectively. The susceptibility in the BALB/c strain is related to development of (Th2)-polarized immune response, genetically characterized by a high production of interleukin (IL)-4 by $CD4^+$ T cells (Sacks and Noben-Trauth, 2002; Mougneau et al., 2011). Conversely, the C57BL/6 strain represents a model for resistance to *L. major*, due to (Th1) polarized immune response, characterized by the production of high amounts of interferon-gamma (IFN-γ) by $CD4^+$ T cells (Sacks and Noben-Trauth, 2002; Mougneau et al., 2011). The differentiation of naïve helper T (Th) cells into Th1 or Th2 cells depends on antigen presentation, timing, and cytokines produced by dendritic cells (DCs) after contact with the parasite (Vieira et al., 1994; Hurdayal and Brombacher, 2014). When DCs express nuclear factors such as STAT6 and secrete IL-4 and IL-10, they instruct naïve Th cells to differentiate into the Th2 phenotype (Dent et al., 1999; Sacks and Noben-Trauth, 2002). DCs expressing the nuclear factors STAT4 (Buxbaum et al., 2002), STAT1, and IL-12, induce the differentiation of naïve Th cells into the Th1 subtype, in turn producing IFN-γ (Stamm et al., 1999; Sacks and Noben-Trauth, 2002; Jayakumar et al., 2008).

The immune responses to other species of *Leishmania* such as *L. braziliensis* and *L. amazonensis* are less well studied than that to *L. major*, and susceptibility mechanisms are not as clearly linked to a Th2 immune response as they are in the *L. major* model. However, it seems to be clear that control of parasite growth is always dependent on IFN-γ and other inflammatory cytokines. In the *L. braziliensis* BALB/c infection model, secretion of IFN-γ and TNF-α, is observed but no Th2 immune response, is induced even in the absence of IL-12 (Souza-Neto et al., 2004; Vargas-Inchaustegui et al., 2008). Also, susceptibility to *L. amazonensis* is related to very low levels of IFN-γ production and low cell proliferation rate in response to its expression of serine phosphate on its membrane and to a high expression of ecto-nucleotidases (Maioli et al., 2004; Franca-Costa et al., 2012).

Parasites including the *Leishmania* species employ mechanisms to escape the immune response, interfering with signaling pathways of antigen-presenting cells (APCs) and with the differentiation of Th cells (Mougneau et al., 2011). An important escape mechanism employed by *Leishmania* may be related to the conversion of trinucleotides to adenosine (Ado). It has been reported that ATP leads mostly to pro-inflammatory signals while Ado acts by limiting the inflammation (Bours et al., 2006; Cekic and Linden, 2016). Our group and others have shown that increased ecto-nucleotidase activity on the surface of these parasites correlates with different virulence levels of the cutaneous form of the disease (Maioli et al., 2004; Marques-da-Silva et al., 2008). *L. amazonensis* has the highest activity of ecto-nucleotidases, which leads to a higher concentration of Ado, decreasing the capacity of DC to present antigens and induce differentiation of Th cells leading to less Th cell proliferation and cytokine production (de Souza et al., 2010; Leite et al., 2012; **Figure 1**).

The complex dynamics of the *Leishmania*-host interaction can be addressed with a certain degree of success by using mathematical and computational modeling. A system of ordinary differential equations (ODEs) was proposed (Nelson and Velasco-Hernandez, 2002) and later expanded (Biswas et al., 2016) to describe the dynamics of macrophages and parasites in the early phase of infection prior to the development of the adaptive immune response. Another approach—agent-based modeling (i.e., a class of discrete computational models; Castiglione, 2009)—has been implemented with *L. major* infection data to describe the dynamics of parasites and macrophages in the later phase of infection (Dancik et al., 2010). The authors found that the decrease in the number of macrophages following peak infection could be explained by their uptake of necrotic tissues. Paradoxically, they also found that a decrease in the parasite reproduction rate might eventually lead to more parasites. In line with these results, a different ODE model showed a negative correlation between parasite load in the initial stage of the infection and the overall number of parasites at the end of the observed time window (Länger et al., 2012). The hypothesis arising from both models is that a smaller reproduction rate elicits a weaker immune response, resulting in higher survival rates of the parasite.

Despite some progress, comprehensive models for *Leishmania*-host interactions and leishmaniasis progression have not been yet fully implemented: most models so far are based only on specific aspects of the disease such as the interaction between macrophages and parasites. To our knowledge, this is the first model of leishmaniasis that covers the general dynamics of the infection and takes into account the importance of purinergic (i.e., adenosine- and ATP-based) signaling. Here we propose a model of cutaneous leishmaniasis caused by different *Leishmania* species, *L. major, L. braziliensis*, and *L. amazonensis*, which aims to establish a minimum set of rules that can describe the development of infection for each species and to test the importance of Ado release as a virulence factor. We created a model composed of the key immune competent cell types ($CD4^+$ Th cells, macrophages, DCs and epithelial cells) and molecules (IL-4, IL-12, IFN-γ, Ado, and nitric oxide, NO) reported in the literature, and the parasite. By modeling such key aspects together, we were able to demonstrate the effect of Ado on the number of parasites and the lesion formation process, thus showing the importance of Ado in the inhibition of inflammatory Th cells in *Leishmania* infection, as well as in the lesion formation processes.

MATERIALS AND METHODS

The Computational Model

One of the first lattice-gas models (Pandey and Stauffer, 1989, 1990) of infectious diseases was constructed with the aim of simulating events occurring at infected sites and draining lymph

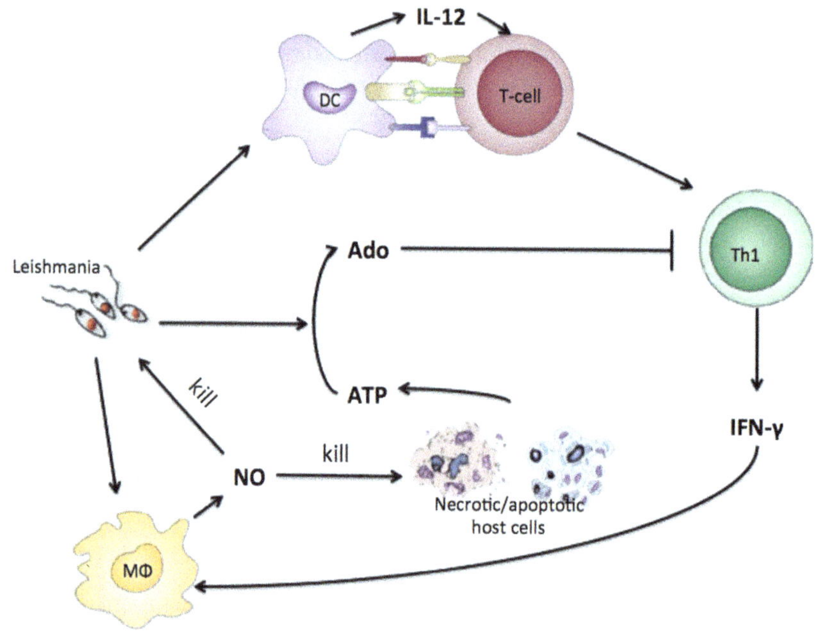

FIGURE 1 | Simplified view of the immune response to *Leishmania* infection with purinergic metabolism. Leishmania antigen will be presented to naïve T-cells by DC. T-cells will differentiate into Th1-cells that will produce INF-gamma. IFN-gamma will instruct macrophages to produce NO that kills parasite and host cells. Necrotic host cells releases high concentrations of ATP and other nucleotides that are converted by leishmania to adenosine which inhibits Th1 cells.

nodes. This type of model comprises a space-representing lattice, where the "sites" on the lattice can take a given number of different states. Evolution of the simulation, i.e., state change at the sites, is done in discrete time steps. In each time step, the state change (or not) at a given site is determined by the state of the site itself and the neighboring sites. Here, a bi-dimensional lattice with six neighbors per lattice-point and periodic boundary conditions was implemented. A representation of a portion of this lattice can be seen in **Figure 2**.

Each lattice site, representing a given volume, contains a combination of cells, cytokines and other molecules (Equations 2–10 and **Table 1**). These entities may be present in *low* or *high* concentration, represented by 0 or 1 respectively. These entities will interact and as a result, their states will change during the simulation steps (**Figure 2**).

In mathematical terms, the whole lattice $L \times L$ is represented by the vector $S(t) = (S_1(t), \ldots, S_{L\times L}(t))$ where each $S_i(t)$, a bit-word representing site i at time t, $S_i(t) = (s_{i,1}(t), \ldots, S_{i,n}(t))$ and $s_{i,k}(t)$ represents the concentration (0 for low and 1 for high) of the entities k, at time t in lattice point i. The binary state of $s_{i,k}(t+1)$ at time $(t+1)$ depends on the state of the neighboring sites, including the site s itself at the previous iteration t,

$$s_{i,k}(t+1) = HS\left(\sum_{j\in I_i} s_{j,k}(t) - \theta_k\right) \tag{1}$$

where I_i is the set of neighbors of lattice point i. The value θ_k is a threshold value that is zero for all entities except for epithelial cells for which it is 2, avoiding the unrealistic scenario of having islands of living cells in the middle of dead ones. The function HS is the Heaviside step function $HS(x) = 1$ for $x > 0$ and 0 for $x \leq 0$.

At any time step t, this value is calculated for all entities $k = 1, \ldots, n$ and lattice points $i = 1, \ldots, L^2$. Then, entities in the same site i interact with each other through Boolean rules representing the reaction rules (Equations 2–10 below). The resulting value $s_{i,k}(t+1)$ represents the new micro-state at time $t+1$. Equation (1) leads to the propagation of the entities on the lattice and together with the reaction rules represents the reaction-diffusion terms (thus including diffusion, creation and annihilation of particles) of the model. A rationale for each of Equations (2)–(9) is provided in this section and further validation from the literature is provided in **Table 1**.

The model considers $n = 9$ particles representing biological entities, namely: IL-12; IL-4; interferon IFN-γ (indicated IFN), activated T-helpers lymphocytes type 1 (Th1) and type 2 (Th2), *Leishmania* parasite (L); nitric oxide and reactive oxygen species (collectively indicated as NO); adenosine (Ado); epithelial cells (E). Besides these, three other entities are implicitly represented: macrophages, DC and naïve T helper cells. In details along the simulation, we consider that each one of these three entities is always present, as in work by Pandey and Stauffer (Pandey and Stauffer, 1989, 1990).

The reaction rules of the model are described as follows. Equations (6)–(8) use the realization of a Bernoulli event $\psi(k_i)$ that takes value 1 with probability k_i; in other words, $\psi(k_i)$ models a chemical reaction as a stochastic event occurring with rate k_i. Values of k_i were selected to agree with those published in the literature (**Table 3**). In the equations below, the symbol "$\vee$"

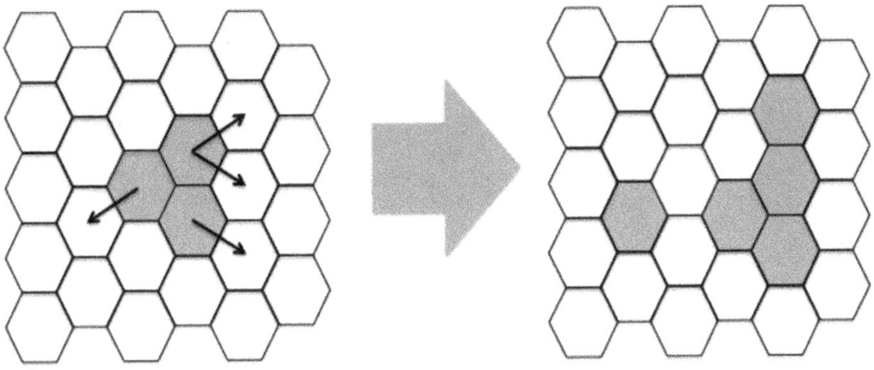

FIGURE 2 | Example of two iterations of a portion of the lattice. White hexagons represent epithelial cells and gray area hexagons shared by *Leishmania* and epithelial cells. Besides these two agents, macrophages, DC and naïve T-cells are assumed to be present everywhere. Notice that the lattice is initialized with three adjacent hexagons containing *Leishmania* and these hexagons propagate randomly modeled by Equations (1) and (9). In latter iterations other players like Th1/2 cells will also be generated.

represents an "OR" logical operator, the symbol "∧" represents an "AND," while "¬" represents a "NOT."

$$IL4 = Th2 \tag{2}$$

$$IFN = Th1 \tag{3}$$

$$IL12 = L \wedge IL4 \tag{4}$$

$$Ado = NO \wedge L \tag{5}$$

$$Th1 = \{[\psi(k_1) \wedge L \wedge (IL12 \vee \phi_{IL12}) \wedge \neg(\psi(k_2) \wedge IL4)] \vee [Th1 \wedge (\psi(k_3) \vee L)]\} \wedge \neg(\psi(k_4) \wedge Ado) \tag{6}$$

$$Th2 = \{(\psi(k_1) \wedge L \wedge \neg(IL12 \vee \phi_{IL12})) \vee [Th1 \wedge (\psi(k_3) \vee L)]\} \wedge \neg(\psi(k_4) \wedge Ado) \tag{7}$$

$$NO = IFN \tag{8}$$

$$L = \psi(k_5) \wedge L \wedge \neg NO \tag{9}$$

$$E = E \wedge \neg NO \tag{10}$$

Equations (2) and (3) show the production of the two antagonistic key cytokines IL-4 and IFN-γ produced respectively by Th2 and Th1 cells (Mougneau et al., 2011; Alexander and Brombacher, 2012).

IL-12 is produced by DCs in the model in response to *Leishmania* (L) and IL-4, represented in Equation (4). The rule of IL-4 instigating the production of IL-12 by DC is established in the literature. For a review see the work of Hochrein et al. (2000). In the case of leishmaniasis, this process has been observed for *L. major* in mice (Biedermann et al., 2001).

Equation (5) describes Ado production after NO and *Leishmania* signals, here being modeled as the conversion of nucleotides to Ado by *Leishmania* ecto-nucleotidase after host cell content released upon injury caused by NO (**Figure 1**) (Marques-da-Silva et al., 2008; de Souza et al., 2010). In this model, Ado represents the ratio between adenosine and ATP (ATP and other nucleotides). We consider that there is always some kind of host cell present in a lattice point. These cells may be the epithelial cells represented explicitly in the model or may be cells from sub-epithelial tissues.

Equations (6) and (7) show the interactions leading to the differentiation and survival of Th1 and Th2 cells. These two equations are very similar and can be broken down into three parts: (1) activation/priming, (2) recruitment/survival, and (3) Ado inhibition.

The leishmania antigen (L) being presented by DC to naïve T-cells is modeled by the terms "$\psi(k_1) \wedge L \wedge (IL12 \vee \phi_{IL12}) \wedge \neg(\psi(k_2) \wedge IL4)$" and "$\psi(k_1) \wedge L \wedge \neg(IL12 \vee \phi_{IL12})$," leading to activation and priming to Th1 or Th2 cells respectively. This process is non-deterministic, with $\psi(k_1)$ the likelihood of finding a T-cell with TCR specific to *leishmania* antigens. As can be observed, IL-12 drives the priming of naïve T-cells to Th1 phenotype (Mougneau et al., 2011) and IL-4 acts as an inhibitor of Th1 priming (Szabo et al., 1997). The ϕ_{IL12} codes for the need of IL-12 for Th1 priming. If ϕ_{IL12} is set to 1 T-cells will be primed to Th1 in spite of IL-12 (Vargas-Inchaustegui et al., 2008). IL-4 does not drive the activation to Th2 in agreement with evidence suggesting that, in the case of leishmaniasis, the Th2 phenotype may be acquired in the absence of IL-4 (Noben-trauth et al., 1996; Mohrs et al., 2000; Stetson et al., 2002). Note that IL-4 inhibition over Th1-cells priming is a probabilistic event with probability k_2.

The term "$Th \wedge (\psi(k_3) \vee L)$," present in both Equations (6) and (7), leads to activated Th-cells expansion. This expansion occurs mainly in the regions where the antigens (L) are present. In the absence of antigen Th-cells die out with a half-life determined by "$\psi(k_3)$." This term accounts for clonal expansion and recruitment (Malherbe et al., 2000; Mougneau et al., 2011). Note that in this term antigen leads to the survival of Th cells, which is also in agreement with the literature (Reckling et al., 2008).

Ado inhibition was modeled by the third part of Equation (6) and (7) ($\neg(\psi(k_4) \wedge Ado)$), letting Ado inhibit activation and survival of Th cells. This process is also probabilistic and higher probabilities represent higher Ado/ATP ratios. For reviews of the effect of Ado on the immune system see the works of Bours et al. (2006) and Cekic and Linden (2016).

TABLE 1 | Rationale for Equations (2)–(10): references reporting experimental evidences for the parameters used in the model.

Equation	Description	Topics	References
2	IFN-γ production	IFN-γ production by Th1-cells	Heinzel et al., 1989; Malherbe et al., 2000; Stetson et al., 2002; Mougneau et al., 2011; Alexander and Brombacher, 2012
3	IL-4 production	IL-4 production by Th2 cells	Heinzel et al., 1989; Malherbe et al., 2000; Stetson et al., 2002; Mougneau et al., 2011; Alexander and Brombacher, 2012
4	IL-12 production	IL-12 production by DCs in response to leishmania	Mougneau et al., 2011; Alexander and Brombacher, 2012; Liu and Uzonna, 2012
		IL-4 instruct IL12 production	Hochrein et al., 2000; Biedermann et al., 2001
		IL-4 instructs IL12 production in *L. major*	Belkaid et al., 2000; Biedermann et al., 2001; Stetson et al., 2002; Ehrchen et al., 2010
		Absence of IL4 instructing production of IL12 in *L. amazonensi/braziliensis*	Souza-Neto et al., 2004; Loffler et al., 2007; Vargas-Inchaustegui et al., 2008
5	Adenosine production	Nucleotide release by necrotic/apoptotic cells	Bours et al., 2006; Cekic and Linden, 2016
		Nucleotide to Adenosine conversion by Ecto-nucleotidase	Bours et al., 2006; Cekic and Linden, 2016
		Leishmania Ecto-nucleotidase	Cohn and Gottlieb, 1997; Berredo-Pinho et al., 2001; Maioli et al., 2004; Marques-da-Silva et al., 2008; de Souza et al., 2010
6 and 7	Th 1/2-cells	DCs presents leishmania antigens to T-cells*	Woelbing et al., 2006; von Stebut, 2007; Mougneau et al., 2011
		IL-12 bias activation to Th1	Woelbing et al., 2006; von Stebut, 2007; Mougneau et al., 2011; Liu and Uzonna, 2012
		IL-4 inhibits Th1 priming	Szabo et al., 1997
		Th-cells clonally expand in response to antigen*	Malherbe et al., 2000; Murphy et al., 2008
		Th-cells seek antigen*	Filipe-Santos et al., 2009; Mougneau et al., 2011
		Antigen promote survival of Th-cells*	Reckling et al., 2008
		Treg inactivate Th-cells*	Alexander and Brombacher, 2012
		Adenosine deactivates Th-cells and activates Treg*	Bours et al., 2006; Cekic and Linden, 2016
		Th2 activation independently of IL-4	Mohrs et al., 2000; Stetson et al., 2002
8	NO/ROS production	Macrophages produce NO/ROS in response to IFN-γ	Mougneau et al., 2011; Alexander and Brombacher, 2012; Duque and Descoteaux, 2014; Podinovskaia and Descoteaux, 2015
9	Leishmania survival	Leishmania reproduces inside macrophages	Mougneau et al., 2011; Duque and Descoteaux, 2014; Podinovskaia and Descoteaux, 2015
		Leishmania killed by NO/ROS	Mougneau et al., 2011; Alexander and Brombacher, 2012; Duque and Descoteaux, 2014; Podinovskaia and Descoteaux, 2015
10	Epithelial cells survival	Host cells (including epithelial cells) are killed by NO/ROS	Mohrs et al., 2000; Murphy et al., 2008

*Concepts that apply to both Th1 and Th2 cells.
Column 1 Equation number, column 2 brief description of the Equation, column 3 key topics and concepts modeled by the Equation, column 4 bibliographical references justifying these topics.

Equation (8) represents macrophage activation by IFN and subsequent NO production (Mougneau et al., 2011; Podinovskaia and Descoteaux, 2015).

Leishmania duplication in Equation (9) depends on the parameter k_5 representing the reproduction of the parasite inside macrophage and its clearance by NO (Mougneau et al., 2011; Podinovskaia and Descoteaux, 2015).

Equation (10) models the way in which epithelial cells will either be killed by NO or survive and multiply (Murphy et al., 2008; Mougneau et al., 2011). Epithelial cells are affected by NO and do not influence any other entity; they were included in the model so that it was possible to simulate a wound.

The lattice is initialized with all lattices containing epithelial cells and just three adjacent points containing leishmania (**Figure 2**).

Animation

The software MATLAB R2012b was used to extract data with the function *grabit* and to create AVI animations (Supplementary Material).

Sensitivity Analysis

Parameter sensitivity was performed by using Latin Hypercube Sampling (LHS a statistical method for generating a near-random sample of parameter values from a multidimensional distribution) on a grid of 243 combinations of the five parameters of the model (k_1 ... k_5). For each combination, the average of three independent runs was taken. Each execution consisted of 480 iterations and the area under the parasite curve was used as a reference. Partial Ranking Correlation Coefficient (PRCC) between the five parameters and the area under the curve was measured with the software R (function *pcc* of the package *sensitivity*). **Table 2** shows the range of values tested.

RESULTS

Predictions are Coherent with Experimental Results in Animal Models

L. major is the most studied *Leishmania* species, mainly in C57BL/6 and BALB/c mice. These models represent aspects of resistance and susceptibility to the disease and provide a good agreement with known facts about the immune response to this infection (Belkaid et al., 2000; Cangussú et al., 2009). Our approach was first to simulate C57BL/6 mouse *L. major* infection to tune the model, and then to try to adapt it to others cutaneous leishmaniasis as those involving *L. braziliensis* and *L. amazonensis*. We first started a process of extracting rules and tuning parameters by searching the literature and comparing simulated results with data from Belkaid et al. (2000) (**Figure 3**).

The set of parameter values ($\psi(k_i)$) were adjusted to agree with the literature data (**Table 3**). Two *L. major* specific parameters were found: k_2 (50% of IL-4 inhibition rate over Th-cell priming), and ϕ_{IL12} (Th1 priming independent of IL-12). The parameter k_4 (Ado inhibition rate over Th-cells) showed the same value in *L. major* and *L. braziliensis* (5%). The three parameter values k_1 [Th-cell activation probability (0.001%)], k_3 [Th-cells survival probability (18%)] and k_5 [*Leishmania* survival probability (35%)] are not specific since these values are the same in the three different species (**Table 3**). So, these shared parameters values can be reused in other *Leishmania* species simulations. Thus, *L. major* was associated with IL-4 inhibition rate over Th-cell priming and Th1 priming independent of IL-12, while Th-cells activation and survival probability and *Leishmania* survival probability are common parameters shared by all these species.

TABLE 2 | Range of values tested in LHS-PRCC (latin hypercube sampling-partial ranking correlation coefficient in the sensitivity analysis).

Parameter	Description	Range
k_1	T-cell activation probability	0.00001–0.01%
k_2	IL-4 inhibition rate over T_h priming	0–100%
k_3	T_h-cells survival probability	0–20%
k_4	Ado inhibition rate over T_h-cells	0–100%
k_5	Leishmania survival probability	30–100%

Changing Parameters Allows Simulation of *L. braziliensis* or *L. amazonensis* Infection

The first point we observed was that there is no evidence of IL-4 or IL-12 priming Th-cells during infection of C57BL/6 mice with *L. amazonensis* or *L. braziliensis*, and the absence of IL-12 does not impair the control of *L. braziliensis* (Maioli et al., 2004). This was simulated by setting ϕ_{IL12} to 1, which permits Th1 priming independent of IL-12. This change completely abrogates IL-4 production and lead to smaller lesions in agreement with observations of *L. braziliensis* infection (**Figures 4, 7**). Notice in **Table 3** that for these types of leishmaniasis the inhibition of IL-4

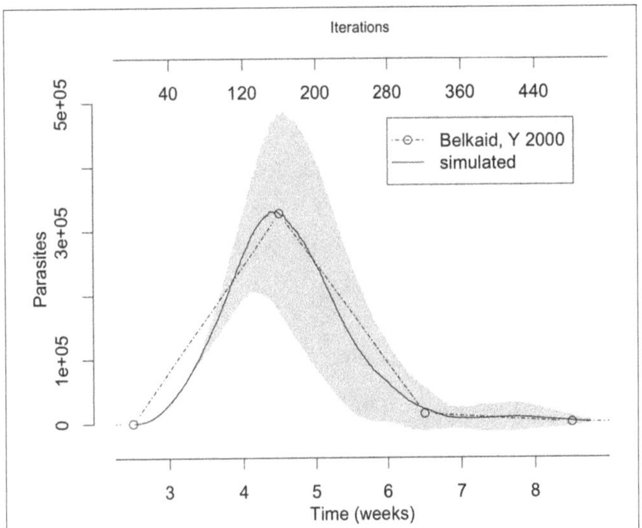

FIGURE 3 | The number of parasites in the lesion in the simulation fits with the number of parasites observed *in vivo* by Belkaid et al. (2000). The gray area represents one standard deviation. Simulation averages and standard deviations were obtained by running the model 10 times with the parameters from column "*L. major*" in **Table 3**.

TABLE 3 | Parameters and values used to simulate each of the three models of cutaneous leishmaniasis.

Parameter	Description	*L. major*	*L. braziliensis*	*L. amazonensis*
k_1	T-cell activation probability	0.001%	0.001%	0.001%
K_2	IL-4 inhibition rate over T_h priming	50%	NA	NA
K_3	T_h-cells survival probability	18%	18%	18%
K_4	Ado inhibition rate over T_h-cells	5%	5%	30%
K_5	Leishmania survival probability	35%	35%	35%
ϕ_{IL12}	Th1 priming independent of IL-12	0	1	1

For some of Leishmania species, the inhibition of IL-4 over Th1 priming is indicated as "not applicable" (NA) since there is no IL-4 production or inhibition.
Column 1: parameter; column 2: parameter description; column 3, 4, 5: values used to simulate L. major, L. braziliensis, L. amazonensis. NA, Not Applicable.

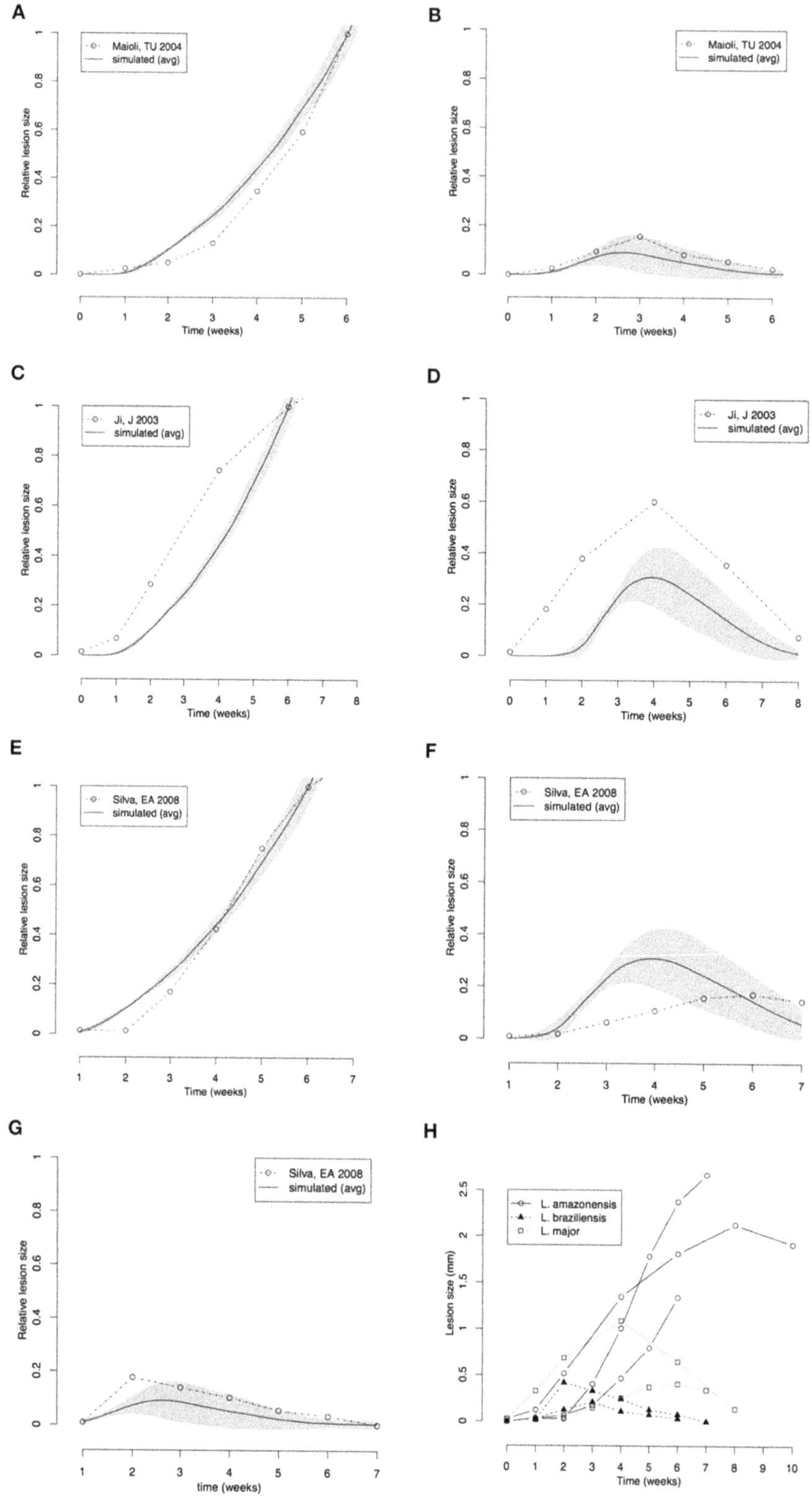

FIGURE 4 | Comparison between lesion sizes in different mouse models of *Leishmania* infection. **(A,B)** Comparison with data extracted from Maioli et al. (2004); *L. amazonensis* **(A)** *L. major* **(B)**. **(C,D)** Comparison with data from Marques-da-Silva et al. (2008); *L. amazonensis* **(C)**, *L. braziliensis* **(D)**. **(E–G)** Comparison with data from Ji et al. (2003); *L. amazonensis* **(E)**, *L. major* **(F)**, *L. braziliensis* **(G)**. **(H)** Comparison between data extracted from the three papers. All simulation and real data **(A–G)** were normalized to the size of the *L. amazonensis* lesion at 6th week. Simulations of the three cutaneous leishmaniasis were conducted with the parameter settings showed in **Table 3**. Each plot **(A–G)** represents the average ± standard deviation (gray area) of 10 simulations.

over Th1 priming is indicated as "not applicable" (NA) since there is no IL-4 production or inhibition (Maioli et al., 2004).

One explanation for the differences between leishmaniasis coming from different species is the parasite ability to metabolize ATP by membrane ecto-nucleotidase enzymes. *L. amazonensis* has higher efficiency than other species in metabolizing purines by membrane ecto-nucleodidase and this increases the Ado concentration in the microenvironment, so a higher Ado/ATP ratio can inhibit immune response (Marques-da-Silva et al., 2008; de Souza et al., 2010). To simulate this, the rate of Ado inhibition (k_4) over Th-cell activation and survival was increased and eventually we found an unresolved disease with thicker lesions full of live parasites in agreement with the expected findings for *L. amazonensis* infection in C57BL/6 mice (Marques-da-Silva et al., 2008; **Figures 4–6**).

Our simulated data was compared with the results of reported time-series for these three models of leishmaniasis (Ji et al., 2003; Maioli et al., 2004; Marques-da-Silva et al., 2008). These papers report time-series for lesion size measured as thickness of footpad or ear swelling in mice. Our models simulate lesion in the form of a superficial wound. However, the general dynamics of the lesion must be the same. The data used in the simulation was normalized to compare with the real lesions (**Figures 4A–G**).

The lesion size time series from the literature (Ji et al., 2003; Maioli et al., 2004; Marques-da-Silva et al., 2008) and the simulated data were normalized by the size of *L. amazonensis* lesion at the 6th week. This normalization allowed checking if the models could simulate lesions with similar relative sizes.

Comparison of our simulated data from models of *L. braziliensis* and *L. amazonensis* infection with footpad thickness measured by Maioli et al. (2004) showed that the models made good predictions for lesion growth and healing (**Figures 4A,B**). The relative size of the lesion caused by *L. braziliensis* with respect to that caused by *L. amazonensis* is also correctly simulated. The time-step length defined in **Figure 3** (80 steps/week) and the starting point of zero weeks post-infection was used.

An agreement between the model and the biological data was observed in the lesion formation induced by *L. amazonensis* and by *L. major* simulations; the peak and recovery time of *L. braziliensis* infection and the growing of lesion in *L. amazonensis* infection were correctly predicted (**Figures 4C,D**).

The predictions made by the model agreed with biological data in the range of the variability (shown in **Figure 4H**). These comparisons indicated that the three models are fine-tuned using correct parameters values, and can simulate the progression and outcome of the lesion size induced by infection with *Leishmania* species.

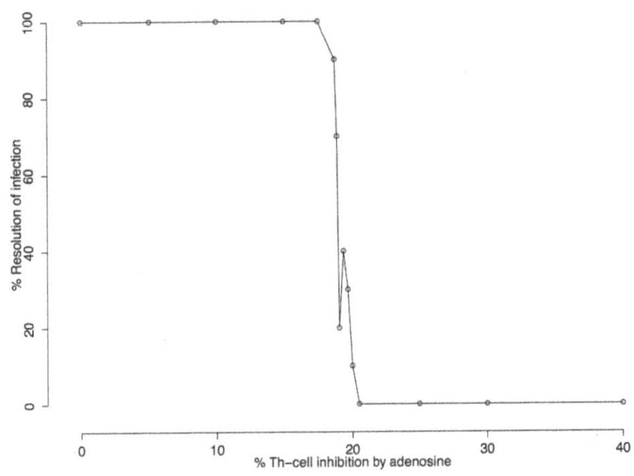

FIGURE 5 | Infection resolution rate as a function of the percentage of adenosine (Ado) inhibition. Simulations were run for 3000 iterations with parameters k1 = 0.001%, k2 = 0%, k3 = 18%, k5 = 35%, ϕ_{IL12} =1 and Ado inhibition rate over Th cells (k4) varying from 0 to 40%. Resolution rates were calculated over 10 independent simulations. Simulated mice were reported as cured (number of parasites equal zero) or non-cured (number of parasites greater than zero) after 3,000 iterations. The figure shows that 20.5% adenosine inhibition rate over Th cell is the critical value beyond which no cures are observed.

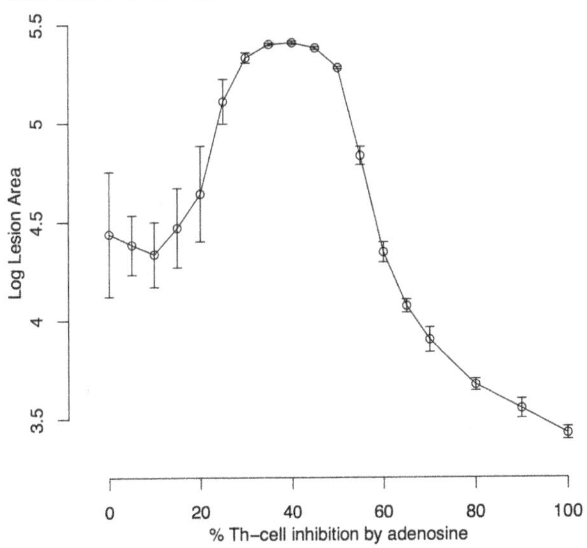

FIGURE 6 | Simulated lesion area with respect to adenosine inhibition over Th cells. Simulations were run for 480 iterations (6 weeks) with the settings k1 = 0.001%, k2 = 0%, k3 = 18%, k5 = 35%, ϕ_{IL12}= 1 and Ado inhibition rate over Th cells (k4) varying from 0 to 100%. Lesion peaks measured as the log of the number of dead epithelial cells were reported. Each dot represents the average ± standard deviation of 10 simulations.

Sensitivity Analysis of the Model

Sensitivity analysis was performed by testing combinations of parameters in the range shown in **Table 2**. The procedure was to vary the parameter values in the broadest range as possible given their restriction. For k_1, which represents the TCR-antigen specificity probability, the value must be small, so the range tested included values from 0.00001 to 0.01%. Values of k_3 above 20% do not make sense, because it would simulate replication and not half-life, and conversely k_5 cannot be below 20%; a minimum of 30% was used for biological fidelity considerations.

Sensitivity analysis reveals that the capacity of Ado to inhibit naïve Th cells activation (k_4) is an important parameter (**Table 4**). This parameter has the largest influence on the number of parasites throughout the simulation, overcoming the parasite

TABLE 4 | Sensitivity analysis performed on parameters k1,...,k5 with Latin Hypercube Sampling (LHS) and Partial Ranking Correlation Coefficient (PRCC) (Gomero, 2012).

Parameter	Description	PRCC
k_1	T-cell activation probability	-0.2401 ± 0.0633
k_2	IL-4 inhibition rate over T_h priming	0.2580 ± 0.0638
k_3	T_h-cells survival probability	-0.1014 ± 0.0781
k_4	Ado inhibition rate over T_h-cells	0.8949 ± 0.0128
k_5	Leishmania survival probability	0.7719 ± 0.0256

The PRCC is shown as average ± standard deviation measured with 200 bootstraps.

growth rate (related to the value k_1). The correlation is positive, showing that Ado increases the susceptibility to leishmania infection. IL-4 also showed a positive correlation with parasite number, which indicates that it is a susceptibility promoter. However, Th cell activation probability and Th cell survival probability (related to Th-cell half-life) showed a negative correlation with parasite number. This makes sense since Th cell activation probability and Th cell survival probability can both be linked to decreasing the probability of parasite survival. A variation of this test was tried in which k_1 was fixed at 0.001%, and it had very similar results. In another variation, IL-12 production was turned off and again the results were similar to those in **Table 4** (data not shown).

Inhibition of Th-Cell Activation by Adenosine Is the Key Factor in the Leishmaniasis Outcome

Following sensitivity analysis that points to the capacity of Ado to inhibit cell activation as the most important parameter, a deeper exploration was performed. **Figure 5** shows the percentage of resolution of the infection in respect to Ado inhibition in Th-cells. These simulations were performed without IL-12 production and with the capacity of Ado to inhibit Th-cell activation (k4) varying between 0 and 40%. Simulated mice were considered cured if after 3,000 iterations the parasite number was equal to zero. The threshold for not curing leishmaniasis is around 20.5% inhibition of Th-cell activation by Ado. The outcome experiments showed that inhibition rate agrees with the phenotype for *L. amazonensis* infection, but we decided to use 30% inhibition instead of 20.5%. Nevertheless, 20.5% inhibition capacity of Ado in Th-cell activation may fit data from infection with less virulent strains of *L. amazonensis.*

The effect of Ado on the number of parasites is intuitive, with the number of parasites growing with as Ado concentration and its capacity to inhibit Th-cells increases. It was evaluated by the size of the lesion measured in terms of the number of "dead" lattice points in respect to the Ado inhibition rate in effector Th-cells (k_4) (**Figure 6**). In this experiment, we let lesions evolve for 480 iterations (6 weeks of simulation). This shows that inhibition in the range of 0–20% does not have a strong effect on the maximum lesion size; inhibition from 20 to 40% inhibition leads to an increase in the lesion size and finally with Ado inhibition over effector Th-cells from 40 to 100%, the lesion size decreased. In this extreme case (>40% of inhibition) the number of parasites continuously increase but immune response is almost completely inhibited, which explains smaller lesions, while in the middle case (20–40%) there is an immune response strong enough to cause lesions but not strong enough to control the parasite growth.

These results indicate that a range of 0–15% in the inhibition in Th-cells' activation by Ado represents the peak of a lesion that eventually heals, while points greater than 20% represents the size of the lesion at the end of simulation since these lesions do not heal and grow continuously. Besides that, lesions with inhibition up to 55% represent a single globular dense wound while points above this threshold represent the sum of several diffuse lesions (Supplementary Material).

A comparison between the pattern of simulated lesions and real lesions is shown in **Figure 7**. In **Figure 7B** it is possible to see the pattern of simulated *L. braziliensis* lesion (**Table 3** column 4) and the comparison with real lesion (**Figure 7A**). We can see the model correctly predicts this wound as the smallest of the tree lesions simulated. **Figure 7D** shows the pattern produced by the simulation of *L. major* infection (**Table 3** column 3) and **Figure 7C** shows the real lesion. Similarly, the simulated lesion of *L. amazonensis* (**Table 3** column 5) is seen in **Figure 7F** and a real lesion in **Figure 7E**. The model correctly predicts that as the largest lesion. Assuming a lattice-point diameter of 10 μm, which is roughly the size of one host cell, the dimension of the entire lattice is about 1 cm^2, which is about the size of a mouse ear. In this respect, we observed that the simulated lesions are comparable in size to real lesions in mice. The evidence above indicates that these models are fine-tuned and can simulate the infection profile with different *Leishmania* species, and different induced immune response and lesion outcome at an equivalent size to what is seen in mouse models of infections.

DISCUSSION

The model we present here was created with the aim to reproduce the behavior of *Leishmania* infection from experimental parasite burden curve related to the immune response developed by the host in the mouse model.

In this model, the time-step length was not predefined by the parameters in Equations (2)–(10) but defined *a posteriori* by superimposing simulated dynamics with real data. In this sense, comparisons with experimental data (Belkaid et al., 2000) serve as a qualitative validation of the model and as a means of extracting values such as time-step length and the starting point of simulation (**Figure 3**). During the fine-tuning, it was found that the key parameter controlling step-size was Th-cell activation probability (k_1). Any value of k_1 in the range of 0.001–100% probability reproduced published data but with markedly differences in the step-size. With a probability of activation of 100% the time step is close to ~80 h (~half a week), while when such probability is 0.001% the time step is 2 h (80 steps/week). The inverse reasoning can be applied to check that it can make perfect sense. In a long period, such as ~80 h of antigen exposure, the probability of finding a Th-cell specific for leishmania antigen will be close to 100%, while for a smaller period (e.g., 2 h) this probability will be very low at least for low dose inoculations.

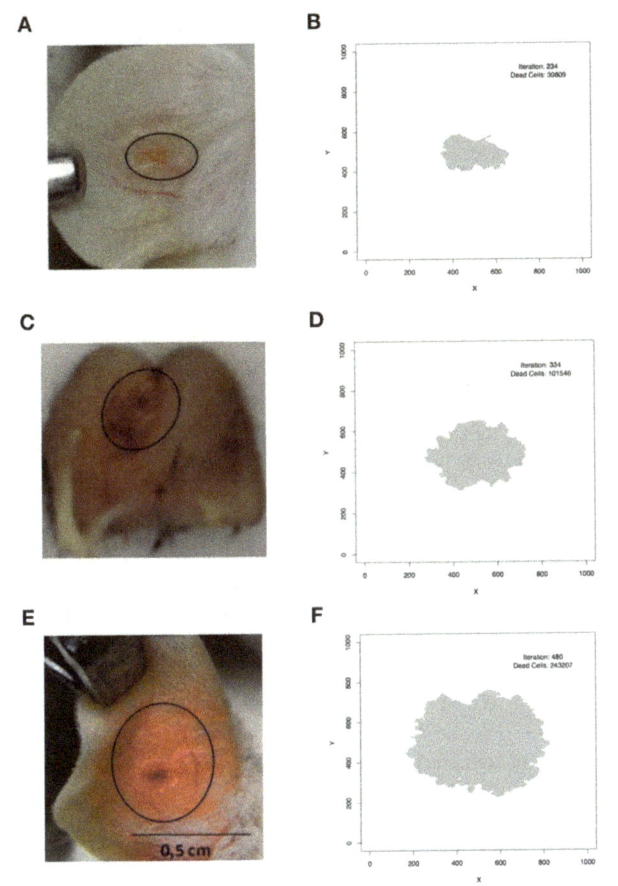

FIGURE 7 | Comparison between simulated and real lesion patterns. **(A,B)** *L. braziliensis*. **(C,D)** *L. major*. **(E,F)** *L. amazonensis*. **(A)** is courtesy of Priscila Guerra (FIOCRUZ, Brazil); **(C)** is from Maioli, TU unpublished data; **(E)** is from Araujo et al. (2014), reproduced in accordance with the policy of the journal. In **(B,D,F)** *iteration* is the step in which the screen shot of the lesion was taken and *dead cells* is the number of lattice-points that contain dead epithelial cells.

The other four parameters had an important bias in the outcome of the disease but they were found not to influence the time-step length. It is interesting to notice that k_2 and k_4 are related to levels of inhibitors (IL-4 and Ado) which do not depend on time while k_1, k_3, and k_5 are related to Th-cell activation, and Th-cell survival probabilities and leishmania replication rate., All these depend on time, but only k_1 affects time-step length.

The parameter Th-cell half-life (k_3) is sensitive to Th-cell activation (k_1). With k_1 high (>10%) the k_3 value is nearly irrelevant but for k_1 low (<0.01) k_3 must have a value greater than zero for a cure to be possible. Biologically, this finding makes sense since Th-cells have half-lives of days (Murphy et al., 2008) and k_1 low and k_3 close to zero would lead to an unrealistically short half-life of hours or minutes. It can be also observed that k_3 correlates negatively with the number of parasites throughout the simulation (**Table 4**). Most experiments used a value of 18% for k_3 (**Table 3**). This value will give a Th-cell half-live, in the absence of antigen, of about 11.5 steps (1 day), which is roughly close to the half-life of these cells *in vivo*. Throughout the simulation, the survival of Th cells will also be influenced by parasite presence and Ado production. Entities representing molecules (cytokines, Ado and NO) were modeled with a lifespan of 1 time step (2 h), in agreement with the fact that these substances have half-lives of minutes to hours (Bocchi, 1991; Loffler et al., 2007).

A broad range of values of k_1 could reproduce qualitatively the profile published by Belkaid (Belkaid et al., 2000): indeed Th-cells activation probability in the range of 10-100% leads to a growth in parasite number of the order of $10–10^2$. The same study reported that the number of parasites, following an injection of 10^2 early developmental stage (amastigotes) parasites, has grown up to 10^5 late developmental stage (promastigotes) parasites within 4.5 weeks (Belkaid et al., 2000). It is to be noted that, according to von Stebut (2007), 90% of parasites injected are killed by the complement within 3 min: this means a $10^3–10^4$-fold increase in the number of parasites. These figures are better reproduced by an activation probability k_1 ~0.001%. The parameter controlling parasite growth rate (k_5) also plays a role in tuning the results to better reproduce literature data. In this work, the pair of values $k_1 = 0.001\%$ and $k_5 = 35\%$ was very successful in reproducing published data.

The comparisons made in **Figure 3** also showed that the simulation starts at 2.5 weeks post-infection. The key reason why it could not simulate the first 2.5 weeks of the disease is that this model is a quadratic approximation of the real phenomenon. As an approximation, it cannot reproduce the whole dynamics but only a certain range, similar to what one would expect with a Taylor linearization over a critical point. Besides that, 3 lattice-points containing parasites can be translated to 10^2 parasites in a mouse which is not very far from the expected value after 2.5 weeks post-infection given that only about 10 of 100 injected parasites survive after 3 min (von Stebut, 2007). A similar approach of only simulating the late phase of *Leishmania* infection was used by Dancik et al. (2010); the simulations in his work start at 3.5 weeks post-infection. Nevertheless, the present model simulates part of the early silent phase of infection that according to Belkaid et al. (2000) lasts for the first 3 or 4 weeks.

It was possible to expand a *L. major* model to simulate other cutaneous leishmaniasis (*L. braziliensis* and *L. amazonensis*). As it can be seen in **Table 3** there is no IL-4 induced production of IL-12 for these other leishmaniasis (for a review on this see Hochrein et al., 2000). This adequately models the finding of Maioli et al. (2004) that no IL-4 producing cells could be detected during *L. braziliensis* or *L. amazonensis* C57BL/6 infection. An increase in Ado concentration to inhibit the activation of Th-cells was used to simulate *L. amazonensis* infection, in agreement with literature reports of incurable lesions in C57BL/6 mice infected with *L. amazonensis*, and with higher ecto-nucleotidase activity in the surface of this parasite (Berredo-Pinho et al., 2001; Ji et al., 2003; Maioli et al., 2004; Marques-da-Silva et al., 2008; de Souza et al., 2010; Gomes et al., 2015). This higher activity may lead to higher Ado and lower ATP concentration at the site of infection.

Notice that for simulation of *L. braziliensis* infection in C57BL/6 mice it was not necessary to tune the parameters of the model, but only to turn ϕ_{IL12} on; this change was nevertheless extracted directly from literature (Souza-Neto et al., 2004; Vargas-Inchaustegui et al., 2008). In the case of *L. amazonensis* only Ado inhibition over Th-cells (k4) was changed.

Comparison of the lesion size modeled in these simulations with experimental data from Marques-da-Silva et al. (2008), Maioli et al. (2004), Ji et al. (2003) (**Figures 4A–G**) showed that the model is capable of simulating different mouse models of cutaneous leishmaniasis. These comparisons not only validate the new simulations (*L. braziliensis* and *L. amazonensis*) but they also serve as a further validation for the *L. major* model. It is interesting to notice that the simulations were fitted to these other published data (**Figures 4A–G**) using the step-size found with Belkaid et al. (2000) comparison (80 steps/week). The appearance of the lesion takes a few weeks in mice. Thus, the starting point had to be changed from 2.5 to zero weeks post-infection. A justification for that is that in Belkaid's article (Belkaid et al., 2000), the infection was induced with a low dose of inoculum (10^2 parasites injected in the ear), while in the other studies in our comparison the infection was induced with high dose inoculum (10^5–10^6 parasites injected in the footpad). It is therefore reasonable to assume a different starting point for the appearance of the lesion. It is interesting that, according to the simulations, the inoculum size does not change the dynamics of late infection.

It is important to highlight that the comparisons in **Figure 4** are only meant to be qualitative, since different lesion metrics (lesion area *vs.* thickness) are used. The aim of these comparisons is to see if the model can capture key aspects of lesion dynamics such as when they appear and disappear and the time when they reach a peak. Data in **Figures 4A–G** were normalized by the size of *L. amazonensis* infection lesion in C57BL/mice at 6 weeks post-infection. This approach made it possible to compare the relative sizes of different cutaneous leishmaniasis lesions. We observed a good agreement between the model and literature with *L. amazonensis* lesions, i.e., the largest lesion, followed by *L. major*, and by *L. braziliensis*, which induces the smallest wounds in C57BL/6 mice.

While k_1 is the key value for setting the time-step length, Ado inhibition over effector cells (k_4) is the most important parameter for simulating the outcome of the disease. This can be observed in the sensitivity analysis (**Table 4**) and in **Figures 5**, **6**. This shows that this parameter has the most influence over the number of parasites throughout the infection and it also controls whether the infection will be cured. These results agree with Marques-da-Silva et al. (2008) and correlate the different outcomes between the three leishmaniasis in this study with ecto-nucleotidase activity on the surface of parasites and a correlation of ecto-nucleotidase activity with the virulence of different strains of *L. amazonensis* (de Souza et al., 2010).

Lesion growth is influenced by Ado concentration as is shown in **Figures 6**, **7**. These results show that this purine has a non-linear relationship with growth. Moderate inhibition of Th-cells activation may lead to the largest lesions, in agreement with Marques-da-Silva et al. (2008), Maioli et al. (2004) and Ji et al. (2003). But high Ado concentration would have a stronger inhibition of Th-cell activation and it may lead to smaller and more diffuse lesions (Supplementary Material). These data may correlate with the different outcomes of *L. amazonensis* infection in humans (Silveira et al., 2009; Hombach and Clos, 2014). It may be the case that for some genetic backgrounds, the immune system responds strongly to Ado with more secretion of IL-10 and TGF-β leading to diffuse cutaneous leishmaniasis outcome. Nevertheless, such effects remain speculative and more studies are needed to fully decipher the influence of Ado in human leishmaniosis.

This model also includes the role of IL-4. This cytokine will induce the production of IL-12 (Hochrein et al., 2000) and at the same time inhibits the action of IL-12 in Th-cells (Szabo et al., 1997). It is reported in the literature that if IL-4 is presented in the earlier phase of leishmaniasis it leads to the production of IL-12 and prime Th1 cells, while if it is presented during Th-cells priming it will lead to Th2 production and will suppress the expression of the IL-12 receptor (Biedermann et al., 2001). Furthermore, Belkaid et al. (2000) showed that IL-4 is produced during the whole infection (weeks 1–22) and that it peaks during the Th-cell priming phase (weeks 4–8) without impairing the Th1 response. The apparent contradiction between these two results can most likely be explained by the dose of IL-4. Biedermann and coworkers (Biedermann et al., 2001) injected 1 μg of IL-4 into the mice, which in a conservative calculation will lead to 10^4 pg/ml of that cytokine, while Belkaid (Belkaid et al., 2000) measures physiological doses of 10–100 pg/ml in the lymph node. The current work simulates physiological conditions that are more in line with what Belkaid (Belkaid et al., 2000) showed. Nevertheless, sensitivity analysis showed that IL-4, despite stimulating the production of IL-12, promotes susceptibility to infection, in accordance with the literature (Biedermann et al., 2001; Cangussú et al., 2009).

It was observed in the animations of *L. major* infection (Supplementary Material) that there is a spatial negative correlation between *L. major* parasites and NO production. This finding agrees with results from (Cangussú et al., 2009).

We have shown how a robust model of cutaneous leishmaniasis has been built and validated. It consists of a minimum set of rules that can describe and differentiate *L. amazonensis*, *L. braziliensis*, and *L. major* infection. The simulator agrees with key experimental results published in the literature such as the antagonism between IL-4 and IFN-γ and brings new lights to the influence of Ado signaling in these infections. We could observe a non-linear relationship between this purine and lesion formation and to confirm that it is the key factor in differentiating cutaneous leishmaniasis. Higher Ado concentration can inhibit Th-cell activation leading to infection outcomes that have been seen in experimental models of leishmaniasis. This model can therefore represent a valuable tool for answering questions regarding cellular and molecular players, inflammatory processes related to these infections and finally exploration of combination therapies involving drugs such as sodium stibogluconate, topical paromomycin preparations, etc.

AUTHOR CONTRIBUTIONS

HR, TM, LF, PT, and FC conceived of the study, HR and FC ran the simulations, all authors contributed to the analysis, wrote the manuscript and finally read and approved the final manuscript.

ACKNOWLEDGMENTS

We thank EU FP7 project MISSION-T2D (600803) Conselho Nacional de Desenvolvimento Científico e Tecnológico (CNPq) and Fundação de Amparo a Pesquisa de Minas Gerais (FAPEMIG) (Brazil) for the fellowships to HR and TM and the Consiglio Nazionale delle Ricerche (CNR—Italy) to support the work. Dr. Luis Carlos Crocco Afonso (Universidade Federal de Ouro Preto—Brazil) is kindly acknowledged for his critical contribution to the work. We also thank Priscila Guerra (Centro de Pesquisas Gonçalo Moniz/FIOCRUZ—Salvador—Brazil) for providing the *L. braziliensis* lesion picture in **Figure 7**. Finally, we thank Clare Sansom for carefully reading the manuscript.

REFERENCES

Alexander, J., and Brombacher, F. (2012). T helper1/T helper2 cells and resistance/susceptibility to *Leishmania* infection : is this paradigm still relevant? *Front. Immunol.* 3:80. doi: 10.3389/fimmu.2012.00080

Alvar, J., Velez, I. D., Bern, C., Herrero, M., Desjeux, P., Cano, J., et al. (2012). Leishmaniasis worldwide and global estimates of its incidence. *PLoS ONE* 7:e35671. doi: 10.1371/journal.pone.0035671

Araujo, M. V., Souza, P. S. O., Queiroz, A. C., Matta, C. B. B., Leite, A. B., Silva, A. E., et al. (2014). Synthesis, leishmanicidal activity and theoretical evaluations of a series of substituted bis-2-Hydroxy-1,4-Naphthoquinones. *Molecules* 19, 15180–15195. doi: 10.3390/molecules190915180

Belkaid, Y., Mendez, S., Lira, R., Kadambi, N., Milon, G., and Sacks, D. (2000). A natural model of *Leishmania* major infection reveals a prolonged "silent" phase of parasite amplification in the skin before the onset of lesion formation and immunity. *J. Immunol.* 165, 969–977. doi: 10.4049/jimmunol.165.2.969

Berredo-Pinho, M., Peres-Sampaio, C. E., Chrispim, P. P. M., Belmont-Firpo, R., Lemos, A. P., Martiny, A., et al. (2001). A Mg-Dependent Ecto-ATPase in *Leishmania* amazonensis and its possible role in adenosine acquisition and virulence. *Arch. Biochem. Biophys.* 391, 16–24 doi: 10.1006/abbi.2001.2384

Biedermann, T., Zimmermann, S., Himmelrich, H., Gumy, A., Egeter, O., Sakrauski, A. K., et al. (2001). IL-4 instructs TH1 responses and resistance to *Leishmania* major in susceptible BALB/c mice. *Nat. Immunol.* 11, 1054–1060. doi: 10.1038/ni725

Biswas, D., Priti Kumar, R., Xue-Zhi, L., Al Basir, F., and Pal, J. (2016). Role of macrophage in the disease dynamics of cutaneous leishmaniasis: a delay induced mathematical Study. *Commun. Math. Biol. Neurosci.* 2016:4.

Bocchi, V. (1991). Interleukins: clinical pharmacokinetics and practical considerations. *Clin. Pharmacokinet.* 21, 274–284. doi: 10.2165/00003088-199121040-00004

Bours, M. J. L., Swennen, E. L. R., Virgilio, F., Di, C., B. N., and Dagnelie, P. C. (2006). Adenosine 5′ -triphosphate and adenosine as endogenous signaling molecules in immunity and inflammation. *Pharmacol. Ther.* 112, 358–404. doi: 10.1016/j.pharmthera.2005.04.013

Buxbaum, L. U., Uzonna, J. E., Goldschmidt, M. H., and Scott, P. (2002). Control of New World cutaneous leishmaniasis is IL-12 independent but STAT4 dependent. *Eur. J. Immunol.* 32, 3206–3215. doi: 10.1002/1521-4141(200211)32:11<3206::AID-IMMU3206>3.0.CO;2-J

Cangussú, S. D., Souza, C. C., Campos, C. F., Vieira, L. Q., Carlos, L., Arantes, R. M. E., et al. (2009). Histopathology of *Leishmania* major infection: revisiting *L.* major histopathology in the ear dermis infection model. *Mem. Inst. Oswaldo Cruz* 104, 918–922. doi: 10.1590/S0074-02762009000600017

Carvalho, E. M., Johnson, W. D., Barreto, E., Marsden, P. D., Costa, J. L., Reed, S., et al. (1985). Cell mediated immunity in American cutaneous and mucosal leishmaniasis. *J. Immunol.* 135, 4144–4148.

Castiglione, F. (2009). "Agent based modeling and simulation, introduction to," in *Encyclopedia of Complexity and Systems Science, Vol. 1*, ed R. Meyers (New York, NY: Springer), 197–200.

Cekic, C., and Linden, J. (2016). Purinergic regulation of the immune system. *Nat. Rev. Immunol.* 16, 177–192. doi: 10.1038/nri.2016.4

Cohn, C. S., and Gottlieb, M. (1997). The acquisition of purines by Trypanosomatids. *Parasitol. Tod.* 13, 231–235. doi: 10.1016/S0169-4758(97)01059-4

Dancik, G. M., Jones, D. E., and Dorman, K. S. (2010). Parameter estimation and sensitivity analysis in an agent-based model of *Leishmania* major infection. *J. Theor. Biol.* 262, 398–412. doi: 10.1016/j.jtbi.2009.10.007

Dent, A. L., Doherty, T. M., Paul, W. E., and Staudt, L. M. (1999). BCL-6-Deficient Mice Reveal an IL-4-Independent, STAT6-dependent pathway that controls susceptibility to infection by *Leishmania* major. *J. Immunol.* 163, 2098–2013.

de Souza, C. M., de Assis, E. A., Gomes, R. S., Silva, E. A. M., Melo, M. N., Fietto, J. L. R., et al. (2010). The influence of ecto-nucleotidases on *Leishmania amazonensis* infection and immune response in C57B/6 mice. *Acta Trop.* 115, 262–269. doi: 10.1016/j.actatropica.2010.04.007

Duque, G. A., and Descoteaux, A. (2014). Macrophage cytokines: involvement in immunity and infectious diseases. *Front. Immunol.* 5:491. doi: 10.3389/fimmu.2014.00491

Ehrchen, J. M., Roebrock, K., Foell, D., Nippe, N., von Stebut, E., Weiss, J. M., et al. (2010). Keratinocytes determine Th1 immunity during early experimental Leishmaniasis. *PLoS Pathog.* 6:e1000871. doi: 10.1371/journal.ppat.1000871

Filipe-Santos, O., Pescher, P., Breart, B., Lippuner, C., Aebischer, T., Glaichenhaus, N., et al. (2009). A Dynamic map of antigen recognition by CD4 T Cells at the site of *Leishmania* major infection. *Cell Host Microbe* 6, 23–33. doi: 10.1016/j.chom.2009.04.014

Franca-Costa, J., Wanderley, M., Deolindo, P., Zarattini, J. B., Barral, A., Borges, V. M., et al. (2012). Exposure of phosphatidylserine on *Leishmania* amazonensis isolates is associated with diffuse cutaneous Leishmaniasis and parasite infectivity. *PLoS ONE* 7:e36595. doi: 10.1371/journal.pone.0036595

Gomero, B. (2012). *Latin Hypercube Sampling and Partial Rank Correlation Coefficient Analysis Applied to an Optimal Control Problem.* Master's thesis, University of Tennessee.

Gomes, R. S., Carvalho, L. C. F., Vasconcellos, R. S., Fietto, J. R. L., and Afonso, L. C. C. (2015). E-NTPase (ecto-nucleotidase trifosfato diphosphohydrolase) of *Leishmania* amazonensis inhibits macrophage activation. *Microbes Infecti.* 17, 295–303. doi: 10.1016/j.micinf.2014.12.009

Heinzel, F. P., Sadick, M. D., Holaday, B. J., Coffmanj, R. L., and And Locksley, R. M. (1989). Reciprocal expression of interferon-y or interleukin 4 during the resolution or progression of murine leishmaniasis evidence for expansion of distinct helper T Cell Subsets. *J. Exp. Med.* 169, 59–72. doi: 10.1084/jem.169.1.59

Hochrein, H., O'Keeffe, M., Luft, T., Vandenabeele, S., Grumont, R. J., Maraskovsky, E., et al. (2000). Interleukin (IL)-4 is a major regulatory cytokine governing bioactive IL-12 production by mouse and human dendritic cells. *J. Exp. Med.* 192, 823–834. doi: 10.1084/jem.192.6.823

Hombach, A., and Clos, J. (2014). No stress - Hsp90 and signal transduction in *Leishmania*. *Parasitology* 141, 1156–1166. doi: 10.1017/S0031182013002151

Hurdayal, R., and Brombacher, F. (2014). The role of IL-4 and IL-13 in cutaneous Leishmaniasis. *Immunol. Lett.* 161, 179–183. doi: 10.1016/j.imlet.2013.12.022

Jayakumar, A., Donovan, M. J., Tripathi, V., Ramalho-ortigao, M., and McDowell, M. A. (2008). Leishmania major Infection Activates NF-k B and interferon regulatory factors 1 and 8 in human dendritic cells. *Infect. Immun.* 76, 2138–2148. doi: 10.1128/IAI.01252-07

Ji, J., Sun, J., and Soong, L. (2003). Impaired expression of inflammatory cytokines and chemokines at early stages of infection with *Leishmania* amazonenses. *Infect. Immun.* 71, 4278–4288. doi: 10.1128/IAI.71.8.4278-4288.2003

Länger, B. M., Pou-barreto, C., González-alcón, C., Valladares, B., Wimmer, B., and Torres, N. V. (2012). Modeling of leishmaniasis infection dynamics: novel application to the design of effective therapies. *BMC Syst. Biol* 6:1. doi: 10.1186/1752-0509-6-1

Leite, P. M., Gomes, R. E., Figueiredo, A. B., Serafim, T. D., Tafuri, W. L., Souza, C. C., et al. (2012). Ecto-nucleotidase activities of promastigotes from Leishmania (Viannia) braziliensis relates to parasite infectivity and disease clinical outcome. *PLoS Negl. Trop. Dis.* 6:e1850. doi: 10.1371/journal.pntd.0001850

Liu, D., and Uzonna, J. E. (2012). The early interaction of *Leishmania* with macrophages and dendritic cells and its influence on the host immune response. *Front. Cell. Infect. Microbiol.* 2:83. doi: 10.3389/fcimb.2012.00083

Loffler, M., Morote-garcia, J. C., Eltzschig, S. A., Coe, I. R., and Eltzschig, H. K. (2007). Physiological roles of vascular nucleoside transporters. *Arterioscler. Thromb. Vasc. Biol.* 27, 1004–1013. doi: 10.1161/ATVBAHA.106.126714

Maioli, T. U., Takane, E., Arantes, R. M. E., Fietto, J. L. R., and Afonso, L. C. C. (2004). Immune response induced by New World *Leishmania* species in C57BL/6 mice. *Parasitol. Res.* 94, 207–212. doi: 10.1007/s00436-004-1193-6

Malherbe, L., Filippi, C., Julia, V., Foucras, G., Moro, M., Appel, H., et al. (2000). Selective activation and expansion of high-affinity cd4+ t cells in resistant mice upon infection with *Leishmania* major. *Immunity* 13, 771–782. doi: 10.1016/S1074-7613(00)00075-3

Marques-da-Silva, E. D. A., Camargos, J., Oliveira, D., and Afonso, C. (2008). Extracellular nucleotide metabolism in *Leishmania*: influence of adenosine in the establishment of infection. *Microb. Infect.* 10, 850–857. doi: 10.1016/j.micinf.2008.04.016

Mohrs, M., Holscher, C. and Brombacher, F. (2000). Interleukin-4 receptor alpha-deficient BALB/c mice show an unimpaired T helper 2 polarization in response to *Leishmania major* infection. *Infect. Immun.* 68, 1773–1780. doi: 10.1128/IAI.68.4.1773-1780.2000

Mougneau, E., Bihl, F., and Glaichenhaus, N. (2011). Cell biology and immunology of *Leishmania. Immunol. Rev.* 240, 286–296. doi: 10.1111/j.1600-065X.2010.00983.x

Murphy, K., Travers, P., Walport, M., and Janeway, C. (2008). *Janeway's Immunobiology*. New York, NY: Garland Science.

Nelson, P., and Velasco-Hernández, J. X. (2002). Modeling the immune response to parasitic infections: Leishmaniasis and Chagas disease. *Com. Theor. Biol.* V6:2.

Noben-trauth, N., Kropf, P., and Mullert, I. (1996). Susceptibility to *Leishmania* major infection in interleukin-4-Deficient mice. *Science* 447, 1994–1997.

Pandey, R. B., and Stauffer, D. (1989). Immune response via interacting three dimensional network of cellular automata. *J. Phys. France* 50, 1–10. doi: 10.1051/jphys:019890050010100

Pandey, R. B., and Stauffer, D. (1990). Metastability with probabilistic cellular automata in an HIV Infection. *J. Stat. Phys.* 61, 235–240. doi: 10.1007/BF01013962

Podinovskaia, M., and Descoteaux, A. (2015). *Leishmania* and the macrophage: a multifaceted interaction. *Fut. Microbiol.* 10, 111–129. doi: 10.2217/fmb.14.103

Reckling, S., Divanovic, S., Karp, C. L., Wojciechowski, S., Belkaid, Y., and Hildeman, D. (2008). Proapoptotic Bcl-2 Family Member Bim Promotes Persistent Infection and Limits Protective Immunity. *Infect. Immun.* 76, 1179–1185. doi: 10.1128/IAI.01093-06

Sacks, D., and Noben-Trauth, N. (2002). The immunology of susceptibility and resistance to *Leishmania* major in mice. *Nat. Rev. Immunol.* 2, 845–858. doi: 10.1038/nri933

Silveira, F. T., Lainson, R., Gomes, C. M. D. E. C., Laurenti, M. D., and Corbett, C. E. P. (2009). Immunopathogenic competences of *Leishmania (V.) braziliensis* and L. (L.) amazonensis in American cutaneous leishmaniasis. *Paras. Immunol.* 31, 423–431. doi: 10.1111/j.1365-3024.2009.01116.x

Souza-Neto, S. M., Carneiro, C. M., Vieira, L. Q., and Afonso, L. C. C. (2004). *Leishmania* braziliensis: partial control of experimental infection by interleukin-12p40 deficient mice. *Mem. Inst. Oswaldo Cruz* 99, 289–294. doi: 10.1590/S0074-02762004000300009

Stamm, L. M., Satoskar, A. A., Ghosh, S. K., David, J. R., and Abhay, R. (1999). STAT-4 mediated IL-12 signaling pathway is critical for the development of protective immunity in cutaneous leishmaniasis. *Eur. J. Immunol.* 29, 2524–2529. doi: 10.1002/(SICI)1521-4141(199908)29:08<2524::AID-IMMU2524>3.0.CO;2-H

Stetson, D. B., Mohrs, M., Mallet-Designe, V., Teyton, L., and Locksley, R. M. (2002). Rapid expansion and IL-4 expression by *Leishmania*-specific naive helper T cells *in vivo*. *Immunity* 17, 191–200. doi: 10.1016/S1074-7613(02)00363-1

Szabo, S. J., Dighe, A. S., Gubler, U., and Murphym, K. M. (1997). Regulation of the interleukin (IL)-12R b2 subunit expression in developing T Helper 1 (Th1) and Th2 cells. *J. Exp. Med.* 185, 817–824. doi: 10.1084/jem.185.5.817

Vargas-Inchaustegui, D. A., Xin L., and Soong L. (2008). *Leishmania braziliensis* infection induces dendritic cell activation, ISG15 transcription, and the generation of protective immune responses. *J. Immunol.* 180, 7537–7545. doi: 10.4049/jimmunol.180.11.7537

Vieira, L. Q., Hondowicz, B. D., Afonso, L. C. C., Wysocka, M., Trinchieri, G., and Scott, P. (1994). Infection with *Leishmania* major induces interleukin-12 production *in vivo*. *Immunol. Lett.* 40, 157–161. doi: 10.1016/0165-2478(94)90187-2

von Stebut, E. (2007). Cutaneous *Leishmania* infection: progress in pathogenesis research and experimental therapy. *Exp. Dermatol.* 16, 340–346. doi: 10.1111/j.1600-0625.2007.00554.x

WHO (2017). *Leishmaniasis. Fact Sheet.* Available online at: http://www.who.int/mediacentre/factsheets/fs375/en/

Woelbing, F., Kostka, S. L., Moelle, K., Belkaid, Y., Sunderkoetter, C., Verbeek, S., et al. (2006). Uptake of Leishmania major by dendritic cells is mediated by Fc-gamma receptors and facilitates acquisition of protective immunity. *J. Exp. Med.* 203, 177–188. doi: 10.1084/jem.20052288

Conflict of Interest Statement: The authors declare that the research was conducted in the absence of any commercial or financial relationships that could be construed as a potential conflict of interest.

9

Th2/1 Hybrid Cells Occurring in Murine and Human Strongyloidiasis Share Effector Functions of Th1 Cells

Cristin N. Bock[1], *Subash Babu*[2,3], *Minka Breloer*[4], *Anuradha Rajamanickam*[2], *Yukhti Boothra*[2], *Marie-Luise Brunn*[4], *Anja A. Kühl*[5], *Roswitha Merle*[6], *Max Löhning*[7,8], *Susanne Hartmann*[1] *and Sebastian Rausch*[1*]

[1] Department of Veterinary Medicine, Institute of Immunology, Freie Universität Berlin, Berlin, Germany, [2] National Institutes of Health-NIRT-International Center for Excellence in Research, Chennai, India, [3] Laboratory of Parasitic Diseases, National Institutes of Allergy and Infectious Diseases, National Institutes of Health, Bethesda, MD, United States, [4] Section for Molecular Biology and Immunology, Bernhard Nocht Institute for Tropical Medicine, Hamburg, Germany, [5] Medical Department, Division of Gastroenterology, Infectiology and Rheumatology/Research Center ImmunoSciences, Charité-University Medicine Berlin, Berlin, Germany, [6] Department of Veterinary Medicine, Institute for Veterinary Epidemiology and Biostatistics, Freie Universität Berlin, Berlin, Germany, [7] Experimental Immunology, Department of Rheumatology and Clinical Immunology, Charité-University Medicine Berlin, Berlin, Germany, [8] Pitzer Laboratory of Osteoarthritis Research, German Rheumatism Research Center (DRFZ), Leibniz Institute, Berlin, Germany

Edited by:
Chang H. Kim,
Purdue University, United States

Reviewed by:
Seung Goo Kang,
Kangwon National University, South Korea
Jee Ho Lee,
La Jolla Institute for Allergy and Immunology, United States

***Correspondence:**
Sebastian Rausch
sebastian.rausch@fu-berlin.de

Infections by the soil-transmitted threadworm *Strongyloides stercoralis* affect 30–100 million people worldwide, predominantly in tropic and sub-tropic regions. Here we assessed the T helper cell phenotypes in threadworm-infected patients and experimental murine infections with focus on CD4$^+$ T cells co-expressing markers of Th2 and Th1 differentiation. We show that mice infected with the close relative *S. ratti* generate strong Th2 responses characterized by the expansion of CD4$^+$ GATA-3$^+$ cells expressing IL-4/-5/-13 in blood, spleen, gut-draining lymph nodes, lung and gut tissue. In addition to conventional Th2 cells, significantly increased frequencies of GATA-3$^+$T-bet$^+$ Th2/1-hybrid cells were detected in all organs and co-expressed Th2- and Th1-cytokines at intermediate levels. Assessing the phenotype of blood-derived CD4$^+$ T cells from South Indian patients infected with *S. stercoralis* and local uninfected control donors we found that GATA-3 expressing Th2 cells were significantly increased in the patient cohort, coinciding with elevated eosinophil and IgE/IgG4 levels. A fraction of IL-4$^+$CD4$^+$ T cells simultaneously expressed IFN-γ hence displaying a Th2/1 hybrid phenotype. In accordance with murine Th2/1 cells, human Th2/1 cells expressed intermediate levels of Th2 cytokines. Contrasting their murine counterparts, human Th2/1 hybrids were marked by high levels of IFN-γ and rather low GATA-3 expression. Assessing the effector function of murine Th2/1 cells *in vitro* we found that Th2/1 cells were qualified for driving the classical activation of macrophages. Furthermore, Th2/1 cells shared innate, cytokine-driven effector functions with Th1 cells. Hence, the key findings of our study are that T helper cells with combined characteristics of Th2 and Th1 cells are integral to immune responses of helminth-infected mice, but also occur in helminth-infected humans and we suggest that Th2/1 cells are poised for the instruction of balanced immune responses during nematode infections.

Keywords: nematode, strongyloides, Th2, hybrid, T-bet, GATA-3, co-expression, cytokines

INTRODUCTION

Infections by helminths affect approximately 2 billion people globally, with soil-transmitted worms being the most prevalent. Infections with the threadworm *S. stercoralis* are currently estimated to afflict approximately 30–100 million people worldwide and are mostly asymptomatic (Puthiyakunnon et al., 2014). However, when unrecognized, the infection bears the risk of developing into a life-threatening condition in states of immune suppression (Weatherhead and Mejia, 2014).

Infections with parasitic nematodes lead to the instruction of type 2 immune responses marked by the differentiation of naïve CD4$^+$ T cells into T helper type 2 (Th2) cells (Anthony et al., 2007). These are characterized by the expression of the lineage-specifying transcription factor GATA-3 resulting in the competence to produce the effector cytokines interleukin (IL)-4, IL-5 and IL-13 (Zheng and Flavell, 1997; Zhu et al., 2010). Animal studies show that Th2 responses are central to the control of enteric helminth infections by orchestrating a broad spectrum of defense mechanisms, such as the production of Th2-driven antibody subclasses, specialized macrophage effector programs and physiological changes like intestinal goblet cell hyperplasia, mucus hyper-secretion and intensified intestinal smooth muscle contractions (Finkelman et al., 2004; Patel et al., 2009; Harris and Gause, 2011; Allen and Sutherland, 2014). While primary infections are often long lasting, the resulting Th2-dominated immunological environment is highly effective in restricting experimental re-infection under laboratory conditions (Dawkins and Grove, 1981; Urban et al., 1991; Finkelman et al., 1997; Anthony et al., 2007; Eschbach et al., 2010). Many species, however, manage to re-infect their host, as exemplified by hookworms (*Necator, Ancylostoma*), whipworms (*Trichuris*), and *Ascaris* repeatedly infecting humans by tissue migrating larvae or the ingestion of infective eggs, respectively (Turner et al., 2003, 2008; Quinnell et al., 2004; Figueiredo et al., 2010). *S. stercoralis* is unique as the parthenogenic larvae are able to develop further into adults in the infected host, leading to multiple and potentially lifelong circles of autoinfection (Weatherhead and Mejia, 2014).

We have previously shown the induction of a stably differentiated hybrid T helper population with combined characteristics of Th2 and Th1 cells at the single cell level, namely the co-expression of GATA-3 and Th2 cytokines together with the lineage-specifying transcription factor and signature cytokine of Th1 cells, T-bet and IFN-γ, in experimental helminth infections. These cells, while being able to support both Th2 and Th1 immune responses, display a quantitatively reduced potential for Th2- as well as Th1-associated effector functions (Peine et al., 2013). We asked whether such Th2/1 cells also occur in helminth-infected patients and hence investigated T helper cell responses in patients infected by *S. stercoralis* in South India. Experimental infections with the murine model *S. ratti* were employed to assess whether the development and proportions of Th2/1 hybrid cells differ depending on parasite burden and phase of infection and to collect more detailed information about the prevalence of Th2/1 hybrid, conventional Th2 and Th1 cells in different organs affected by the parasite during its life cycle. Furthermore, we aimed to assess if Th2/1, similar to Th1 cells present in higher numbers, may serve as a source for IFN-γ sufficient for the instruction of classical macrophage activation.

We show that Th2/1 hybrid cells co-expressing IL-4 and IFN-γ are not restricted to a considerable range of murine helminth infections, but are also detectable in *S. stercoralis* infected patients. In mice, the proportion of Th2/1 hybrids within Th2 cells was independent of worm burden or phase of infection, but Th2/1 cells were most prominent in spleen and small intestine. To our knowledge, we show for the first time that human Th2/1 hybrid cells are marked by high IFN-γ and low GATA-3 expression, contrasting the IFN-γ/GATA-3 intermediate phenotype of their murine counterparts. Functionally, murine Th2/1 hybrid cells shared effector aspects with Th1 cells in producing IFN-γ in response to cytokine triggers and the ability to drive classical macrophage activation.

MATERIALS AND METHODS

Ethics Statement and Study Population

All individuals were examined as part of a natural history study protocol approved by Institutional Review Boards of the National Institute of Allergy and Infectious Diseases, USA and the National Institute for Research in Tuberculosis, India (ClinicalTrials.gov identifiers NCT00375583, and NCT00001230), and informed written consent was obtained from all participants.

We studied a total of 74 individuals comprising 34 clinically asymptomatic, *S. stercoralis*-infected individuals (Inf) and 40 uninfected, healthy individuals with endemic normal status (EN) in Tamil Nadu, South India (**Tables 1, 2**). All individuals were recruited from a rural population by screening of individuals for helminth infection by stool microscopy and serology. Inclusion criteria were age of 18 to 65 years and willingness to give blood and stool samples for examination; exclusion criteria were past anthelmintic treatment, other helminth infections, or HIV infection. Strongyloides infection was diagnosed by the presence of IgG antibodies to the recombinant *Strongyloides* antigen, NIE,

TABLE 1 | Demographic profile of infected and uninfected cohorts.

Parameter	Value for the group	
	Infected (n = 34)	**Uninfected (n = 40)**
No. of male subjects	16	21
No. of female subjects	18	19
Mean age (range [year])	34 (19–58)	33 (18–60)
Clinical status	Healthy	Healthy
Symptom(s)	None	None
Socioeconomic status	Rural workers	Rural workers
NIE ELISA result	Positive	Negative
Results of stool examination for *S. stercoralis*	Positive	Negative
Presence of other helminth infections	Negative	Negative

TABLE 2 | Hematological profile of infected and uninfected cohorts.

Factor[a]	GM (range) for the group		
	Infected (n = 34)	Uninfected (n = 40)	P-value[b]
Hb (g/dL)	13.07 (7.6–16.9)	51.77 (8.7–174)	NS
RBC (10^6 /μl)	4.68 (3.7–6)	4.80 (3.5–6.46)	NS
WBC (10^3 /μl)	8.51 (5.1–13.8)	8.55 (5.3–13.3)	NS
HCT (%)	39.47 (25–51)	40.35 (27–54)	NS
PLT (10^3 /μl)	267.5 (159–413)	287.1 (137–446)	NS

[a]*Hb, hemoglobin; RBC, red blood cells; WBC, white blood cells; HCT, hematocrit; PLT, platelets.*
[b]*NS, not significant.*

as described previously (Bisoffi et al., 2014; Buonfrate et al., 2015). None of the individuals had lymphatic filariasis verified with TropBio Og4C3 enzyme-linked immunosorbent assay (ELISA) (Trop Bio Pty. Ltd., Townsville, Queensland, Australia) or other intestinal helminths (based on stool microscopy). None of the tested individuals suffered from acute tuberculosis, analyzed via QuantiFERON TB Gold-in-Tube enzyme-linked immunosorbent assay (ELISA) (Cellestis).

All infected individuals were treated with single doses of ivermectin and albendazole. All uninfected individuals were anti-*Strongyloides* NIE negative and negative for filarial and other intestinal helminths as well as acute tuberculosis.

Hematological Parameters

Hemograms were performed on all individuals using the Act-5 Diff hematology analyzer (Beckman Coulter, Brea, CA, USA).

PBMC Isolation and *In vitro* Culture

Heparinized blood was centrifuged at 400 × g for 10 min, plasma separated and stored at 4°C. Samples were refilled with RPMI-1640 and PBMC isolated by Ficoll diatrizoate gradient centrifugation (LSM; ICN Biomedicals). Cells were then washed, resuspended in freezing medium (RPMI 1640, 10% DMSO, 45% heat inactivated FCS, Harlan Bioproducts) and stored in liquid nitrogen until usage. For *in vitro* culture the cryopreserved cells were thawed gently, washed twice and cultured with RPMI 1640 medium supplemented with penicillin-streptomycin (100 U and 100 μg/ml, respectively), L-glutamine (2 mM), 1% NEAA MEM (all from PAN-Biotech, Aidenbach, Germany) and 5% heat inactivated AB human serum (Biochrom, Berlin, Germany). For stimulations and intracellular staining cells were counted using trypan blue and adjusted to 1×10^7 cells/ml. 2×10^6 cells/well were placed on round-bottom 96 well tissue culture plates, stimulated with phorbol 12-myristate 13-acetate (PMA) and ionomycin (both Sigma-Aldrich, MO, USA) at concentrations of 25 ng/ml and 0.5 μg/ml or media alone and incubated for 4 h at 37°C. Brefeldin A solution (10 μg/ml, eBioscience, CA, USA) was added after 30 min. After 4 h cells were washed, stained and analyzed as given below.

Elisa

Plasma levels of total IgE, IgG1, IgG3, and IgG4 were evaluated using Ready-Set-Go! ELISA kits (eBioscience) according to the manufacturer's instructions. All samples were run in duplicates.

Animal Experimentation, Mice and Parasites

Animal experiments were performed in accordance with the National Animal Protection Guidelines and approved by Federal Health Authorities of the States of Hamburg (permission number 55/13). The *S. ratti* life cycle was maintained in Wistar rats purchased from Charles River (Sulzfeld, Germany) as described earlier (Eschbach et al., 2010). Female C57BL/6 mice were bred in house at the Bernhard Nocht Institute Hamburg, Germany. Mice were kept in individually ventilated cages under specific pathogen-free (SPF) condition, infected by 200 or 2,000 *S. ratti* iL3 in the hind footpad and sacrificed by isoflurane inhalation followed by cervical dislocation at day 10 or 20 post infection at 8–10 weeks of age. Parasite burdens were examined at day 6 post infection in faces via quantification of *S. ratti* 28S ribosomal RNA using real-time quantitative PCR as described elsewhere (Nouir et al., 2012).

Preparation of Single Cell Suspension

Spleens and mesenteric lymph nodes (mLN) were isolated and placed in cold RPMI 1640 wash medium containing 1% FCS, 100 U/ml penicillin and 100 μg/ml streptomycin (all from PAN - Biotech, Aidenbach, Germany) and then forced through 70 μm cell strainers (BD Bioscience, San Jose, CA) to obtain single cell suspensions. Erythrocytes in spleen cell suspension were lysed using ACK buffer containing 150 mM NH_4Cl, 0.1 mM $KHCO_3$ and 0.1 mM Na_2EDTA, pH 7.2 for 5 min on ice followed by two washing steps. Small intestinal lamina propria (siLP) cells were isolated as described earlier (Strandmark et al., 2016).

Lungs were perfused and rinsed with 0.9% NaCl until the tissue turned white before isolation of single cells. The lung was rinsed in ice-cold RPMI 1640 containing 10% FCS. Tissue was then transferred onto petri dishes, cut in small pieces (~ 2 mm) and subsequently added to 10 ml PBS containing 0.1265 U/ml collagenase D and DNase (0.15 mg/ml, both Sigma-Aldrich, Steinheim, Germany) followed by incubation in a tube shaker water bath (250 rpm, 37°C) for 1 h. Digested lung tissues were forced through 40 μm cell strainers, washed twice and erythrocytes lysed using ACK buffer followed by two washing steps.

For the isolation of PBMC, whole blood was diluted 2:1 with RPMI 1640 containing 10% FCS and layered onto Pancoll (density of 1.077 g/ml, PAN-Biotech, Aidenbach, Germany), centrifuged and washed twice with PBS.

Cells of all tissues were resuspended in RPMI 1640 containing 10% FCS, counted using a CASY automated cell counter (Roche-Innovatis, Reutlingen, Germany) and were adjusted to 1×10^7 cells/ml. Cells were plated on round-bottom 96 well tissue culture plates (Costar, Corning Inc., NY, USA), stimulated with PMA and ionomycin at concentrations of 50 ng/ml and 1 μg/ml and incubated for 30 min at 37°C, followed by addition of Brefeldin A (10 μg/ml) and further stimulation for 2.5 h.

Flow Cytometry

Human cells were stained with fixable viability dyes (eFluor780 or eFluor506 eBioscience), fixed and permeabilized using the eBioscience Foxp3 staining kit and stained intracellularly for the following markers: CD3 (BV510, clone OKT3), CD4 (PerCP, clone SK3), CD45RO (FITC, clone UCHL1), IL-4 (PE, MP4-25D2), IL-5 (PE, clones MP4-25D2, TRFK5), IL-13 (FITC, clone PVM13-1), IFN-γ, (eF450, clone 4S.B3), GATA-3 (eF660, clone TWAJ) and T-bet (PE-Cy7, clone eBio4B10). Murine cells were stained with fixable viability dye (eFluor780, eBioscience) and subsequently fixed and permeabilized using the Foxp3 staining kit and stained intracellularly for the following markers: CD4 (PerCP, clone RM4-5), GATA-3 (eFluor660, clone TWAJ), T-bet (PE-Cy7, clone eBio4B10), IL-4 (PE, clone 11B11), IL-13 (Alexa488, clone eBio13A), IL-5 (PE, clone TRFK5), IFN-γ (eFluor450, clone XMG1.2). All antibodies were from eBioscience, BioLegend and BD Biosciences.

In vitro T Helper Subset Differentiation

Cells from spleens and peripheral lymph nodes of naïve C57BL/6 mice were stained for CD4 (BrilliantViolet 510, clone RM4-5), CD62-L (APC-eFluor780, clone MEL-14), CD44 (PE, clone IM7) and CD25 (APC, clone 61.5) (all antibodies from eBioscience and BioLegend) and naïve $CD4^{+}CD25^{-}CD62\text{-}L^{high}CD44^{neg}$ cells were isolated on a FACS Aria cell sorter (BD Bioscience). Cells were plated on 48 well plates (Costar) coated with anti-CD3/anti-CD28 antibodies (1 μg/ml each, clones 145-2C11 and 37.51, from BD Biosciences). Th1 differentiation was induced by addition of recombinant murine IFN-γ and IL-12 (10 ng/ml each, PeproTech) and 10 μg/ml anti-IL-4 (clone 11B11, BioLegend, San Diego, CA, USA). Th2 development was induced by addition of 30 ng/ml recombinant murine IL-4 (PeproTech) and anti-IFN-γ/anti-IL12/23 p40 antibodies (clones AN18, C17.8, BioLegend, 10 μg/ml each). Th2/1 hybrids were generated by addition of IFN-γ, IL-12 and IL-4 in the concentrations given above. Recombinant human IL-2 (10 ng/ml, PeproTech) was added to all cultures and replaced in fresh medium on day 3. Cells were analyzed for expression of T-bet, GATA-3, IFN-γ IL-4 and IL-13 after 5 to 6 days by intracellular antibody staining.

T Helper Cell Innate Function

Cells isolated from mice infected with *S. ratti* for 10 days were stimulated with the following recombinant murine cytokines (all from PeproTech, Hamburg) or monoclonal antibodies (from BD Biosciences) for 6 h: IL-33 (100 ng/ml) and IL-7 (10 ng/ml), IL-18 and IL-12 (both 10 ng/ml), anti-CD3 (clone 145-2C11) and anti CD28 antibodies (clone 37.51, both 2 μg/ml). Controls were left untreated. Brefeldin A (10 μg/ml) was added after 30 min. Cells were then stained for CD4, GATA-3, T-bet, IL-13 and IFN-γ.

Macrophage/T Cell Co-cultures and Nitric Oxide Assay

Peritoneal cells were isolated from naïve C57BL/6 mice by flushing the peritoneal cavity with ice-cold PBS (20 mM EDTA, 0.2% BSA) followed by washing in RPMI. 3×10^5 cells were plated on 96 well round-bottom plates (Costar) in 200 μl in RPMI and incubated at 37°C for 1 h. Non-adhering cells were removed by 3 washing steps with warm RPMI. 1×10^5 *in vitro* generated Th1, Th2 or Th2/1 cells were added and co-cultured in 200 μl for 24 h. Lipopolysaccharide (LPS, L5529, Sigma) was added for co-stimulation at 0.5 μg/ml to some wells. Control cultures received 1 or 10 ng/ml recombinant murine IFN-γ. Nitrite concentrations in culture media were quantified by the Griess reaction.

Histology

Proximal small intestinal tissue samples were fixed in formalin and histochemically stained with hematoxylin and eosin (H&E) to assess histomorphology and with periodic acid Schiff (PAS) for goblet cell quantification.

Enteritis was scored as described earlier (Rausch et al., 2009). Images were acquired using the AxioImager Z1 microscope (Carl Zeiss MicroImaging, Inc., Jena, Germany) at 100× magnification. All evaluations were performed in a blinded manner.

Statistical Analyses

All data were assessed for Gaussian distribution. Statistically significant differences between two groups were analyzed by using Student's *t*-test (parametric) or Mann-Whitney *U*-test (non-parametric) using GraphPad Prism 7 software (San Diego, CA). For multiple comparisons, the Kruskal-Wallis test with Dunn's correction was performed. *P*-values $\leq$ 0.05 were considered to indicate statistical significance.

The regression analyses were carried out using SAS 9.4. Quantitative variables were tested for normality (PROC UNIVARIATE) and when necessary transformed to logarithmic values. After graphic assessment of the assumption of linear relationships (PROC GPLOT) and assessment of correlations between variables (PROC CORR) associations between variables were investigated by multivariable linear models with the procedure PROC REG. Models with different independent factors were compared by using the adjusted R^2 and the global F-statistics. The variable "group" as well as the main variable of the respecting analyses were always kept in the model, but other factors were removed in a backward selection according to the *p*-value and the change of R^2. Model diagnostics included residues assessment (normality), test for multicollinearity and variance inflation. Observations with great influence (according to leverage hat-values or Cook's D) were excluded, if the model changed significantly after removing the observation. *P*-values $\leq$ 0.05 were considered to indicate statistical significance.

RESULTS

S. ratti Infection Results in Th2 Induction

In order to assess the immune response to *S. ratti*, mice were infected with 200 or 2,000 infective stage 3 larvae and dissected at day 10 or 20 post infection (**Figure 1A**). Worm burdens were assessed at day 6 by quantification of *Strongyloides* DNA in faces. Expectedly and as shown before, mice infected with 2,000 larvae displayed significantly higher worm burdens than mice inoculated with 200 larvae (**Figure 1B**; Eschbach et al., 2010). Histological examination of proximal small intestinal tissue samples showed that the infection did not result in immunopathological changes by day 10, while some mice

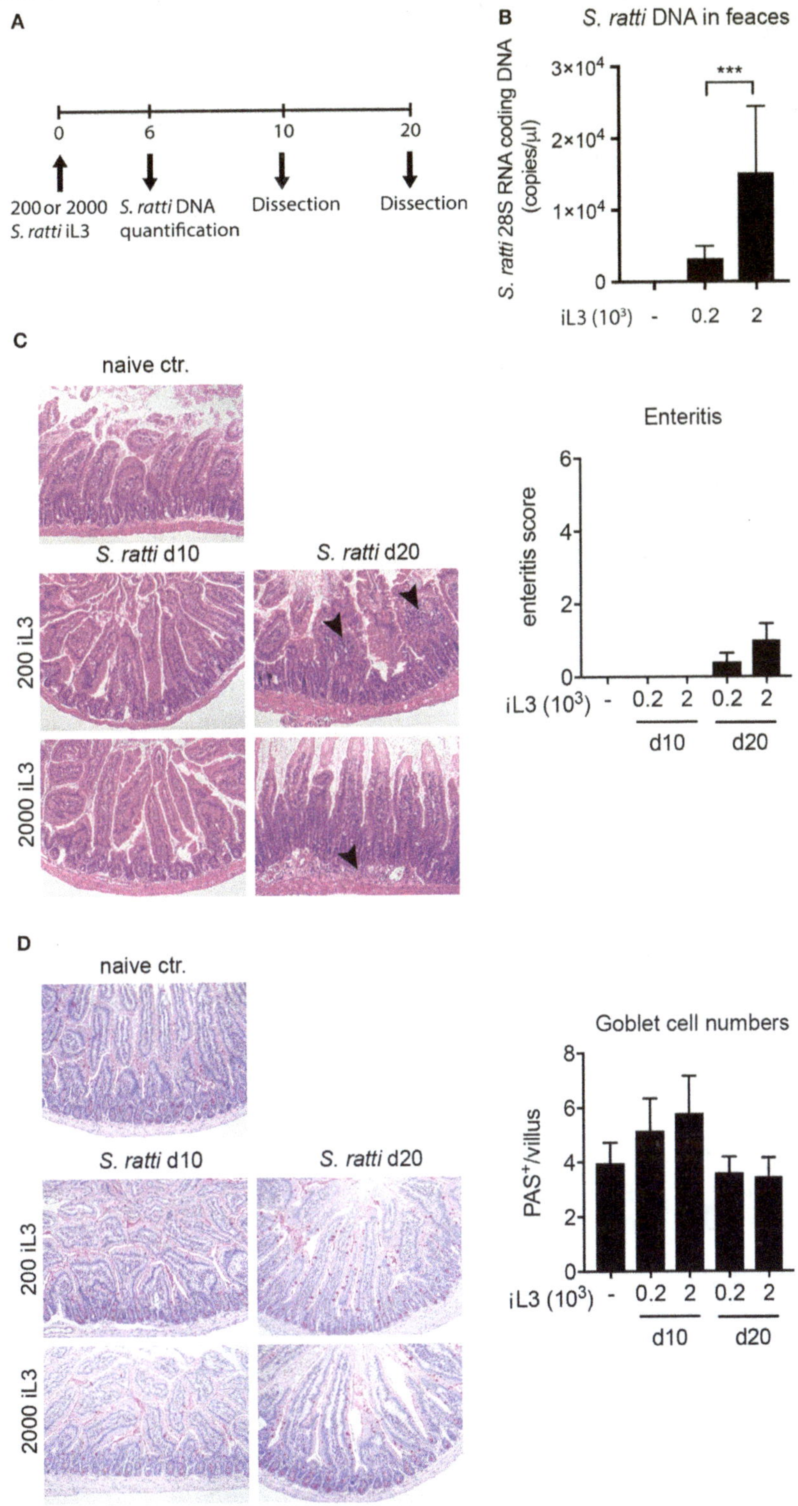

FIGURE 1 | *S. ratti* infection leads to mild immunopathology in mice. **(A)** Experimental time line. C57BL/6 mice were infected with 200 or 2,000 *S. ratti* stage 3 larvae and dissected 10 or 20 days post infection. **(B)** Quantification of *Strongyloides* DNA at day 6 post infection. **(C)** Exemplary pictures of H&E stained proximal small intestinal cross sections. Magnification × 100. Mild cellular infiltrates in the lamina propria at day 20 are marked by arrow heads. Bar graph depicts enteritis scores of experimental groups. **(D)** Exemplary pictures of PAS stained proximal small intestinal cross sections. Magnification × 100. Mucus filled goblet cells appear magenta. Bar graph depicts quantification of goblet cells per villus in small intestinal cross sections. Mean + SD of $n = 6$ (naïve ctr.) and 5 (infected) mice is shown. Data originate from one out of two experiments with similar results. $^{***}p < 0.005$.

displayed mild signs of cellular infiltration at day 20 post infection (**Figure 1C**). Numbers of mucus-producing goblet cells were at best mildly and transiently, but not significantly increased by day 10 post infection (**Figure 1D**).

Expectedly, infected mice displayed significantly increased frequencies of $CD4^+$ T cells expressing GATA-3 and IL-4 in spleen, gut-draining mesenteric lymph nodes (mLN) and small intestinal lamina propria (siLP) when compared to uninfected controls (**Figures 2A–D**). Th2 cells were also elevated in blood and lung tissue of infected mice (SI Figures 1A,B). $T\text{-bet}^+$ Th1 cells tended to increase in the spleen of infected mice, reaching significance at day 20 post infection, while IFN-γ expression by $CD4^+$ T cells from spleens was transiently elevated at day 10 (**Figures 2E,F**). Frequencies of T-bet expressing cells in mLN, siLP and other organs were similar in all groups (**Figures 2G,H** and SI Figures 1C,D) while IFN-γ responses in the small intestine were significantly reduced in infected mice (**Figure 2H**).

Collectively, *S. ratti* infection led to local and systemic Th2 responses confirming previous studies (Eschbach et al., 2010; Blankenhaus et al., 2011), while transiently elevated IFN-γ production and expansion of T-bet expressing Th1 cells was restricted to the spleen. Pathological changes and Th2-driven increases of goblet cells in the small intestine were only mild, pointing out the relatively asymptomatic nature of *S. ratti* infection in mice.

Th2/1 Hybrid Cells Occur in Mice Infected with *S. ratti*

Asking whether infections with *S. ratti* led to the expansion of Th2/1 cells as previously shown for other helminth infections (Peine et al., 2013), we screened the organs of naïve and infected mice for $CD4^+$ T cells simultaneously expressing GATA-3 and T-bet. We detected significantly increased frequencies of $GATA\text{-}3^+T\text{-bet}^+$ Th2/1 cells in all organs of infected mice (**Figures 3A–D** and SI Figures 2A,B). The proportions of T-bet co-expressing Th2/1 cells within the total $GATA\text{-}3^+CD4^+$ population were highest in spleen and siLP of *S. ratti* infected mice (**Figure 3E**). T-bet/IFN-γ co-expressing cells were detected in similar proportions within IL-4 and IL-13 producers from spleens of mice infected for 10 days (**Figure 3F**) and the frequencies of $IFN\text{-}\gamma^+$ Th2/1 hybrids in Th2 cytokine producing populations were similar when comparing day 10 and 20 post infection (**Figure 3G**).

As shown previously (Peine et al., 2013), Th2/1 hybrid cells expressed lower levels of GATA-3 and IL-4 than conventional Th2 cells (**Figure 3H**) and IFN-γ production was significantly decreased compared to Th1 cells (**Figure 3I**). Notably, T-bet expression by Th2/1 cells was significantly elevated compared to infection-derived Th1 cells (**Figure 3I**), which might reflect the acute activation status of the Th2/1 cells.

Thereby, our previous demonstration of the induction of Th2/1 hybrid cells in nematode and Schistosome infections (Peine et al., 2013) can be generalized to mice infected with different doses of threadworms.

Human Study Population Characteristics

To evaluate whether $CD4^+$ T cells with combined characteristics of Th2 and Th1 cells also occur in human helminth-infected patients we investigated blood samples of patients infected with *S. stercoralis* and endemic uninfected control donors. The demographic profile of the cohorts is given in **Table 1**. No differences in age range, gender and socio-economic status were observed between the two studied groups. All individuals were healthy and free of symptoms. Hematological features of both cohorts are depicted in **Table 2**. No differences concerning hemoglobin levels, red and white blood cell counts, hematocrit or platelet counts were observed between the groups. The frequencies of lymphocytes and eosinophils were significantly elevated in the infected cohort (SI Figures 3A,D), while neutrophil frequencies were significantly lower in *S. stercoralis* infected patients (SI Figure 3B). Blood monocyte and basophil frequencies were not different between the groups (SI Figures 3C,E).

Human *S. stercoralis* Infection Is Associated with Increased Th2 Responses

To compare the immune status of helminth-infected individuals and uninfected control subjects, PBMC from *S. stercoralis*-infected donors and healthy endemic controls were stimulated with PMA/ionomycin and assessed for markers of Th1 and Th2 differentiation by flow cytometry. The *S. stercoralis*-infected group displayed significantly elevated frequencies of $CD3^+CD4^+GATA\text{-}3^+$ Th2 cells compared to the uninfected control group (**Figures 4A,B**) and a higher ratio of Th2:Th1 cells (SI Figure 4). While frequencies of IL-4 and IL-5 expressing T cells were similar in both cohorts, the *S. stercoralis*-infected group displayed significantly increased levels of IL-13 expressing cells (**Figure 4B**). Linear regression analysis confirmed a significant effect of the group in terms of IL-13 levels ($p = 0.0407$) and showed that increased GATA-3 expression was associated with increased IL-13 expression ($p = 0.0279$) (SI Figure 5A). Furthermore, levels of IL-4, IL-13 and IFN-γ significantly increased with age ($p = 0.0030$, $p = 0.0062$, and $p = 0.0407$, respectively, data not shown).

No differences were observed for Th1 cells expressing T-bet and IFN-γ between the cohorts (**Figure 4C**), but increased T-bet expression levels were associated with higher IFN-γ expression ($p < 0.0001$) (SI Figure 5B).

Hence, *S. stercoralis* infection in humans is marked by Th2 differentiation, while frequencies of Th1 cells are indistinguishable from healthy controls.

Th2/1 Hybrid Cells Are Detectable in Blood of *S. stercoralis* Infected Patients

We next asked whether hybrid Th2/1 cells sharing characteristics of Th2 and Th1 cells were detectable in blood samples of the study cohorts. We detected $CD3^+CD4^+$ T cells distinctly co-expressing IL-4 and IFN-γ in the infected as well as the healthy control group (**Figures 4A,D**). Furthermore, the *S. stercoralis*-infected cohort displayed significantly increased frequencies of $CD3^+CD4^+$ T cells co-expressing GATA-3 and T-bet compared to healthy

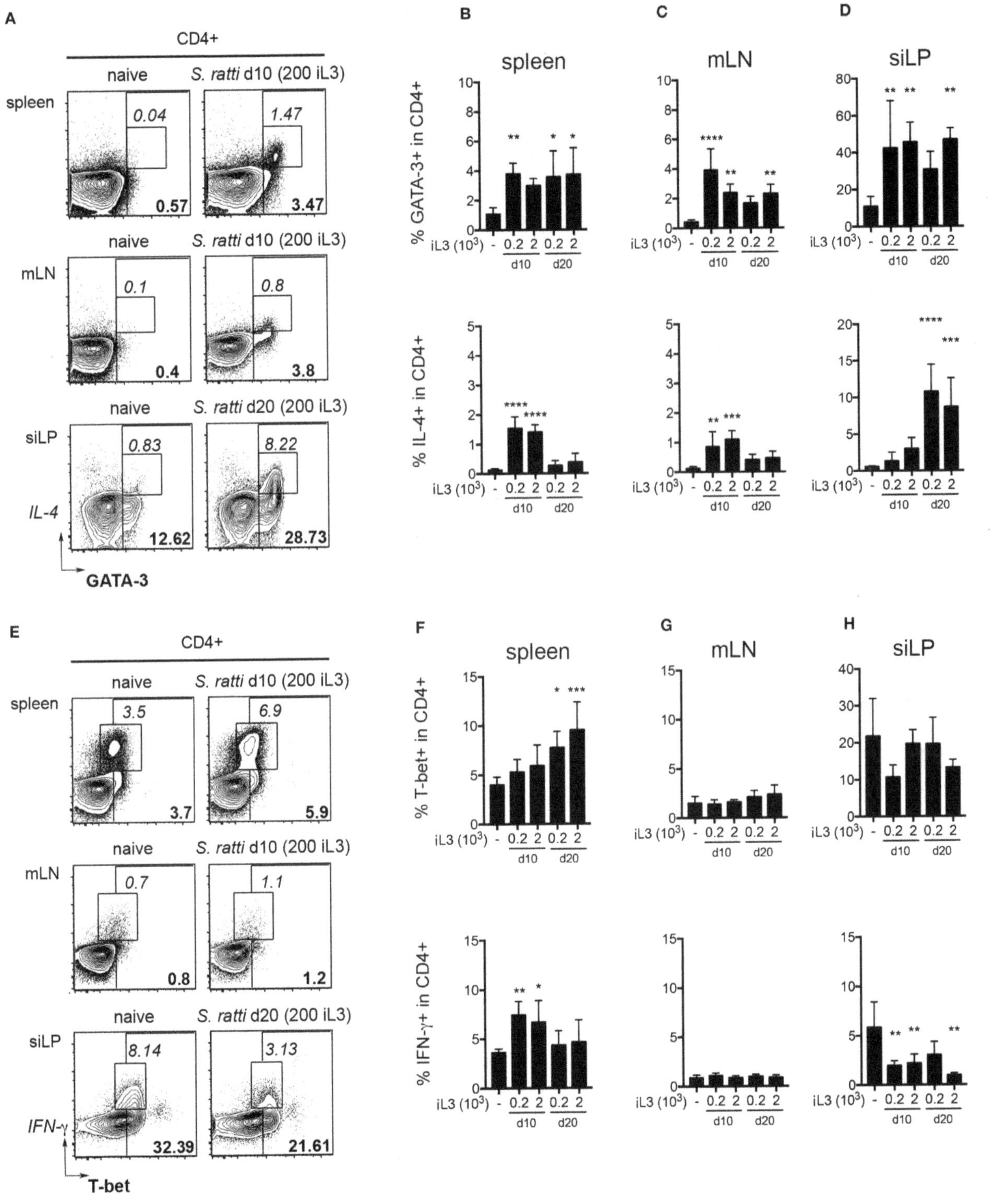

FIGURE 2 | *S. ratti* infection leads to systemic and local Th2 response. Phenotypes of $CD4^+$ T cells were assessed in mice infected with 200 or 2,000 *S. ratti* stage 3 larvae. **(A)** Exemplary flow cytometry plots of live $CD4^+$ T cells derived from spleen, mesenteric lymph nodes (mLN) and small intestinal lamina propria (siLP) of an uninfected control and *S. ratti* infected mouse (200 iL3) at the depicted days post infection. Bold numbers report frequencies of GATA-3 expressing cells, italic numbers report frequencies of GATA-3^+IL-4^+ cells. **(B–D)** Frequencies of GATA-3^+ cells (top) and IL-4^+ cells (bottom) within live $CD4^+$ T cells isolated from spleen **(B)**, mLN **(C)** and siLP **(D)** as detected after 4h of PMA/ionomycin stimulation. **(E)** Exemplary flow cytometry plots of live $CD4^+$ T cells as described in **(A)**. Bold numbers report frequencies of T-bet expressing cells, italic numbers report frequencies of IFN-γ^+ cells. **(F–H)** Frequencies of T-bet^+ cells (top) and IFN-γ^+ cells (bottom) within live $CD4^+$ T cells isolated from spleen **(F)**, mLN **(G)** and siLP **(H)** detected after 4 h of PMA/ionomycin stimulation. Mean + SD of n = 5–6 (naïve ctr.) and 4–5 (infected) mice. Data from one out of two experiments with similar results are shown. $^*p < 0.05$, $^{**}p < 0.01$, $^{***}p < 0.005$, $^{****}p < 0.001$ comparing infected to naïve controls.

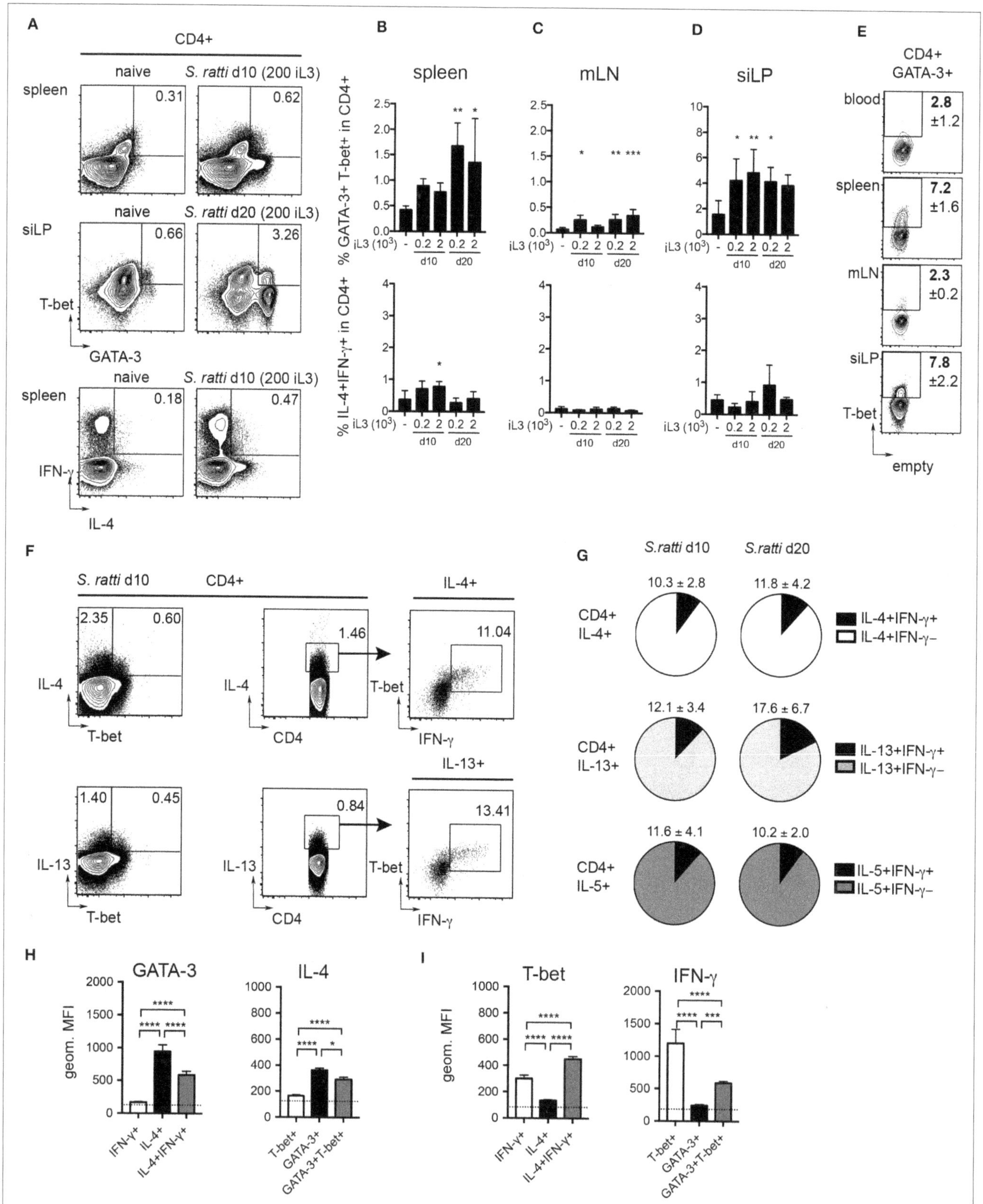

FIGURE 3 | Th2/1 cells with combined Th2 and Th1 features are induced during *S. ratti* infection. Mice infected with 200 or 2,000 *S. ratti* stage 3 larvae were screened for Th2/1 cells co-expressing Th2 and Th1 lineage transcription factors and cytokines. **(A)** Exemplary flow cytometry plots of live CD4^{+} T cells derived from

(Continued)

FIGURE 3 | Continued
spleen (top and bottom) and small intestinal lamina propria (middle) of an uninfected control and *S. ratti* infected mouse at the depicted days post infection. Numbers indicate frequencies of GATA-3$^+$T-bet$^+$ and IL-4$^+$IFN-γ$^+$ cells, respectively. **(B–D)** Frequencies of GATA-3$^+$T-bet$^+$ cells (top) and IL-4$^+$IFN-γ$^+$ cells (bottom) within live CD4$^+$ T cells isolated from spleen **(B)**, mLN **(C)** and siLP **(D)** as detected after 4h of PMA/ionomycin stimulation. Significance was tested comparing infected and naïve controls. **(E)** Exemplary plots depicting frequencies of T-bet expressing cells in CD4$^+$GATA-3$^+$ T cells derived from peripheral blood, spleen, mLN and siLP of mice infected for 10 days (200 iL3) stained directly *ex vivo*. Numbers indicate mean values and SD of 4-5 mice. **(F)** Concatenated plots depicting IL-4 single and IL-4/T-bet co-expressing cells (top left) and IL-13 single and IL-13/T-bet co-expressing cells (bottom left) in CD4 cells isolated from spleens of 5 mice infected for 10 days with *S. ratti* (200 iL3). Center and right plots show detection of T-bet$^+$ IFN-γ producing cells in the IL-4 and IL-13 producing populations. **(G)** Pie charts depict proportions of IFN-γ$^+$ Th2/1 cells (black) within the IL-4 (white), IL-13 (light gray) and IL-5 (dark gray) producing CD4$^+$GATA-3$^+$ T cell derived from spleens of mice infected with *S. ratti* (200 iL3) for 10 (left) and 20 days (right). Mean and SD of $n = 5$ mice is shown. **(H,I)** Geometric mean fluorescence intensity (MFI) of GATA-3 and IL-4 **(H)** and T-bet and IFN-γ signals **(I)** of the depicted CD4$^+$ subpopulations derived from mice infected with *S. ratti* (200 iL3) for 10 days. The MFI of IL-4$^-$IFN-γ$^-$ and GATA-3$^-$T-bet$^-$ cells is depicted by a dotted line. Mean and SD of $n = 5$ mice. Data originate from one out of two experiments with similar results. $^*p < 0.05$, $^{**}p < 0.01$, $^{***}p < 0.005$, $^{****}p < 0.001$.

controls (**Figure 4D**). Expectedly, IL-4 single producing cells clustered in the GATA-3$^+$ population, while some, but not all IFN-γ$^+$ cells expressed elevated levels of T-bet (**Figure 4E**). IL-4$^+$IFN-γ$^+$ Th2/1 hybrid cells, however, featured a GATA-3^{low}T-bet^{high} phenotype and clustered with the fraction of IFN-γ$^+$ cells expressing the highest levels of T-bet (**Figure 4E**). Investigating the proportions of IFN-γ$^+$ cells within the total IL-4$^+$ population confirmed that the proportions of Th2/1 cells were similar in uninfected controls and *S. stercoralis* infected patients, hence the ratios of Th2:Th2/1 cells were similar in both cohorts (**Figure 4F**). However, higher values of conventional Th2 cells (IL-4+, IL-13+ or IL-5+) correlated with increased Th2/1 hybrid cell frequencies co-expressing IFN-γ and the respective Th2 cytokines ($p < 0.0001$) irrespective of the *Strongyloides* infection status (SI Figure 6).

Assessing the expression levels of GATA-3, T-bet, IL-4 and IFN-γ by mean fluorescence intensities (MFI) confirmed that human IL-4$^+$IFN-γ$^+$ Th2/1 hybrid cells expressed significantly lower levels of GATA-3 and IL-4 than IL-4 (or IL-13, not shown) single producers (**Figure 4G**). The mean expression levels of T-bet and IFN-γ, however, were similar for IFN-γ single and IL-4$^+$IFN-γ$^+$ double producing cells (**Figure 4G**).

Taken together, CD4$^+$ T cells with a Th2/1 hybrid phenotype marked by the co-expression of IL-4 and IFN-γ were detectable in *Strongyloides*-infected patients and healthy controls. The frequencies of Th2/1 cells were positively influenced by the magnitude of the overall Th2 response. In contrast to murine Th2/1 hybrids expressing intermediate levels of GATA-3, IL-4 and IFN-γ (**Figure 3**), human Th2/1 hybrid cells were marked by high IFN-γ production and low GATA-3 expression.

S. stercoralis Infection Is Associated with a Distinct Serum Antibody Profile

Next, we assessed if *S. stercoralis* infection was marked by changes in the serum antibody profile. The infected cohort displayed significantly increased total levels of the Th2-associated antibody classes IgE and IgG4 compared to the uninfected control group (**Figures 5A,B**). IgE levels were positively correlated with IL-13 levels ($p = 0.0011$, data not shown). Interestingly, also the level of IgG3 was significantly increased in the *S. stercoralis*-infected group, while the levels of IgG1, a subclass associated with Th1 responses in humans, were similar in both cohorts (**Figures 5C,D**).

Th2/1 Cells Share Effector Functions with Th1 Cells

T helper cells not only produce effector cytokines in response to T cell receptor (TCR) triggering by their cognate antigen, but may also react to combinations of IL-1 cytokine family members and STAT activators (Guo et al., 2012). Th2 cells have been shown to produce IL-5 and IL-13 in response to the combined stimulation by IL-33 and IL-7 (Guo et al., 2015), while stimulation by IL-18 and IL-12 results in IFN-γ production by Th1 cells (Robinson et al., 1997; Yoshimoto et al., 1998). We thus asked if Th2/1 hybrid cells induced in helminth infections share innate effector functions with Th2 and Th1 cells. To this end, we isolated CD4$^+$ T cells from mice acutely infected with *S. ratti* to compare their TCR-independent and TCR-induced effector responses. In response to IL-33 and IL-7, both Th2 cells and Th2/1 cells failed to produce significant amounts of IL-13 (**Figures 6A,B**) despite the expression of the IL-33 receptor ST2 (**Figure 6C**). After stimulation with IL-18 and IL-12, we detected similar IFN-γ responses of by Th1 and Th2/1 hybrid cells (**Figures 6A,D**).

We next compared *in vitro* generated murine Th1 and Th2/1 cells for their efficiency in macrophage activation. As shown previously (Peine et al., 2013), naïve cells stimulated in presence of IL-4, IFN-γ and IL-12 differentiated into a homogenous population of Th2/1 hybrids co-expressing GATA-3 and T-bet, many of which co-produced IL-4 and IFN-γ in response to re-stimulation (**Figures 7A,B**). Similar to Th2/1 cells induced *in vivo* (**Figure 3**), *in vitro*-generated Th2/1 hybrid cells produced significantly lower levels of IFN-γ than Th1 cells (**Figure 7C**), despite similar expression levels of T-bet (**Figure 7A**). In co-cultures with peritoneal macrophages, spontaneous IFN-γ secretion by Th1 cells triggered similar levels of nitric oxide (NO) production by macrophages as induced by IFN-γ added exogenously (**Figure 7D**). Th2/1 hybrid cells induced approximately 10-fold lower NO-responses (**Figure 7D**), consistent with their lower IFN-γ production upon stimulation (**Figure 7C**), while classic Th2 cells failed to trigger an NO response (**Figure 7D**). However, when macrophages where additionally stimulated with lipopolysaccharide (LPS), the limited amount of IFN-γ produced by Th2/1 cells was sufficient to significantly enhance NO-production over the levels produced in response to the LPS-trigger alone (**Figure 7E**).

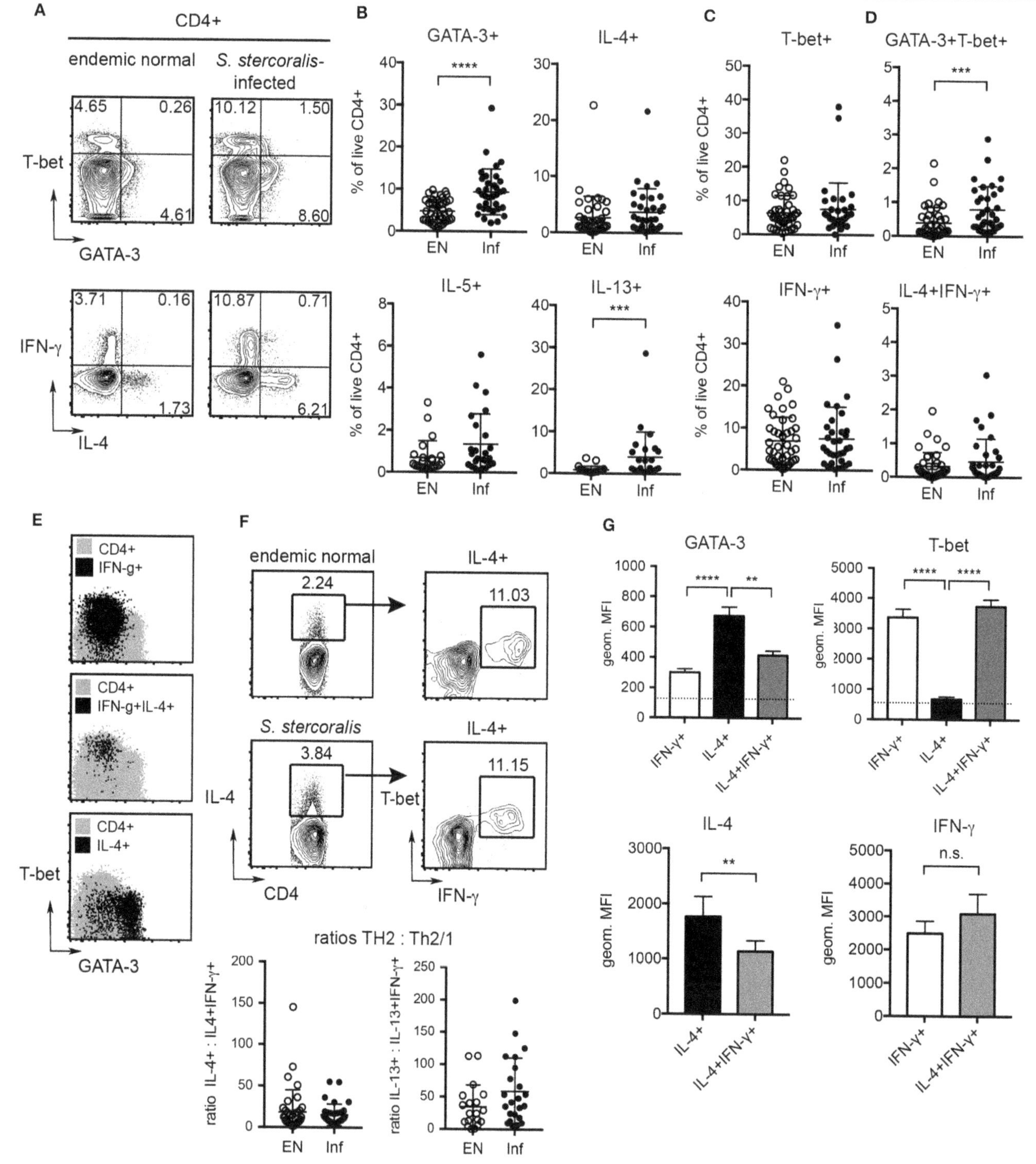

FIGURE 4 | Detection of increased Th2 responses in *S. stercoralis*-infected patients and characterization of human Th2/1 hybrid cells. PBMC where stimulated with PMA/ionomycin and cytokine responses and expression of GATA-3 and T-bet were detected by intracellular staining. **(A)** Exemplary plots of GATA-3 and T-bet (top) and IL-4 and IFN-γ expression (bottom) by $CD4^+$ T cells from an uninfected endemic control and a *S. stercoralis* infected donor. **(B)** Frequencies of GATA-3, IL-4, IL-5, and IL-13 expressing Th2 cells as detected in the endemic normal control group (EN) and *S. stercoralis*-infected group (Inf). **(C)** Frequencies of T-bet and IFN-γ expressing Th1 cells. **(D)** Frequencies of GATA-3^+T-bet^+ and IL-4^+IFN-γ^+ Th2/1 hybrid cells. Mean, SD and individual values are shown. **(E)** Backgating of IFN-γ^+ Th1, IFN-γ^+IL-4^+ Th2/1 and IL-4^+ Th2 cells (black) on GATA-3 and T-bet expression of total $CD4^+$ cells (gray). Exemplary plots of a *S. stercoralis*-infected donor are shown. **(F)** Detection of IFN-γ co-producing cells in the total IL-$4^+$$CD4^+$ population of a control and *S. stercoralis*-infected patient and ratios of IL-4 single producing:IL-4^+IFN-γ^+ cells and IL-13 single producing:IL-13^+IFN-γ^+ cells within the cohorts. **(G)** Expression levels of GATA-3 and T-bet in IFN-γ^+ Th1, IL-4^+ Th2 and IL-4^+IFN-γ^+ Th2/1 cells (top). The MFI of IL-4^-IFN-γ^- cells is depicted by a dotted line. Bottom: Expression levels of IL-4 in Th2 vs. Th2/1 cells and IFN-γ in Th1 vs. Th2/1 cells. Data (mean and SD) are derived from samples of 5 *S. stercoralis* infected donors comprising >100 IL-4^+IFN-γ^+ cells assessed in two independent experiments. $^{**}p < 0.01$, $^{***}p < 0.005$, $^{****}p < 0.001$.

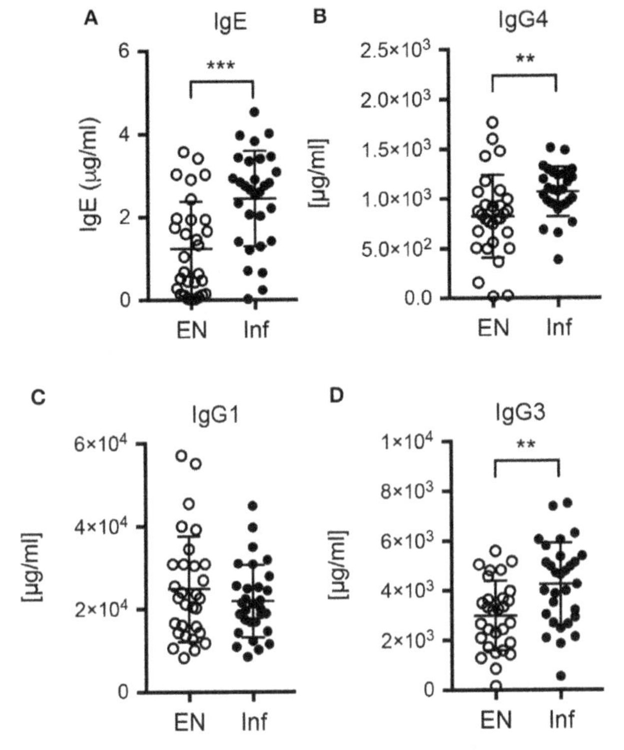

FIGURE 5 | Antibody levels in plasma samples of endemic controls and *S. stercoralis* infected patients. Serum levels of **(A)** total IgE, **(B)** total IgG4, **(C)** total IgG1 and **(D)** total IgG3. $^{**}p < 0.01$, $^{***}p < 0.005$.

In conclusion, Th2/1 hybrid cells induced in helminth infection are reactive to cytokine triggers leading to TCR-independent IFN-γ production. IFN-γ produced by Th2/1 hybrid cells is sufficient for the classical activation of macrophages under appropriate conditions.

DISCUSSION

Here we confirm that experimental murine and natural human infections by threadworms are predominantly associated with Th2 responses (Chiuso-Minicucci et al., 2010; Anuradha et al., 2015; Breloer and Abraham, 2016). Mice infected with *S. ratti* displayed locally and systemically increased frequencies of Th2 cells and only low signs of intestinal immunopathology, which is in line with the mostly asymptomatic course of threadworm infections in human patients (Siddiqui and Berk, 2001; Vadlamudi et al., 2006; Montes et al., 2010). *S. stercoralis* infected patients displayed elevated frequencies of blood eosinophils, Th2 cells, IgE and IgG4, while frequencies of Th1 cells expressing T-bet and IFN-γ were similar to uninfected controls.

Previously we have shown that infections with two helminth species, *H. polygyrus* and *S. mansoni*, lead to the differentiation of Th2/1 hybrid cells stably co-expressing GATA-3 and T-bet as well as Th2 and Th1 effector cytokines. This phenotype was maintained after clearance of infection and progression to memory cells, arguing against a transient Th2/1 state (Peine et al., 2013). Here we show that Th2/1 cells also occur in murine experimental threadworm infections, suggesting that Th2/1 hybrid cells are an integral part of the immune response to a wide range of helminth infections.

Th2 and Th1 differentiation have long been considered as mutually exclusive, as cells differentiated under polarizing conditions express distinct patterns of the lineage defining transcription factors GATA-3 and T-bet and the respective cytokines (Zheng and Flavell, 1997; Szabo et al., 2000; Löhning et al., 2002). Furthermore, positive feedback mechanisms and reciprocal inhibition of the developmental programs reinforce and assure the efficient and mutually exclusive differentiation under the appropriate conditions (Ouyang et al., 2000; Afkarian et al., 2002; Jenner et al., 2009). However, not only mice infected with helminths leading to strong Th2 reactions, but also human patients infected with *S. stercoralis* displayed Th2/1 cells co-expressing Th2 and Th1 cytokines, albeit at low levels. To date, we cannot exclude that reprogramming of Th1 cells and/or Th2 cells by opposing signals (Hegazy et al., 2010; Panzer et al., 2012) contributes to Th2/1 generation during helminth infections.

Our murine experimental data show that the proportion of Th2/1 cells within the total GATA-3 expressing Th2 population differed depending on the body compartment. The highest proportions of Th2/1 cells were detected in spleen and small intestinal tissue, while their proportions were lower in gut-draining lymph nodes and blood. We hence speculate that the low frequencies of Th2/1 cells detected in blood of threadworm-infected patients may not necessarily reflect the proportion of Th2/1 cells in other compartments of the human body. Whether Th2/1 hybrids and conventional Th2 cells differ in their proliferative behavior, survival, and reaction to chemokines remains to be established. Further studies are also needed to assess if the preferential location of helminth-induced Th2/1 cells in spleen and the parasite-afflicted organ is associated with specific effector functions.

Our data show that human and murine Th2/1 cells clearly differed phenotypically: while murine Th2/1 hybrids were readily detectable by the coexpression of GATA-3 and T-bet, human Th2/1 cells expressed rather low levels of GATA-3, but were detectable by coexpression of IL-4 and IFN-γ. As not all GATA-3^{+}T-bet^{+} cells from helminth-infected mice coproduced Th2 cytokines and IFN-γ simultaneously when restimulated *in vitro* it is important to note that the detection of human hybrids based on the coexpression of cytokines may lead to an underestimation of the proportion of Th2/1 cells in humans. Human and murine Th2/1 cells also differed functionally with respect to IFN-γ production: while human Th2/1 hybrids were marked by high expression levels of IFN-γ, murine Th2/1 hybrids expressed significantly lower levels than Th1 cells. T-bet expression was similar in human Th2/1 cells and Th1 cells, and T-bet expression of murine Th2/1 hybrids even exceeded the levels detected in Th1 cells, which may be explained by differential activation states of the cells. Still, only murine Th2/1 cells were restricted in IFN-γ production, which at least in murine Th1 cells is largely driven and quantitatively controlled by T-bet expression amounts (Szabo et al., 2000; Helmstetter et al., 2015). This functional difference in human vs. murine Th2/1 hybrids might be explained by the finding that human Th2/1 hybrid cells (characterized as

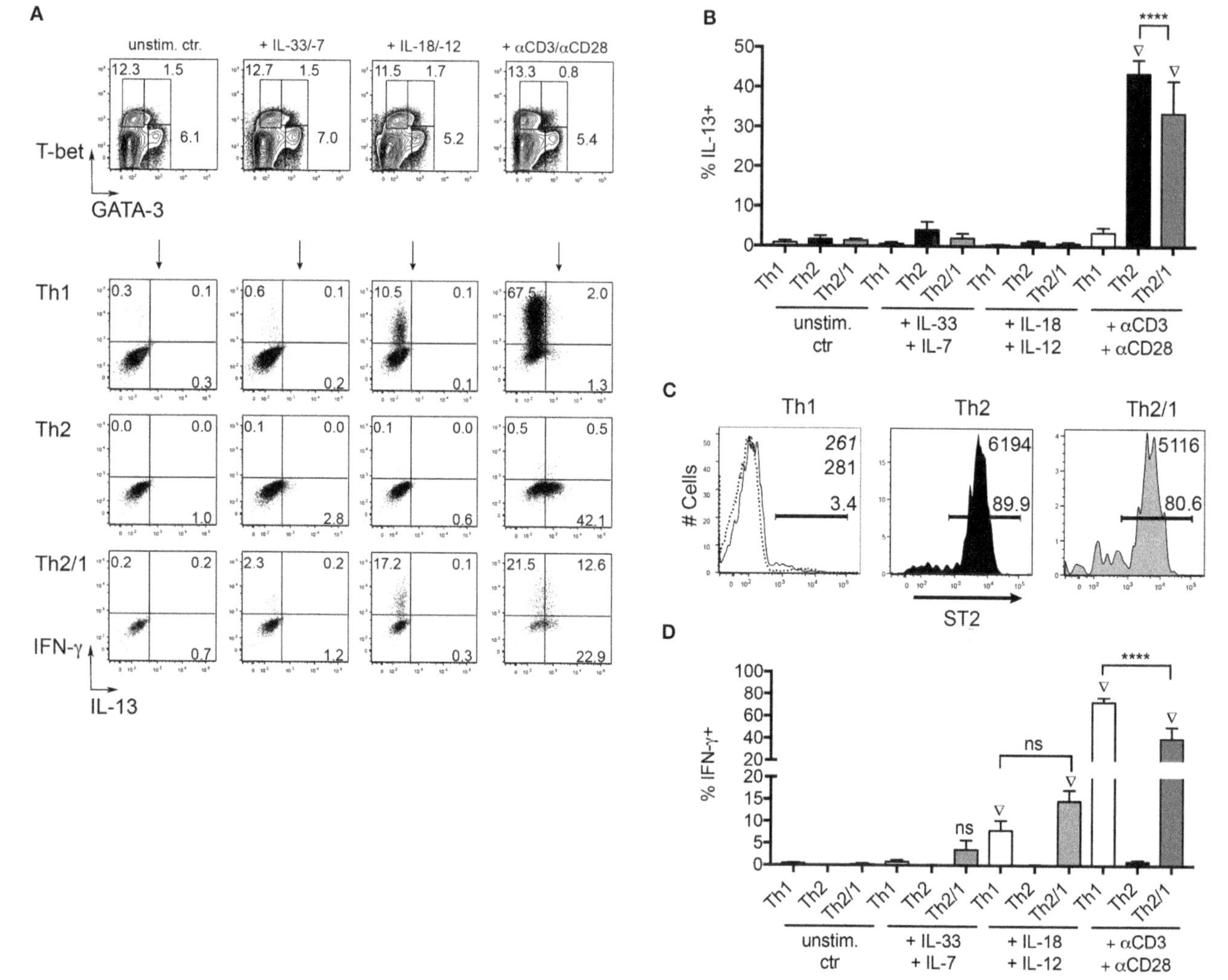

FIGURE 6 | Th2/1 cells share innate function with Th1 cells. **(A)** $CD4^+$ cells isolated from *S. ratti*-infected C57BL/6 mice at day 10 post infection with 200 iL3 were stained for GATA-3 and T-bet (top row) after stimulation with IL-33 and IL-7, IL18 and IL-12 or anti-CD3/anti-CD28 antibodies. $T\text{-}bet^+$ Th1, $GATA\text{-}3^+$ Th2 and $GATA\text{-}3^+T\text{-}bet^+$ Th2/1 cells were assessed for IFN-γ and IL-13 production in response to stimulation (2nd–4th row). Plots are concatenated from five mice. **(B)** Frequencies of IL-13 producers in response to cytokine and TCR-triggering. Mean and SD of 5 *S. ratti*-infected mice is shown. **(C)** ST2 expression by Th1, Th2 and Th2/1 cells from *S. ratti*-infected mice. Mean fluorescence intensities of the populations are given in the right top corner. Dashed line and italic number relate to $CD4^+T\text{-}bet^-GATA\text{-}3^-$ cells. **(D)** Frequencies of IFN-γ producers in response to cytokine and TCR-triggering. Data are representative for two independent experiments. $^{****}p < 0.001$. Diamond symbols indicate values significantly different from the respective unstimulated control samples.

IL-4/IFN-γ co-producing cells) displayed rather low levels of GATA-3 expression. It hence seems likely that the lack of GATA-3-driven counter-regulation of T-bet functions allows unabated IFN-γ production by human Th2/1 cells (Chang and Aune, 2007; Jenner et al., 2009). Yet we can only speculate on how human Th2/1 cells retain their (reduced) production of IL-4 and other Th2 cytokines in face of low GATA-3 expression. In mice, conditional deletion of GATA-3 from established Th2 cells diminishes Th2 cell maintenance and IL-5 and IL-13, but not IL-4 production (Pai et al., 2004; Zhu et al., 2004). Whether other factors such as c-Maf expression allow human hybrids to express Th2 cytokines in a setting of low GATA-3 expression remains to be investigated (Kim et al., 1999). Similarly, it remains to be established if murine and human $CD4^+$ T cell co-expressing Th2 and Th1 cytokines differ in other regulatory elements of effector functions and if their relatively high proportion in the spleen has functional relevance.

An interesting finding in our patient survey was that not only Th2-associated antibody classes (IgE, IgG4) were elevated in threadworm-infected patients, but also IgG3 was significantly increased in the infected cohort. IgG3 is a potent pro-inflammatory antibody with high affinity to the activating Fcγ receptor I (FcγRI), the latter being central for the control of bacterial infections (Ioan-Facsinay et al., 2002; Vidarsson et al., 2014). Both IgG3 class switching by B cells and FcRI expression by human myeloid cells are positively regulated by IFN-γ (Erbe et al., 1990; Snapper et al., 1992). Hence IFN-γ expression by Th2/1 cells in reactive lymph nodes or the

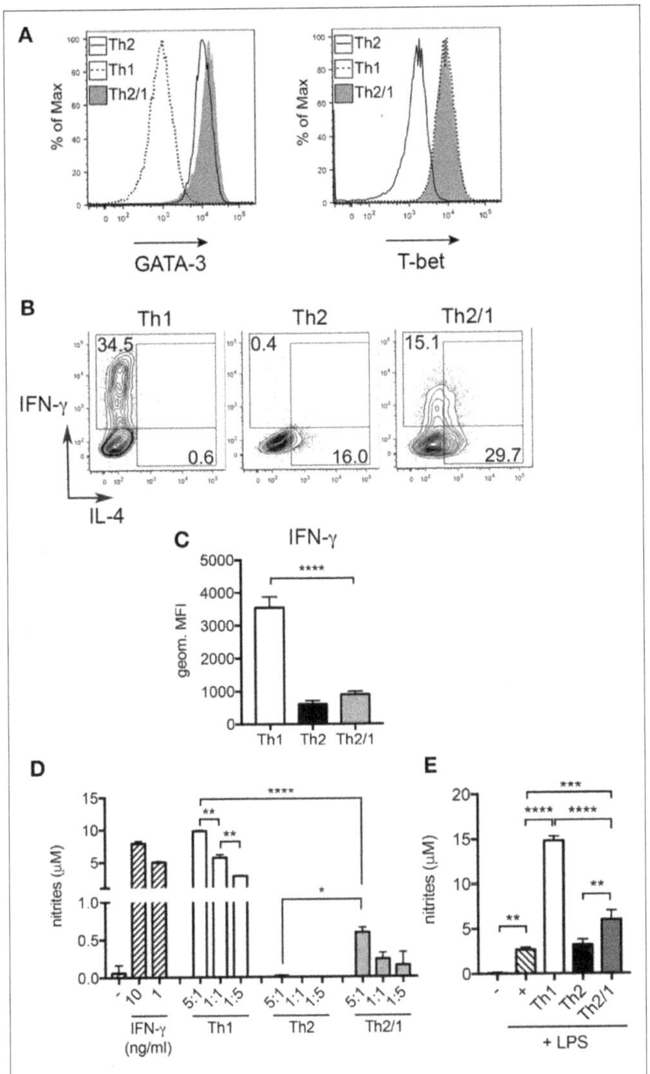

FIGURE 7 | Th2/1 cells are capable of supporting classical macrophage effector function. Murine Th1, Th2, and Th2/1 hybrid cells were generated from naïve $CD4^{+}$ T cells *in vitro* and surveyed for **(A)** GATA-3 (left) and T-bet (right) expression. **(B)** IL-4 and IFN-γ expression by *in vitro*-generated Th1, Th2, and Th2/1 cells in response to PMA/ionomycin stimulation. **(C)** Geometric mean fluorescence intensity of IFN-γ in Th1, Th2, and Th2/1 hybrid cells. **(D)** Nitrite accumulation in supernatant of peritoneal macrophages left untreated (–), stimulated with recombinant IFN-γ or incubated with Th1, Th2, and Th2/1 cells in the depicted T cell:macrophage ratios for 24 h. **(E)** Nitrite concentrations in supernatant of macrophages left untreated (–), stimulated with LPS or co-cultured with T cells (1:1 ratio) in presence of LPS. Mean and SD of five cultures is shown. Data are representative for three independent experiments. $^{*}p < 0.05$, $^{**}p < 0.01$, $^{***}p < 0.005$, $^{****}p < 0.001$.

spleen, where their proportion is relatively high, might contribute to the diversification of antibody responses and assure that antibodies primarily involved in opsonization of pathogens or their secreted components do not go short in Th2-associated infections mainly driving IgE and IgG4 production by B cells.

We found that murine Th2/1 cells not only co-express IFN-γ and Th2 cytokines in response to TCR-triggering, but also responded to the combination of the STAT activator IL-12 and IL-1 family member IL-18 with production of IFN-γ. It is tempting to speculate that the differentiation of Th2/1 cells in response to helminths inducing strong Th2 reactions, such as *S. ratti*, *H. polygyrus* and *S. mansoni*, may provide an advantage to the infected host in preventing an overtly and exclusively Th2-biased immune set-up. It is critical for the immune system to quickly respond to rapidly replicating microbes controlled by Th1 responses and classically activated macrophages. Similar to e.g. enhanced IFN-γ production by NK cells sensing IL-18 and IL-12 during infection with the protozoan *Toxoplasma gondii* (Cai et al., 2000), Th2/1 cells co-induced with conventional Th2 cells during helminth infections and co-infiltrating the infected organs may contribute to early IFN-γ production in response to cytokine triggers produced upon protozoan, bacterial and viral infections. Although most likely subordinate to Th1 cells in this regard, their activated state during ongoing helminth infection may facilitate IFN-γ responses by Th2/1 cells in response to cytokine triggers and hence help in supporting adequate Th1 reactions in face of ongoing Th2 responses.

There is experimental evidence that nitric oxide is toxic for *Strongyloides* parasites and limits worm fecundity as well as autoinfection in mice (Ruano et al., 2012, 2015). We show that murine Th2/1 cells are, expectedly, subordinate to Th1 cells in driving NO production by macrophages, coinciding with their limited IFN-γ production. However, in conjunction with TLR triggering, the limited IFN-γ production of Th2/1 cells was sufficient to stimulate significant NO production. Hence Th2/1 cells may be important to ensure that the helminth-infected host is able to quickly and adequately react to co-infections where an unabated IFN-γ response is crucial. Furthermore, IFN-γ production by Th2/1 cells generated during helminth infection often including tissue migratory larval stages may be advantageous in preventing bacterial dissemination facilitated by tissue damage (Pesce et al., 2008), especially upon parasite re-exposure of organs densely seeded with Th2 memory cells (Steinfelder et al., 2017). We currently assess if Th2/1 cells constitute a considerable source of IFN-γ and of other factors affecting the immune response to the parasite and, possibly, coinfecting pathogens.

Taken together we provide evidence that Th2/1 cells developing during helminth infections are not a feature restricted to the murine host, but also occur in humans. Especially human Th2/1 cells seem to be able to produce IFN-γ in similar amounts as Th1 cells, posing the question whether they may efficiently counter-regulate an overt Th2 bias in helminth infections and allergic diseases. By sharing effector functions with Th1 cells they may act as a provision against hampered responses to co-infecting pathogens in face of a strongly Th2-biased immune status.

AUTHOR CONTRIBUTIONS

CB and SR performed all the experiments. SH and SR conceptualized and designed the research. SB, AR and YB recruited and classified human subjects. CB, MLB, AK, and RM analyzed the data. CB, MB, SH, and SR wrote the manuscript. All authors approved the final version of the manuscript.

FUNDING

This work was funded by the Deutsche Forschungsgemeinschaft (IRTG 1673, CB, SH, SR and GRK 2046, SH, SR) and the Karl-Enigk-Stiftung (CB), and, in part, by the Division of Intramural Research, NIAID, USA. MB is funded by the DFG BR 3754/2-2.

ACKNOWLEDGMENTS

The excellent support by the technicians Y. Weber, B. Sonnenburg, M. Müller, C. Palissa, and S. Spieckermann is acknowledged gratefully.

REFERENCES

Afkarian, M., Sedy, J. R., Yang, J., Jacobson, N. G., Cereb, N., Yang, S. Y., et al. (2002). T-bet is a STAT1-induced regulator of IL-12R expression in naïve CD4+ T cells. *Nat. Immunol.* 3, 549–557. doi: 10.1038/ni794

Allen, J. E., and Sutherland, T. E. (2014). Host protective roles of type 2 immunity: parasite killing and tissue repair, flip sides of the same coin. *Semin. Immunol.* 26, 329–340. doi: 10.1016/j.smim.2014.06.003

Anthony, R. M., Rutitzky, L. I., Urban, J. F. Jr., Stadecker, M. J., and Gause, W. C. (2007). Protective immune mechanisms in helminth infection. *Nat. Rev. Immunol.* 7, 975-987 doi: 10.1038/nri2199

Anuradha, R., Munisankar, S., Dolla, C., Kumaran, P., Nutman, T. B., and Babu, S. (2015). Parasite antigen-specific regulation of Th1, Th2, and Th17 responses in *Strongyloides stercoralis* infection. *J. Immunol.* 195, 2241–2250. doi: 10.4049/jimmunol.1500745

Bisoffi, Z., Buonfrate, D., Sequi, M., Mejia, R., Cimino, R. O., Krolewiecki, A. J., et al. (2014). Diagnostic accuracy of five serologic tests for *Strongyloides stercoralis* infection. *PLoS Negl. Trop. Dis.* 8:e2640. doi: 10.1371/journal.pntd.0002640

Blankenhaus, B., Klemm, U., Eschbach, M. L., Sparwasser, T., Huehn, J., Kühl, A. A., et al. (2011). *Strongyloides ratti* infection induces expansion of Foxp3+ regulatory T cells that interfere with immune response and parasite clearance in BALB/c mice. *J. Immunol.* 186, 4295–4305. doi: 10.4049/jimmunol.1001920

Breloer, M., and Abraham, D. (2016). *Strongyloides* infection in rodents: immune response and immune regulation. *Parasitology* 144, 295–315. doi: 10.1017/S0031182016000111

Buonfrate, D., Sequi, M., Mejia, R., Cimino, R. O., Krolewiecki, A. J., Albonico, M., et al. (2015). Accuracy of five serologic tests for the follow up of *Strongyloides stercoralis* infection. *PLoS Negl. Trop. Dis.* 9:e0003491. doi: 10.1371/journal.pntd.0003491

Cai, G., Kastelein, R., and Hunter, C. A. (2000). Interleukin-18 (IL-18) enhances innate IL-12-mediated resistance to *Toxoplasma gondii*. *Infect. Immun.* 68, 6932–6938. doi: 10.1128/IAI.68.12.6932-6938.2000

Chang, S., and Aune, T. M. (2007). Dynamic changes in histone-methylation 'marks' across the locus encoding interferon-gamma during the differentiation of T helper type 2 cells. *Nat. Immunol.* 8, 723–731. doi: 10.1038/ni1473

Chiuso-Minicucci, F., Marra, N. M., Zorzella-Pezavento, S. F., França, T. G., Ishikawa, L. L., Amarante, M. R., et al. (2010). Recovery from *Strongyloides* venezuelensis infection in Lewis rats is associated with a strong Th2 response. *Parasite Immunol.* 32, 74–78. doi: 10.1111/j.1365-3024.2009.01160.x

Dawkins, H. J., and Grove, D. I. (1981). Kinetics of primary and secondary infections with *Strongyloides ratti* in mice. *Int. J. Parasitol.* 11, 89–96. doi: 10.1016/0020-7519(81)90031-X

Erbe, D. V., Collins, J. E., Shen, L., Graziano, R. F., and Fanger, M. W. (1990). The effect of cytokines on the expression and function of Fc receptors for IgG on human myeloid cells. *Mol. Immunol.* 27, 57–67. doi: 10.1016/0161-5890(90)90060-D

Eschbach, M. L., Klemm, U., Kolbaum, J., Blankenhaus, B., Brattig, N., and Breloer, M. (2010). *Strongyloides ratti* infection induces transient nematode-specific Th2 response and reciprocal suppression of IFN-gamma production in mice. *Parasite Immunol.* 32, 370–383. doi: 10.1111/j.1365-3024.2010.01199.x

Figueiredo, C. A., Barreto, M. L., Rodrigues, L. C., Cooper, P. J., Silva, N. B., Amorim, L. D., et al. (2010). Chronic intestinal helminth infections are associated with immune hyporesponsiveness and induction of a regulatory network. *Infect. Immun.* 78, 3160–3167. doi: 10.1128/IAI.01228-09

Finkelman, F. D., Shea-Donohue, T., Goldhill, J., Sullivan, C. A., Morris, S. C., Madden, K. B., et al. (1997). Cytokine regulation of host defense against parasitic gastrointestinal nematodes: lessons from studies with rodent models. *Annu. Rev. Immunol.* 15, 505–533. doi: 10.1146/annurev.immunol.15.1.505

Finkelman, F. D., Shea-Donohue, T., Morris, S. C., Gildea, L., Strait, R., Madden, K. B., et al. (2004). Interleukin-4- and interleukin-13-mediated host protection against intestinal nematode parasites. *Immunol. Rev.* 201, 139–155. doi: 10.1111/j.0105-2896.2004.00192.x

Guo, L., Huang, Y., Chen, X., Hu-Li, J., Urban, J. F. Jr., and Paul, W. E. (2015). Innate immunological function of TH2 cells *in vivo*. *Nat. Immunol.* 6, 1051–1059. doi: 10.1038/ni.3244

Guo, L., Junttila, I. S., and Paul, W. E. (2012). Cytokine-induced cytokine production by conventional and innate lymphoid cells. *Trends Immunol.* 33, 598–606. doi: 10.1016/j.it.2012.07.006

Harris, N., and Gause, W. C. (2011). To B or not to B: B cells and the Th2-type immune response to helminths. *Trends Immunol.* 32, 80–88. doi: 10.1016/j.it.2010.11.005

Hegazy, A. N., Peine, M., Helmstetter, C., Panse, I., Fröhlich, A., Bergthaler, A., et al. (2010). Interferons direct Th2 cell reprogramming to generate a stable GATA-3^{+}T-bet^{+} cell subset with combined Th2 and Th1 cell functions. *Immunity* 32, 116–128. doi: 10.1016/j.immuni.2009.12.004

Helmstetter, C., Flossdorf, M., Peine, M., Kupz, A., Zhu, J., Hegazy, A. N., et al. (2015). Individual T helper cells have a quantitative cytokine memory. *Immunity* 42, 108–122. doi: 10.1016/j.immuni.2014.12.018

Ioan-Facsinay, A., de Kimpe, S. J., Hellwig, S. M., van Lent, P. L., Hofhuis, F. M., van Ojik, H. H., et al. (2002). FcgammaRI (CD64) contributes substantially to severity of arthritis, hypersensitivity responses, and protection from bacterial infection. *Immunity* 16, 391–402. doi: 10.1016/S1074-7613(02)00294-7

Jenner, R. G., Townsend, M. J., Jackson, I., Sun, K., Bouwman, R. D., Young, R. A., et al. (2009). The transcription factors T-bet and GATA-3 control alternative pathways of T-cell differentiation through a shared set of target genes. *Proc. Natl. Acad. Sci. U.S.A.* 106, 17876–17881. doi: 10.1073/pnas.0909357106

Kim, J. I., Ho, I. C., Grusby, M. J., and Glimcher, L. H. (1999). The transcription factor c-Maf controls the production of interleukin-4 but not other Th2 cytokines. *Immunity* 10, 745–751. doi: 10.1016/S1074-7613(00)80073-4

Lohning, M., Richter, A., and Radbruch, A. (2002). Cytokine memory of T helper lymphocytes. *Adv. Immunol.* 80, 115–181. doi: 10.1016/S0065-2776(02)80014-1

Montes, M., Sawhney, C., and Barros, N. (2010). *Strongyloides stercoralis*: there but not seen. *Curr. Opin. Infect. Dis.* 23, 500–504. doi: 10.1097/QCO.0b013e32833df718

Nouir, N. B., Eschbach, M. L., Piédavent, M., Osterloh, A., and Kingsley, M. T., Erttmann, K., et al. (2012).Vaccination with *Strongyloides ratti* heat shock protein 60 increases susceptibility to challenge infection by induction of Th1 response. *Vaccine* 30, 862–871. doi: 10.1016/j.vaccine.2011.11.110

Ouyang, W., Löhning, M., Gao, Z., Assenmacher, M., Ranganath, S., Radbruch, A., et al. (2000). Stat6-independent GATA-3 autoactivation directs IL-4-independent Th2 development and commitment. *Immunity* 12, 27–37. doi: 10.1016/S1074-7613(00)80156-9

Pai, S. Y., Truitt, M. L., and Ho, I. C. (2004). GATA-3 deficiency abrogates the development and maintenance of T helper type 2 cells. *Proc. Natl. Acad. Sci. U.S.A.* 101, 1993–1998. doi: 10.1073/pnas.0308697100

Panzer, M., Sitte, S., Wirth, S., Drexler, I., Sparwasser, T., and Voehringer, D. (2012). Rapid *in vivo* conversion of effector T cells into Th2 cells during helminth infection. *J. Immunol.* 188, 615–623. doi: 10.4049/jimmunol.1101164

Patel, N., Kreider, T., Urban, J. F. Jr., and Gause, W. C. (2009). Characterisation of effector mechanisms at the host:parasite interface during the immune response to tissue-dwelling intestinal nematode parasites. *Int. J. Parasitol.* 39, 13–21. doi: 10.1016/j.ijpara.2008.08.003

Peine, M., Rausch, S., Helmstetter, C., Fröhlich, A., Hegazy, A. N., Kühl, A. A., et al. (2013). Stable T-bet$^+$GATA-3$^+$ Th1/Th2 hybrid cells arise *in vivo*, can develop directly from naive precursors, and limit immunopathologic inflammation. *PLoS Biol.* 11:e1001633. doi: 10.1371/journal.pbio.1001633

Pesce, J. T., Liu, Z., Hamed, H., Alem, F., Whitmire, J., Lin, H., et al. (2008). Neutrophils clear bacteria associated with parasitic nematodes augmenting the development of an effective Th2-type response. *J. Immunol.* 180, 464–474. doi: 10.4049/jimmunol.180.1.464

Puthiyakunnon, S., Boddu, S., Li, Y., Zhou, X., Wang, C., Li, J., et al. (2014). *Strongyloidiasis*—an insight into its global prevalence and management. *PLoS Negl. Trop. Dis.* 8:e3018. doi: 10.1371/journal.pntd.0003018

Quinnell, R. J., Pritchard, D. I., Raiko, A., Brown, A. P., and Shaw, M. A. (2004). Immune responses in human necatoriasis: association between interleukin-5 responses and resistance to reinfection. *J. Infect. Dis.* 190, 430–438. doi: 10.1086/422256

Rausch, S., Huehn, J., Loddenkemper, C., Hepworth, M. R., Klotz, C., Sparwasser, T., et al. (2009). Establishment of nematode infection despite increased Th2 responses and immunopathology after selective depletion of Foxp3+ cells. *Eur. J. Immunol.* 39, 3066–3077. doi: 10.1002/eji.200939644

Robinson, D., Shibuya, K., Mui, A., Zonin, F., Murphy, E., Sana, T., et al. (1997). IGIF does not drive Th1 development but synergizes with IL-12 for interferon-gamma production and activates IRAK and NFkappaB. *Immunity* 7, 571–581. doi: 10.1016/S1074-7613(00)80378-7

Ruano, A. L., López-Abán, J., Fernández-Soto, P., de Melo, A. L., and Muro, A. (2015). Treatment with nitric oxide donors diminishes hyperinfection by *Strongyloides* venezuelensis in mice treated with dexamethasone. *Acta Trop.* 152, 90–95. doi: 10.1016/j.actatropica.2015.08.019

Ruano, A. L., López-Abán, J., Gajate, C., Mollinedo, F., De Melo, A. L., and Muro, A. (2012). Apoptotic mechanisms are involved in the death of *Strongyloides* venezuelensis after triggering of nitric oxide. *Parasite Immunol.* 34, 570–580. doi: 10.1111/pim.12004

Siddiqui, A. A., Berk, S. L. (2001). Diagnosis of *Strongyloides stercoralis* Infection. *Clin. Infect. Dis.* 33, 1040–1047. doi: 10.1086/322707

Snapper, C. M., McIntyre, T. M., Mandler, R., Pecanha, L. M., Finkelman, F. D., Lees, A., et al. (1992). Induction of IgG3 secretion by interferon gamma: a model for T cell-independent class switching in response to T cell-independent type 2 antigens. *J. Exp. Med.* 175, 1367–1371. doi: 10.1084/jem.175.5.1367

Steinfelder, S., Rausch, S., Michael, D., Kühl, A. A., and Hartmann, S. (2017). Intestinal helminth infection induces highly functional resident memory CD4+ T cells in mice. *Eur. J. Immunol.* 47, 353–363. doi: 10.1002/eji.201646575

Strandmark, J., Steinfelder, S., Berek, C., Kühl, A. A., Rausch, S., and Hartmann, S. (2016). Eosinophils are required to suppress Th2 responses in Peyer's patches during intestinal infection by nematodes. *Mucosal Immunol.* 10, 661–672. doi: 10.1038/mi.2016.93.

Szabo, S. J., Kim, S. T., Costa, G. L., Zhang, X., Fathman, C. G., and Glimcher, L. H. (2000). A novel transcription factor, T-bet, directs Th1 lineage commitment. *Cell* 100, 655–669. doi: 10.1016/S0092-8674(00)80702-3

Turner, J. D., Faulkner, H., Kamgno, J., Cormont, F., Van Snick, J., Else, K. J., et al. (2003). Th2 cytokines are associated with reduced worm burdens in a human intestinal helminth infection. *J. Infect. Dis.* 188, 1768–1775. doi: 10.1086/379370

Turner, J. D., Jackson, J. A., Faulkner, H., Behnke, J., Else, K. J., Kamgno, J., et al. (2008). Intensity of intestinal infection with multiple worm species is related to regulatory cytokine output and immune hyporesponsiveness. *J. Infect. Dis.* 197, 1204–1212. doi: 10.1086/586717

Urban, J. F.Jr., Katona, I. M., Paul, W. E., and Finkelman, F. D. (1991). Interleukin 4 is important in protective immunity to a gastrointestinal nematode infection in mice. *Proc. Natl. Acad. Sci. U.S.A.* 88, 5513–5517. doi: 10.1073/pnas.88.13.5513

Vadlamudi, R. S., Chi, D. S., and Krishnaswamy, G. (2006). Intestinal *strongyloidiasis* and hyperinfection syndrome. *Clin. Mol. Allergy* 4:8. doi: 10.1186/1476-7961-4-8

Vidarsson, G., Dekkers, G., and Rispens, T. (2014). IgG subclasses and allotypes: from structure to effector functions. *Front. Immunol.* 5:520. doi: 10.3389/fimmu.2014.00520

Weatherhead, J. E., and Mejia, R. (2014). Immune response to infection with *Strongyloides stercoralis* in patients with infection and hyperinfection. *Curr. Trop. Med. Rep.* 1, 229–233. doi: 10.1007/s40475-014-0032-9

Yoshimoto, T., Takeda, K., Tanaka, T., Ohkusu, K., Kashiwamura, S., Okamura, H., et al. (1998). IL-12 up-regulates IL-18 receptor expression on T cells, Th1 cells, and B cells: synergism with IL-18 for IFN-gamma production. *J. Immunol.* 161, 3400–3407.

Zheng, W., and Flavell, R. A. (1997). The transcription factor GATA-3 is necessary and sufficient for Th2 cytokine gene expression in CD4 T cells. *Cell* 89, 587–596. doi: 10.1016/S0092-8674(00)80240-8

Zhu, J., Min, B., Hu-Li, J., Watson, C. J., Grinberg, A., Wang, Q., et al. (2004). Conditional deletion of Gata3 shows its essential function in T_H1-T_H2 responses. *Nat. Immunol.* 5, 1157–1165. doi: 10.1038/ni1128

Zhu, J., Yamane, H., and Paul, W. E. (2010). Differentiation of effector CD4 T cell populations (*). *Annu. Rev. Immunol.* 28, 445–489. doi: 10.1146/annurev-immunol-030409-101212

10

MALDI-TOF MS Profiling-Advances in Species Identification of Pests, Parasites, and Vectors

*Jayaseelan Murugaiyan * and Uwe Roesler*

Institute of Animal Hygiene and Environmental Health, Centre for Infectious Medicine, Freie Universität Berlin, Berlin, Germany

Edited by:
Anton Aebischer,
Robert Koch-Insitute, Germany

Reviewed by:
Joshua D. Shrout,
University of Notre Dame, USA
Maria Hadjifrangiskou,
Vanderbilt University Medical Center, USA

***Correspondence:**
Jayaseelan Murugaiyan
jayaseelan.murugaiyan@fu-berlin.de

Invertebrate pests and parasites of humans, animals, and plants continue to cause serious diseases and remain as a high treat to agricultural productivity and storage. The rapid and accurate species identification of the pests and parasites are needed for understanding epidemiology, monitoring outbreaks, and designing control measures. Matrix-assisted laser desorption ionization time-of-flight mass spectrometry (MALDI-TOF MS) profiling has emerged as a rapid, cost effective, and high throughput technique of microbial species identification in modern diagnostic laboratories. The development of soft ionization techniques and the release of commercial pattern matching software platforms has resulted in the exponential growth of applications in higher organisms including parasitology. The present review discusses the proof-of-principle experiments and various methods of MALDI MS profiling in rapid species identification of both laboratory and field isolates of pests, parasites and vectors.

Keywords: MALDI MS typing, MALDI TOF MS, intact protein profiling, pests, parasites, species, spectra reference databases

INTRODUCTION

Invertebrate pests and parasites of plants, mammals, birds, amphibians, and reptiles account for increased losses in the agricultural sector and continue to play a considerable role in the spread of infectious diseases (Paini et al., 2016; Poulin et al., 2016). Accurate and rapid species identification of pests and parasites is extremely important for initiating species-specific treatment procedures, understanding the epidemiology, monitoring of outbreaks, and designing control measures (Gibson, 2009; Furlong, 2015). Traditionally, trained taxonomists or entomologists visually examine or observe microscopically the morphological characteristics for species determination. However, in addition to being time-consuming, misidentification possibilities, distinguishing immature or development stages, damaged samples, cryptic species, and species differing by minor morphological characteristics make identification challenging and often impossible (McKeand, 1998). Molecular methods, whichever available, are accurate and applicable to any development stages. On the other hand, these methods are also labor intensive, expensive, time consuming, and difficult to apply for species for which sequences are not available (Wong et al., 2014). Furthermore, in certain cases such as *Leishmania* subtyping, which is crucial for treatment, identification generally requires several weeks for performing complex and expensive analyses (Roelfsema et al., 2011). In recent years, proteome based linear matrix-assisted laser desorption/ionization time-of-flight mass spectrometry (MALDI-TOF MS profiling or MALDI MS typing), which is a well-established technique for microbial species identification, has also been successfully applied to a variety of parasites and their vectors (Seng et al., 2009; Bizzini and Greub, 2010; Patel, 2013; Nomura, 2015; Karger, 2016; Singhal et al., 2016; Yssouf et al., 2016). The popularity of the method is due to its rapidness, easy to use, high throughput analysis, accuracy, reliability equal to that of the molecular methods of species identification and cost-effectiveness despite the initial cost of the machine (Dhiman et al., 2011; Neville et al., 2011; Tran et al., 2015; Ge et al., 2016). The technique involves generation of MALDI MS spectra for a given species and pattern matching with that of the spectra database of the well-defined species to deduce the species information (Welker and Moore, 2011; Nagy et al., 2012; Suarez et al., 2013). The spectra pattern matching is carried out using automated commercial software suites, such as Bruker Biotyper (Bruker Daltonics, Bremen, Germany), VITEK MS (BioMérieux, Nuertingen, Germany: earlier Axima (Shimadzu)-SARAMIS (AnagnosTec) systems), Andromas (Andromas SAS), or MicrobeLynx (Waters) (Sogawa et al., 2011; Bille et al., 2012; Patel, 2013; Cassagne et al., 2016). The commercial software tools are usually integrated with their own spectra reference database, and utilize a unique algorithm for spectra processing, pattern matching, and result interpretation.

The manufacturer-provided database is limited only in terms of reference spectra for available microbial species, and currently the reference information for pests and parasites are not included. The software generally includes the possibility to create reference spectra for any organism to be integrated within the existing database. The database extension has been utilized to create additional reference spectra to enhance the identification confidence and to include reference spectra of the missing species, including higher organisms (Bohme et al., 2012; Murugaiyan et al., 2012, 2014; Hoppenheit et al., 2013). Several reviews have been dedicated to the recent developments of MALDI MS typing of plant nematodes and organisms related to parasitology (Ahmad and Babalola, 2014; Karger, 2016; Singhal et al., 2016; Yssouf et al., 2016). Therefore, the focus of this review is on the various approaches reported for MALDI MS typing based species identification of pests, parasites, and their vectors ranging from laboratory isolates to that of field samples.

MALDI MS BASIS OF SPECIES IDENTIFICATION

MALDI MS based species identification involves three steps:

(1) Sample spotting onto a specially designed metal plate called the target plate,
(2) MALDI TOF MS measurments and
(3) Species deduction through pattern matching of the spectra with the database of spectra derived from known and/or well-defined species.

A small portion of biological substances e.g., microbial colonies or a drop of intact/crude protein extracted using simple procedures is directly added to the target plate and allowed to air dry. Then, the sample spot is overlaid with a drop of an excess concentration of UV-absorbing small organic compounds, referred to as a matrix. There are several choices of matrix such as α-cyano-4-hydroxycinnamic acid (HCCA/CHCA), sinapinic acid (3, 5- dimethoxy-4-hydroxycinnamic acid) (SA), and 2,5-dihydroxybenzoic acid (DHB). HCCA is most frequently reported matrix; however, there is no universally recommended matrix.

In the MALDI instrument, a small region of the crystalline sample-matrix spot (usually 0.05–0.2 mm in diameter) is irradiated using a pulsed beam of a laser, generally a nitrogen beam with a wavelength of 337 nm is used in most commercial machines. The matrix absorbs the laser energy, and rapidly heats up resulting in desorption (vaporization) or structural decomposition of the proteins and protonation to form a hot dense plume of ablated gases and ions (Clark et al., 2013). Using an electric field, the ions are accelerated into a vacuum tube that terminates in an ion detector. The ions are usually of single charge and the acceleration voltage results in the same kinetic energy applied to every single charged ions, which results in separation of ions based on mass/charge (m/z) ration in the drift or vacuum tube.

The time of flight "TOF" of ions is recorded as MALDI spectra where the x-axis represents *m/z* ratio and the y-axis represents the intensity (or number) of same/similar ions. MALDI MS ions are singly charged, representing the non-fragmented parent ion mass, the resulting spectra is simple, and therefore, the species of unknown samples can be easily deduced after data processing and direct pattern matching with that of the spectra established from well-defined species compiled as a database. The identity of spectral peaks or protein sequence information is not important, as the species deduced by matching the protein profiles usually at a range of 2–20 kDa (2,000–20,000 m/z) (Evason et al., 2001; Sauer and Kliem, 2010; Welker and Moore, 2011; Karlsson et al., 2015; Cassagne et al., 2016).

ADVANCES IN INVERTEBRATE PESTS, PARASITE, AND VECTOR PROFILING

In the past 16 years (**Figure 1**), MALDI MS profiling has been successfully applied for species identification of different pests, parasites and vectors such as nematodes, protozoa, and arthropods.

Proof of Principle Experiments

The early proof of principle experiments were focused on identification of biomarker peaks, standardization of sample preparation, matrixes and measurement optimization.

Protozoans and Unicellular Parasites

The first report of MALDI MS typing of protozoa was demonstrated using *Cryptosporidium* spp. associated with human infections. The species-specific spectra were reported from oocytes of *C. parvum* and *C. muris* isolated from feces of experimentally inoculated mice, lysed by freeze-thaw cycle, and spotted with HCCA as matrix (Magnuson et al., 2000). Later, it was shown that incubation of intact oocytes and purified sporozoites for 45 min with the matrix was critical for generating mass spectra with a large number of reproducible

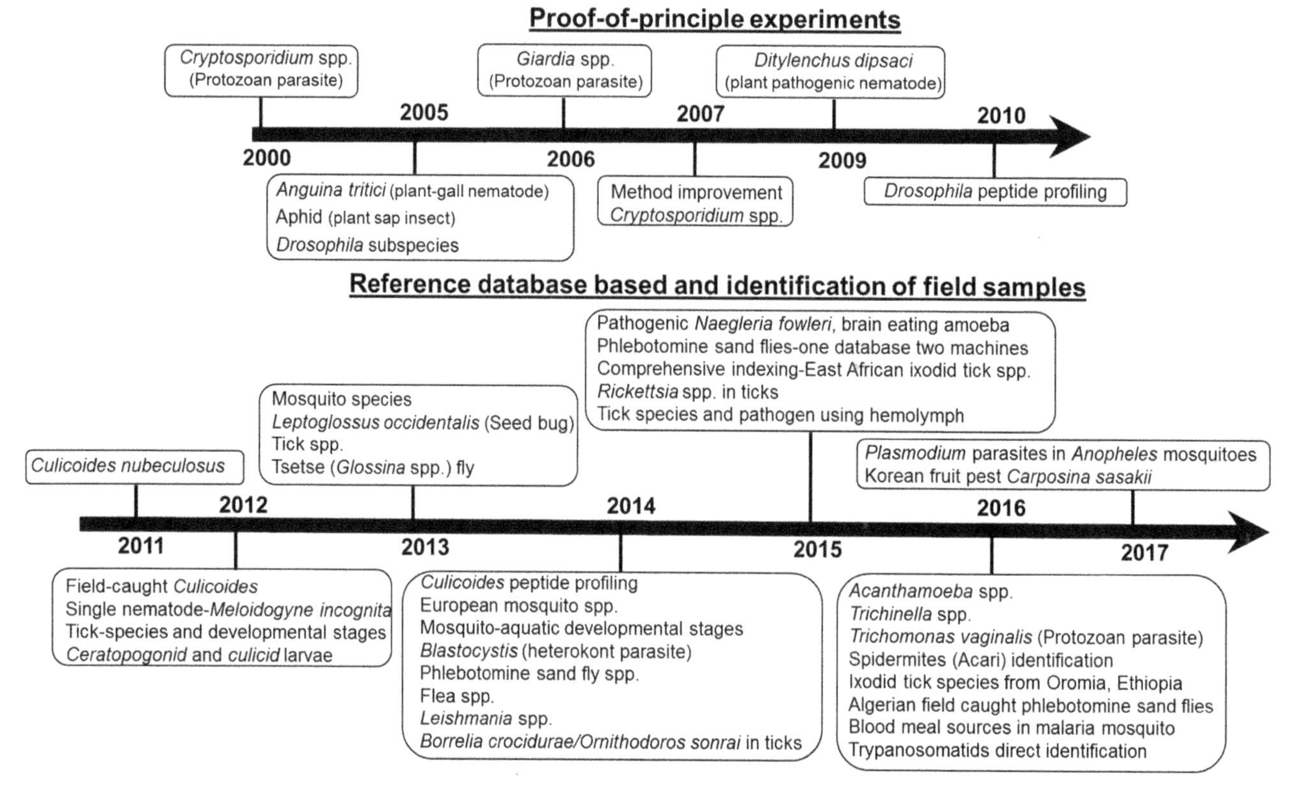

FIGURE 1 | Time line on MALDI profiling application of pests, parasites, and vector species identification.

peaks for *C. parvum* oocysts (Glassmeyer et al., 2007). Subsequently, direct application of whole spores, spore shells, and soluble fractions of spore-forming unicellular parasites such as microsporidia, *Encephalitozoon cuniculi*, *Encephalitozoon hellem*, *Encephalitozoon intestinalis*, and *Brachiola algerae* isolated from humans and propagated on monolayers of Vero monkey kidney (E6) cells, displayed species-specific markers in the mass range of 2,000–8,000 Da (Moura et al., 2003). Later, species-specific peaks in the range of *m/z* 3,000–19,000 was reported for the water-borne protozoan parasite, *Giardia* spp., the causative agent of giardiasis. The cysts, cyst walls, and trophozoites of *G. lamblia* and *G. muris* isolated from feces of experimentally challenged mice, were washed, mixed with an equal volume of sinnapinic acid, incubated, and spotted for MALDI MS analysis (Villegas et al., 2006).

Insects and Pests

Although not a pest or parasite, *Drosophila* has been used as a model for insect profiling possibilities. Protein extraction by simple grinding of adult whole insect in water was shown to generate species-specific spectra capable of distinguishing sibling species of *Drosophila* sub-species. The insect sex and matrix was not found to influence the spectra (Campbell, 2005). Likewise, species-specific peaks of varying intensities in a range of 3,000–25,000 *m/z* have been reported for three different aphids (plant phloem sap-feeding insects), green peach aphid *Myzus persicae* Sulzer, cowpea aphid *Aphis craccivora* Koch, and blue-green aphid (blue alfalfa aphid) *Acyrthosiphon kondoi* Shinji, independent of their dietary host plants (Perera et al., 2005).

Nematodes and Developmental Stage Discrimination

Species-specific and diagnostic peaks have also been reported for simple extracts of three plant nematodes, *Anguina tritici* (wheat seed-gall nematode), its closely *Anguina funesta* (ryegrass nematode), and *Meloidogyne javanica* (root-knot nematode that infects horticultural and vegetable crops; Perera et al., 2005). Several years later, direct crushing of the root-knot nematode, *Meloidogyne incognita* was shown to be useful in rapid discrimination between the harmless and harmful J_2 developmental stages and adult nematode (Ahmad et al., 2012).

Peptide Profiling

In this approach, also referred as shotgun mass mapping or SMM, whole body protein extracts were subjected to trypsin digestion without purification or fractionation steps, and the resulting peptides were utilized for generation of MALDI MS spectra for insect vector species such as *Drosophila* (Feltens et al., 2010) and biting midges (Uhlmann et al., 2014). Feltens et al. had applied nano-high performance liquid chromatography coupled with electrospray ionization mass spectrometry for identification of some of the MALDI MS profiles and revealed that most of the proteins were of muscles and mitochondria. However, SMM is time-consuming and handling large set of samples is challenging.

Data Independent Analysis and Clinical Sample Survey

The data independent species discrimination or grouping of microorganism is based on the visual examination for the presence or absence of peaks. This technique is very similar to those analyses performed before the days of the implementation of software with automated pattern matching algorithms; however, a different algorithm is used for rapid determination of the presence or absence of peaks for identification or discrimination. For example, this technique has been reported for the discrimination of the *Leishmania* subgenus *Viannia* or *Leishmania* exclusively based on the presence of 2 pairs of peaks (Mouri et al., 2014), as well as differentiation of protozoan parasitic *Entamoeba histolytica* and *Entamoeba dispar* (Azian et al., 2006).

Database-Based Enabled Rapid Species Identification Extended to Field Samples

MALDI MS typing based rapid species identification is usually achieved through pattern-matching of the unknown samples with that of a spectral reference library (database) created from known organisms. The main concerns at the proteome level are differences between the various developmental stages and complexity associated with various body parts. As listed in **Table 1**, vector related reference spectra were reported using commercial MALDI instrument-software suites. The proteins were extracted through homogenization and the parameters recommended for microbial species identification was followed. HCCA and SA were reported as the most utilized matrices for Bruker Biotyper and SARAMIS (Vitex MS), respectively. Despite the success of the procedures, these reference spectra remain *in-house* databases. Following the compilation of vector-specific reference spectra databases, the method proved to be rapid (~2–5 min/sample) as in the case of microbial species identification.

Parasites

In every reported case of parasite database approaches, Bruker BioTyper software tool and formic acid/acetonitrile extraction was applied. In the first such study, 56 clinical specimens belonging to 23 species of *Leishmania* were cultured, and promastigote pellets were utilized for database construction (Cassagne et al., 2014). Among 69 clinical isolates used for testing, only three samples were not identified. In a similar study, a database was constructed from four reference strains and the two clinical isolate were identified as *L. infantum* (Culha et al., 2014). In another study, using 19 enteric parasite *Blastocystis* isolates from 19 patients, a database for five subtypes was created and the remaining specimens were identified by matching (Martiny et al., 2014). Likewise, the differentiation of *E. histolytica* and *E. dispar* was demonstrated after establishment of the reference spectra and discriminating peaks were matched with the proteins identified through SDS-PAGE MALDI TOF MS based protein identification approach (Calderaro et al., 2015). Bruker BioTyper based database compilation were also reported for the food nematode *Trichinella* (Mayer-Scholl et al., 2016), *Trichomonas vaginalis* (Calderaro et al., 2016), *Acanthamoeba* spp.(Del Chierico et al., 2016) using a database for direct identification of trypanosomatids (Avila et al., 2016).

Toward "Vector Spectra Reference Database"

Kaufmann et al., were the first to report on utilization of SARAMIS premium software to create a reference database for two laboratory-reared *C. nubeculosus* biting midges (Kaufmann et al., 2011), and which was then extended to a larvae-specific database, screening of field collected samples, and applied for entomological surveys in Senegal, Africa. It was further reported as a means for discrimination of cryptic *Anopheles*, and demonstrated that the usefulness of mosquito eggs in species identification of field collected samples (Schaffner et al., 2014; Yssouf et al., 2014a). The Bruker Biotyper database has since been utilized to create a comprehensive "Vector specific reference spectra database" that includes spectra from leg proteins of 6 tick species, 30 mosquito species, one louse, one triatomine, one bed bug, and five flea species (Yssouf et al., 2013a,b, 2014b, 2015a). In addition, the package has been used to establish an aquatic developmental stage database starting from the larva stage to pupa of 6 mosquito species and detection of host blood meal and the presence of parasites (Niare et al., 2016; Laroche et al., 2017).

Pests

Despite the earlier proof of concept experiments for pests, the database approach was reported for only one plant pest in which Biotyper was utilized to distinguish evolutionary and morphologically close species of spider mites. Female adults of the Kanzawa (*Tetranychus kanzawai*), the two-spotted (*T. urticae*) spider mites and three other related species, namely *T. phaselus* Ehara (Tp), the bean red spider mite (*T. ludeni* Zacher) (Tl), and the tomato red spider mite (*T. evansi* Baker & Pritchard) (Te) were shown to be distinguishable. On the other hand, male adults and nymphs were reported to be non-distinguishable. Direct lysing of a single intact mite on target plates using double side carbon tape was also shown to generate spectra comparable to that of the extracts from 10 pooled individuals (Kajiwara et al., 2016). Recently, it was demonstrated that using MALDI MS, Tinkerbell LT, and its associated software MicroIDSys (ASTA Inc. Suwon, Korea), the larvae of the Korean apple pest, *Carposina sasakii*, could be effectively discriminated in about 15 min. Without such rapid identification methods, the export of these fruits might be hampered or rejected due to time-consuming pre-export inspection (Jeon et al., 2017).

DUAL IDENTIFICATION OF VECTORS, PARASITES, AND MEAL SOURCE

MALDI MS profiling has also been shown to be an effective method for simultaneous identification of vectors and parasite species, as in case of simultaneous identification of *Borrelia crocidurae/Ornithodoros sonrai* and *Rickettsia* spp. in ticks (Fotso et al., 2014; Yssouf et al., 2015b). Direct spotting of haemolymph from a dissected tick leg allows for the simultaneous and direct species identification of ticks and associated pathogens, and useful in species identification of parasites and vector while leaving the vector remains available

TABLE 1 | Reference database based species identification of parasite vectors.

S. No	Organisms	Sample/database	Protein extraction †	Matrix*	Software and database ≠		Comment	References
					Bruker BioTyper±	SARAMIS¥		
1	*Culicoides* biting midges	Whole insects or thoraxes	(1) Water and (2) FA (5-50%)	SA, DHB		+	Two laboratory reared -*C. nubeculosus*, better spectra with SA, recommended removal of abdomen, ethanol storage, and high concentration of formic acid influenced spectra	Kaufmann et al., 2011
2		Thoraxes with head, wings, and legs	10% FA	SA		+	first field study, better results with fresh samples compared to ethanol stored	Kaufmann et al., 2012
3						+	Ethanol preserved larvae, Spectra differed with development stage	Steinmann et al., 2013
4				HCCA		+	field survey at Senegal, Africa	Sambou et al., 2015
5	Mosquitoes	head and thorax		SA		+	Several months of ethanol preserved	Muller et al., 2013
6		legs	70% FA and 50% ACN	HCCA	+		Proteins extracted from legs is sufficient	Yssouf et al., 2013b
7					+		European mosquito species identification	Yssouf et al., 2014a
8					+		Mosquitos' species and midgut microbial species identification after culturing	Tandina et al., 2016
9		Whole specimen	70% FA		+		Culicidae juvenile database-aquatic developmental stages	Dieme et al., 2014
10		Eggs		SA		+	Eggs as source for species surveillance	Schaffner et al., 2014
11		Abdomen	70% FA and 50% AC	HCCA	+		Blood mean source identification in malaria mosquito	Niare et al., 2016
12		Head and thorax	Water		+		Plasmodium parasite identification in *Anopheles*	Laroche et al., 2017
13	Ticks	Whole tick, nymphs, and larvae	Sonication with 6-M guanidinium chloride solution, acidified with TFA and eluted with 0.1% TFA/75% ACN	HCCA	+		Developmental stages for 7 tick species	Karger et al., 2012
14		Legs	70% FA and 50% ACN		+		Proteins extracted from legs is sufficient	Yssouf et al., 2013a
16			25% FA	SA		+	comprehensive indexing of East African ixodid tick species	Rothen et al., 2016
17		1 Spirochetes spotted directly 2 tick legs	70% FA and 50% ACN	HCCA	+		*Borrelia crocidurae* /*Ornithodoros sonrai* in ticks.	Fotso et al., 2014
18		1 Hemolymph from leg 2 *R. c. conorii* strain extracte	70% FA and 100% ACN		+		*Rh. sanguineus* specimens infected by *R. c. conorii* and *A. variegatum* specimens infected by *R. africae*	Yssouf et al., 2015a
19		1 Tick legs 2 Cultured and purified Rickettsia species			+		*Rickettsia* spp in Ticks	Yssouf et al., 2015b
20	Flea	Abdomen excised whole specimen	70% FA and 50% ACN		+		Five flea species	Yssouf et al., 2014b

(Continued)

TABLE 1 | Continued

S. No	Organisms	Sample/database	Protein extraction†	Matrix*	Software and database ≠		Comment	References
					Bruker BioTyper±	SARAMIS¥		
21	*Glossina*. spp Tsetse fly	Whole insect and dissected body parts	70% FA and 100% ACN		+		Five lab reared *Glossina*. spp. Wings is sufficient	Hoppenheit et al., 2013
22	Phlebotomine sand flies	Thoraxes	(1) water and (2) 25% FA	SA	+		Discrimination of five Mediterranean species, Water extract yielded superior result to that of formic acid extract	Dvorak et al., 2014
23		Thoraxes, wings, and legs	70% FA and 50% ACN	HCCA	+		Six species caught from Algeria.	Lafri et al., 2016
24		Thoraxes with wings and legs	10% FA	SA, DHB		+	1. Ultraflex III MALDI TOF mass spectrometer measurement and an in-house phyton script to transfer mzXML files in to SARAMIS software. 2. Spectra measurement using Axima Confidence to create a reference spectra database for 20 species	Mathis et al., 2015

*†Protein extraction by homogenization: FA, Formic acid; ACN, acetonitrile; TFA, Trifluroacetic acid; *Matrix: HCCA, α-Cyano-4-hydroxycinnamic acid; SA, Sinapinic acid; DHB, 2,5-Dihydroxybenzoic acid; Software and database:≠ Plus symbol indicates the commercial software in which the database was created and incorporated,± BioTyper™—software from Bruker Daltonics, Bremen, Germany. ¥-SARAMIS™ software (Spectral. ARchive And Microbial Identification System, originally developed by AnagnosTec, Potsdam-Golm, Germany and now acquired and redeveloped as Vitek-MS by bioMérieux, Marcy L'Etoile, France).*

for other laboratory investigations (Fotso et al., 2014). MALDI MS profiling has further been successfully applied to determine the feeding patterns of mosquitoes up to 24 h post-blood meal (Niare et al., 2016). A future goal for the application of MALDI MS profiling in pest/parasites will be the rapid species identification of vectors, parasites and blood meal either through individual analysis or through simultaneous monitoring processes. The recent demonstration of rapid distinguishing of the *Plasmodium* infection status among *Anopheles stephensi* mosquitoes underscores that MALDI MS typing could be useful in entomological surveys including species-specific infection status (Laroche et al., 2017).

UNIVERSAL DATABASE AND FIELD SAMPLES

All the reported parasitology associated databases were developed as in-house databases and usually not accessable by other researchers, although several authors have agreed to supply the reference spectra upon request to other scientists possessing the same instrumentation and software tools. However, beyond a few initiations such as SpectraBank, there is no universal reference database such as protein database Swissprot/Uniprot for the purpose of species identification (Bohme et al., 2012). Recently, it was shown that the spectra generated from two different commercial MALDI MS instruments (Axima Confidence and Bruker Ultraflex III MS) could be analyzed in a single database (SARAMIS) in which a database was constructed for 20 species of phlebotomine sand flies based on measurements with Axima Confidence MS (Mathis et al., 2015). This underscores the possibilities of creation of online public reference databases that might be useful for any type of MALDI MS machines or spectral data formats. The online public database for parasitology is of great importance in terms of economy, time, and rapid analysis of samples collected from different geographical regions or hosts. The open source reference spectra database demands standardization of influencing parameters/processes affecting the sampling, such as developmental stage, specimen storage conditions, sample preparation/extraction methods, variations due to the spotting, instrumental, and post-measurement software settings.

CONCLUSION

Despite the achievements of MALDI TOF MS in microbial species identification, the application in parasitology remains limited to *in-house* databases integrated into commercial software. There is no commercial software tool or reference database available for parasitology, however, most of the successful reports were based on the principles, procedures, software, and databases best described for microorganisms. The crucial factors influencing parasitology MALDI MS typing includes: specimen associated parameters (age, developmental stage, sex, differing body parts, fed state), sample preparation procedures (sample storage, protein extraction solvents, and methods, sample spotting method, and matrix), and measurement parameters. MALDI MS typing of field specimens will be helpful in creating a distribution map and evaluation of the spread of parasites associated with disease. Few reports describe the spectral differences among the geographically different populations (Dieme et al., 2014; Dvorak et al., 2014; Hoppenheit et al., 2014). However, one should remain cautious, as the reliability of MALDI TOF MS in phylogenetic analysis is yet to be proven. The establishment of open source software and databases might be useful in future parasitological surveys and for rapid assessment of real time infection status.

AUTHOR CONTRIBUTIONS

JM conceived and wrote the manuscript. UR reviewed the manuscript.

ACKNOWLEDGMENTS

We would like to thank Karsten Tedin, Freie Universitaet Berlin, Germany and Vanessa Kowbel, University of Manitoba, Canada for their assistance of skillful grammatical corrections.

REFERENCES

Ahmad, F., and Babalola, O. O. (2014). Application of mass spectrometry as rapid detection tool in plant nematology. *Appl. Spectrosc. Rev.* 49, 1–10. doi: 10.1080/05704928.2013.798799

Ahmad, F., Gopal, J., and Wu, H. F. (2012). Rapid and highly sensitive detection of single nematode via direct MALDI mass spectrometry. *Talanta* 93, 182–185. doi: 10.1016/j.talanta.2012.02.009

Avila, C. C., Almeida, F. G., and Palmisano, G. (2016). Direct identification of trypanosomatids by matrix-assisted laser desorption ionization-time of flight mass spectrometry (DIT MALDI-TOF MS). *J. Mass Spectrom.* 51, 549–557. doi: 10.1002/jms.3763

Azian, M. Y. N., Hakim, S. L., and Maslawaty, M. N. (2006). Use of molecular tools to distinguish *Entamoeba histolytica* and *Entamoeba dispar* infection among the aborigines in Cameron Highlands. *Trop. Biomed.* 23, 31–36.

Bille, E., Dauphin, B., Leto, J., Bougnoux, M. E., Beretti, J. L., Lotz, A., et al. (2012). MALDI-TOF MS Andromas strategy for the routine identification of bacteria, mycobacteria, yeasts, *Aspergillus* spp. and positive blood cultures. *Clin. Microbiol. Infect.* 18, 1117–1125. doi: 10.1111/j.1469-0691.2011.03688.x

Bizzini, A., and Greub, G. (2010). Matrix-assisted laser desorption ionization time-of-flight mass spectrometry, a revolution in clinical microbial identification. *Clin. Microbiol. Infect.* 16, 1614–1619. doi: 10.1111/j.1469-0691.2010.03311.x

Bohme, K., Fernandez-No, I. C., Barros-Velazquez, J., Gallardo, J. M., Canas, B., and Calo-Mata, P. (2012). Spectrabank: an open access tool for rapid microbial identification by MALDI-TOF MS fingerprinting. *Electrophoresis* 33, 2138–2142. doi: 10.1002/elps.201200074

Calderaro, A., Piergianni, M., Buttrini, M., Montecchini, S., Piccolo, G., Gorrini, C., et al. (2015). MALDI-TOF mass spectrometry for the detection and differentiation of *Entamoeba histolytica* and *Entamoeba dispar*. *PLoS ONE* 10:e0122448. doi: 10.1371/journal.pone.0122448

Calderaro, A., Piergianni, M., Montecchini, S., Buttrini, M., Piccolo, G., Rossi, S., et al. (2016). MALDI-TOF mass spectrometry as a potential tool for *Trichomonas vaginalis* identification. *BMC Infect. Dis.* 16:261. doi: 10.1186/s12879-016-1594-z

Campbell, P. M. (2005). Species differentiation of insects and other multicellular organisms using matrix-assisted laser desorption/ionization time of flight mass spectrometry protein profiling. *Syst. Entomol.* 30, 186–190. doi: 10.1111/j.1365-3113.2004.00279.x

Cassagne, C., Normand, A. C., L'ollivier, C., Ranque, S., and Piarroux, R. (2016). Performance of MALDI-TOF MS platforms for fungal identification. *Mycoses* 59, 678–690. doi: 10.1111/myc.12506

Cassagne, C., Pratlong, F., Jeddi, F., Benikhlef, R., Aoun, K., Normand, A. C., et al. (2014). Identification of *Leishmania* at the species level with matrix-assisted laser desorption ionization time-of-flight mass spectrometry. *Clin. Microbiol. Infect.* 20, 551–557. doi: 10.1111/1469-0691.12387

Clark, A. E., Kaleta, E. J., Arora, A., and Wolk, D. M. (2013). Matrix-assisted laser desorption ionization-time of flight mass spectrometry: a fundamental shift in the routine practice of clinical microbiology. *Clin. Microbiol. Rev.* 26, 547–603 doi: 10.1128/CMR.00072-12

Culha, G., Akyar, I., Yildiz Zeyrek, F., Kurt, O., Gunduz, C., Ozensoy Toz, S., et al. (2014). Leishmaniasis in Turkey: determination of *Leishmania* species by matrix-assisted laser desorption ionization time-of-flight mass spectrometry (MALDI-TOF MS). *Iran. J. Parasitol.* 9, 239–248.

Del Chierico, F., Di Cave, D., Accardi, C., Santoro, M., Masotti, A., D'alfonso, R., et al. (2016). Identification and typing of free-living *Acanthamoeba* spp. by MALDI-TOF MS Biotyper. *Exp. Parasitol.* 170, 82–89. doi: 10.1016/j.exppara.2016.09.007

Dhiman, N., Hall, L., Wohlfiel, S. L., Buckwalter, S. P., and Wengenack, N. L. (2011). Performance and cost analysis of matrix-assisted laser desorption ionization-time of flight mass spectrometry for routine identification of yeast. *J. Clin. Microbiol.* 49, 1614–1616. doi: 10.1128/JCM.02381-10

Dieme, C., Yssouf, A., Vega-Rua, A., Berenger, J. M., Failloux, A. B., Raoult, D., et al. (2014). Accurate identification of Culicidae at aquatic developmental stages by MALDI-TOF MS profiling. *Parasit. Vectors* 7:544. doi: 10.1186/s13071-014-0544-0

Dvorak, V., Halada, P., Hlavackova, K., Dokianakis, E., Antoniou, M., and Volf, P. (2014). Identification of phlebotomine sand flies (Diptera: Psychodidae) by matrix-assisted laser desorption/ionization time of flight mass spectrometry. *Parasit. Vectors* 7:21. doi: 10.1186/1756-3305-7-21

Evason, D. J., Claydon, M. A., and Gordon, D. B. (2001). Exploring the limits of bacterial identification by intact cell-mass spectrometry. *J. Am. Soc. Mass Spectrom.* 12, 49–54. doi: 10.1016/S1044-0305(00)00192-6

Feltens, R., Gorner, R., Kalkhof, S., Groger-Arndt, H., and Von Bergen, M. (2010). Discrimination of different species from the genus *Drosophila* by intact protein profiling using matrix-assisted laser desorption ionization mass spectrometry. *BMC Evol. Biol.* 10:95. doi: 10.1186/1471-2148-10-95

Fotso, A. F., Mediannikov, O., Diatta, G., Almeras, L., Flaudrops, C., Parola, P., et al. (2014). MALDI-TOF mass spectrometry detection of pathogens in vectors: the *Borrelia crocidurae/Ornithodoros sonrai* Paradigm. *PloS Negl. Trop. Dis.* 8:e2984. doi: 10.1371/journal.pntd.0002984

Furlong, M. J. (2015). Knowing your enemies: integrating molecular and ecological methods to assess the impact of arthropod predators on crop pests. *Insect Sci.* 22, 6–19. doi: 10.1111/1744-7917.12157

Ge, M. C., Kuo, A. J., Liu, K. L., Wen, Y. H., Chia, J. H., Chang, P. Y., et al. (2016). Routine identification of microorganisms by matrix-assisted laser desorption ionization time-of-flight mass spectrometry: success rate, economic analysis, and clinical outcome. *J. Microbiol. Immunol. Infect.* S1684–S1182, 30063–30069. doi: 10.1016/j.jmii.2016.06.002

Gibson, W. (2009). Species-specific probes for the identification of the African tsetse-transmitted trypanosomes. *Parasitology* 136, 1501–1507. doi: 10.1017/S0031182009006179

Glassmeyer, S. T., Ware, M. W., Schaefer, F. W. III, Shoemaker, J. A., and Kryak, D. D. (2007). An improved method for the analysis of *Cryptosporidium parvum* oocysts by matrix-assisted laser desorption/ionization time of flight mass spectrometry. *J. Eukaryot. Microbiol.* 54, 479–481. doi: 10.1111/j.1550-7408.2007.00287.x

Hoppenheit, A., Murugaiyan, J., Bauer, B., Clausen, P. H., and Roesler, U. (2014). Analysis of *Glossina palpalis gambiensis* and *Glossina tachinoides* from two distant locations in Burkina Faso using MALDI TOF MS. *Parasitol. Res.* 113, 723–726 doi: 10.1007/s00436-013-3701-z

Hoppenheit, A., Murugaiyan, J., Bauer, B., Steuber, S., Clausen, P. H., and Roesler, U. (2013). Identification of Tsetse (*Glossina* spp.) using matrix-assisted laser desorption/ionisation time of flight mass spectrometry. *PLoS Negl. Trop. Dis.* 7:e2305. doi: 10.1371/journal.pntd.0002305

Jeon, J. H., Oh, H., Yun, C. S., Byun, B., Park, J., Park, H. S., et al. (2017). Rapid and reliable species identification of *Carposina sasakii* from its morphological homologues, by MALDI-TOF mass spectrometry. *J. Asia Pac. Entomol.* 20, 411–415. doi: 10.1016/j.aspen.2017.02.013

Kajiwara, H., Hinomoto, N., and Gotoh, T. (2016). Mass fingerprint analysis of spider mites (Acari) by matrix-assisted laser desorption/ionization time-of-flight mass spectrometry for rapid discrimination. *Rapid Commun. Mass Spectrom.* 30, 1037–1042. doi: 10.1002/rcm.7534

Karger, A. (2016). Current developments to use linear MALDI-TOF spectra for the identification and typing of bacteria and the characterization of other cells/organisms related to infectious diseases. *Proteomics Clin. Appl.* 10, 982–993. doi: 10.1002/prca.201600038

Karger, A., Kampen, H., Bettin, B., Dautel, H., Ziller, M., Hoffmann, B., et al. (2012). Species determination and characterization of developmental stages of ticks by whole-animal matrix-assisted laser desorption/ionization mass spectrometry. *Ticks Tick Borne Dis.* 3, 78–89. doi: 10.1016/j.ttbdis.2011.11.002

Karlsson, R., Gonzales-Siles, L., Boulund, F., Svensson-Stadler, L., Skovbjerg, S., Karlsson, A., et al. (2015). Proteotyping: proteomic characterization, classification and identification of microorganisms - A prospectus. *Syst. Appl. Microbiol.* 38, 246–257. doi: 10.1016/j.syapm.2015.03.006

Kaufmann, C., Schaffner, F., Ziegler, D., Pfluger, V., and Mathis, A. (2012). Identification of field-caught *Culicoides* biting midges using matrix-assisted laser desorption/ionization time of flight mass spectrometry. *Parasitology* 139, 248–258. doi: 10.1017/S0031182011001764

Kaufmann, C., Ziegler, D., Schaffner, F., Carpenter, S., Pfluger, V., and Mathis, A. (2011). Evaluation of matrix-assisted laser desorption/ionization time of flight mass spectrometry for characterization of *Culicoides nubeculosus* biting midges. *Med. Vet. Entomol.* 25, 32–38. doi: 10.1111/j.1365-2915.2010.00927.x

Lafri, I., Almeras, L., Bitam, I., Caputo, A., Yssouf, A., Forestier, C. L., et al. (2016). Identification of Algerian field-caught Phlebotomine sand fly vectors by MALDI-TOF MS. *PLoS Negl. Trop. Dis.* 10:e0004351. doi: 10.1371/journal.pntd.0004351

Laroche, M., Almeras, L., Pecchi, E., Bechah, Y., Raoult, D., Viola, A., et al. (2017). MALDI-TOF MS as an innovative tool for detection of *Plasmodium* parasites in Anopheles mosquitoes. *Malar. J.* 16:5. doi: 10.1186/s12936-016-1657-z

Magnuson, M. L., Owens, J. H., and Kelty, C. A. (2000). Characterization of *Cryptosporidium* parvum by matrix-assisted laser desorption ionization-time of flight mass spectrometry. *Appl. Environ. Microbiol.* 66, 4720–4724. doi: 10.1128/AEM.66.11.4720-4724.2000

Martiny, D., Bart, A., Vandenberg, O., Verhaar, N., Wentink-Bonnema, E., Moens, C., et al. (2014). Subtype determination of Blastocystis isolates by matrix-assisted laser desorption/ionisation time-of-flight mass spectrometry (MALDI-TOF MS). *Eur. J. Clin. Microbiol. Infect. Dis.* 33, 529–536. doi: 10.1007/s10096-013-1980-z

Mathis, A., Depaquit, J., Dvorak, V., Tuten, H., Banuls, A. L., Halada, P., et al. (2015). Identification of phlebotomine sand flies using one MALDI-TOF MS reference database and two mass spectrometer systems. *Parasit. Vectors* 8:266. doi: 10.1186/s13071-015-0878-2

Mayer-Scholl, A., Murugaiyan, J., Neumann, J., Bahn, P., Reckinger, S., and Nockler, K. (2016). Rapid identification of the foodborne pathogen *Trichinella* spp. by Matrix-Assisted Laser Desorption/Ionization Mass Spectrometry. *PLoS ONE* 11:e0152062. doi: 10.1371/journal.pone.0152062

McKeand, J. B. (1998). Molecular diagnosis of parasitic nematodes. *Parasitology* 117(Suppl.), S87–S96.

Moura, H., Ospina, M., Woolfitt, A. R., Barr, J. R., and Visvesvara, G. S. (2003). Analysis of four human microsporidian isolates by MALDI-TOF mass spectrometry. *J. Eukaryot. Microbiol.* 50, 156–163. doi: 10.1111/j.1550-7408.2003.tb00110.x

Mouri, O., Morizot, G., Van Der Auwera, G., Ravel, C., Passet, M., Chartrel, N., et al. (2014). Easy identification of leishmania species by mass spectrometry. *PLoS Negl. Trop. Dis.* 8:e2841. doi: 10.1371/journal.pntd.0002841

Muller, P., Pfluger, V., Wittwer, M., Ziegler, D., Chandre, F., Simard, F., et al. (2013). Identification of cryptic Anopheles mosquito species by molecular protein profiling. *PLoS ONE* 8:e57486. doi: 10.1371/journal.pone.0057486

Murugaiyan, J., Ahrholdt, J., Kowbel, V., and Roesler, U. (2012). Establishment of a matrix-assisted laser desorption ionization time-of-flight mass spectrometry database for rapid identification of infectious achlorophyllous green micro-algae of the genus *Prototheca*. *Clin. Microbiol. Infect.* 18, 461–467. doi: 10.1111/j.1469-0691.2011.03593.x

Murugaiyan, J., Walther, B., Stamm, I., Abou-Elnaga, Y., Brueggemann-Schwarze, S., Vincze, S., et al. (2014). Species differentiation within the *Staphylococcus* intermedius group using a refined MALDI-TOF MS database. *Clin. Microbiol. Infect.* 20, 1007–1014. doi: 10.1111/1469-0691.12662

Nagy, E., Becker, S., Kostrzewa, M., Barta, N., and Urban, E. (2012). The value of MALDI-TOF MS for the identification of clinically relevant anaerobic bacteria in routine laboratories. *J. Med. Microbiol.* 61, 1393–1400. doi: 10.1099/jmm.0.043927-0

Neville, S. A., Lecordier, A., Ziochos, H., Chater, M. J., Gosbell, I. B., Maley, M. W., et al. (2011). Utility of matrix-assisted laser desorption ionization-time of flight mass spectrometry following introduction for routine laboratory bacterial identification. *J. Clin. Microbiol.* 49, 2980–2984. doi: 10.1128/JCM.00431-11

Niare, S., Berenger, J. M., Dieme, C., Doumbo, O., Raoult, D., Parola, P., et al. (2016). Identification of blood meal sources in the main African malaria mosquito vector by MALDI-TOF MS. *Malar. J.* 15:87. doi: 10.1186/s12936-016-1152-6

Nomura, F. (2015). Proteome-based bacterial identification using matrix-assisted laser desorption ionization-time of flight mass spectrometry (MALDI-TOF MS): a revolutionary shift in clinical diagnostic microbiology. *Biochim. Biophys. Acta* 1854, 528–537. doi: 10.1016/j.bbapap.2014.10.022

Paini, D. R., Sheppard, A. W., Cook, D. C., De Barro, P. J., Worner, S. P., and Thomas, M. B. (2016). Global threat to agriculture from invasive species. *Proc. Natl. Acad. Sci. U.S.A.* 113, 7575–7579. doi: 10.1073/pnas.1602205113

Patel, R. (2013). Matrix-assisted laser desorption ionization-time of flight mass spectrometry in clinical microbiology. *Clin. Infect. Dis.* 57, 564–572. doi: 10.1093/cid/cit247

Perera, M. R., Vanstone, V. A., and Jones, M. G. K. (2005). A novel approach to identify plant parasitic nematodes using matrix-assisted laser desorption/ionization time-of-flight mass spectrometry. *Rapid Commun. Mass Spectrom.* 19, 1454–1460. doi: 10.1002/rcm.1943

Poulin, R., Besson, A. A., Morin, M. B., and Randhawa, H. S. (2016). Missing links: testing the completeness of host-parasite checklists. *Parasitology* 143, 114–122. doi: 10.1017/S0031182015001559

Roelfsema, J. H., Nozari, N., Herremans, T., Kortbeek, L. M., and Pinelli, E. (2011). Evaluation and improvement of two PCR targets in molecular typing of clinical samples of Leishmania patients. *Exp. Parasitol.* 127, 36–41. doi: 10.1016/j.exppara.2010.06.024

Rothen, J., Githaka, N., Kanduma, E. G., Olds, C., Pfluger, V., Mwaura, S., et al. (2016). Matrix-assisted laser desorption/ionization time of flight mass spectrometry for comprehensive indexing of East African ixodid tick species. *Parasit. Vectors* 9:151. doi: 10.1186/s13071-016-1424-6

Sambou, M., Aubadie-Ladrix, M., Fenollar, F., Fall, B., Bassene, H., Almeras, L., et al. (2015). Comparison of matrix-assisted laser desorption ionization-time of flight mass spectrometry and molecular biology techniques for identification of Culicoides (Diptera: ceratopogonidae) biting midges in senegal. *J. Clin. Microbiol.* 53, 410–418. doi: 10.1128/JCM.01855-14

Sauer, S., and Kliem, M. (2010). Mass spectrometry tools for the classification and identification of bacteria. *Nat. Rev. Microbiol.* 8, 74–82. doi: 10.1038/nrmicro2243

Schaffner, F., Kaufmann, C., Pfluger, V., and Mathis, A. (2014). Rapid protein profiling facilitates surveillance of invasive mosquito species. *Parasit. Vectors* 7:142. doi: 10.1186/1756-3305-7-142

Seng, P., Drancourt, M., Gouriet, F., La Scola, B., Fournier, P. E., Rolain, J. M., et al. (2009). Ongoing revolution in bacteriology: routine identification of bacteria by matrix-assisted laser desorption ionization time-of-flight mass spectrometry. *Clin. Infect. Dis.* 49, 543–551. doi: 10.1086/600885

Singhal, N., Kumar, M., and Virdi, J. S. (2016). MALDI-TOF MS in clinical parasitology: applications, constraints and prospects. *Parasitology* 143, 1491–1500. doi: 10.1017/S0031182016001189

Sogawa, K., Watanabe, M., Sato, K., Segawa, S., Ishii, C., Miyabe, A., et al. (2011). Use of the MALDI BioTyper system with MALDI-TOF mass spectrometry for rapid identification of microorganisms. *Anal. Bioanal. Chem.* 400, 1905–1911. doi: 10.1007/s00216-011-4877-7

Steinmann, I. C., Pfluger, V., Schaffner, F., Mathis, A., and Kaufmann, C. (2013). Evaluation of matrix-assisted laser desorption/ionization time of flight mass spectrometry for the identification of ceratopogonid and culicid larvae. *Parasitology* 140, 318–327. doi: 10.1017/S0031182012001618

Suarez, S., Ferroni, A., Lotz, A., Jolley, K. A., Guerin, P., Leto, J., et al. (2013). Ribosomal proteins as biomarkers for bacterial identification by mass spectrometry in the clinical microbiology laboratory. *J. Microbiol. Methods* 94, 390–396. doi: 10.1016/j.mimet.2013.07.021

Tandina, F., Almeras, L., Kone, A. K., Doumbo, O. K., Raoult, D., and Parola, P. (2016). Use of MALDI-TOF MS and culturomics to identify mosquitoes and their midgut microbiota. *Parasit. Vectors* 9:495. doi: 10.1186/s13071-016-1776-y

Tran, A., Alby, K., Kerr, A., Jones, M., and Gilligan, P. H. (2015). Cost savings realized by implementation of routine microbiological identification by matrix-assisted laser desorption ionization-time of flight mass spectrometry. *J. Clin. Microbiol.* 53, 2473–2479. doi: 10.1128/JCM.00833-15

Uhlmann, K. R., Gibb, S., Kalkhof, S., Arroyo-Abad, U., Schulz, C., Hoffmann, B., et al. (2014). Species determination of Culicoides biting midges via peptide profiling using matrix-assisted laser desorption ionization mass spectrometry. *Parasit. Vectors* 7:392. doi: 10.1186/1756-3305-7-392

Villegas, E. N., Glassmeyer, S. T., Ware, M. W., Hayes, S. L., and Schaefer, F. W. III. (2006). Matrix-assisted laser desorption/ionization time-of-flight mass spectrometry-based analysis of *Giardia lamblia* and *Giardia muris*. *J. Eukaryot. Microbiol.* 53(Suppl. 1), S179–S181. doi: 10.1111/j.1550-7408.2006.00223.x

Welker, M., and Moore, E. R. (2011). Applications of whole-cell matrix-assisted laser-desorption/ionization time-of-flight mass spectrometry in systematic microbiology. *Syst. Appl. Microbiol.* 34, 2–11. doi: 10.1016/j.syapm.2010.11.013

Wong, S. S., Fung, K. S., Chau, S., Poon, R. W., Wong, S. C., and Yuen, K. Y. (2014). Molecular diagnosis in clinical parasitology: when and why? *Exp. Biol. Med.* 239, 1443–1460. doi: 10.1177/1535370214523880

Yssouf, A., Almeras, L., Berenger, J. M., Laroche, M., Raoult, D., and Parola, P. (2015a). Identification of tick species and disseminate pathogen using hemolymph by MALDI-TOF MS. *Ticks Tick Borne Dis.* 6, 579–586. doi: 10.1016/j.ttbdis.2015.04.013

Yssouf, A., Almeras, L., Raoult, D., and Parola, P. (2016). Emerging tools for identification of arthropod vectors. *Future Microbiol.* 11, 549–566. doi: 10.2217/fmb.16.5

Yssouf, A., Almeras, L., Terras, J., Socolovschi, C., Raoult, D., and Parola, P. (2015b). Detection of *Rickettsia* spp in ticks by MALDI-TOF MS. *PLoS Negl. Trop. Dis.* 9:e0003473. doi: 10.1371/journal.pntd.0003473

Yssouf, A., Flaudrops, C., Drali, R., Kernif, T., Socolovschi, C., Berenger, J. M., et al. (2013a). Matrix-assisted laser desorption ionization-time of flight mass spectrometry for rapid identification of tick vectors. *J. Clin. Microbiol.* 51, 522–528. doi: 10.1128/JCM.02665-12

Yssouf, A., Parola, P., Lindstrom, A., Lilja, T., L'ambert, G., Bondesson, U., et al. (2014a). Identification of European mosquito species by MALDI-TOF MS. *Parasitol. Res.* 113, 2375–2378. doi: 10.1007/s00436-014-3876-y

Yssouf, A., Socolovschi, C., Flaudrops, C., Ndiath, M. O., Sougoufara, S., Dehecq, J. S., et al. (2013b). Matrix-assisted laser desorption ionization–time of flight mass spectrometry: an emerging tool for the rapid identification of mosquito vectors. *PLoS ONE* 8:e72380. doi: 10.1371/journal.pone.0072380

Yssouf, A., Socolovschi, C., Leulmi, H., Kernif, T., Bitam, I., Audoly, G., et al. (2014b). Identification of flea species using MALDI-TOF/MS. *Comp. Immunol. Microbiol. Infect. Dis.* 37, 153–157. doi: 10.1016/j.cimid.2014.05.002

11

Toxoplasma Co-infection Prevents Th2 Differentiation and Leads to a Helminth-Specific Th1 Response

Norus Ahmed[1], Timothy French[2], Sebastian Rausch[1], Anja Kühl[3], Katrin Hemminger[1], Ildiko R. Dunay[2], Svenja Steinfelder[1†] and Susanne Hartmann[1†]*

[1] Department of Veterinary Medicine, Institute of Immunology, Freie Universität Berlin, Berlin, Germany, [2] Institute of Inflammation and Neurodegeneration, Otto-von-Guericke University, Magdeburg, Germany, [3] Division of Gastroenterology, Medical Department, Infection and Rheumatology, Research Center ImmunoSciences, Berlin, Germany

Edited by:
Slobodan Paessler, University of Texas Medical Branch, United States

Reviewed by:
Patricia Talamás-Rohana, Center for Research and Advanced Studies of the National Polytechnic Institute (CINVESTAV), Mexico
Georgia Perona-Wright, University of Glasgow, United Kingdom

***Correspondence:**
Susanne Hartmann
susanne.hartmann@fu-berlin.de

[†] These authors have contributed equally to this work.

Nematode infections, in particular gastrointestinal nematodes, are widespread and co-infections with other parasites and pathogens are frequently encountered in humans and animals. To decipher the immunological effects of a widespread protozoan infection on the anti-helminth immune response we studied a co-infection with the enteric nematode *Heligmosomoides polygyrus* in mice previously infected with *Toxoplasma gondii.* Protective immune responses against nematodes are dependent on parasite-specific Th2 responses associated with IL-4, IL-5, IL-13, IgE, and IgG1 antibodies. In contrast, *Toxoplasma gondii* infection elicits a strong and protective Th1 immune response characterized by IFN-γ, IL-12, and IgG2a antibodies. Co-infected animals displayed significantly higher worm fecundity although worm burden remained unchanged. In line with this, the Th2 response to *H. polygyrus* in co-infected animals showed a profound reduction of IL-4, IL-5, IL-13, and GATA-3 expressing T cells. Co-infection also resulted in the lack of eosinophilia and reduced expression of the Th2 effector molecule RELM-β in intestinal tissue. In contrast, the Th1 response to the protozoan parasite was not diminished and parasitemia of *T. gondii* was unaffected by concurrent helminth infection. Importantly, *H. polygyrus* specific restimulation of splenocytes revealed *H. polygyrus*-reactive CD4$^+$ T cells that produce a significant amount of IFN-γ in co-infected animals. This was not observed in animals infected with the nematode alone. Increased levels of *H. polygyrus*-specific IgG2a antibodies in co-infected mice mirrored this finding. This study suggests that polarization rather than priming of naive CD4$^+$ T cells is disturbed in mice previously infected with *T. gondii*. In conclusion, a previous *T. gondii* infection limits a helminth-specific Th2 immune response while promoting a shift toward a Th1-type immune response.

Keywords: Th2, Th1, *Toxoplasma gondii*, *Heligmosomoides polygyrus*, co-infection, helminth

INTRODUCTION

Gastrointestinal nematode infections affect around 24% of the human population (WHO, 2017 last modified January, 2017 http://www.who.int/mediacentre/factsheets/fs366/en/; Horton, 2003). These parasites are not necessarily fatal though they cause high morbidity including malnourishment, intestinal inflammation and anemia in both acutely and chronically infected patients. In particular, school children are affected hindering their mental and physical development. Moreover, individuals living in endemic areas get frequently re-infected and immunity only develops after several decades (Mosmann and Coffman, 1989). Most areas endemic for nematodes are co-endemic for various diseases, such as malaria, tuberculosis, toxoplasmosis (Bahia-Oliveira et al., 2009), leishmaniasis and salmonellosis (Hotez and Kamath, 2009). Every pathogen should be encountered by a tailored immune response engaging a certain set of effector molecules, however this is a problem for the immune system during co-infections. Seroprevalence of *Toxoplasma gondii* reaches up to 70% in certain areas with high chances of co-infection with different pathogens among the human population (Bahia-Oliveira et al., 2009; Pappas et al., 2009). High prevalence of *T. gondii* is found in tropical regions, such as Latin America, Middle East, Africa and Southeast Asia. On the other hand *T. gondii* infection evokes and is controlled by a very different immune response compared to helminth infections. Detailed experimental studies are required to unravel how acute or chronic infections with certain pathogens affect the immune system, when faced with new challenges by unrelated infections.

Helminth infections are typically characterized by the activation and expansion of $CD4^+$ T helper 2 (Th2) cells, which express the transcription factor GATA-3 and secrete interleukin (IL)-4, IL-5, IL-9, and IL-13, leading to IgG1 and IgE antibody production. In addition, the Th2 response leads to eosinophilia, enhanced mucus production, specific granuloma-formation around larvae, as well as specific priming of innate cells, such as macrophages. This immune response can directly, or via upregulation of effector molecules, such as RELM-β produced by goblet cells, reduce worm fecundity and enhance parasite expulsion (Artis et al., 2004; Owyang et al., 2006).

Helminths evade the host immune responses due to host-parasite interactions (McSorley and Maizels, 2012) whereby the Th2 immune responses are actively regulated by the worm (Yazdanbakhsh et al., 2001). Thus, the Th2 response is accompanied by the emergence of parasite-induced regulatory cells, such as regulatory B-cells (Breg) (Hussaarts et al., 2011), regulatory T-cells (Treg) (Taylor et al., 2012) and alternatively activated macrophages (AAM) (Gordon and Martinez, 2010), which are known to limit parasite-specific and unspecific immune responses (Steinfelder et al., 2016). *Heligmosomoides polygyrus* is a well-studied strictly intestinal helminth of mice featuring all of the aforementioned characteristics (Reynolds et al., 2012). In addition to this, it is a widespread natural infection of wild mice (Maaz et al., 2016). The parasites are orally taken up as infective stage 3 larvae (L3), which subsequently embed themselves into the small intestinal wall to develop into L4. They then emerge as adults into the lumen, where they prevail for weeks before being expelled, depending on the mouse strain (Bansemir and Sukhdeo, 1994; Reynolds et al., 2012).

In contrast, *T. gondii* is an obligate intracellular protozoan parasite, which orally infects warm-blooded vertebrate hosts. After an initial intestinal phase, *T. gondii* spreads systemically and converts into a dormant stage in muscle and brain tissues (Dubey, 2008). Human infections with *T. gondii* are common and are mostly asymptomatic in immunocompetent individuals (Ho-Yen and Joss, 1992), although they may trigger basal inflammation (Parlog et al., 2015). Here, IFN-γ plays an important role in the containment of *T. gondii* (Ely et al., 1999). However, a previous latent infection in immunocompromised humans can reactivate and cause life threating encephalitis if left untreated (Luft et al., 1984; Montoya and Liesenfeld, 2004). During *T. gondii* infection a T helper 1 (Th1) immune response is elicited. This provides a strong, protective immune response and is characterized by dendritic cells (DC) producing IL-12. The production of IL-12 leads to the differentiation of $CD4^+$ T cells into Th1 cells expressing the transcription factor T-bet and the secretion of IFN-γ. Additionally, innate cells, such as neutrophils, NK-cells and innate lymphoid cells provide other early sources of IFN-γ (Gazzinelli et al., 1994; Sturge et al., 2013; Klose et al., 2014).

Differentiation of Th1 and Th2 cells has been well documented in the literature. *In vitro*-based studies have shown that Th1 or Th2 polarizing conditions cause differentiated cells to lose their ability to completely switch phenotype after increased cell division (Murphy et al., 1996; Grogan et al., 2001). However, other studies have shown that Th subsets have the flexibility to produce non-lineage-specific cytokines (Murphy and Stockinger, 2010; O'Garra et al., 2011; Coomes et al., 2013). Furthermore, we have previously reported a subset of Th hybrid cells expressing both transcription factors T-bet and GATA-3, as well as producing IFN-γ and IL-4 at intermediate levels during helminth infections (Peine et al., 2013).

Studies on *H. polygyrus* and *T. gondii* co-infection in mice have so far focused on a previous infection with helminths and have shown that initially $CD4^+$ and $CD8^+$ T cell immunity against *T. gondii* is suppressed in mice. At later stages the *T. gondii*-specific $CD4^+$ T cell response recovers whereas the $CD8^+$ response remains disrupted (Khan et al., 2008). In line with this, other studies have shown that prior infection with *H. polygyrus* induced suppression of IL-12 dependent differentiation of effector $CD8^+$ T cells as well as IFN-γ production against *T. gondii*. Interestingly, IL-4 and IL-10 deficiency was necessary to reverse the obstructing effect of *H. polygyrus* infection on the $CD8^+$ T cell response toward *Toxoplasma* (Marple et al., 2017). The majority of co-infection studies despite being protozoan, viral or bacterial infection, have focused on infections with helminth first due to their ability to downmodulate immune responses (Rousseau et al., 1997; Liesenfeld et al., 2004; Chen et al., 2005, 2006; Graham et al., 2005; Su et al., 2005, 2014a,b; Weng et al., 2007; Khan et al., 2008; Noland et al., 2008; Miller et al., 2009; Frantz et al., 2010; Dias et al., 2011; Potian et al., 2011; Kolbaum et al., 2012; du Plessis et al., 2013; Osborne et al., 2014; Budischak et al., 2015; Coomes et al., 2015; Gondorf et al., 2015; Rafi et al., 2015; Obieglo et al., 2016). In light of the fact, that Th2 immunity against helminths is an ongoing challenge in humans and livestock, we aimed to investigate how a previous protozoan infection affects the development of Th2 responses in $CD4^+$ T cells and protection against helminths.

We observed that a previous *T. gondii* infection leads to an overall suppression of *H. polygyrus*-specific Th2 immunity and enables *H. polygyrus*-specific $CD4^+$ T cells to produce IFN-γ.

MATERIALS AND METHODS

Animals

Female NMRI and C57BL/6 mice (8 weeks old; purchased from Janvier, Saint Berthevin, France) were bred under specific pathogen-free (SPF) conditions at the Institute of Medical Microbiology, Universitätsklinikum Magdeburg, Germany or at the Institute of Immunology, Department of Veterinary Medicine, Freie Universität Berlin. The experiments performed followed the National Animal Protection Guidelines and were approved by the German Animal Ethics Committee for the protection of animals.

Isolation of *T. gondii* Tissue Cysts and Oral *T. gondii* Infection

Female NMRI mice were infected orally (p.o.) with type II ME49 strain *T. gondii* cysts. After 8–10 months, tissue cysts were collected from the brains of chronically infected mice. After perfusion, brains were mechanically homogenized in 1 mL sterile PBS. Cysts were quantified using a light microscope and 8–10 weeks old female C57BL/6 mice were infected with 2-tissue cysts p.o. by oral gavage in a total volume of 200 μl/mouse (Möhle et al., 2016)

H. polygyrus Infection

The parasite *Heligmosomoides polygyrus* was retained by serial passage in C57BL/6 mice as described previously (Rausch et al., 2008). Mice aged 8–10 weeks old were infected by oral gavage with 200 L3 larvae in drinking water. On day 14 post infection (p.i.) mice were sacrificed by isofluorane inhalation.

Detection of *T. gondii* Parasitemia by PCR

Toxoplasma gondii burden was determined using Roche FastStart Essential DNA Green Master kit with manufacturer's protocol. TgB1 (TIBMolbiol, Berlin, Germany) was used as a target gene and Mm.ASL (TIBMolbiol, Berlin, Germany) as a reference (Heimesaat et al., 2014). Target/reference ratios were all calculated using the LightCycler® 480 Software release 1.5.0 (Roche, Germany).

Worm Fecundity and Worm Burden

Adult worms were isolated from the small intestine and counted. Female worms were subsequently kept individually (8 per mouse) in a 96 well round-bottom plate containing RPMI, 200 U/ml penicillin and 200 μg/ml streptomycin (all from PAA, Austria) at 37°C. After 24 h female *H. polygyrus* adults were removed from the wells and fecundity was determined by counting the eggs shed per female worm using a binocular microscope.

Preparation of Parasite Antigen

Heligmosomoides polygyrus antigen (HpAg) was prepared from adults worms that were kept in culture containing 100 U/ml penicillin and 100 μg/ml streptomycin for 24 h as described before (Rausch et al., 2008).

Cell Culture

Cells were cultured in complete RPMI 1640 medium (cRPMI) containing 10% FCS 200 U/ml penicillin, 200 μg/ml streptomycin (all from PAA, Austria) in an incubator at 37°C and 5% CO_2.

Single Cell Suspension Preparation

Spleen and mesenteric lymph nodes (mLN) were isolated from mice, homogenized and filtered through 70 μm cell strainers (BD Bioscience, San Jose, CA) to obtain single cell suspensions. The cells were then washed and re-suspended in cRPMI. Cells were counted using a CASY automated cell counter (Roche-Innovatis, Reutlingen, Germany). Small intestinal lamina propria (siLP) and epithelium (siE) cells were isolated by the removal of the whole small intestine that was then stored on ice in cold HBSS (w/o Ca^{2+} Mg^{2+}) (PAA, Pasching, Austria) containing 2% FCS and 10 mM HEPES (PAA, Pasching, Austria). Small intestines were washed through with 20 ml cold buffer using a 20G needle. After washing, mesenteric fat and Peyer's patches were removed. The small intestines were then cut open longitudinally and mucus scraped off with forceps. Additionally adult *H. polygyrus* worms were removed and counted using forceps. Small intestines were then washed in HBSS/FCS/HEPES and cut in 1 cm pieces and stored in 20 ml HBSS/FCS/HEPES containing 0.154 mg/ml DTE (Sigma-Aldrich, St. Louis, MO). The 1 cm pieces were incubated in a tube shaker water bath (200 rpm, 37°C) for 15 min. This step was repeated twice and then the intestinal pieces were transferred into 20 ml HBSS/FCS/HEPES containing 5 mM EDTA and agitated at room temperature for 15 min, repeated three times. Intestinal pieces were put into fresh 20 ml HBSS/FCS/HEPES and the cell suspension containing epithelium and intraepithelial lymphocytes retrieved for density gradient isolation. Intestinal pieces were washed in RPMI to remove residual EDTA and then placed in 10 ml 37°C complete RPMI 1640 medium containing 0.1 mg/ml Liberase (Roche, Basel, Switzerland) and 0.1 mg/ml DNAse (Sigma-Aldrich, St. Louis, MO, USA). Intestinal pieces were then incubated at 37°C, 200 rpm for 30 min. After incubation, tubes containing intestinal pieces were vortexed vigorously to disturb remaining intestinal pieces. The intestinal pieces were then forced up and down through an 18G needle. Suspensions were then filtered over a 70 μm cell strainer and washed twice with HBSS/HEPES. The cell suspensions from siLP and siE were added on a percoll gradient (GE healthcare life sciences, Sweden). Lamina propria and epithelial cells were collected from the 40%/70% interface after centrifugation. Cells were washed in cRPMI and counted using Neubauer chambers (C-Chip, Biochrom GmbH, Berlin, Germany).

Generation and Antigen Loading of Bone Marrow-Derived Dendritic Cells

Naïve female C57BL/6 mice were used for isolation of bone marrow from the femur and tibia. Bone marrow cells were washed in RPMI medium and 1×10^6 cells/ml were cultured in 10 ml/petri dish for 6 days in cRPMI containing 10 ng/ml recombinant murine GM-CSF (PeproTech, Hamburg, Germany). On day 3, 10 ml of cRPMI with 10 ng/ml GM-CSF was added. On day 6 BmDC were counted, seeded at 1×10^5 cells/well in a 96 well plate and stimulated with 50 μg/ml of

H. polygyrus antigen (HpAg) for 24 h. Cells were then washed and used for the co-culture experiment.

Antigen-Specific Restimulation of CD4$^+$ Splenocytes

1×10^6 splenocytes were co-cultured with 1×10^5 BmDC pulsed overnight with HpAg for 5 h in the presence of 3 μg/ml Brefeldin A (eBioscience, San Diego, CA, USA) followed by intracellular staining for CD154 and cytokines.

Cell Proliferation Assay

Spleen cells were isolated and stained with CFSE (Carboxyfluorescein succinimidyl ester). 1×10^6 CFSE labeled cells were cultured with 20 μg/ml *H. polygyrus* antigen. Cells were cultured for 6 days and restimulated with 1 μg/ml PMA and 1 μg/ml Ionomycin (both Sigma-Aldrich, St. Louis, MO, USA) in the presence of 3 μg/ml Brefeldin A (eBioscience, San Diego, CA, USA) followed by intracellular staining.

Realtime PCR

RNA was isolated from intestinal tissue sections previously stored at −80°C via homogenization in RNA lysis buffer. The tissue supernatant was processed with a innuPREP RNA kit (Analytik Jena, Jena, Germany) following manufacturer's instructions. 2 μg of RNA was reverse transcribed to cDNA using the High Capacity RNA to cDNA kit (Applied Biosystems, Foster City, CA). The relative expression of β-actin, resistin-like molecule-beta (Relm-β), IL-12 and IFN-γ, was determined by Real Time PCR using 10 ng of cDNA and the FastStart Universal SYBR Green Master Mix (Roche, Basel, Switzerland). Primer pairs used for gene amplification were as follows: β-actin forward: GGCTGTATTCCCCTCCATCG, reverse: CCAGTTGGTAAC AATGCCATGT, Relm-β (Retnlb) forward: GGCTGTGGATCG TGGGATAT, reverse: GAGGCCCAGTCCATGACTGA. IL-12 forward: ATGGCCATGTGGGAGCTGGAGAAAG, reverse: GTGGAGCAGCAGATGTGAGTGGCT. IFN-γ forward: ATg AACgCTACACACTgCATC, reverse: CCATCCTTTTgCCAg TTCCTC. Primer pair efficiency was determined via a standard curve. The mRNA expression was normalized to the β-actin housekeeping gene and calculated by Roche Light Cycler 480 software.

Cytokine Detection by ELISA

3.5×10^5 splenocytes were stimulated with 20 μg/ml *H. polygyrus* antigen or 2 μg/ml anti-CD3 and anti-CD28 (both eBioscience, San Diego, CA, USA) for 6 days. Supernatants were analyzed for IL-4, and IFN-γ using Ready-Set-Go Elisa Kits (eBioscience, San Diego, CA, USA) according to the manufacturer's instructions.

Antibody Isotype Detection by ELISA

Heligmosomoides polygyrus-specific IgG1 and IgG2a were measured in serum. 96 well microtiter plates coated with 10 μg/ml *H. polygyrus* antigen were incubated with serum diluted 1:100 with 3% BSA in PBS. Bound antibody isotypes were detected using alkaline phosphatase conjugated anti-mouse IgG1 and IgG2a antibodies diluted 1:5000 each (Rockland, PA, USA) and para-nitrophenylphosphate (Sigma, Steinheim am Albuch, Germany). All samples were run in duplicates. Arbitrary units were calculated using pooled samples as reference.

Flow Cytometry

For surface and intracellular staining, the monoclonal antibodies listed were used: CD4 (PerCP) (RM4-5); CD192 (CCR2) (Alexa 647) (SA203G11) all from BioLegend (Biozol); CD8 (53-6.7); IL-4 (PE-Cy7) (11B11); IL-5 (PE) (TRFK5); IL-13 (Alexa 488) (eBio13A); IFN-γ (eFluor 450) (XMG1.2); CD154 (PE) (MR1); Foxp3 Alexa 488 (FJK-16s); GATA3 (eFluor 660) (TWAJ); Dead Cell Exclusion Marker (DCE) (efluor 780); DCE (efluor 506); Siglec F (PE) (E50-2440); T-bet (PE) (eBio4B10); IL-13 (eFluor 660) (eBio13A); CD11b (PE) (M1/70); F4/80 (PerCP-Cy5.5) (BM8); Ly-6G (Gr-1) (PE-Cy7) (RB6-8c5); Ly-6C (eFluor 450) (HK1.4); TNF-α (Alexa488) (MP6-XT22) all from eBioscience, San Diego, CA, USA.

For intracellular staining of cytokines and transcription factors cells were fixed and permeabilized using the fix/perm buffer kit (eBioscience, San Diego, CA, USA). FACSCantoII flow cytometer and FACSAriaIII sorter (both BD Bioscience, Heidelberg, Germany) were used for cell analysis. FlowJo software 10.2 was used for final analysis (Tree star Inc., Ashland, OR, USA).

Statistics

Experiments were performed as shown and displayed as mean ± SD or mean ± SEM as indicated. Statistical analysis was performed using GraphPad Prism software (La Jolla, CA, USA). The level of significance was determined using the Mann Whitney *U*-test or Kruskal-Wallis with Dunn's multiple comparison test.

RESULTS

Prior Infection with *T. gondii* Results in Increased Fecundity of *H. polygyrus* in Co-infection

We investigated whether infection with *T. gondii* affects the control of helminth parasites in the small intestine (**Figure 1A**). Mice infected with *T. gondii* for 14 days followed by *H. polygyrus* infection did not show altered parasitemia of *T. gondii* in the heart compared to mice infected with *T. gondii* alone (**Figure 1B**). Similarly, co-infected mice did not show a significant difference in *H. polygyrus* adult worm burden compared to *H. polygyrus* single infection (**Figure 1C**). However, female worms retrieved from co-infected mice showed a significantly higher fecundity compared to worms from *H. polygyrus* single infection (**Figure 1D**). Thus, a previous and on-going infection with the protozoan parasite *T. gondii* leads to a decline of anti-helminthic control in terms of fecundity leading to enhanced egg production.

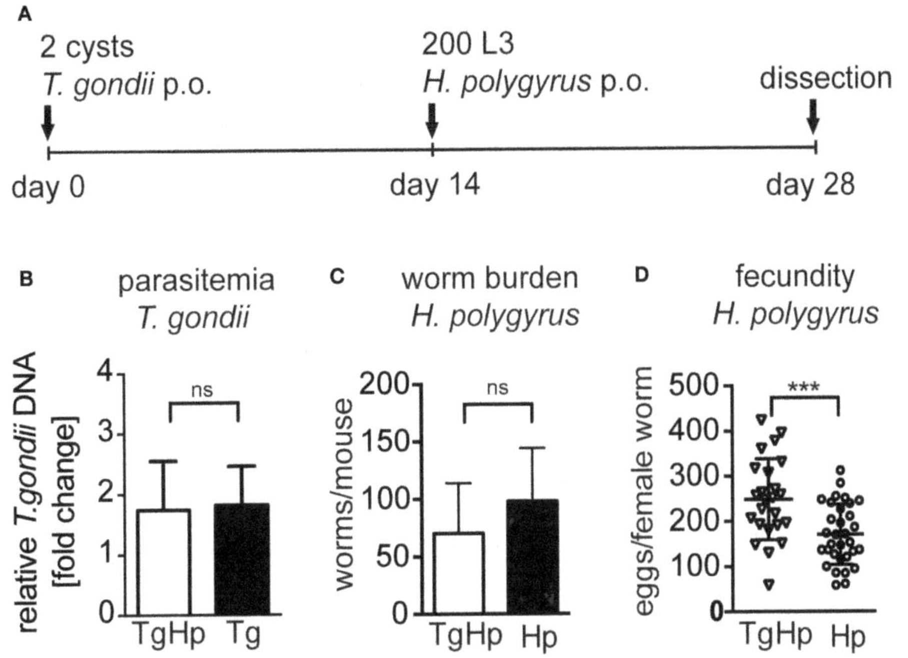

FIGURE 1 | Experimental design **(A)**, C57BL/6 mice were infected with 2 ME49 *T. gondii* tissue cysts and/or 200 *H. polygyrus* L3 larvae. **(B)** Parasitemia of *T. gondii* in the heart, pooled from two independent experiments, fold change compared to uninfected, data shown as mean ± SEM, $n = 6$–7 **(C)** *H. polygyrus* worm burden. **(D)** Fecundity of female worms. Panels **(C,D)** are representative of three independent experiments with $n = 4$. Data shown as mean ± SD; statistical analysis was performed using the Mann-Whitney test, $^{***}P \leq 0.001$.

Previous Infection with *T. gondii* Selectively Restricts Th2 Polarization in Response to Helminth Infection

The increased fecundity in co-infected mice, described as number of eggs produced per female worm *ex vivo*, might be due to insufficient Th2 immune pressure. To test this we compared systemic and local immune responses in co-infected and single infected groups. To differentiate between the contrasting immune responses the Th2-lineage marker GATA3 (Zheng and Flavell, 1997) and the Th1-lineage marker T-bet (Szabo et al., 2000) were used. GATA3 is also present on a subset of regulatory T cells that also express Foxp3. Regulatory T cells were excluded using their expression of Foxp3 (**Figure 2A**; Wohlfert et al., 2011).

The frequency of $GATA3^+Foxp3^-CD4^+$ was drastically reduced in the spleen, small intestinal lamina propria (siLP) and small intestinal epithelial layer (siE) in co-infected mice compared to mice infected with *H. polygyrus* only. The reduction in GATA3 was similar to levels found in uninfected mice (**Figure 2B**). Furthermore, histology of the small intestine of co-infected mice showed no GATA-3 expression compared to *H. polygyrus* infected mice (**Figure 2E**). On the contrary, the Th1-lineage marker T-bet in $CD4^+$ T cells was expressed in co-infected mice with higher levels to *T. gondii* alone in all compartments (**Figure 2C**). In addition to this, $T\text{-bet}^+$ expression in $CD8^+$ T cells was higher in siLP, siEL and mLN in co-infected mice compared to mice infected with *T. gondii* alone (**Figure 2D**).

Co-infection Leads to Suppression of Th2 Cytokine Responses in $CD4^+$ T Cells

The lack of GATA3 expression prompted us to investigate whether the failure to differentiate into Th2 cells (**Figure 2**) extends to the inability to secrete Th2 cytokines. $CD4^+$ T cells were restimulated with PMA/Ionomycin and cytokine expression was assessed (**Figure 3A**). The frequency of $CD4^+$ cells producing IL-4 in spleen, siLP and mLN showed a marked reduction in co-infected mice compared to the *H. polygyrus* single-infected group. However, only a trend in the reduction of IL-4 was observed in siEL (**Figure 3B**). Also, the frequency of IL-5 and IL-13 in spleen, siLP, siEL, and mLN showed a significant reduction in co-infected mice in comparison to *H. polygyrus* infection alone (**Figures 3C,D**). This observation shows that the Th2 immune responses are suppressed locally as well as systemically in mice previously infected with *T. gondii*. On the contrary, $CD4^+$ cells producing the Th1 cytokine IFN-γ showed an increase in the co-infected group compared to mice infected with *T. gondii* alone (**Figure 3E**), mirroring the enhanced T-bet expression found in the same cell population (**Figure 2C**). Similarly, T-bet and IFN-γ expression in $CD8^+$ T cells were comparable in mice single and co-infected with *T. gondii* (Figure S1). To further investigate this finding, splenocytes were stimulated with anti-CD3/28 to evaluate the ability of these

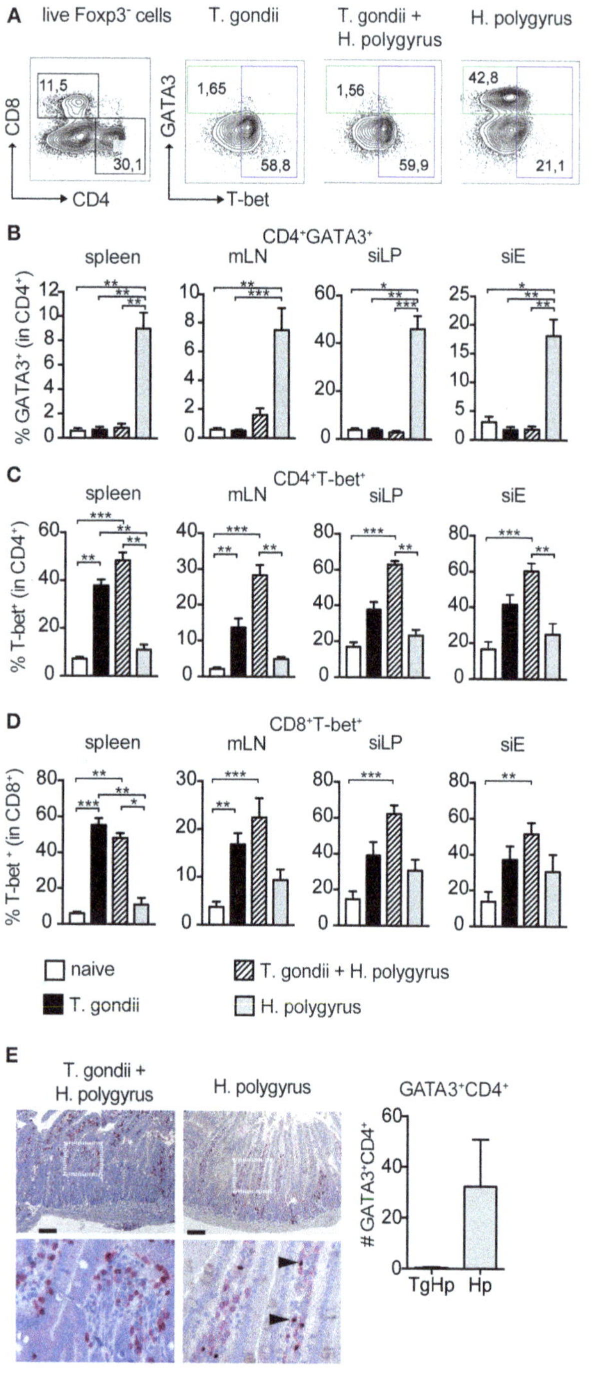

FIGURE 2 | Restricted Th2 responses in co-infected mice. Cells from spleen, mesenteric lymph nodes (mLN), small intestinal lamina propria (siLP) and small intestinal epithelium (siE) were isolated and stimulated with PMA and ionomycin in the presence of Brefeldin A followed by intranuclear staining for the lineage transcription factors GATA3 and T-bet. Gating strategy shown in **(A)**, Bar graphs showing frequencies of CD4$^+$ T cells expressing GATA3 **(B)**, T-bet **(C)**, and T-bet expression in CD8$^+$ T cells **(D)**. GATA3 expression in the duodeunum of the small intestine with scale bar of 100 μm **(E)**, data shown as mean ± SEM pooled from 2 independent experiments $n = 6$, statistical analysis was performed using the Mann-Whitney test. **(B–D)** shown as mean ± SEM, pooled from two independent experiments with $n = 8$–10. Statistical analysis was performed using the Kruskal-Wallis with Dunn's multiple comparison test, $^*P \leq 0.05$, $^{**}P \leq 0.01$, and $^{***}P \leq 0.001$.

cells to produce the Th2 cytokine IL-4 (**Figure 3F**). The co-infected group did not show any IL-4 production compared to the *H. polygyrus*-infected group whereas IFN-γ was produced in all groups.

Next, we evaluated effector mechanisms that are downstream of a Th2 response. As the appearance of Th2 cytokines in helminth infection is associated with eosinophilia, we tested the influence of a co-infection on the number of eosinophil granulocytes. Consistent with the lack of Th2 cytokine secretion (**Figure 3**), co-infected mice showed a significant reduction in the frequency of eosinophils in spleen (**Figure 4A**) compared to *H. polygyrus* single infection. Similarly, in mice infected with both *T. gondii* and *H. polygyrus* there was reduction in RELM-β expression in small intestinal tissue compared to *H. polygyrus* single infection (**Figure 4B**). This indicates that effector cells and molecules normally elicited by helminth infection are directly affected by the absence of Th2 cytokines in a co-infection setting. In contrast, no changes were observed in the frequency of inflammatory monocytes (F4/80$^+$GR1$^+$Ly6C$^+$) in both single and co-infected mice (**Figures 4C,D**). However, a significant reduction was observed in the production of TNF-α in inflammatory monocytes of co-infected mice in comparison to *T. gondii* single infected mice (**Figure 4E**),. In addition to this, co-infected mice showed a drastic reduction in *H. polygyrus* specific IgG1 compared to *H. polygyrus* single infection, which showed a prominent parasite-specific IgG1 response (**Figure 4F**). In contrast, helminth-specific IgG2a is increased in co-infected mice compared to mice infected with helminths alone. Thus, this data indicates that effector cells, effector molecules and the respective antibody response normally elicited by helminth infections are drastically altered in mice previously infected with *T. gondii*.

Co-infection Results in a Helminth-Specific Th1 Profile

The lack of the Th2 immune responses in co-infection may suggest that the CD4$^+$ T cells are not responding to *H. polygyrus* infection. Thus, we aimed to identify helminth antigen-specific CD4$^+$ T cells in co-infected mice. For this we generated bone marrow derived dendritic cells (BmDC) from naïve animals pulsed with *H. polygyrus* antigen (HpAg) and co-cultured them with splenocytes from single and co-infected animals. The antigen-reactive CD4$^+$ cells were subsequently detected by the activation marker CD154 (CD40L) (**Figure 5A**; Frentsch et al., 2005). We observed a reduction in IL-4 and IL-13 in activated CD154$^+$CD4$^+$ cells in the co-infected group compared to the *H. polygyrus* infected group. Interestingly, despite being unable to produce Th2 cytokines, significant numbers of CD154$^+$CD4$^+$ T cells from the co-infected group were able to produce IFN-γ in response to HpAg, which was not observed in the *H. polygyrus*-single infected group (**Figure 5B**). CFSE staining can be used to identify proliferating cells due to halving of CFSE in daughter cells during proliferation. Here, we assessed the proliferation of splenocytes from single and co-infected animals in response to HpAg by gating on CFSE$^-$ cells. Interestingly, while CD4$^+$ T cells from both groups proliferated based on CFSE-staining, the Th2

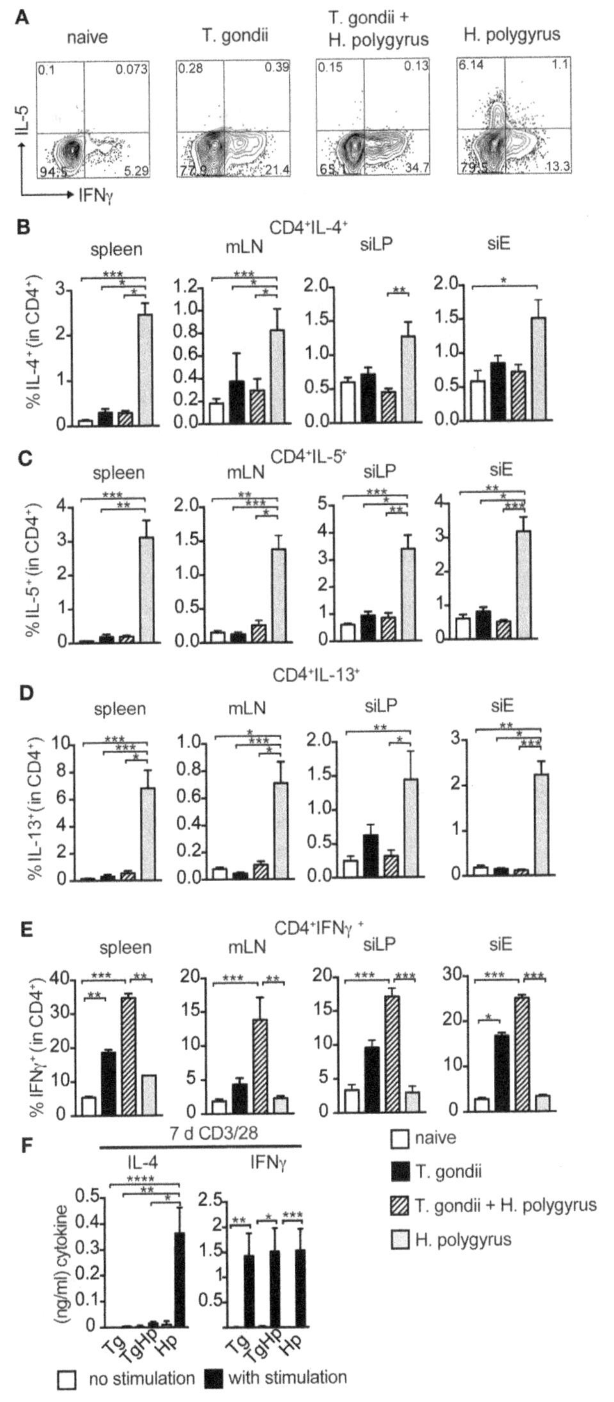

FIGURE 3 | Th2 but not Th1 immune responses are absent in co-infected mice. Cells from spleen, mLN, siLP, and siE of single and co-infected animals were isolated and stimulated with PMA and ionomycin in the presence of Brefeldin A followed by intracellular cytokine staining. Gating strategy for the cytokines IL-5 and IFN-γ in $CD4^+$ cells isolated from spleen **(A)**. Bar graphs showing frequencies of $CD4^+$ T cells expressing IL-4 **(B)**, IL-5 **(C)**, IL-13 **(D)**, and IFN-γ **(E)** in spleen, mLN, siLP, and siE. **(F)** IL-4 and IFN-γ production detected by ELISA in supernatant from 3×10^5 splenocytes stimulated with (black bars) and without (white bars) anti-CD3/CD28 antibodies. **(B–F)** Data shown as mean ± SEM, pooled from two independent experiments with $n = 8$–9 Statistical analysis was performed using the Kruskal-Wallis with Dunn's multiple comparison test, $^*P \leq 0.05$, $^{**}P \leq 0.01$, and $^{***}P \leq 0.001$.

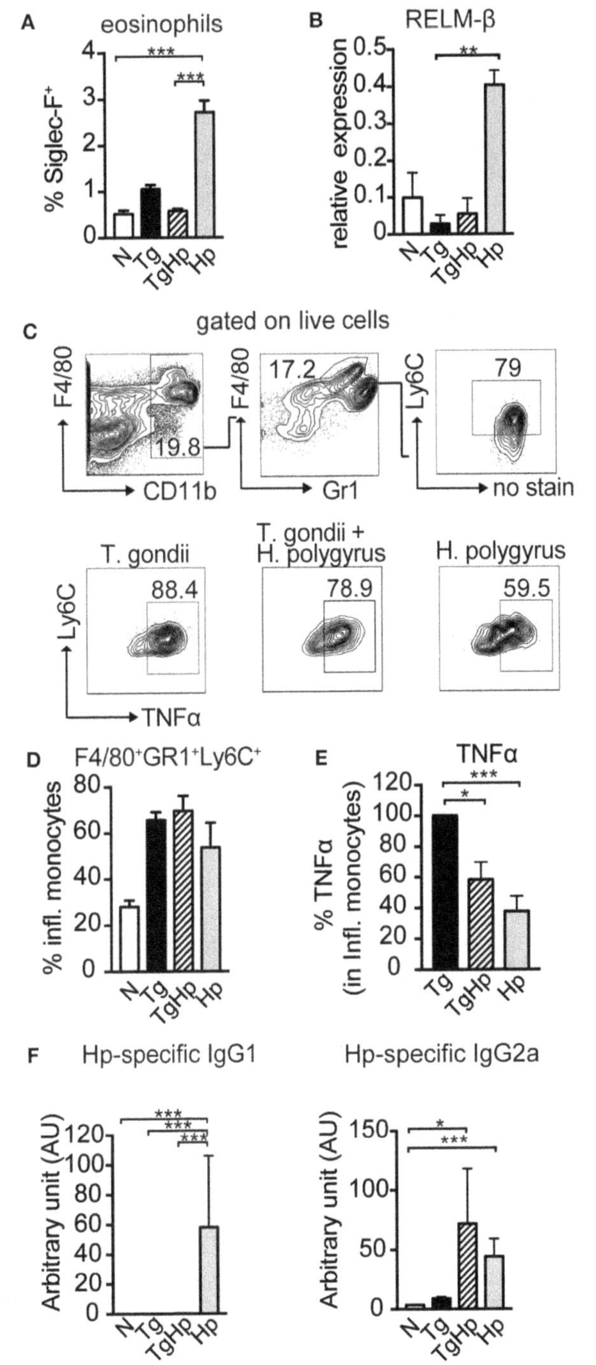

FIGURE 4 | Impact of co-infection on Th1- and Th2-dependent effector cells, effector molecules and antibody isotypes. **(A)** Bar graph showing the frequency of Siglec-F^+ eosinophils in the spleen, pooled from 2 independent experiments $n = 7$–8. **(B)** Relative Gene Expression of RELM-β compared to housekeeping gene β-actin (pooled from two experiments, $n = 5$–8). **(C,D)** Gating strategy and bar graphs showing frequency of inflammatory monocytes ($F4/80^+GR1^+Ly6C^+$) in spleen stimulated with LPS (pooled from two experiments, $n = 8$). **(E)** Percentage of TNFα, with the response of the *T. gondii* infected group represented as 100%, stimulated with LPS, pooled from two experiments, $n = 9$. **(F)** *H. polygyrus* specific IgG1 and IgG2a detected by ELISA, $n = 7$–8 pooled from two independent experiments. Data shown as mean ± SEM. Statistical analysis was performed using the Kruskal-Wallis with Dunn's multiple comparison test, $^*P \leq 0.05$, $^{**}P \leq 0.01$, and $^{***}P \leq 0.001$.

cytokine IL-4 was reduced in co-infected animals compared to helminth single infection. On the other hand, IFN-γ production in response to HpAg was increased in co-infected animals (**Figure 5C**). Additionally, *in vitro* stimulation of splenocytes with HpAg showed similar results. Here, significant amounts of IL-4 and IL-10 could be detected in supernatants from mice infected with *H. polygyrus* only, while IFN-γ was significantly increased in co-infected animals (**Figure 5D**). Hence, this data supports the observation that helminth-specific $CD4^+$ T cells from co-infected animals are unable to commit to the Th2 lineage but produce the Th1 cytokine IFN-γ in response to a helminth infection instead.

DISCUSSION

In this study a previous low-dose oral infection with *T. gondii* prevented the establishment of local and systemic Th2 responses normally induced by infection with *H. polygyrus*. Neither Th2 cytokines nor the transcription factor GATA3 as well as features triggered by IL-4 (IgG1 antibodies, RELM-ß) or IL-5 (eosinophilia) could be detected in co-infected animals. The observed increase in female worm fecundity in co-infected animals is a likely consequence of a lack in Th2 responses due to the reduced antibody levels and effector molecule RELM-ß, as both were shown to influence *H. polygyrus* fecundity (Owyang et al., 2006; McCoy et al., 2008). Interestingly the Th1 response to *T. gondii* was not diminished in $CD4^+$ and $CD8^+$ T cells in co-infected animals, since both subsets were able to produce similar amounts of IFN-γ in contrast to other studies, where the helminth infection precedes the protozoan infection (Khan et al., 2008; Marple et al., 2017). This observation is in line with unaltered parasitemia of *T. gondii* during chronic phase of infection. Furthermore, inflammatory monocytes expressing Ly6C infiltrate the brain to control *T. gondii* via the production of pro-inflammatory mediators, such as TNF-α, IL-1-α IL-1-β and nitric oxide synthase (Dunay et al., 2008, 2010; Biswas et al., 2015). In co-infected animals the frequency of inflammatory monocytes was not altered, but the capacity to produce TNF-α in response to LPS was reduced. However, this had no effect on parasitemia of *T. gondii*.

The observation of an apparent reduction in Th2 responses might be due to abolished priming and polarization events that occur at various stages, such as insufficient priming of naïve $CD4^+$ helper T cells, altered function of dendritic cells (DC) leading to aberrant polarization, or the local cytokine milieu present at the time of helminth infection. Moreover, a recent study has shown that systemic *T. gondii* infection leads to a long-term defect in the generation and function of naive T lymphocytes (Kugler et al., 2016). However, our findings suggest that in a low-dose infection with *T. gondii,* this effect is not as drastic,since helminth-specific $CD4^+$ T cells were shown to proliferate and respond to antigen as seen in **Figure 5**.

The differentiation between Th1 and Th2 cells requires positive feedback loops and cross-inhibition of other lineages for uniform Th cell differentiation (Mosmann and Coffman, 1989; Paul and Seder, 1994). In addition to this the transcription factor specific for Th1, T-bet, has the ability to suppress the Th2 transcription factor GATA-3. This might provide an explanation for the cross-regulation of cytokines in Th cell differentiation (Hwang et al., 2005). During *T. gondii* infection T-bet can suppress IL-4 and GATA-3 expression, thus, preventing endogenous Th2 cell associated programming (Zhu et al., 2012). In our study, the observed up-regulation of T-bet was in line with the significant reduction of GATA-3 in spleen, siLP and siEL. The reduction in GATA-3 expression followed the absent Th2 cytokine production observed in co-infection with *T. gondii*. Our study is in line with other studies showing suppression in the Th2 responses against helminths, when another pathogen is involved prior or at the same time during infection (Liesenfeld et al., 2004; Lass et al., 2013; Nel et al., 2014). Interestingly, the frequencies of $CD4^+$ T-cells from co-infected animals producing either T-bet or IFN-γ are similar to mice infected with *T. gondii* alone or even higher. This suggests that $CD4^+$ T cells expressing T-bet and IFN-γ in coinfected animals consist of pre-existing *T. gondii*-specific T cells and *H. polygyrus*-specific T-cells able to produce T-bet and IFN-γ in this coinfection setting.

In general, helminths are shown to actively induce a Th2 program that requires the programming of dendritic cells (DCs) (Steinfelder et al., 2009). DCs from skin LN exposed to *Nippostrongylus brasiliensis* showed transcriptional changes of different DC subsets (Connor et al., 2017). Generally, DCs are pivotal in eliciting Th2 cell responses *in vivo*. A depletion of the $CD11c^+$ DCs subset during infection with *S. mansoni* led to an abolished Th2 response and an increase in the production of IFN-γ (Phythian-Adams et al., 2010). This reduced Th2 response was also observed in *H. polygyrus* infection when mice were depleted of $CD11c^+$ DCs (Smith et al., 2011). However, during *T. gondii* infection, the induced Th1 immune response is dependent on early IL-12 production by APCs (Scanga et al., 2002). DCs prime naïve T cells, but are also a target of effector cytokines produced by previously polarized effector T cells and innate cells. In our study it is most likely that DCs are affected by the previous and ongoing infection with *T. gondii* and the ensuing cytokine milieu. The presence of IL-12 and IFN-γ at the time point and site of infection as shown in Figure S2 might impact the ability of local DCs to be able to prime naïve T cells for Th2 differentiation. Future studies should investigate the underlying mechanisms and involvement of DCs, such as $CD8\alpha^+$ DCs that are a source of IL-12 during *T. gondii* infection (Mashayekhi et al., 2011).

Dendritic cells can also be primed in response to epithelium-derived cytokines known as alarmins. These cytokines are released during epithelial tissue damage (Swamy et al., 2010). Thymic stromal lymphopoietin (TSLP) plays an important role in mounting a Th2 response in *H. polygyrus* infection (Massacand et al., 2009). Also IL-33 is an alarmin and it has been shown that when DCs are treated with IL-33 they polarize CD4 T cells to produce Th2 cytokines (Besnard et al., 2011; Eiwegger and Akdis, 2011). Another tissue derived cytokine; IL-25 has been demonstrated to be involved in Th2 cytokine responses and *N. brasiliensis* expulsion. However, this cytokine has not been described to directly act on DCs (Fallon et al., 2006;

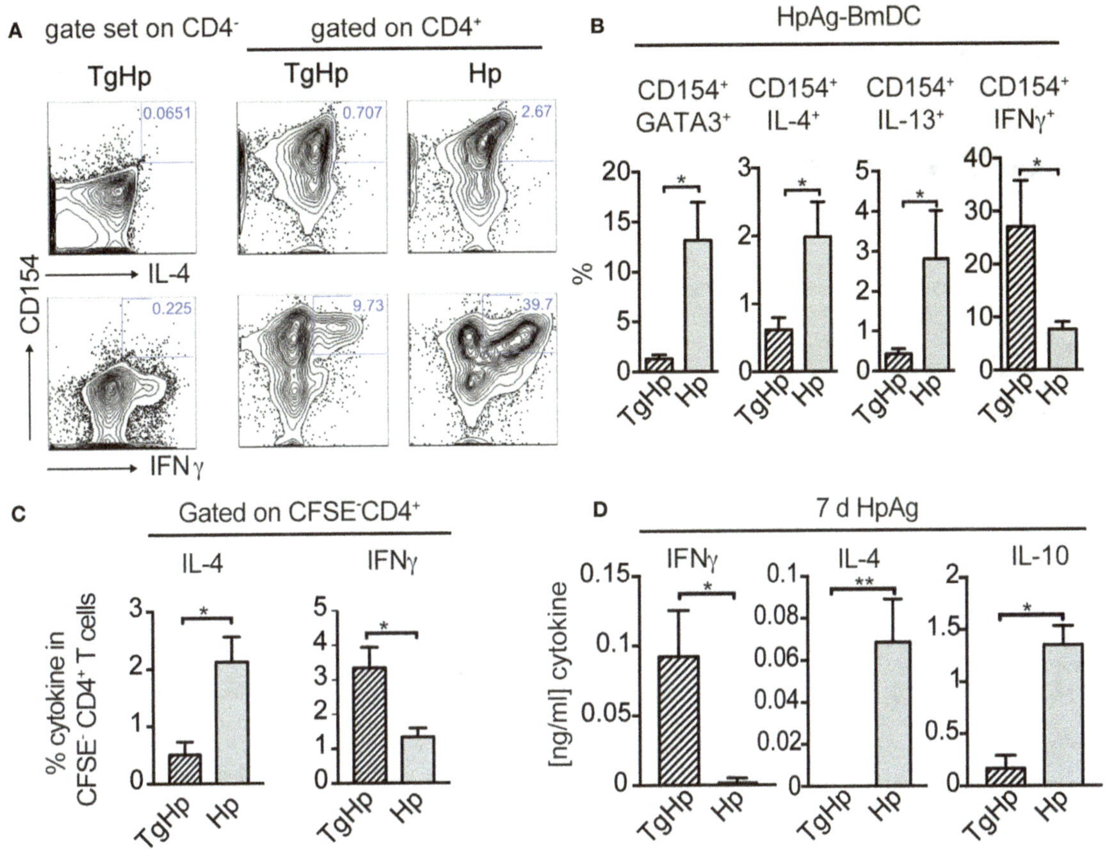

FIGURE 5 | Helminth-reactive CD4$^+$ T cells from co-infected mice show enhanced production of IFN-γ. BmDC (1×10^5) were pulsed with 50 μg/ml H. polygyrus antigen (HpAg) and cultured with 1×10^6 splenocytes from single or co-infected animals for 5 h followed by intracellular staining for CD154 and cytokines. Gating strategy is shown in **(A)** whereby the gate for cells coexpressing CD154 and IL-4, IL-13, or IFN-γ was set using CD4$^-$ cells. **(B)** Bar graphs showing frequencies of CD154$^+$GATA3$^+$, CD154$^+$IL-4$^+$, CD154$^+$IL-13$^+$, and CD154$^+$IFN-γ$^+$ in CD4$^+$ T cells. Data shown as mean ± SD and representative of two independent experiments with $n = 4$–5. **(C)** CFSE labeled CD4$^+$ spleen cells were stimulated for 6 days with 20 μg/ml HpAg. Proliferating spleen cells were gated on (CFSE-CD4+). CD4$^+$ cells were re-stimulated with PMA/Ionomycin and stained for intracellular cytokines IL-4, and IFN-γ; data shown as mean ± SD and is representative for two independent experiments $n = 4$. **(D)** Bar graphs show detection of IFN-γ, IL-4 and IL-10 by ELISA from collected supernatant of 3×10^5 splenocytes stimulated with *H. polygyrus* antigen for 6 days; representative of two independent experiments $n = 4$–5, mean ± SD. Statistical analysis was performed using the Mann-Whitney test, $^*P \leq 0.05$, $^{**}P \leq 0.01$.

Wang et al., 2007). Since early Th2 polarization is dependent on the release of these cytokines that act as alarmins it might be fruitful to investigate these cytokines very early after infection with *H. polygyrus* in previously infected *T. gondii* mice.

Importantly, we show that while helminth-reactive CD4$^+$ T cells are unable to produce Th2 cytokines in a co-infection, they still express significant amounts of IFN-γ after restimulation with helminth antigen. We identified IFN-γ producing *H. polygyrus* antigen (HpAg)-reactive T cells in co-infected animals using the activation marker CD154 and a short stimulation protocol (Frentsch et al., 2005; Chattopadhyay et al., 2006). We also saw this in CFSE$^-$CD4$^+$ T cells that expanded in response to HpAg. In line with our findings, Coomes et al. have shown that a co-infection with *Plasmodium chabaudi* and *H. polygyrus* led to a reduction in Th2 responses. Furthermore, they observed up-regulation of IFN-γ when Th2 cells from *H. polygyrus*-infected mice were adoptively transferred into *Rag1*$^{-/-}$ mice infected with *P. chabaudi*. However, blocking of IL-12 and IFN-γ only partially preserved Th2 immunity in response to *H. polygyrus* (Coomes et al., 2015).

In summary, our data on helminth-antigen specific restimulation of CD4$^+$ T cells suggest that naïve CD4$^+$ T cells harboring a cognate TCR for helminth antigen fail to commit to the Th2 lineage and are polarized toward a Th1 phenotype in mice previously infected with *Toxoplasma*. This switch in cytokine expression leads to the absence of effector features downstream of the Th2 response and consequently to higher worm fecundity in co-infected animals. Recent studies emphasized the importance of bystander activation and concurrent infections on the outcome of the immune response to unrelated pathogens or vaccines (Reese et al., 2016; Tao and Reese, 2017). In regards to the differences in the development of protective Th2 immunity observed in our study and by others in both mice and humans, it is important to focus on infections not only in a "clean" host but also in the context of individual infection history as well as co-infections.

AUTHOR CONTRIBUTIONS

NA, SS, SR, TF, and KH performed all the experiments. SH, ID, and SS conceptualized and designed the research. NA, SS, and SH wrote the manuscript. All authors approved the final version of the manuscript.

FUNDING

This study was funded by the German Research Foundation: GRK 2046 to SH and SS. Norus Ahmed received a stipend of the GRK 2046.

ACKNOWLEDGMENTS

The authors thank Yvonne Weber, Marion Müller, Bettina Sonnenburg, Christiane Palissa, and Beate Anders for providing their excellent technical support.

REFERENCES

Artis, D., Wang, M. L., Keilbaugh, S. A., He, W., Brenes, M., Swain, G. P., et al. (2004). RELMbeta/FIZZ2 is a goblet cell-specific immune-effector molecule in the gastrointestinal tract. *Proc. Natl. Acad. Sci. U.S.A.* 101, 13596–13600. doi: 10.1073/pnas.0404034101

Bahia-Oliveira, L. M., da Silva, J. A., Peixoto-Rangel, A. L., Boechat, M. S. B., Oliveira, A. M. W. A., Massara, C. L., et al. (2009). Host immune response to *Toxoplasma gondii* and *Ascaris lumbricoides* in a highly endemic area: evidence of parasite co-immunomodulation properties influencing the outcome of both infections. *Mem. Inst. Oswaldo Cruz* 104, 273–280. doi: 10.1590/S0074-02762009000200021

Bansemir, A. D., and Sukhdeo, M. V. (1994). The food resource of adult *Heligmosomoides polygyrus* in the small intestine. *J. Parasitol.* 80, 24–28. doi: 10.2307/3283340

Besnard, A.-G., Togbe, D., Guillou, N., Erard, F., Quesniaux, V., and Ryffel, B. (2011). IL-33-activated dendritic cells are critical for allergic airway inflammation. *Eur. J. Immunol.* 41, 1675–1686. doi: 10.1002/eji.201041033

Biswas, A., Bruder, D., Wolf, S. A., Jeron, A., Mack, M., Heimesaat, M. M., et al. (2015). LY6C(high) monocytes control cerebral toxoplasmosis. *J. Immunol.* 194, 3223–3235. doi: 10.4049/jimmunol.1402037

Budischak, S. A., Sakamoto, K., Megow, L. C., Cummings, K. R., Urban, J. F., and Ezenwa, V. O. (2015). Resource limitation alters the consequences of co-infection for both hosts and parasites. *Int. J. Parasitol.* 45, 455–463. doi: 10.1016/j.ijpara.2015.02.005

Chattopadhyay, P. K., Yu, J., and Roederer, M. (2006). Live-cell assay to detect antigen-specific $CD4^+$ T-cell responses by CD154 expression. *Nat. Protoc.* 1, 1–6. doi: 10.1038/nprot.2006.1

Chen, C.-C., Louie, S., McCormick, B. A., Walker, W. A., and Shi, H. N. (2006). Helminth-primed dendritic cells alter the host response to enteric bacterial infection. *J. Immunol.* 176, 472–483. doi: 10.4049/jimmunol.176.1.472

Chen, C.-C., Louie, S., McCormick, B., Walker, W. A., and Shi, H. N. (2005). Concurrent infection with an intestinal helminth parasite impairs host resistance to enteric *Citrobacter rodentium* and enhances *Citrobacter*-induced colitis in mice. *Infect. Immun.* 73, 5468–5481. doi: 10.1128/IAI.73.9.5468-5481.2005

Connor, L. M., Tang, S.-C., Cognard, E., Ochiai, S., Hilligan, K. L., Old, S. I., et al. (2017). Th2 responses are primed by skin dendritic cells with distinct transcriptional profiles. *J. Exp. Med.* 214, 125–142. doi: 10.1084/jem.201 60470

Coomes, S. M., Pelly, V. S., and Wilson, M. S. (2013). Plasticity within the $\alpha\beta^+CD4^+$ T-cell lineage: when, how and what for? *Open Biol.* 3:120157. doi: 10.1098/rsob.120157

Coomes, S. M., Pelly, V. S., Kannan, Y., Okoye, I. S., Czieso, S., Entwistle, L. J., et al. (2015). IFN-γ and IL-12 restrict Th2 responses during Helminth/*Plasmodium* co-infection and promote IFN-γ from Th2 cells. *PLoS Pathog.* 11:e1004994. doi: 10.1371/journal.ppat.1004994

Dias, A. T., de Castro, S. B. R., Alves, C. C. S., Rezende, A. B., Rodrigues, M. F., Machado, R. R. P., et al. (2011). Lower production of IL-17A and increased susceptibility to *Mycobacterium bovis* in mice coinfected with *Strongyloides venezuelensis*. *Mem. Inst. Oswaldo Cruz* 106, 617–619. doi: 10.1590/S0074-02762011000500015

du Plessis, N., Kleynhans, L., Thiart, L., van Helden, P. D., Brombacher, F., Horsnell, W. G. C., et al. (2013). Acute helminth infection enhances early macrophage mediated control of mycobacterial infection. *Mucosal Immunol.* 6, 931–941. doi: 10.1038/mi.2012.131

Dubey, J. P. (2008). The history of *Toxoplasma gondii*–the first 100 years. *J. Eukaryot. Microbiol.* 55, 467–475. doi: 10.1111/j.1550-7408.2008.00345.x

Dunay, I. R., Damatta, R. A., Fux, B., Presti, R., Greco, S., Colonna, M., et al. (2008). $Gr1^+$ inflammatory monocytes are required for mucosal resistance to the pathogen *Toxoplasma gondii*. *Immunity* 29, 306–317. doi: 10.1016/j.immuni.2008.05.019

Dunay, I. R., Fuchs, A., and Sibley, L. D. (2010). Inflammatory monocytes but not neutrophils are necessary to control infection with *Toxoplasma gondii* in mice. *Infect. Immun.* 78, 1564–1570. doi: 10.1128/IAI.00472-09

Eiwegger, T., and Akdis, C. A. (2011). IL-33 links tissue cells, dendritic cells and Th2 cell development in a mouse model of asthma. *Eur. J. Immunol.* 41, 1535–1538. doi: 10.1002/eji.201141668

Ely, K. H., Kasper, L. H., and Khan, I. A. (1999). Augmentation of the CD8+ T cell response by IFN-gamma in IL-12-deficient mice during *Toxoplasma gondii* infection. *J. Immunol.* 162, 5449–5454.

Fallon, P. G., Ballantyne, S. J., Mangan, N. E., Barlow, J. L., Dasvarma, A., Hewett, D. R., et al. (2006). Identification of an interleukin (IL)-25-dependent cell population that provides IL-4, IL-5, and IL-13 at the onset of helminth expulsion. *J. Exp. Med.* 203, 1105–1116. doi: 10.1084/jem.20051615

Frantz, F. G., Rosada, R. S., Peres-Buzalaf, C., Perusso, F. R. T., Rodrigues, V., Ramos, S. G., et al. (2010). Helminth coinfection does not affect therapeutic effect of a DNA vaccine in mice harboring tuberculosis. *PLoS Negl. Trop. Dis.* 4:e700. doi: 10.1371/journal.pntd.0000700

Frentsch, M., Arbach, O., Kirchhoff, D., Moewes, B., Worm, M., Rothe, M., et al. (2005). Direct access to $CD4^+$ T cells specific for defined antigens according to CD154 expression. *Nat. Med.* 11, 1118–1124. doi: 10.1038/nm1292

Gazzinelli, R. T., Wysocka, M., Hayashi, S., Denkers, E. Y., Hieny, S., Caspar, P., et al. (1994). Parasite-induced IL-12 stimulates early IFN-gamma synthesis and resistance during acute infection with *Toxoplasma gondii*. *J. Immunol.* 153, 2533–2543.

Gondorf, F., Berbudi, A., Buerfent, B. C., Ajendra, J., Bloemker, D., Specht, S., et al. (2015). Chronic filarial infection provides protection against bacterial sepsis by functionally reprogramming macrophages. *PLoS Pathog.* 11:e1004616. doi: 10.1371/journal.ppat.1004616

Gordon, S., and Martinez, F. O. (2010). Alternative activation of macrophages: mechanism and functions. *Immunity* 32, 593–604. doi: 10.1016/j.immuni.2010.05.007

Graham, A. L., Lamb, T. J., Read, A. F., and Allen, J. E. (2005). Malaria-filaria coinfection in mice makes malarial disease more severe unless filarial infection achieves patency. *J. Infect. Dis.* 191, 410–421. doi: 10.1086/426871

Grogan, J. L., Mohrs, M., Harmon, B., Lacy, D. A., Sedat, J. W., and Locksley, R. M. (2001). Early transcription and silencing of cytokine genes underlie polarization of T helper cell subsets. *Immunity* 14, 205–215. doi: 10.1016/S1074-7613(01)00103-0

Heimesaat, M. M., Dunay, I. R., Schulze, S., Fischer, A., Grundmann, U., Alutis, M., et al. (2014). Pituitary adenylate cyclase-activating polypeptide ameliorates experimental acute ileitis and extra-intestinal sequelae. *PLoS ONE* 9:e108389. doi: 10.1371/journal.pone.0108389

Horton, J. (2003). Human gastrointestinal helminth infections: are they now neglected diseases? *Trends Parasitol.* 19, 527–531. doi: 10.1016/j.pt.2003.09.007

Hotez, P. J., and Kamath, A. (2009). Neglected tropical diseases in sub-saharan Africa: review of their prevalence, distribution, and disease burden. *PLoS Negl. Trop. Dis.* 3:e412. doi: 10.1371/journal.pntd.0000412

Ho-Yen, D. O., and Joss, A. W. L. (1992). *Human Toxoplasmosis, 1st Edn.* Oxford; New York, NY: Oxford University Press.

Hussaarts, L., van der Vlugt, L. E. P. M., Yazdanbakhsh, M., and Smits, H. H. (2011). Regulatory B-cell induction by helminths: implications for allergic disease. *J. Allergy Clin. Immunol.* 128, 733–739. doi: 10.1016/j.jaci.2011.05.012

Hwang, E. S., Szabo, S. J., Schwartzberg, P. L., and Glimcher, L. H. (2005). T helper cell fate specified by kinase-mediated interaction of T-bet with GATA-3. *Science* 307, 430–433. doi: 10.1126/science.1103336

Khan, I. A., Hakak, R., Eberle, K., Sayles, P., Weiss, L. M., and Urban, J. F. (2008). Coinfection with *Heligmosomoides polygyrus* fails to establish CD8$^+$ T-cell immunity against *Toxoplasma gondii*. *Infect. Immun.* 76, 1305–1313. doi: 10.1128/IAI.01236-07

Klose, C. S. N., Flach, M., Möhle, L., Rogell, L., Hoyler, T., Ebert, K., et al. (2014). Differentiation of type 1 ILCs from a common progenitor to all helper-like innate lymphoid cell lineages. *Cell* 157, 340–356. doi: 10.1016/j.cell.2014.03.030

Kolbaum, J., Eschbach, M.-L., Steeg, C., Jacobs, T., Fleischer, B., and Breloer, M. (2012). Efficient control of *Plasmodium yoelii* infection in BALB/c and C57BL/6 mice with pre-existing *Strongyloides ratti* infection. *Parasite Immunol.* 34, 388–393. doi: 10.1111/j.1365-3024.2012.01369.x

Kugler, D. G., Flomerfelt, F. A., Costa, D. L., Laky, K., Kamenyeva, O., Mittelstadt, P. R., et al. (2016). Systemic toxoplasma infection triggers a long-term defect in the generation and function of naive T lymphocytes. *J. Exp. Med.* 213, 3041–3056. doi: 10.1084/jem.20151636

Lass, S., Hudson, P. J., Thakar, J., Saric, J., Harvill, E., Albert, R., et al. (2013). Generating super-shedders: co-infection increases bacterial load and egg production of a gastrointestinal helminth. *J. R. Soc. Interface* 10:20120588. doi: 10.1098/rsif.2012.0588

Liesenfeld, O., Dunay, I. R., and Erb, K. J. (2004). Infection with *Toxoplasma gondii* reduces established and developing Th2 responses induced by *Nippostrongylus brasiliensis* infection. *Infect. Immun.* 72, 3812–3822. doi: 10.1128/IAI.72.7.3812-3822.2004

Luft, B. J., Brooks, R. G., Conley, F. K., McCabe, R. E., and Remington, J. S. (1984). Toxoplasmic encephalitis in patients with acquired immune deficiency syndrome. *JAMA* 252, 913–917. doi: 10.1001/jama.1984.03350070031018

Maaz, D., Rausch, S., Richter, D., Krücken, J., Kühl, A. A., Demeler, J., et al. (2016). Susceptibility to ticks and Lyme disease spirochetes is not affected in mice co-infected with nematodes. *Infect. Immun.* 84, 1274–1286. doi: 10.1128/IAI.01309-15

Marple, A., Wu, W., Shah, S., Zhao, Y., Du, P., Gause, W. C., et al. (2017). Cutting edge: helminth coinfection blocks effector differentiation of CD8 T cells through alternate host Th2- and IL-10–mediated responses. *J. Immunol.* 198, 634–639. doi: 10.4049/jimmunol.1601741

Mashayekhi, M., Sandau, M. M., Dunay, I. R., Frickel, E. M., and Khan, A. (2011). CD8α$^+$ dendritic cells are the critical source of interleukin-12 that controls acute infection by *Toxoplasma gondii* Tachyzoites.*Immunity* 35, 249–259. doi: 10.1016/j.immuni.2011.08.008

Massacand, J. C., Stettler, R. C., Meier, R., Humphreys, N. E., Grencis, R. K., Marsland, B. J., et al. (2009). Helminth products bypass the need for TSLP in Th2 immune responses by directly modulating dendritic cell function. *Proc. Natl. Acad. Sci. U.S.A.* 106, 13968–13973. doi: 10.1073/pnas.0906367106

McCoy, K. D., Stoel, M., Stettler, R., Merky, P., Fink, K., Senn, B. M., et al. (2008). Polyclonal and specific antibodies mediate protective immunity against enteric helminth infection. *Cell Host Microbe* 4, 362–373. doi: 10.1016/j.chom.2008.08.014

McSorley, H. J., and Maizels, R. M. (2012). Helminth infections and host immune regulation. *Clin. Microbiol. Rev.* 25, 585–608. doi: 10.1128/CMR.05040-11

Miller, C. M. D., Smith, N. C., Ikin, R. J., Boulter, N. R., Dalton, J. P., and Donnelly, S. (2009). Immunological interactions between 2 common pathogens, Th1-inducing protozoan *Toxoplasma gondii* and the Th2-inducing helminth *Fasciola hepatica*. *PLoS ONE* 4:e5692. doi: 10.1371/journal.pone.0005692

Möhle, L., Israel, N., Paarmann, K., Krohn, M., Pietkiewicz, S., Müller, A., et al. (2016). Chronic *Toxoplasma gondii* infection enhances β-amyloid phagocytosis and clearance by recruited monocytes. *Acta Neuropathol. Commun.* 4:25. doi: 10.1186/s40478-016-0293-8

Montoya, J. G., and Liesenfeld, O. (2004). Toxoplasmosis. *Lancet Lond. Engl.* 363, 1965–1976. doi: 10.1016/S0140-6736(04)16412-X

Mosmann, T. R., and Coffman, R. L. (1989). TH1 and TH2 cells: different patterns of lymphokine secretion lead to different functional properties. *Annu. Rev. Immunol.* 7, 145–173. doi: 10.1146/annurev.iy.07.040189.001045

Murphy, E., Shibuya, K., Hosken, N., Openshaw, P., Maino, V., Davis, K., et al. (1996). Reversibility of T helper 1 and 2 populations is lost after long-term stimulation. *J. Exp. Med.* 183, 901–913.

Murphy, K. M., and Stockinger, B. (2010). Effector T cell plasticity: flexibility in the face of changing circumstances. *Nat. Immunol.* 11, 674–680. doi: 10.1038/ni.1899

Nel, H. J., du Plessis, N., Kleynhans, L., Loxton, A. G., van Helden, P. D., and Walzl, G. (2014). *Mycobacterium bovis* BCG infection severely delays *Trichuris muris* expulsion and co-infection suppresses immune responsiveness to both pathogens. *BMC Microbiol.* 14:9. doi: 10.1186/1471-2180-14-9

Noland, G. S., Urban, J. F., Fried, B., and Kumar, N. (2008). Counter-regulatory anti-parasite cytokine responses during concurrent *Plasmodium yoelii* and intestinal helminth infections in mice. *Exp. Parasitol.* 119, 272–278. doi: 10.1016/j.exppara.2008.02.009

O'Garra, A., Gabryšová, L., and Spits, H. (2011). Quantitative events determine the differentiation and function of helper T cells. *Nat. Immunol.* 12, 288–294. doi: 10.1038/ni.2003

Obieglo, K., Feng, X., Bollampalli, V. P., Dellacasa-Lindberg, I., Classon, C., and Österblad, M. (2016). Chronic gastrointestinal nematode infection mutes immune responses to Mycobacterial infection distal to the gut. *J. Immunol.* 196, 2262–2271. doi: 10.4049/jimmunol.1500970

Osborne, L. C., Monticelli, L. A., Nice, T. J., Sutherland, T. E., Siracusa, M. C., Hepworth, M. R., et al. (2014). Coinfection. virus-helminth coinfection reveals a microbiota-independent mechanism of immunomodulation. *Science* 345, 578–582. doi: 10.1126/science.1256942

Owyang, A. M., Zaph, C., Wilson, E. H., Guild, K. J., McClanahan, T., Miller, H. R. P., et al. (2006). Interleukin 25 regulates type 2 cytokine-dependent immunity and limits chronic inflammation in the gastrointestinal tract. *J. Exp. Med.* 203, 843–849. doi: 10.1084/jem.20051496

Pappas, G., Roussos, N., and Falagas, M. E. (2009). Toxoplasmosis snapshots: global status of *Toxoplasma gondii* seroprevalence and implications for pregnancy and congenital toxoplasmosis. *Int. J. Parasitol.* 39, 1385–1394. doi: 10.1016/j.ijpara.2009.04.003

Parlog, A., Schlüter, D., and Dunay, I. R. (2015). *Toxoplasma gondii*-induced neuronal alterations. *Parasite Immunol.* 37, 159–170. doi: 10.1111/pim.12157

Paul, W. E., and Seder, R. A. (1994). Lymphocyte responses and cytokines. *Cell* 76, 241–251. doi: 10.1016/0092-8674(94)90332-8

Peine, M., Rausch, S., Helmstetter, C., Fröhlich, A., Hegazy, A. N., Kühl, A. A., et al. (2013). Stable T-bet$^+$GATA-3$^+$ Th1/Th2 hybrid cells arise *in vivo*, can develop directly from naive precursors, and limit immunopathologic inflammation. *PLoS Biol.* 11:e1001633. doi: 10.1371/journal.pbio.1001633

Phythian-Adams, A. T., Cook, P. C., Lundie, R. J., Jones, L. H., Smith, K. A., Barr, T. A., et al. (2010). CD11c depletion severely disrupts Th2 induction and development *in vivo*. *J. Exp. Med.* 207, 2089–2096. doi: 10.1084/jem.20100734

Potian, J. A., Rafi, W., Bhatt, K., McBride, A., Gause, W. C., and Salgame, P. (2011). Preexisting helminth infection induces inhibition of innate pulmonary anti-tuberculosis defense by engaging the IL-4 receptor pathway. *J. Exp. Med.* 208, 1863–1874. doi: 10.1084/jem.20091473

Rafi, W., Bhatt, K., Gause, W. C., and Salgame, P. (2015). Neither primary nor memory immunity to *Mycobacterium tuberculosis* infection is compromised in mice with chronic enteric helminth infection. *Infect. Immun.* 83, 1217–1223. doi: 10.1128/IAI.03004-14

Rausch, S., Huehn, J., Kirchhoff, D., Rzepecka, J., Schnoeller, C., Pillai, S., et al. (2008). Functional analysis of effector and regulatory T cells in a parasitic nematode infection. *Infect. Immun.* 76, 1908–1919. doi: 10.1128/IAI.01233-07

Reese, T. A., Bi, K., Kambal, A., Filali-Mouhim, A., Beura, L. K., Bürger, M. C., et al. (2016). Sequential Infection with common pathogens promotes human-like immune gene expression and altered vaccine response. *Cell Host Microbe* 19, 713–719. doi: 10.1016/j.chom.2016.04.003

Reynolds, L. A., Filbey, K. J., and Maizels, R. M. (2012). Immunity to the model intestinal helminth parasite *Heligmosomoides polygyrus*. *Semin. Immunopathol.* 34, 829–846. doi: 10.1007/s00281-012-0347-3

Rousseau, D., Le Fichoux, Y., Stien, X., Suffia, I., Ferrua, B., and Kubar, J. (1997). Progression of visceral leishmaniasis due to Leishmania infantum in BALB/c mice is markedly slowed by prior infection with *Trichinella spiralis*. *Infect. Immun.* 65, 4978–4983.

Scanga, C. A., Aliberti, J., Jankovic, D., Tilloy, F., Bennouna, S., Denkers, E. Y., et al. (2002). Cutting edge: MyD88 is required for resistance to *Toxoplasma gondii* Infection and regulates parasite-induced IL-12 production by dendritic cells. *J. Immunol.* 168, 5997–6001. doi: 10.4049/jimmunol.168.12.5997

Smith, K. A., Hochweller, K., Hämmerling, G. J., Boon, L., MacDonald, A. S., and Maizels, R. M. (2011). Chronic helminth infection promotes immune regulation *in vivo* through dominance of CD11cloCD103- dendritic cells. *J. Immunol.* 186, 7098–7109. doi: 10.4049/jimmunol.1003636

Steinfelder, S., Andersen, J. F., Cannons, J. L., Feng, C. G., Joshi, M., Dwyer, D., et al. (2009). The major component in schistosome eggs responsible for conditioning dendritic cells for Th2 polarization is a T2 ribonuclease (omega-1). *J. Exp. Med.* 206, 1681–1690. doi: 10.1084/jem.20082462

Steinfelder, S., O'Regan, N. L., and Hartmann, S. (2016). Diplomatic assistance: can helminth-modulated macrophages act as treatment for inflammatory disease? *PLoS Pathog.* 12:e1005480. doi: 10.1371/journal.ppat.1005480

Sturge, C. R., Benson, A., Raetz, M., Wilhelm, C. L., Mirpuri, J., Vitetta, E. S., et al. (2013). TLR-independent neutrophil-derived IFN-γ is important for host resistance to intracellular pathogens. *Proc. Natl. Acad. Sci. U.S.A.* 110, 10711–10716. doi: 10.1073/pnas.1307868110

Su, L., Qi, Y., Zhang, M., Weng, M., Zhang, X., Su, C., et al. (2014a). Development of fatal intestinal inflammation in MyD88 deficient mice co-infected with helminth and bacterial enteropathogens. *PLoS Negl. Trop. Dis.* 8:e2987. doi: 10.1371/journal.pntd.0002987

Su, L., Su, C., Qi, Y., Yang, G., Zhang, M., Cherayil, B. J., et al. (2014b). Coinfection with an intestinal helminth impairs host innate immunity against *Salmonella enterica* serovar Typhimurium and exacerbates intestinal inflammation in mice. *Infect. Immun.* 82, 3855–3866. doi: 10.1128/IAI.02023-14

Su, Z., Segura, M., Morgan, K., Loredo-Osti, J. C., and Stevenson, M. M. (2005). Impairment of protective immunity to blood-stage malaria by concurrent nematode infection. *Infect. Immun.* 73, 3531-3539. doi: 10.1128/IAI.73.6.3531-3539.2005

Swamy, M., Jamora, C., Havran, W., and Hayday, A. (2010). Epithelial decision makers: in search of the "epimmunome." *Nat. Immunol.* 11, 656–665. doi: 10.1038/ni.1905

Szabo, S. J., Kim, S. T., Costa, G. L., Zhang, X., Fathman, C. G., and Glimcher, L. H. (2000). A novel transcription factor, T-bet, directs Th1 lineage commitment. *Cell* 100, 655–669. doi: 10.1016/S0092-8674(00)80702-3

Tao, L., and Reese, T. A. (2017). Making mouse models that reflect human immune responses. *Trends Immunol.* 38, 181–193. doi: 10.1016/j.it.2016.12.007

Taylor, M. D., van der Werf, N., and Maizels, R. M. (2012). T cells in helminth infection: the regulators and the regulated. *Trends Immunol.* 33, 181–189. doi: 10.1016/j.it.2012.01.001

Wang, Y.-H., Angkasekwinai, P., Lu, N., Voo, K. S., Arima, K., Hanabuchi, S., et al. (2007). IL-25 augments type 2 immune responses by enhancing the expansion and functions of TSLP-DC-activated Th2 memory cells. *J. Exp. Med.* 204, 1837–1847. doi: 10.1084/jem.20070406

Weng, M., Huntley, D., Huang, I.-F., Foye-Jackson, O., Wang, L., Sarkissian, A., et al. (2007). Alternatively activated macrophages in intestinal helminth infection: effects on concurrent bacterial colitis. *J. Immunol.* 179, 4721–4731. doi: 10.4049/jimmunol.179.7.4721

WHO (2017). *Soil-Transmitted Helminth Infections*. Available online at: http://www.who.int/mediacentre/factsheets/fs366/en/

Wohlfert, E. A., Grainger, J. R., Bouladoux, N., Konkel, J. E., Oldenhove, G., Ribeiro, C. H., et al. (2011). GATA3 controls Foxp3^{+} regulatory T cell fate during inflammation in mice. *J. Clin. Invest.* 121, 4503–4515. doi: 10.1172/JCI57456

Yazdanbakhsh, M., van den Biggelaar, A., and Maizels, R. M. (2001). Th2 responses without atopy: immunoregulation in chronic helminth infections and reduced allergic disease. *Trends Immunol.* 22, 372–377. doi: 10.1016/S1471-4906(01)01958-5

Zheng, W., and Flavell, R. A. (1997). The transcription factor GATA-3 is necessary and sufficient for Th2 cytokine gene expression in CD4 T cells. *Cell* 89, 587–596. doi: 10.1016/S0092-8674(00)80240-8

Zhu, J., Jankovic, D., Oler, A. J., Wei, G., Sharma, S., Hu, G., et al. (2012). The transcription factor T-bet is induced by multiple pathways and prevents an endogenous Th2 cell program during Th1 cell responses. *Immunity* 37, 660–673. doi: 10.1016/j.immuni.2012.09.007

12

Increased *Plasmodium falciparum* Parasitemia in Non-splenectomized *Saimiri sciureus* Monkeys Treated with Clodronate Liposomes

Janaiara A. Cunha[1†], Leonardo J. M. Carvalho[1†], Cesare Bianco-Junior[1], Márcia C. R. Andrade[2], Lilian R. Pratt-Riccio[1], Evelyn K. P. Riccio[1], Marcelo Pelajo-Machado[3], Igor J. da Silva[3], Pierre Druilhe[4] and Cláudio Tadeu Daniel-Ribeiro[1]*

[1] Laboratório de Pesquisa em Malária, Instituto Oswaldo Cruz, Fundação Oswaldo Cruz (Fiocruz), Rio de Janeiro, Brazil, [2] Instituto de Ciência e Tecnologia em Biomodelos, Fiocruz, Rio de Janeiro, Brazil, [3] Laboratório de Patologia, Instituto Oswaldo Cruz, Fiocruz, Rio de Janeiro, Brazil, [4] Vac4All Initiative, Pepinière Paris Biotech Santé, Paris, France

Edited by:
Kai Matuschewski,
Humboldt-Universität zu Berlin,
Germany

Reviewed by:
Ashley Vaughan,
Center for Infectious Disease Research, United States
Jodi L. McGill,
Kansas State University, United States

***Correspondence:**
Cláudio Tadeu Daniel-Ribeiro
malaria@fiocruz.br

† These authors have contributed equally to this work.

A major constraint in the study of *Plasmodium falciparum* malaria, including vaccine development, lies on the parasite's strict human host specificity and therefore the shortage of animal experimental models able to harbor human plasmodia. The best experimental models are neo-tropical primates of the genus Saimiri and Aotus, but they require splenectomy to reduce innate defenses for achieving high and consistent parasitemias, an important limitation. Clodronate-liposomes (CL) have been successfully used to deplete monocytes/macrophages in several experimental models. We investigated whether a reduction in the numbers of phagocytic cells by CL would improve the development of *P. falciparum* parasitemia in non-splenectomized *Saimiri sciureus* monkeys. Depletion of *S. sciureus* splenocytes after *in vitro* incubation with CL was quantified using anti-CD14 antibodies and flow cytometry. Non-infected and *P. falciparum*-infected *S. sciureus* were injected intravenously twice a week with either CL at either 0.5 or 1 mL (5 mg/mL) or phosphate buffered saline (PBS). Animals were monitored during infection and treated with mefloquine. After treatment and euthanasia, spleen and liver were collected for histological analysis. *In vitro* CL depleted *S. sciureus* splenic monocyte/macrophage population in a dose- and time-dependent manner. *In vivo*, half of *P. falciparum*-infected *S. sciureus* treated with CL 0.5 mL, and two-thirds of those treated with CL 1 mL developed high parasitemias requiring mefloquine treatment, whereas all control animals were able to self-control parasitemia without the need for antimalarial treatment. CL-treated infected *S. sciureus* showed a marked decrease in the degree of splenomegaly despite higher parasitemias, compared to PBS-treated animals. Histological evidence of partial monocyte/macrophage depletion, decreased hemozoin phagocytosis and decreased iron recycling was observed in both the spleen and liver of CL-treated infected *S. sciureus*. CL is capable of promoting higher parasitemia in *P. falciparum*-infected *S. sciureus*, associated with evidence of partial macrophage depletion in the spleen and liver. Macrophage depletion by CL is therefore a practical and viable alternative to surgical splenectomy in this experimental model.

Keywords: malaria, *Plasmodium falciparum*, *Saimiri sciureus*, clodronate liposomes, macrophages, spleen, liver

INTRODUCTION

According to the World Health Organization (WHO) estimates, 212 million cases of malaria occurred in 2015, with 429,000 deaths (WHO, 2016). Among the *five* Plasmodium species capable of causing human malaria, *Plasmodium falciparum* is associated with more severe and lethal forms of the disease (Rowe et al., 2009; Quintero et al., 2011). Due to increasing parasite resistance to currently available antimalarial drugs (Chrubasik and Jacobson, 2010; Dondorp et al., 2010), development of an effective vaccine against malaria is urgently needed. Currently, *one* of the promising vaccine candidates (RTS,S/AS01) is being tested in a Phase III clinical trial in Africa in order to inform a decision regarding its deployment (Clemens and Moorthy, 2016; Olotu et al., 2016; Otieno et al., 2016). Another candidate, the MSP3 experimental vaccine, had a promising performance in African children in a double-blind follow-up of a preliminary Phase I study (Sirima et al., 2011). However, there is no assurance that these candidates will become indeed effective vaccines in the near future. Continued evaluation of potential vaccines is therefore expected and necessary.

Animal models for pre-clinical studies are an important component in vaccine development, but the limited availability of experimental models that can harbor human malaria is a critical constraint. The neo-tropical primates of the genus Saimiri and Aotus are experimental models recommended by WHO for pre-clinical testing of malaria vaccine candidates (WHO, 2004). Studies using the *Saimiri sciureus* model showed that immunization against *P. falciparum* blood stage vaccine candidate antigens such as the glutamate-rich protein (GLURP), the merozoite surface protein-3 (MSP3), or the SE36 antigen, using different adjuvants, may induce potent antibody responses and elicit partially protective immunity upon challenge (Carvalho et al., 2004, 2005; Tougan et al., 2013). Besides being susceptible to *P. vivax* and to *P. falciparum* infection (Gysin and Fandeur, 1983; Carvalho et al., 2000, 2002, 2004, 2005; Contamin et al., 2000; Herrera et al., 2002; Collins et al., 2005), these primates are abundant in nature and can be easily handled in captivity due to their relatively small size. Furthermore, they are able to reproduce clinical and pathological manifestations of human malaria such as thrombocytopenia, changes in leukocyte counts and anemia, offering an appropriate model to study the immunopathogenesis of malaria (Contamin et al., 2000; Carvalho et al., 2003). The limited availability of immunological tools to study the immune response in these animals imposes some constraints, but human reagents can be used to some extent and specific Saimiri reagents have been generated (Garraud et al., 1998; Contamin et al., 2005; Alves et al., 2010; Riccio et al., 2015). However, these models also have disadvantages. One of the major constraints is the need for splenectomy to achieve high and consistent parasitemias (Collins, 1992). The immune response against the erythrocytic forms of the parasite is largely mediated by resident cells in the spleen (Criswell et al., 1971; Achtman et al., 2003; Leisewitz et al., 2004) and this organ has critical roles in the immune response during malarial infections. Therefore, radical surgical splenectomy poses a strong limitation for testing malaria vaccines, as the very immune responses the vaccines are intended to elicit may be affected by the intervention. Therefore, alternative approaches to allow increased *P. falciparum* parasitemias in *S. sciureus* without the need for surgical splenectomy are necessary for proper evaluation of potential vaccines.

Liposomes containing a toxic chemical induce macrophage "suicide," depleteing phagocytes in specific tissues. Clodronate, a bisphosphonate drug that activates apoptosis, has been the most widely employed compound in this respect. It has been demonstrated in several animal models, including mice, dogs, and pigs, that macrophages ingest the liposome particles by phagocytosis and are destroyed or become functionally inactivated (van Rooijen and van Nieuwmegen, 1984; Mathes et al., 2006; Kim et al., 2008). The spleen is a site of important macrophage activity and destruction of blood-borne microorganisms including Plasmodium, senescent red blood cells, and clodronate-encapsulated liposomes (van Rooijen and van Nieuwmegen, 1984; van Rooijen and Kors, 1989; van Rooijen et al., 1990; van Rooijen and van Kesteren-Hendrikx, 2002; Abbas et al., 2008). Chemical "splenectomy" by clodronate liposomes is expected to induce higher *P. falciparum* parasitemias as it depletes monocyte/macrophages in large numbers while preserving spleen structure and functions. Indeed, in immunocompromised mice lacking B, T, and NK cells, *P. falciparum* growth was fully controlled by macrophages. Conversely, *P. falciparum* could successfully replicate at very high parasite densities for several weeks when macrophage populations were controlled by repeated administration of clodronate-encapsulated liposomes (Badell et al., 2000; Arnold et al., 2010, 2011). If the same system can be used in *P. falciparum* infections in *S. sciureus* monkeys, it can provide a much improved model for testing malaria vaccines. In such a system, the phagocytic activity of monocytes/macrophages would be decreased allowing increased parasitemia in naive animals, but it is expected that effective vaccines inducing protective adaptative immune responses, in a scenario of preserved spleen structure and function, will be able to contain parasite growth.

In this study, we investigated whether a decrease in the number of monocytes/macrophages by using clodronate-encapsulated liposomes would favor the development of consistent *P. falciparum* parasitemias in *S. sciureus* monkeys without the need for surgical splenectomy, through a "chemical splenectomy." This procedure would also be more respectful of ethical considerations than surgery, because of its transient nature resulting in fast restitutio ad integrum.

MATERIALS AND METHODS

Animals

The animals used in this study were male and female *S. sciureus*, karyotype 14-7, ranging in age from 3 to 19 years and in weight from 0.548 to 0.926 kg. The monkeys, non-splenectomized and malaria-naïve, were obtained from the breeding colony of the Primatology Service (CECAL/Fiocruz), Rio de Janeiro, Brazil. In total, 34 animals were used in *three* independent experiments (**Table 1**). This study was carried out in accordance

TABLE 1 | Number of *Saimiri sciureus* monkeys used per experiment.

	Exp 1	Exp 2	Exp 3	Total
NInf PBS	–	2	1	3
NInf 0.5 mL CL	–	2	1	3
NInf 1.0 mL CL	–	2	1	3
Inf PBS	3	2	3	8
Inf 0.5 mL CL	–	3	4	7
Inf 1.0 mL CL	3	3	4	10
TOTAL	6	14	14	34

Exp, experiment; NInf, non-infected animals; Inf, P. falciparum-infected animals; CL, Clodronate-encapsulated liposomes.

with the recommendations and approved by the Fiocruz Ethics Committee on Animal Use (CEUA Licences L-0062/08 and LW-9/14).

Clodronate-Encapsulated Liposomes

Clodronate-encapsulated liposomes (CL, 5 mg/mL clodronate) were obtained from ClodronateLiposome.org (Department of Molecular Cell Biology and Immunology of the Vrije Universiteit Medisch Centrum - University Amsterdam, VUmc - Netherlands).

Evaluation of Clodronate-Liposome on Macrophages/Monocytes *in Vitro*

Cryopreserved Saimiri splenocytes obtained during splenectomy of *three* naïve animals were thawed, washed twice with pure RPMI medium (Gibco, Grand Island, New York, EUA), resuspended in RPMI supplemented with 10% fetal bovine serum (FBS, Invitrogen, Grand Island, New York, EUA) at a concentration of 5×10^5 cells/ 500 μL and incubated in 5 mL culture tubes (Falcon, BD Biosciences, San Jose, CA, EUA) in RPMI medium containing 15 mM glutamine (Gibco), 10 mM Hepes (Sigma-Aldrich, St. Louis, MO, EUA), 200 U/mL penicillin (Gibco), 200 μg/mL streptomycin (Gibco), 3 mg/mL gentamicin (Sigma-Aldrich) and 2 g/L sodium bicarbonate (Sigma-Aldrich) supplemented with 10% inactivated fetal bovine serum (Invitrogen). CL suspension was added at concentrations of 1, 10, and 100 μg/mL and incubated for 4, 8, 16, or 24 h at 37°C and 5% CO_2. After culture, cells were labeled with anti-CD14-APC antibody (clone 61D3, eBioscience, Science Center Dr. San Diego, CA, EUA), a marker of macrophages and monocytes, and quantified by flow cytometry in the CyAn cell analyser (Dako Cytomation Inc., Carpinteria, CA, EUA) by counting 60,000 events. Data were analyzed using the software Summit (Dako Cytomation).

Evaluation of Clodronate-Liposome *in Vivo*

Plasmodium falciparum FUP strain (Carvalho et al., 2004) was recovered from cryostabilates and the parasitized red blood cells (pRBCs) were passaged by intravenous inoculation in a splenectomized donor monkey. pRBCs from the passage animal were used to infect the experimental group animals intravenously with an inoculum of 10^6 pRBC. The animals were divided into *six* groups, *three* with infected (Inf) animals and *three* control, non-infected (NInf) groups: (1) NInf receiving 1 mL of phosphate buffered saline (PBS - Sigma-Aldrich); (2) NInf receiving 0.5 mL of clodronate-encapsulated liposome (CL); (3) NInf receiving 1 mL of CL; (4) Inf receiving 1 mL of PBS; (5) Inf receiving 0.5 mL of CL; (6) Inf receiving 1 mL of CL. CL injections were performed intravenously *two* times a week, from day 0 of infection. *Three* independent experiments were performed using a total of 34 animals (**Table 1**).

The follow up of infection included a daily evaluation of parasitemia by thin Giemsa-stained blood films, hematocrit (microhematocrit method) and hemoglogin levels twice a week (using the HemoCue Hb301 system, HemoCue AB, Ängelholm, Sweden) as well as daily measurement of body (rectal) temperature. Blood monocyte count was done, twice a week starting from day 0 of infection, by flow cytometry using anti-CD14-APC antibody (clone 61D3, eBioscience) in a CyAn cell analyser (Dako Cytomation) and the data were analyzed using the software Summit (Dako Cytomation). An experienced veterinarian performed daily clinical examinations. Monkeys were treated with mefloquine (15 mg/kg—Biomanguinhos, Fiocruz, Rio de Janeiro, RJ, Brazil) when parasitemia reached 20% or above or in case the hematocrit reached 20% or below or when the monkeys presented manifestations of severe disease (prostration, anorexia). Monkeys that spontaneously controlled their parasitemia also received mefloquine on day 17 to ensure complete parasite clearance. *Four* days after mefloquine treatment, with animals no longer presenting patent parasitemia, all animals (including the uninfected controls) received a last injection of CL (or PBS) and were euthanized 24 h later. The animals were euthanized with 7 mg/kg thiopental (Cristália, Itapira, SP, Brazil) inoculated directly into the heart muscle, after being anesthesized with ketamine (Cristália) 100 mg/kg plus midazolam (União Química, Embu-Guaçu, SP, Brazil) 10 mg/kg. After the death of the animal, liver and spleen were harvested for histological analysis.

Spleen and Liver Analysis

Immediately after liver and spleen harvest, macroscopic evaluation was performed and the spleen was weighted. Samples of the liver and spleen were fixed using a 4% formaldehyde solution (Merk - Darmstadt, Germany) in Millonig's buffer (0.1 M sodium hydroxide, 0.13 M sodium phosphate monobasic—Sigma-Aldrich) and later processed for histology. Paraffin-embedded sections (5 μm) were stained with hematoxylin and eosin (HE), Giemsa or Prussian blue. The slides were analyzed with the aid of a microscope (AxioImager A2, Zeiss, Oberkochen, Germany) and images were captured using an Axiocam HRM (Zeiss) and the software AxionVision Release 4.8.2 (Zeiss).

For hemozoin quantitation in the spleen, the histology slices were dyed with Nuclear Fast Red and mounted with coverslips. Each slide was then completely scanned using VSlide (Metasystems, Germany), generating high definition images (0.8 NA) of all the slices. Because the original images were too big, they were divided into *three* parts for analysis, by using ImageJ, where the red (nuclei) and brown/black (hemozoin) colors were separated with the color threshold function. The hemozoin areas and the total tissue area in each image were measured in square pixels. These results were then used to estimate the relative hemozoin area in each slide.

Statistical Analysis

The significance of the differences between the results or means of all variables was examined by the nonparametric Kruskal-Wallis analysis followed by Dunn test (GraphPad Prism 6, GraphPad Software Inc., San Diego, CA, USA). Results were considered to be statistically significant when $p < 0.05$.

RESULTS

Effect of Clodronate-Encapsulated Liposomes on *S. sciureus* Monocytes *in Vitro*

Even though CL has been used as a rapid inducer of apoptosis of monocytes/macrophages *in vivo* and *in vitro*, especially in mice, there are no available data on the effect of CL in *S. sciureus* monocytes. *In vitro* incubation of *S. sciureus* splenocytes with CL induced death of CD14+ cells (monocyte/macrophage) in a dose-dependent manner, with marked depletion at 100 μg/mL (**Figure 1**).

Effect of Clodronate-Encapsulated Liposomes on *P. falciparum* Infection in *S. sciureus* Monkeys

Parasitemia

Saimiri sciureus monkeys infected with *P. falciparum* and receiving PBS showed variable courses of parasitemia (**Figure 2A**). The maximum parasite density varied between 4.8 and 17.7% (peak average 8.1%). Most animals kept parasitemia below 10%, and one showed extremely low parasitemia throughout the follow up. The peak parasitemia was reached between days 11 and 15. All animals were able to control parasitemia without the need for antimalarial drug treatment. The infected animals receiving 0.5 mL CL also showed variable courses of parasitemia, which reached peak levels between days 10 and 15, with parasite densities ranging between 3.9 and 26.7%

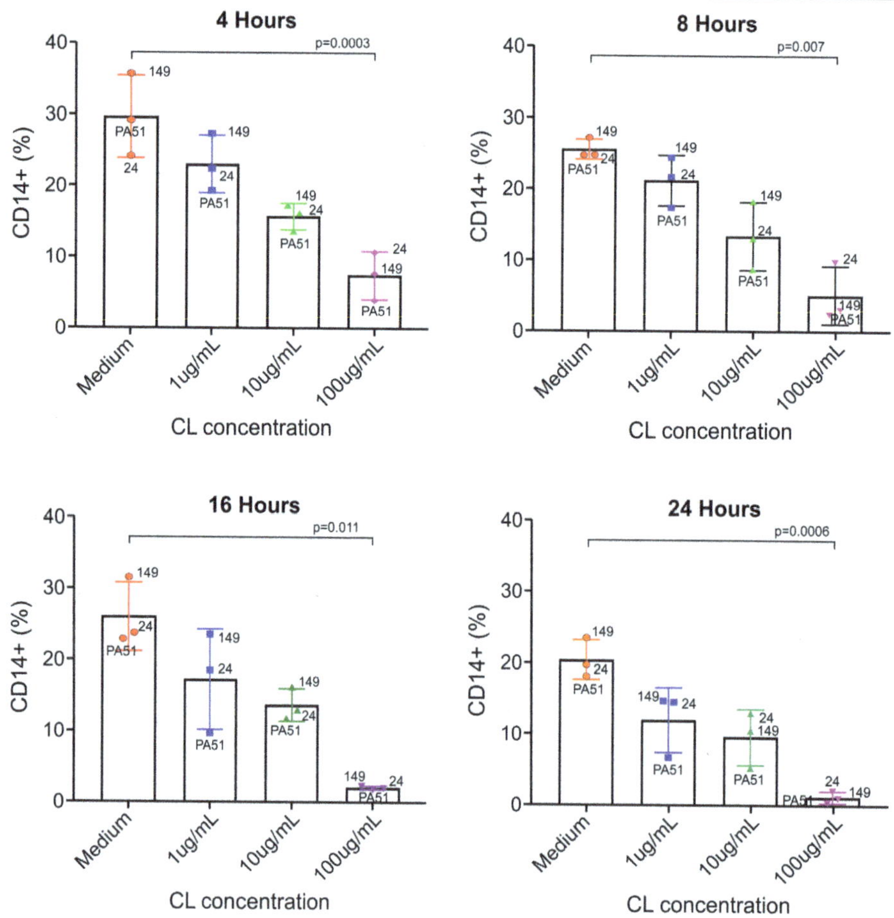

FIGURE 1 | Effect of CL on *S. sciureus* splenocyte viability *in vitro*. CL induced dose-dependent cytotoxicity in monocytes/macrophages. 24, 149, and PA51 refer to *S. sciureus* identification. Medium vs. 100 μg/ml: 4 h ($p = 0.0003$), 8 h ($p = 0.007$), 16 h ($p = 0.011$), and 24 h ($p = 0.0006$). %: percentage of CD14+ cells in total number of splenocytes.

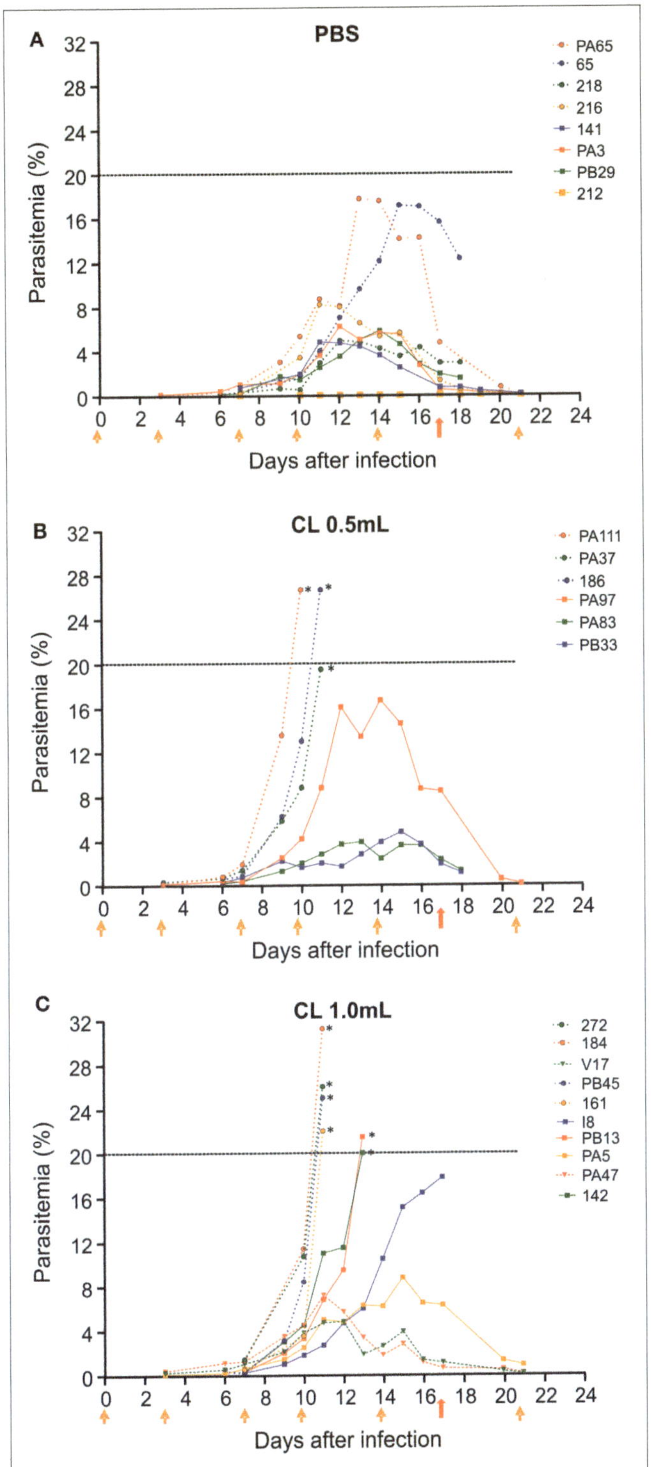

FIGURE 2 | Course of parasitemia after infection of *S. sciureus* with 10^6 pRBC/mL by FUP strain of *P. falciparum*. Parasitemia is shown for animals that received PBS (controls) **(A)**; clodronate liposomes (CL) 0.5 mL **(B)**; or CL 1.0 mL **(C)**. Data are from three separate experiments, with 6–9 animals per group. Orange arrows indicate the timepoints when PBS or CL was given to the animals. Red arrows indicate treatment with mefloquine. Dashed line represents the limit of parasitemia established for treatment (20%) with mefloquine. *Animals that received treatment with mefloquine before day 17 for reaching 20% parasitemia.

(average 16.4%) (**Figure 2B**). Of the *six* animals in this group, *three* (50%) required treatment with mefloquine due to high parasitemia (26.7, 19.5, and 26.7%). In the group of infected animals receiving 1 mL CL the maximum parasite density varied between 4.7 and 31.2% (average 18.5%) and peak parasitemia was reached between days 11 and 15. Of the *nine* animals in the group, *six* (66.6%) required antimalarial treatment due to high parasitemia (22; 26; 31.2; 25; 20, and 21.5%). Depending on the need for treatment and treatment time, animals received a minimum of *four* and a maximum of seven CL injections.

CD14+ Cell Count in Peripheral Blood

There was no apparent effect of *P. falciparum* infection or CL injections on circulating monocytes, as verified by CD14+ cell counts in peripheral blood (**Figure 3**).

Anemia and Other Clinical Parameters

In *P. falciparum*-infected animals, hemoglobin concentration and hematocrit decreased reaching minimum values during or after parasite clearance (**Figure 4**). No weight loss greater than 10% was observed. Body temperature increased 1–2°C during infection and decreased after antimalarial treatment (data not shown). Some animals showed loss of appetite and prostration at the time of peak parasitemia. *Two* animals that received CL 1 mL and presented high parasitemias showed hematuria at the time of peak parasitemia that reversed after mefloquine treatment. Results of experiments 1, 2, and 3 showing the data of parasitemia, CD14 counting, hematocrit, hemoglobin and rectal temperature are shown in **Supplemental Table 1**.

Changes in the Structure of the Spleen and Liver

All infected animals that developed parasitemia over 20% were treated with mefloquine between days 11 and 13 of infection, whereas all other infected animals were treated on day 17. All uninfected and infected-treated animals received a last injection of CL (or PBS) *four* days after mefloquine treatment, when parasitemia had cleared, and were euthanized 24 h later. Spleen and liver were harvested and processed for histological analysis.

Spleen

Treatment of uninfected *S. sciureus* with CL caused no perceivable changes in spleen weight in relation to uninfected animals that received PBS (**Figure 5**). *Plasmodium falciparum* infection, as expected, led to splenomegaly, with an average 5-fold increase in spleen/body weight ratios compared to uninfected animals. Treatment of *P. falciparum*-infected *S. sciureus* with CL 1 mL led to substantial reduction (average of 55%) in the degree of splenomegaly compared to infected animals that received only PBS (**Figure 5** and **Supplemental Table 1**). The decrease in spleen/body weight ratios in animals treated with CL 0.5 mL was less prominent and did not reach significance compared to PBS-treated animals, although the lack of significance is likely due to the small sample size.

The spleen of uninfected, control animals that received PBS showed typical *S. sciureus* splenic architecture, with well-defined limits between the red and white pulps, resting T cell areas, mostly resting follicles, and in some cases with phase I and

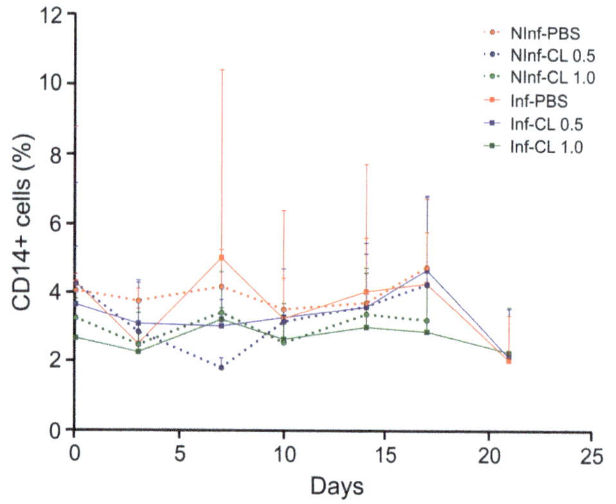

FIGURE 3 | Changes in blood monocyte counts during *P. falciparum* infection and CL administration. Monocyte quantification was performed by flow cytometry using anti-CD14-APC antibodies. Solid lines represent the mean and standard deviation. %: percentage of CD14+ cells in total number of peripheral blood monocuclear cells (PBMC). NInf, non-infected control groups; Inf, *P. falciparum*-infected groups.

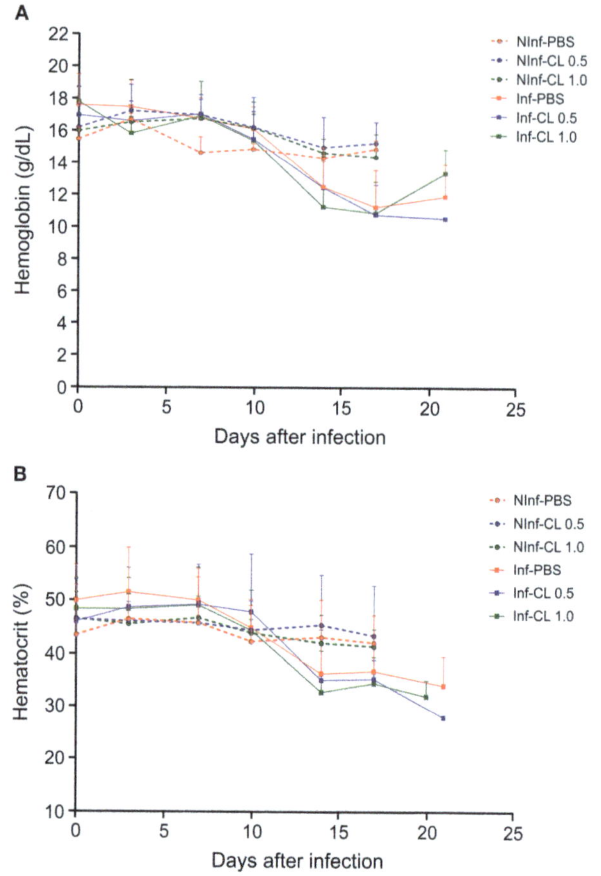

FIGURE 4 | Hemoglobin concentration in the blood **(A)** and hematocrit **(B)** of *S. sciureus*. NInf, non-infected control groups; Inf, *P. falciparum*-infected groups. Solid lines represent the mean and standard deviation.

phase II germinal centers containing a few apoptotic centers, absence of pigment and plasmacytes, and areas of monocyte accumulation in the marginal zone and the red pulp (**Figure 6A**), as previously described (Alves et al., 2015). Uninfected animals that received CL (0.5 or 1 mL) showed decreased number of clusters of monocyte/macrophages in red pulp and of apoptotic centers in the follicles compared to animals that received PBS (**Figure 6B**).

Infected animals that received PBS showed phagocitosed malarial pigment (hemozoin) throughout the red pulp (**Figure 6C**). Erythroid precursors and plasmacytes were observed, and the marginal zone was in disarray (**Figure 6C**). Infected animals that received CL 1 mL showed substantial reduction in the accumulation of malarial pigment in the red pulp (**Figure 6D**), despite the fact that these animals in general showed much higher parasitemias (average 18.5%) as compared to infected animals that received PBS (average 8.1%), although for shorter periods of time (**Figure 2**).

The analysis of spleen sections stained with Perls, which shows ferric iron (Fe^{3+}) within macrophages and can be used not only to observe the physiology of iron recycling but also to estimate the distribution of these cells, revealed that uninfected, control animals showed clusters of iron-containing macrophages distributed throughout the red pulp, and mild staining within follicles (**Figure 7A**). Uninfected, control animals that received CL 0.5 and 1 mL showed reduced amounts of iron-containing macrophages (**Figure 7B**).

Infected animals treated with PBS showed iron staining in the red pulp, but substantially less than uninfected controls (**Figure 7C**). However, as mentioned above (**Figure 6C**), large numbers of hemozoin-containing macrophages were observed. As a rule, there was little or absent colocalization of iron

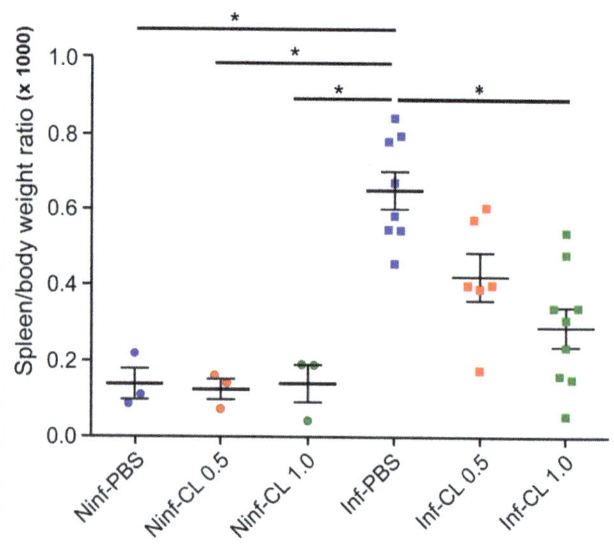

FIGURE 5 | Effect of *P. falciparum* infection and/or CL administration on spleen/body weight ratios. Solid lines represent the mean and standard deviation. *$P < 0.05$.

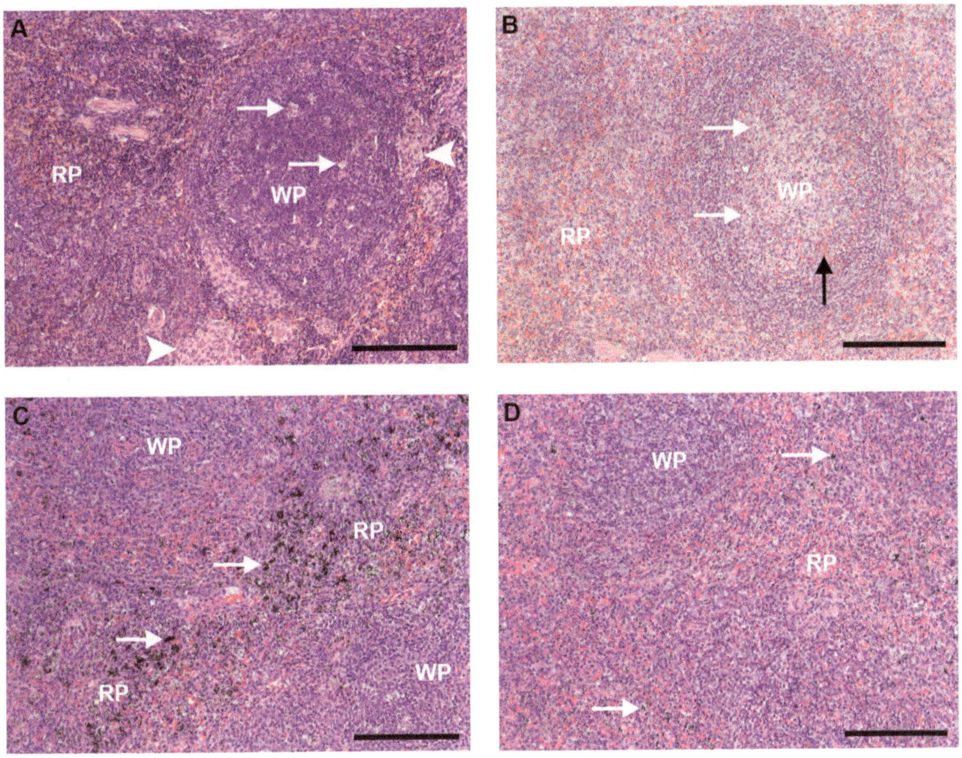

FIGURE 6 | Spleen sections HE staining (bar: 200 μm). **(A)** Spleen of an uninfected, control animal that received PBS (code PA11). **(A)** B-cell follicle (WP, white pulp) is shown, with a few apoptotic centers (arrows); clusters of monocyte/macrophages, typical of Saimiri spleens, are present (arrowheads). The red pulp (RP) shows typical architecture, densily populated with small-nuclei, dark-stained cells, and red blood cells (red stain) flowing through. **(B)** Spleen of an uninfected Saimiri inoculated with CL 1 mL (code V3). In general, the splenic structure was preserved, but cell density was apparently smaller as compared to animals that received PBS, with predominance of cells with light-stained nuclei; penetration of red blood cells inside B-cell follicle was observed (black arrow); apoptotic centers (arrows), which are dependent on macrophages, and clusters of monocyte/macrophages were decreased (clusters of monocytes absent in this image). **(C)** Spleen of a *P. falciparum*-infected Saimiri that received PBS (code 141: treated at day 17, with 0.69% parasitemia, killed 5 days later). Emphasis is given to the distribution of hemozoin (seen as dark, granulated stain - arrows), which could be found throughout the red pulp (RP); loss of well-defined limits between the RP and the white pulp (WP) was observed. **(D)** Spleen of a *P. falciparum*-infected Saimiri that received CL 1 mL (code 272: treated at day 11, with 22 % parasitemia, killed 5 days later). The amount of hemozoin (arrows) was substantially decreased compared to infected animals that received PBS, and seen as small black dots. As in **(C)**, loss of well-defined limits between the red pulp (RP) and the white pulp (WP) was observed.

staining and hemozoin (macrophages showed only *one* staining, **Figure 7C**). Infected animals treated with CL showed less iron staining as compared to animals that received PBS, and also less hemozoin staining (**Figures 7D, 10**).

Liver

With HE staining, livers of uninfected control animals that received PBS showed typical structure, with healthy hepatocytes and absence of necrosis or vacuolization and Kupffer cells without pigment (**Figure 8A** and **Supplemental Figure 1A**). Mononuclear cell infiltrates in the portal space were occasionally observed. Livers of animals that received CL 0.5 or 1 mL showed either no significant changes or, in some cases, evidence of hepatocyte vacuolization. **Figure 8B** shows *one* of these areas of hepatocyte vacuolization, an event that was only occasionally found but may indicate some degree of toxicity induced by CL treatment.

Infected animals that received PBS showed large numbers of mononuclear cells and also erythroid cells, neutrophils and plasmacytes within sinusoids, mononuclear cell infiltration in the portal space, and Kupffer cells containing malarial pigment (**Figure 8C** and **Supplemental Figures 1B–D**). Diffuse vacuolization of hepatocytes was observed in *two* thirds of the animals. Infected animals that received CL showed areas of intense hepatocyte vacuolization, and there were apparently fewer Kupffer cells with malarial pigment than in infected animals that received PBS (**Figure 8D**).

Perls staining of liver sections revealed that uninfected animals that received PBS showed strong iron staining throughout the organ, with granules within hepatocytes and Kupffer cells (**Figure 9A**). Iron staining in liver sections of uninfected animals that received CL 0.5 or 1 mL was less intense than in those that received PBS (**Figure 9B**).

Infected animals that received PBS showed large amounts of hemozoin. Iron staining was weak throughout the organ, but still present in hepatocytes and isolated Kupffer cells or adherent macrophages within sinusoids, with little or no colocalization with hemozoin (**Figure 9C** and **Supplemental Figures 2A,B**).

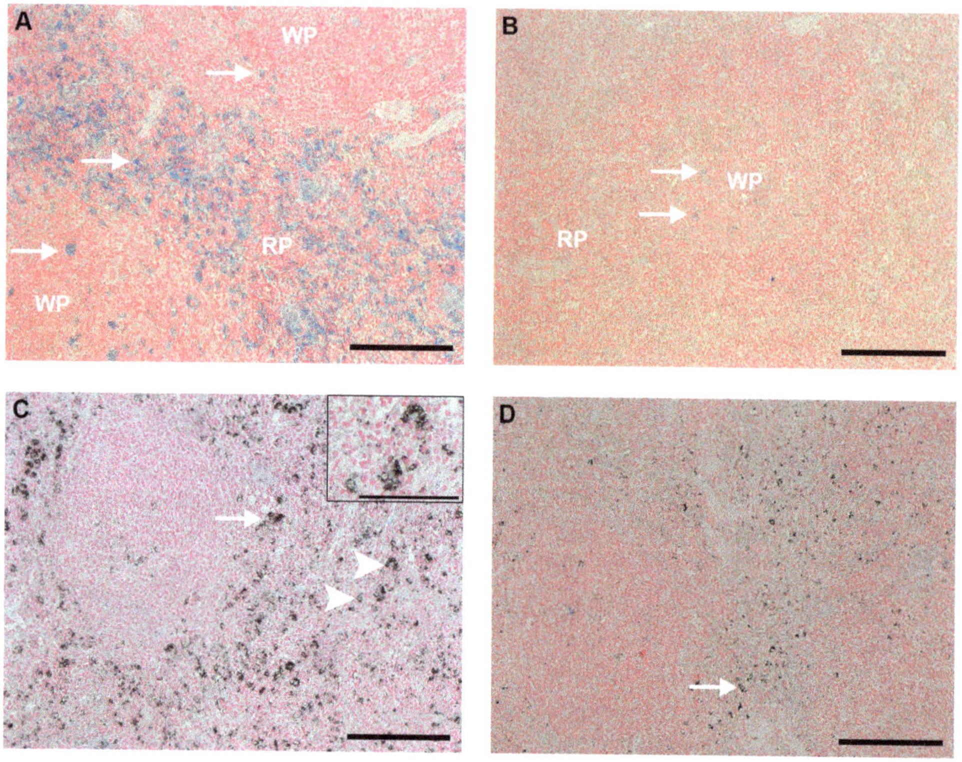

FIGURE 7 | Spleen sections Perls staining (bar: 200 μm, except in **C**, bar: 100 μm). **(A)** Spleen of an uninfected, control animal that received PBS (code PA11). Large amounts of ferric iron-containing macrophages (blue staining) were observed throughout the red pulp (RP), and also sparsed in follicles (arrows). **(B)** Spleen of an uninfected Saimiri inoculated with CL 1 mL (code PB75). Blue staining, representing ferric iron-containing macrophages, nearly disappeared from the red pulp (RP), and was faint in follicles (arrows). **(C)** Spleen of a *P. falciparum*-infected Saimiri that received PBS (code 216: treated at day 17, with 1,3% parasitemia, killed 5 days later). Blue staining, representing ferric iron-containing macrophages, was much fainter in the spleen of infected, compared to uninfected, *S. sciureus*; on the other hand, macrophages were laden with hemozoin (arrow); only few macrophages showed colocalization of iron staining and hemozoin (arrowheads and magnified insert on top right). **(D)** Spleen of a *P. falciparum*-infected Saimiri that received CL 1 mL (code 272: treated at day 11, with 22% parasitemia, killed 5 days later). Presence of iron staining was nearly absent, and presence of hemozoin (arrow) was much decreased in relation to **(C)**.

Infected animals that received CL 0.5 or 1 mL showed less intense hemozoin and iron staining, and Kupffer cells or macrophages with strong iron staining were rarely observed or not at all (**Figure 9D**).

Estimating the Efficacy of CL Treatment in Depleting Macrophages through Splenic Hemozoin Quantification

Qualitative analysis of spleen and liver, as shown in **Figures 6–9**, and decreased spleen/body weight ratios (**Figure 5**) indicated that CL treatment led to a decrease in macrophage population in these organs. Attempts to quantify macrophages using immunostaining with anti-human CD14, CD68, and HAM-56 monoclonal antibodies were unsucessful, probably due to the prolonged period in formalin. The effect of CL treatment on splenic macrophage numbers was therefore further estimated by quantifying hemozoin accumulation in this organ, which increases with increasing parasitemia (Sullivan et al., 1996), and hemozoin-laden macrophages remain in the spleen for several weeks (Frita et al., 2012). Although, CL-treated monkeys showed about half the splenic hemozoin accumulation as compared to PBS-treated animals (**Figure 10A**), this difference did not reach statistical significance due to small sample size and to some degree of variation between animals. However, when hemozoin concentration was adjusted to the level of parasitemia (hemozoin concentration/peak parasitemia, **Figure 10B**; hemozoin concentration/area under the curve of parasitemia, **Figure 10C**), marked differences were observed between the *two* groups, indicating that despite sustaining much higher parasite loads CL-treated animals showed less hemozoin accumulation in the spleen. These data indicate that splenic macrophages of CL-treated animals are either markedly decreased in numbers, as also suggested by HE staining and spleen weights, or are functionally impaired, in any case resulting in decreased capacity to phagocytose parasitized red blood cells.

DISCUSSION

Saimiri monkeys are susceptible to infection by *Plasmodium falciparum* and, together with Aotus, constitute unique experimental models for malaria (WHO, 2004), making these animals particularly useful in preclinical trials of potential

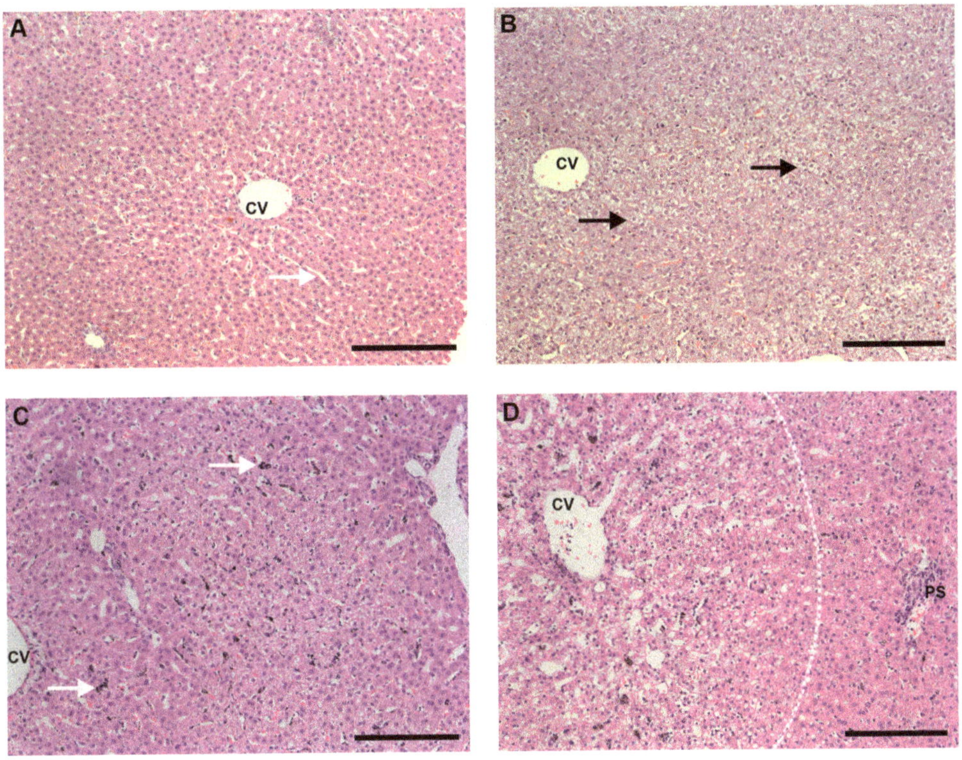

FIGURE 8 | Liver sections HE staining (bar: 200 μm). **(A)** Liver of an uninfected, control animal that received PBS (code PA67), showing typical architecture, healthy hepatocytes and clean synusoids (arrows); CV, centrilobular vein. **(B)** Liver of an uninfected Saimiri inoculated with CL 1 mL (code PB75). The general aspect of most sections was rather normal (similar to the pattern of **A**), but eventually areas of hepatocyte vacuolization, as depicted, were observed; CV, centrilobular vein. **(C)** Liver of a *P. falciparum*-infected Saimiri that received PBS (code 141: treated at day 17, with 0.69 % parasitemia, killed 5 days later). Kupffer cells laden with hemozoin (arrow); CV, centrilobular vein. **(D)** Liver of a *P. falciparum*-infected Saimiri that received CL 1 mL (code 161: treated at day 11, with 22% parasitemia, killed 5 days later). Intense hepatocyte vacuolization was observed, evidenced particularly in the left half of the image, closer to the centrilobular vein (CV) and away from the portal space (PS) (more vacuolized area and more preserved area separated by a dashed line).

malaria vaccines and for studies on pathogenesis (Carvalho et al., 2000, 2004, 2005). Pre-clinical evaluation of vaccines in these experimental models can provide valuable information about the immunogenicity, efficacy and safety of a variety of formulations, facilitating selection for humans trials. Since access to this valuable resource is restricted, with limited number of animals available for research, optimization of the model is needed to allow the design of experiments with reduced sample sizes. This goal faces *two* important limitations regarding the use of non-splenectomized animals: (1) they usually develop low parasitemias, which makes it more difficult to detect the effect of interventions, such as vaccines, on the course of infection; and (2) there is substantial interindividual variability in the levels of parasitemias (Contamin et al., 2000). These *two* factors underscore the need to increase sample sizes in experiments using these animals. The alternative to overcome these limitations has been the use of splenectomized animals, which achieve higher and more consistent parasitemias, allowing smaller experimental groups to be formed. However, this strategy also faces important setbacks: (a) the spleen plays a central role in immunity against plasmodial infections and (b) non-human primates (NHP) are chosen as models for experimental studies with human plasmodia, mainly vaccines, because of their close filogenetic relationship to man. Splenectomy pushes back the model from the natural human situation. For these reasons, splenectomy constitutes a severe handicap especially in immunity and vaccine studies. The use of the "chemical (temporary) splenectomy" described here offers therefore an animal model closer to the target population condition.

In plasmodial infections, the spleen helps to control parasite burden through innate and adaptative immune responses (Yazdani et al., 2006; Portillo et al., 2012; Gazzinelli et al., 2014). Splenic macrophages are major players in this system, clearing parasitized red blood cells through phagocytic activity. Because *S. sciureus* are not *P. falciparum's* natural host, splenic clearance seems to be particularly effective, preventing higher parasitemias. We asked whether partial depletion of the macrophage population in the spleen and other sites would result in higher and more consistent parasitemias in *S. sciureus* while maintaining not only the structure but also the function of the spleen. Together, our results indicate that this goal was largely achieved in this study.

Saimiri sciureus monkeys infected with *Plasmodium falciparum* and treated with periodic intravenous injections of clodronate-encapsulated liposomes (CL) in general developed higher parasitemias requiring antimalarial treatment than

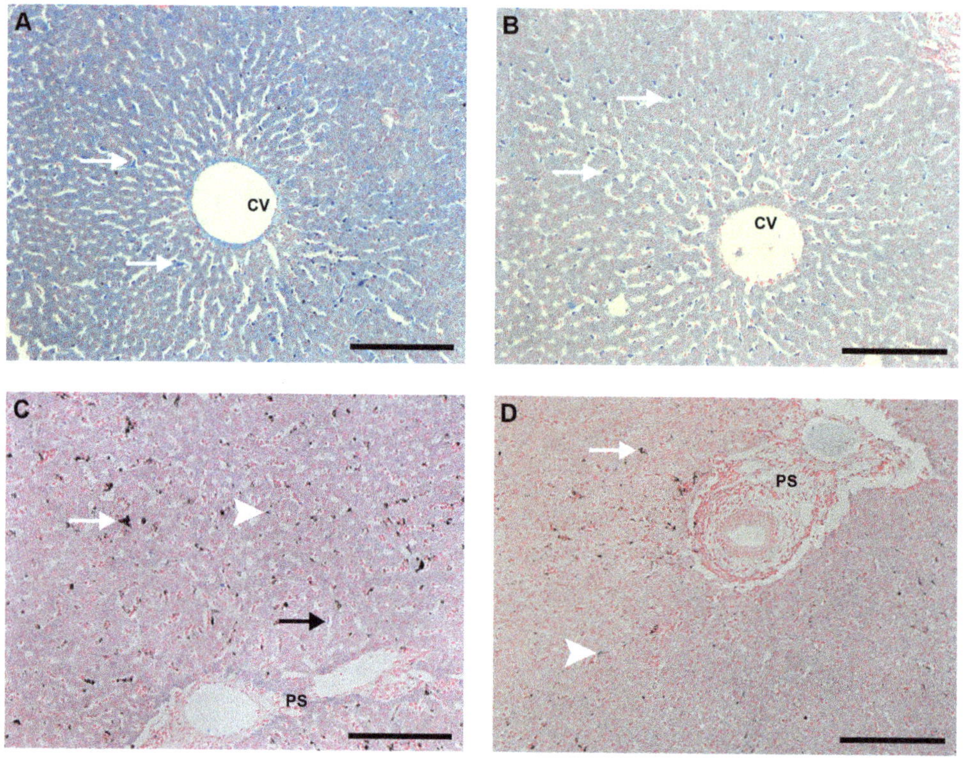

FIGURE 9 | Liver sections Perls staining (bar: 200 μm). **(A)** Liver of an uninfected, control animal that received PBS (code PA11), showing blue staining throughout the hepatocytes, with stronger staining in Kupffer cells (arrows); CV: centrilobular vein **(B)** Liver of an uninfected Saimiri inoculated with CL 1 mL (code V3). The blue stainingwas lighter, especially in hepatocytes, with Kupffer cells still showing more pronounced staining (arrows). CV, centrilobular vein. **(C)** Liver of a *P. falciparum*-infected Saimiri that received PBS (code 216: treated at day 17, with 1,3% parasitemia, killed 5 days later). Iron staining was lighter than **(A)** in both hepatocytes and Kupffer cells, but still visible; Kupffer cells were laden with hemozoin (arrow); in only sporadic cases colocalization of hemozoin and iron staining was observed in Kupffer cells (arrowhead). PS: portal space. **(D)** Liver of a *P. falciparum*-infected Saimiri that received CL 1 mL (code 161: treated at day 11, with 22% parasitemia, killed 5 days later). Both iron staining (arrowhead) and hemozoin (arrow) were decreased in relation to **(C)**. PS: portal space.

infected monkeys treated with PBS. It is not clear why this effect was not observed in *three* out of 9 (33.3%) infected *S. sciureus* treated with CL 1 mL, as they were able to self-control parasitemia, behaving closer to PBS-treated animals. *Three* independent experiments were performed, and these *three* animals were from the same experiment, suggesting that the lot of CL used may not have been optimal. Alternatively, this result would confirm that there is some degree of individual animal variation, either in the efficacy of CL treatment or in the pre-existing state of non-adaptive immunity. It is likely that the number of macrophages will vary from *one* animal to the other. It is advisable that each lot of CL be assayed *in vitro* for monocyte killing capacity prior to the conduction of *in vivo* experiments.

In any case, the efficacy of CL 1 mL treatment was evident, as *two* thirds (6 out of 9) of the treated animals developed parasitemias over 20% requiring mefloquine treatment, whereas all *eight* PBS-treated animals self-controled their parasitemias. Administration of a smaller amount of CL (0.5 mL) also resulted in higher parasitemias overall, with half (3 out of 6) of the animals showing parasitemias over 20%. Results are in agreement with those recorded with *P. falciparum* in immunocompromised mice grafted with human RBCs (Badell et al., 2000; Arnold et al., 2010). Thus, it is very likely that higher CL doses would result in improved macrophage control, and thereby in higher parasitemias. This remains to be investigated in future experiments.

From an ethical point of view CL treatment offers the paramount advantage of avoiding heavy surgery and allowing full recovery of animals. It thus constitutes a major improvement from a scientific as well as from an ethical viewpoint over splenectomy.

Plasmodium falciparum infection and/or CL treatment had little effect on peripheral blood monocyte counts, which is not a surprise as young monocytes have limited phagocytic activity and CL targets preferentially large and active macrophages, which ingest a larger number of liposomes per cell. Indeed, CL injections resulted in marked effects in the spleen and the liver. In uninfected animals, no evident effect of CL injections was observed in spleen/body weight ratios, but the number and distribution of ferric iron-containing cells in the spleen were markedly reduced. Macrophages are involved in senescent red blood cell phagocytosis and iron recycling, and therefore CL injections largely depleted this cell population in the spleen. In *Plasmodium falciparum*-infected animals, CL injections resulted in milder splenomegaly and this effect was associated histologically with marked

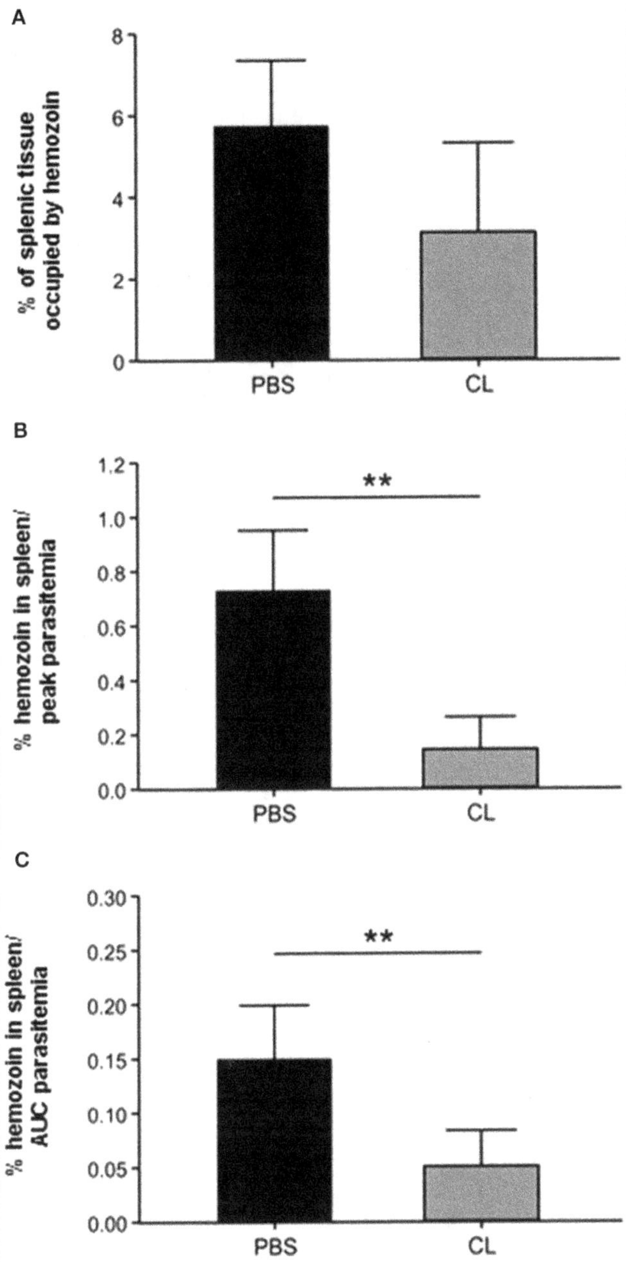

FIGURE 10 | Estimation of the effect of CL treatment on splenic macrophage population through hemozoin quantification. **(A)** Percentage of the splenic tissue occupied by hemozoin in PBS-treated and CL-treated infected animals. **(B,C)** Amount of splenic hemozoin adjusted by parasitemia in PBS-treated and CL-treated infected animals. The percentage of splenic tissue occupied by hemozoin (as in **A**) was divided by the peak parasitemia **(B)** or by the area under the curve (AUC) of parasitemia **(C)** of each animal. $^{**}P < 0.01$.

reductions in hemozoin-containing cells and further reductions in iron-containing cells. Efforts to further substantiate the histological findings by specific macrophage staining with commercially available anti-human CD14, CD68, and HAM-56 monoclonal antibodies were unsucessful, probably due to the prolonged period the biological material was kept in formalin.

Our results also indicate that *P. falciparum* infection in *S. sciureus* causes impaired iron-recycling by macrophages. Infected animals showed large numbers of hemozoin-containing macrophages but decreased numbers of ferric iron-containing cells in the spleen. An effect on iron homeostasis was also observed in the liver. It is known that macrophages are very important actors in controlling the iron upload and metabolism in hepatocytes, mostly via hepcidin. Therefore, it is possible that the reduction in iron staining in hepatocytes after CL treatment resulted from the instability of the hepcidin production due to Kupffer cell destruction (Fleming, 2005; Makui et al., 2005). However, additional studies are needed in order to clarify the mechanisms behind this phenomenon. In addition, colocalization of hemozoin and iron was a rare event, indicating that phagocytes were busy processing hemozoin from infected red blood cells and their capacity to carry out phagocytosis of uninfected red blood cells was impaired. Although the dark and gross pattern of hemozoin might actually prevent visualization of the light blue iron staining and therefore colocalization might be underestimated, some facts suggest that iron uptake by macrophages was impaired: (i) even macrophages with little, sparse amount of hemozoin showed no iron staining; (ii) colocalization was observed in some cells heavily laden with hemozoin. Since it has been shown that hemozoin may persist for weeks to months after parasite clearance (Frita et al., 2012; Alves et al., 2015), it may negatively impact the immune responses and iron recycling of the affected individuals for long periods of time after treatment has been implemented and therefore, contribute significantly to increasing malaria morbidity. Interestingly, in infected animals, Kupffer cells and sinusoidal macrophages heavily laden with iron were observed. This finding may indicate that young cells from the bone marrow repopulate the liver in an effort to restore iron recycling and other functions.

Depletion of macrophages by CL shows a number of advantages over surgical splenectomy for the study of malaria vaccines in Saimiri monkeys. However, macrophages are very important in the immune responses against *P. falciparum* through direct infected red blood cell phagocytosis or antibody-mediated parasite opsonization or inhibition (Bouharoun-Tayoun et al., 1990; Buffet et al., 2011). Therefore, sharp decreases in macrophage numbers might affect the antiplasmodial immune responses a given pre-clinical vaccine trial may be attempting to evaluate. The same limitation can be considered for dendritic cells, which also play relevant roles in antiplasmodial immunity (Urban et al., 1999, 2001). Indeed, phagocytic marginal dendritic cells but not interdigitating dendritic cells are known to be depleted by CL treatment (Leenen et al., 1998), which can affect immune responses to particulate antigens (Delemarre et al., 1990). These limitations need to be taken into account when using CL treatment as the strategy to induce higher *P. falciparum* parasitemias.

It has been shown that plasmodial infections in humans (Urban et al., 2005), Saimiri (Alves et al., 2015) and mice (Achtman et al., 2003; Carvalho et al., 2007; Martins et al., 2009) induce disarray of the spleen and other lymphoid organs, with disturbance of germinal center architecture. This finding was confirmed in the present study in *S. sciureus*, and CL administration had no apparent effect on this event. The splenic changes observed in *P. falciparum*-infected, saline-treated Saimiri 5 days after mefloquine treatment were similar to those recently reported for *P. falciparum*-infected Saimiri at peak parasitemia before antimalarial treatment (Alves et al., 2015). These changes included the presence of large numbers of phagocytes in the red pulp heavily laden with malaria pigment, disarray of B-cell follicles, blurred limits between the red and white pulps, and penetration of RBCs into follicles. In that study, 14 days after chloroquine treatment, spleens showed better white pulp organization and persistence of hemozoin in the red pulp but with a different pattern with more compacted, less granulous pigment (Alves et al., 2015). Therefore, the pattern of splenic changes observed in infected animals 5 days after mefloquine treatment in the present study was more similar to the changes observed at peak parasitemia prior to antimalarial treatment than after an extended period (2 weeks) after antimalarial treatment. This finding suggests that 5 days following antimalarial drug treatment is insufficient to reverse the pathological changes in spleen structure induced by *P. falciparum* infection.

Finally, infected animals that received CL showed more intense hepatocyte vacuolization. This effect was most likely a result of a combination of CL injection with higher parasitemias in these animals, because both uninfected animals receiving CL and infected animals receiving PBS showed some degree of hepatocyte vacuolization, milder than when the events were combined.

In conclusion, these results indicate that CL depleted splenic macrophages leading to decreased parasite phagocytosis, decreased splenic congestion, and increased parasitemias. CL administration is therefore a practical and viable alternative to surgical splenectomy in this experimental model.

AUTHOR CONTRIBUTIONS

JC participated in study design, carried out the experiments and helped LC in drafting the manuscript; CBJ participated in study design and carried out the experiments, MA, LP-R, ER, and MP carried out the experiments and reviewed the manuscript; IdS carried out the experiments; LC, CD-R, and PD conceived the study, participated in its design and coordination, and reviewed the manuscript. All authors have read and approved the final manuscript.

FUNDING

This study was supported by Coordenação de Aperfeiçoamento de Pessoal de Nível Superior (CAPES), Conselho Nacional de Desenvolvimento Científico e Tecnológico (CNPq, Brazil), Fundação Carlos Chagas Filho de Apoio de Amparo à Pesquisa do Estado do Rio de Janeiro (FAPERJ, Brazil), Instituto Oswaldo Cruz (FIOCRUZ, Brazil) and Programa de Apoio a Núcleos de Excelência-PRONEX (DECIT/CNPq/FAPERJ). CD-R and LC are recipients of Research Productivity fellowships from CNPq and are supported by FAPERJ as "Cientistas do Nosso Estado."

SUPPLEMENTARY MATERIAL

Supplemental Figure 1 | Liver sections, HE (bar: 100 μm). **(A)** Liver of an uninfected, control animal that received PBS (code PA67), in higher magnification than **Figure 8A**, showing Kupffer cells (arrows). **(B–D)** Liver of a *P. falciparum*-infected Saimiri that received PBS (code 141: treated at day 17, with 0.69% parasitemia, killed 5 days later), in greater detail compared to **Figure 8C**. Portal infiltrates (black arrow), increased cellularity in sinusoids with presence of mononuclear cells (white arrowhead), erythroid cells (thin arrow) and plasma cells (black arrowhead).

Supplemental Figure 2 | Liver sections, Perls (bar: 100 μm). **(A,B)** Liver of a *P. falciparum*-infected Saimiri that received PBS (code 216: treated at day 17, with 1.3% parasitemia, killed 5 days later), in greater detail compared to **Figure 9C**. Intrasinusoidal macrophages, circulating or attached to the sinusoidal wall, laden with malarial pigment (white arrows). There was little or no colocalization of hemozoin and iron staining (black arrow).

Supplemental Table 1 | Results of experiments 1, 2, and 3 showing the data of parasitemia, CD14 counting, hematocrit, hemoglobin, rectal temperature, weight and spleen/body weight ratios.

REFERENCES

Abbas, A. K., Lichtman, A. H., and Pillai, S. (2008). *Imunologia Celular e Molecular, 6th Edn.* Rio de Janeiro: Elsevier.

Achtman, A. H., Khan, M., MacLennan, I. C., and Langhorne, J. (2003). Plasmodium chabaudi chabaudi infection in mice induces strong B cell responses and striking but temporary changes in splenic cell distribution. *J. Immunol.* 171, 317–324. doi: 10.4049/jimmunol.171.1.317

Alves, F. A., Pelajo-Machado, M., Totino, P. R., Souza, M. T., Gonçalves, E. C., Schneider, M. P., et al. (2015). Splenic architecture disruption and parasite-induced splenocyte activation and anergy in *Plasmodium falciparum*-infected *Saimiri sciureus* monkeys. *Malar. J.* 14:128. doi: 10.1186/s12936-015-0641-3

Alves, F. A., Souza, M. T., Gonçalves, E. C., Schneider, M. P., Marinho, A. M., Muniz, J. A., et al. (2010). DNA sequencing of 13 cytokine gene fragments of *Aotus infulatus* and *Saimiri sciureus,* two non-human primate models for malaria. *Cytokine* 52, 151–155. doi: 10.1016/j.cyto.2010.09.004

Arnold, L., Tyagi, R. K., Mejia, P., Swetman, C., Gleeson, J., Perignon, J. L., et al. (2011). Further improvements of the *P. falciparum* humanized mouse model. *PLoS ONE* 6:e18045. doi: 10.1371/journal.pone.0018045

Arnold, L., Tyagi, R. K., Mejia, P., van Rooijen, N., Perignon, J. L., and Druilhe, P. (2010). Analysis of innate defences against *Plasmodium falciparum* in immunodeficient mice. *Malar. J.* 9:197. doi: 10.1186/1475-2875-9-197

Badell, E., Oeuvray, C., Moreno, A., Soe, S., van Rooijen, N., Bouzidi, A., et al. (2000). Human malaria in immunocompromised mice: an *in vivo* model to study defense mechanisms against *Plasmodium falciparum. J. Exp. Med.* 192, 1653–1659. doi: 10.1084/jem.192.11.1653

Bouharoun-Tayoun, H., Attanath, P., Sabchareon, A., Chongsuphajaisiddhi, T., and Druilhe, P. (1990). Antibodies that protect humans against *Plasmodium falciparum* blood stages do not on their own inhibit parasite growth and invasion *in vitro,* but act in cooperation with monocytes. *J. Exp. Med.* 172, 1633–1641.

Buffet, P. A., Safeukui, I., Deplaine, G., Brousse, V., Prendki, V., Thellier, M., et al. (2011). The pathogenesis of *Plasmodium falciparum* malaria in humans: insights from splenic physiology. *Blood* 117, 381–392. doi: 10.1182/blood-2010-04-202911

Carvalho, L. J., Ferreira-da-Cruz, M. F., Daniel-Ribeiro, C. T., Pelajo-Machado, M., and Lenzi, H. L. (2007). Germinal center architecture disturbance during *Plasmodium berghei* ANKA infection in CBA mice. *Malar. J.* 16:59. doi: 10.1186/1475-2875-6-59

Carvalho, L. J. M., Alves, F. A., Bianco-Jr, C., Oliveira, S. G., Zanini, G. M., Soe, S., et al. (2005). Immunization of *Saimiri sciureus* monkeys with a recombinant hybrid protein derived from the *Plasmodium falciparum* antigens glutamate-rich protein and merozoite surface protein-3 can induce partial protection with Freund's and Montanide ISA720 adjuvants. *Clin. Diagn. Lab. Immunol.* 12, 242–248. doi: 10.1128/CDLI.12.2.242-248.2005

Carvalho, L. J., Alves, F. A., de Oliveira, S. G., do Valle, R. R., Fernandes, A. A., Muniz, J. A., et al. (2003). Severe anemia affects both splenectomized and non-splenectomized *Plasmodium falciparum*-infected Aotus infulatus monkeys. *Mem. Inst. Oswaldo Cruz.* 98, 679–686. doi: 10.1590/S0074-0276200 3000500016

Carvalho, L. J. M., Daniel-Ribeiro, C. T., and Goto, H. (2002). Malaria vaccine: candidate antigens, mechanisms, constraints and prospects. *Scand. J. Immunol.* 56, 327–343. doi: 10.1046/j.1365-3083.2002.01160.x

Carvalho, L. J. M., Oliveira, S. G., Alves, F. A., Brígido, M. C. O., Muniz, J. A. P. C., and Daniel-Ribeiro, C. T. (2000). Aotus infulatus is susceptible to *Plasmodium falciparum* infection and may constitute an alternative experimental model for malaria. *Mem. Inst. Oswaldo Cruz* 95, 363–365. doi: 10.1590/S0074-02762000000300011

Carvalho, L. J. M., Oliveira, S. G., Theisen, M., Alves, F. A., Andrade, M. C. R., Zanini, G. M., et al. (2004). Immunization of *Saimiri sciureus* monkeys with *Plasmodium falciparum* merozoite surface protein-3 and glutamate-rich protein suggests that protection is related to antibody levels. *Scand. J. Immunol.* 59, 363–372. doi: 10.1111/j.0300-9475.2004.01409.x

Chrubasik, C., and Jacobson, R. L. (2010). The development of artemisinin resistance in malaria: reasons and solutions. *Phytother. Res.* 24, 1104–1106. doi: 10.1002/ptr.3133

Clemens, J., and Moorthy, V. (2016). Implementation of RTS,S/AS01 malaria vaccine – the need for further evidence. *N. Engl. J. Med.* 374, 2596–2597. doi: 10.1056/NEJMe1606007

Collins, W. (1992). South american monkeys in the development and testing of malaria vaccines. *Mem. Inst. Oswaldo Cruz* 87(Suppl. 3), 401–406. doi: 10.1590/S0074-02761992000700068

Collins, W. E., Galland, G. G., Barnwell, J. W., Udhayakumar, V., Sullivan, J. S., Nace, D., et al. (2005). Preliminary observations on the efficacy of a recombinant multistage *Plasmodium falciparum* vaccine in Aotus nancymai monkeys. *Am. J. Trop. Med. Hyg.* 73, 686–693.

Contamin, H., Behr, C., Mercereau-Puijalon, O., and Michel, J. C. (2000). *Plasmodium falciparum* in the squirrel monkey (*Saimiri sciureus*): infection of nonsplenectomised animals as a model for exploring clinical manifestations of malaria. *Microbes Infect.* 2, 945–954. doi: 10.1016/S1286-4579(00)00401-9

Contamin, H., Loizon, S., Bourreau, E., Michel, J. C., Garraud, O., Mercereau-Puijalon, O., et al. (2005). Flow cytometry identification and characterization of mononuclear cell subsets in the neotropical primate *Saimiri sciureus* (squirrel monkey). *J. Immunol. Methods* 297, 61–71. doi: 10.1016/j.jim.2004.11.019

Criswell, B. S., Butler, W. T., Rossen, R. D., and Knight, V. (1971). Murine malaria: the role of humoral factors and macrophages in destruction of parasitized erythrocytes. *J. Immunol.* 107, 212–221.

Delemarre, F. G., Kors, N., and van Rooijen, N. (1990). Elimination of spleen and of lymph node macrophages and its difference in the effect on the immune response to particulate antigens. *Immunobiology* 182, 70–78. doi: 10.1016/S0171-2985(11)80584-X

Dondorp, A. M., Yeung, S., White, L., Nguon, C., Day, N. P., Socheat, D., et al. (2010). Artemisinin resistance: current status and scenarios for containment. *Nat. Rev. Microbiol.* 9, 272–280. doi: 10.1038/nrmicro2331

Fleming, R. E. (2005). The iron sensor: macrophage, hepatocyte, both? *Blood* 106, 1893–1894. doi: 10.1182/blood-2005-07-2673

Frita, R., Carapau, D., Mota, M. M., and Hänscheid, T. (2012). *In vivo* hemozoin kinetics after clearance of Plasmodium berghei infection in mice. *Malar. Res. Treat.* 2012:373086. doi: 10.1155/2012/373086

Garraud, O., Contamin, H., Perraut, R., Behr, C., and Gysin, J. (1998). Analysis on reactivity of human lymphocyte and monocyte-specific antibodies with peripheral blood mononuclear cells from squirrel monkeys (*Saimiri sciureus*). *J. Med. Primatol.* 73, 686–693. doi: 10.1111/j.1600-0684.1998.tb00074.x

Gazzinelli, R. T., Kalantari, P., Fitzgerald, K. A., and Golenbock, D. T. (2014). Innate sensing of malaria parasites. *Nat. Rev. Immunol.* 14, 744–757. doi: 10.1038/nri3742

Gysin, J., and Fandeur, T. (1983). *Saimiri sciureus* (karyotype 14-7): an alternative experimental model of *Plasmodium falciparum* infection. *Am. J. Trop. Med. Hyg.* 32, 461–467. doi: 10.4269/ajtmh.1983.32.461

Herrera, S., Perlaza, B. L., Bonelo, A., and Arévalo-Herrera, M. (2002). Aotus monkeys: their great value for anti-malaria vaccines and drug testing. *Int. J. Parasitol.* 32, 1625–1635. doi: 10.1016/S0020-7519(02)00191-1

Kim, H. M., Lee, Y. W., Lee, K. J., Kim, H. S., Cho, S. W., van Rooijen, N., et al. (2008). Alveolar macrophages are indispensable for controlling influenza viruses in lungs of pigs. *J. Virol.* 82, 4265–4274. doi: 10.1128/JVI.02602-07

Leenen, P. J., Radosević, K., Voerman, J. S., Salomon, B., van Rooijen, N., Klatzmann, D., et al. (1998). Heterogeneity of mouse spleen dendritic cells: *in vivo* phagocytic activity, expression of macrophage markers, and subpopulation turnover. *J. Immunol.* 160, 2166–2173.

Leisewitz, A. L., Rockett, K. A., Gumede, B., Jones, M., Urban, B., and Kwiatkowski, D. P. (2004). Response of the splenic dendritic cell population to malaria infection. *Infect. Immun.* 72, 4233–4239. doi: 10.1128/IAI.72.7.4233-4239.2004

Makui, H.;, Soares, R. J.;, Jiang, W., Constante, M., and Santos, M. M. (2005). Contribution of Hfe expression in macrophages to the regulation of hepatic hepcidin levels and iron loading. *Blood* 106, 2189–2195. doi: 10.1182/blood-2005-02-0629

Martins, Y. C., Smith, M. J., Pelajo-Machado, M., Werneck, G. L., Lenzi, H. L., Daniel-Ribeiro, C. T., et al. (2009). Characterization of cerebral malaria in the outbred Swiss Webster mouse infected by *Plasmodium berghei* ANKA. *Int. J. Exp. Pathol.* 90, 119–130. doi: 10.1111/j.1365-2613.2008.00622.x

Mathes, M., Jordan, M., and Dowa, S. (2006). Evaluation of liposomal clodronate in experimental spontaneous autoimmune hemolytic anemia in dogs. *Exp. Hematol.* 34, 1393–1402. doi: 10.1016/j.exphem.2006.05.014

Olotu, A., Fegan, G., Wanbua, J., Nyangweso, G., Leach, A., and Lievens, M. (2016). Seven-years efficacy of RTS,S/AS01 malaria vaccine among young african children. *N. Engl. J. Med.* 374, 2519–2529. doi: 10.1056/NEJMoa1515257

Otieno, L., Oneko, M., Otieno, W., Abuodha, J., Owino, E., Odero, C., et al. (2016). Safety and immunogenicity of RTS,S/AS01 malaria vaccine in infants and children with WHO stage 1 or 2 HIV disease: a randomised, double-blind, controlled trial. *Lancet Infect. Dis.* 16, 1134–1144. doi: 10.1016/S1473-3099(16)30161-X

Portillo, H. A., Ferrer, M., Brugat, T., Martin-Jaular, L., Langhorne, J., Lacerda, M. V. G., et al. (2012). The role of the spleen in malaria. *Cell. Microbiol.* 14, 343–355. doi: 10.1111/j.1462-5822.2011.01741.x

Quintero, J. P., Siqueira, A. M., Tobón, A., Blair, S., Moreno, A., Arévalo-Herrera, M., et al. (2011). Malaria-related anaemia: a Latin American perspective. *Mem. Inst. Oswaldo Cruz* 106(Suppl. 1), 91–104. doi: 10.1590/S0074-02762011000900012

Riccio, E. K., Pratt-Riccio, L. R., Bianco-Junior, C., Sanchez, V., Totino, P. R., and Carvalho, L. J. (2015). Molecular and immunological tools for the evaluation of the cellular immune response in the neotropical monkeys *Saimiri sciureus*, a non-human primate model for malaria research. *Malar. J.* 14:166. doi: 10.1186/s12936-015-0688-1

Rowe, J. A., Claessens, A., Corrigan, R. A., and Arman, M. (2009). Adhesion of *Plasmodium falciparum* infected erythrocytes to human cells: molecular mechanisms and therapeutic implications. *Expert Rev Mol. Med.* 11:e16. doi: 10.1017/S1462399409001082

Sirima, S. B., Cousens, S., and Druilhe, P. (2011). Protection against malaria by MSP3 candidate vaccine. *N. Engl. J. Med.* 365, 1062–1064. doi: 10.1056/NEJMc1100670

Sullivan, A. D., Ittarat, I., and Meshnick, S. R. (1996). Patterns of haemozoin accumulation in tissue. *Parasitology* 112(Pt 3), 285–294.

Tougan, T., Aoshi, T., Coban, C., Katakai, Y., Kai, C., Yasutomi, Y., et al. (2013). TLR9 adjuvants enhance immunogenicity and protective efficacy of the SE36/AHG malaria vaccine in nonhuman primate models. *Hum. Vaccin. Immunother.* 9, 283–290. doi: 10.4161/hv.22950

Urban, B. C., Ferguson, D. J., Pain, A., Willcox, N., Plebanski, M., Austyn, J. M., et al. (1999). *Plasmodium falciparum*-infected erythrocytes modulate the maturation. *Nature* 400, 73–77.

Urban, B. C., Willcox, N., and Roberts, D. J. (2001). A role for CD36 in the regulation of dendritic cell function. *Proc. Natl. Acad. Sci. U.S.A.* 98, 8750–8755. doi: 10.1073/pnas.151028698

Urban, B. C., Hien, T. T., Day, N. P., Phu, N. H., Roberts, R., Pongponratn, E., et al. (2005). Fatal *Plasmodium falciparum* malaria causes specific patterns of splenic architectural disorganization. *Infect. Immun.* 73, 1986–1994. doi: 10.1128/IAI.73.4.1986-1994.2005

van Rooijen, N., and Kors, N. (1989). Effects of intracellular diphosphonates on cells of the mononuclear phagocyte system: *in vivo* effects of liposome-encapsulated diphosphonates on different macrophage subpopulations in the spleen. *Calcif. Tis. Int.* 45, 153–156. doi: 10.1007/BF02556058

van Rooijen, N., Kors, N., vd Ende, M., and Dijkstra, C. D. (1990). Depletion and repopulation of macrophages in spleen and liver of rat after intravenous treatment with liposome-encapsulated dichloromethylene diphosphonate. *Cell Tis. Res.* 260, 215–222.

van Rooijen, N., and van Kesteren-Hendrikx, E. (2002). Clodronate liposomes: perspectives in research and therapeutics. *J. Liposome Res.* 12, 81–94. doi: 10.1081/LPR-120004780

van Rooijen, N., and van Nieuwmegen, R. (1984). Elimination of phagocytic cells in the spleen after intravenous injection of liposome-encapsulated dichloromethylene diphosphonate. an enzyme-histochemical study. *Cell Tis. Res.* 238, 355–358.

WHO (2004). *MALVAC Meeting 2004: Evaluation of Malaria Vaccines. Pre-clinical Evaluation Group: Optimizing the Developmental Pathway from the Lab to the Clinic.* Report from a technical consultation at WHO/IVR Malaria Vaccine Advisory Committee meeting Montreux; 2004.

WHO (2016). *World Malaria Report 2016.* World Health Organization: 2015. Available online at: http://www.who.int/malaria/publications/world-malaria-report-2016/report/en/

Yazdani, S. S., Mukherjee, P., Chauhan, V. S., and Chitnis, C. E. (2006). Immune response to asexual blood-stages of malaria parasites. *Curr. Mol. Med.* 6, 187–203. doi: 10.2174/156652406776055212

13

Interaction between *Plasmodium* Glycosylphosphatidylinositol and the Host Protein Moesin Has No Implication in Malaria Pathology

Josefine Dunst[1,2]*, Nahid Azzouz[1,3], Xinyu Liu[4], Sachiko Tsukita[5], Peter H. Seeberger[1,3] and Faustin Kamena[1,2]*

[1] Institute of Chemistry and Biochemistry, Free University Berlin, Berlin, Germany, [2] Parasitology Unit, Max Planck Institute for Infection Biology, Berlin, Germany, [3] Department of Biomolecular Systems, Max Planck Institute for Colloids and Interfaces, Potsdam, Germany, [4] Department of Chemistry, University of Pittsburgh, Pittsburgh, PA, USA, [5] Department of Frontier Biosciences, Graduate School of Frontier Biosciences, Osaka University, Osaka, Japan

Edited by:
Anton Aebischer,
Robert Koch-Institute, Germany

Reviewed by:
Nyssa Drinkwater,
Monash University, Australia
Sabrina Absalon,
Boston Children's Hospital, USA

****Correspondence:***
Josefine Dunst
dunstj@zedat.fu-berlin.de
Faustin Kamena
kamena@zedat.fu-berlin.de

Glycosylphosphatidylinositol (GPI) anchor of *Plasmodium falciparum* origin is considered an important toxin leading to severe malaria pathology through stimulation of pro-inflammatory responses from innate immune cells. Even though the GPI-induced immune response is widely described to be mediated by pattern recognition receptors such as TLR2 and TLR4, previous studies have revealed that these two receptors are dispensable for the development of severe malaria pathology. Therefore, this study aimed at the identification of potential alternative *Plasmodium* GPI receptors. Herein, we have identified the host protein moesin as an interaction partner of *Plasmodium* GPI *in vitro*. Given previous reports indicating the relevance of moesin especially in the LPS-mediated induction of pro-inflammatory responses, we have conducted a series of *in vitro* and *in vivo* experiments to address the physiological relevance of the moesin-*Plasmodium* GPI interaction in the context of malaria pathology. We report here that although moesin and *Plasmodium* GPI interact *in vitro,* moesin is not critically involved in processes leading to *Plasmodium*-induced pro-inflammatory immune responses or malaria-associated cerebral pathology.

Keywords: GPI, ERM, moesin, *Plasmodium*, cerebral malaria

INTRODUCTION

Malaria still causes a devastatingly high number of deaths and new infections each year and is thereby a major contributor to the global burden of infectious diseases (WHO, 2016). This disease is caused by human host-adapted *Plasmodium* species and transmitted by the bite of an infective *Anopheles* mosquito. During *Plasmodium* infection, an immune response is mounted by the host in order to limit parasite expansion and mediate clearance. Consequently, blood stage infection is accompanied by a systemic pro-inflammatory immune response resulting in classical symptoms of mild malaria such as fever (Stevenson and Riley, 2004). However, some individuals progress to a severe course of malaria, partly owing to an imbalance in the pro- and anti-inflammatory immune response (Langhorne et al., 2008), resulting in malaria-associated mortality which is largely attributed to *P. falciparum* infections (WHO, 2016). One of the major complications of severe malaria is cerebral malaria (CM) which manifests with retinal abnormalities (Storm and Craig, 2014) as well as impaired consciousness or coma (Cunnington et al., 2013). The symptoms of CM are attributable to sequestration of infected erythrocytes and inflammatory leukocyte subsets, endothelial dysfunction, and inflammation (Storm and Craig, 2014), and these processes are mutually dependent and have synergetic effects (Cunnington et al., 2013). However, the precise molecular mechanisms underlying CM are not yet fully understood.

The induction of innate pro-inflammatory cytokine responses is mediated by germline-encoded pattern-recognition receptors, such as toll-like receptors (TLR), which recognize conserved microbial structures, i.e., pathogen-associated molecular patterns (PAMP) (Kawai and Akira, 2011). Among the malaria PAMP, glycosylphosphatidylinositols (GPI) are considered the main pathogenicity factor (Gowda, 2007). While GPI structure is conserved among *Plasmodium* species, human and *Plasmodium* GPI differ considerably (Boutlis et al., 2005). GPI serve as membrane anchors for certain cell surface proteins such as circumsporozoite protein and merozoite surface protein 1, and are also abundantly present free of protein attachment in membranes of pathogenic protozoa (Gowda, 2007; Gazzinelli et al., 2014). *P. falciparum* GPI have been found to induce the production of nitric oxide, tumor necrosis factor (TNF), and interleukin 1β (IL-1β) in murine macrophages *in vitro* (Schofield and Hackett, 1993; Tachado et al., 1996) and a synthetic malarial GPI glycan was demonstrated to be immunogenic *in vivo* (Schofield et al., 2002). Together, these findings point toward a role for *Plasmodium* GPI in malaria pathogenesis. Notably, *Plasmodium* GPI were described to be primarily recognized by TLR2 or heterodimers of TLR2/1 and TLR2/6 (Krishnegowda et al., 2005), yet TLR-deficiency did not protect mice from experimental cerebral malaria (ECM) (Togbe et al., 2007; Lepenies et al., 2008), indicating that TLR-mediated pro-inflammatory immune responses are not critical in the development of ECM. Since elucidating molecular mechanisms leading to malaria pathology might allow specific modulation of innate immune activation to prevent detrimental immune responses, this study was designed to identify potential *Plasmodium* GPI receptors. Using synthetic GPI affinity chromatography, we have identified the host protein moesin as an interaction partner of *P. falciparum* GPI and further addressed the functional relevance of this interaction in the development of malaria pathology. Moesin is a member of the ezrin-radixin-moesin (ERM) family of intracellular proteins which link actin filaments to transmembrane proteins (Louvet-Vallee, 2000) and interact with proteins involved in key signaling events, such as phosphatidylinositide 3-kinase, protein kinase A, or Rho-specific GDP dissociation inhibitors (Ivetic and Ridley, 2004; Niggli and Rossy, 2008; Ponuwei, 2016). Additionally, moesin cell surface translocation has been described upon lipopolysaccharide (LPS) stimulation *in vitro* (Iontcheva et al., 2004; Takamatsu et al., 2009), pointing toward a role for moesin in PAMP recognition. Moreover, we reasoned that moesin may play a role in the immune response to *Plasmodium* infection via its ability to interact with *Plasmodium* GPI as well as in malaria pathology due to its ability to modulate immunological synapse and endothelial paracellular gap formation (Itoh et al., 2002; Koss et al., 2006; Parameswaran and Gupta, 2013). Therefore, the capability of moesin to translocate to the cell surface upon *Plasmodium* GPI stimulation as well as the impact of moesin-deficiency on malaria PAMP-mediated cytokine induction and phagocytosis of *P. berghei* was analyzed *in vitro*. Additionally, *P. berghei* ANKA-infected moesin-deficient mice were used as a model to study the role of moesin in the host immune response to *Plasmodium* and in the development of cerebral pathology *in vivo*. We report here that despite the interaction between *Pf*GPI and moesin *in vitro*, moesin does not translocate to the cell surface in response to malaria PAMP in human and murine macrophages. Moreover, moesin-deficiency did not impair *Plasmodium*-induced cytokine responses *in vitro* and *in vivo* and did not protect mice infected with *P. berghei* ANKA from development of ECM.

Abbreviations: BMDC, bone-marrow derived dendritic cells; BMDM, bone-marrow derived macrophages; CM, cerebral malaria; DC, dendritic cells; ECM, experimental cerebral malaria, ERM, ezrin-radixin-moesin; FCS, fetal calf serum; FMO, fluorescence-minus-one; GPI, glycosylphosphatidylinositol; IFN, interferon; IL, interleukin; LPS, lipopolysaccharide; PAMP, pathogen-associated molecular pattern, *PbS*, *Plasmodium* berghei schizonts; *PbSE*, *Plasmodium* berghei schizont extract; *PfSE*, *Plasmodium falciparum* schizont extract; PMA, phorbol 12-myristate 13-acetate; TLR, toll-like receptor; TNF, tumor necrosis factor

MATERIALS AND METHODS

GPI Affinity Chromatography and Mass Spectrometry

GPI glycans were synthesized with a terminal sulfhydryl-containing linker (Kwon et al., 2005; Liu et al., 2005) to be covalently immobilized on SulfoLink® coupling gel (Pierce, Rockford, IL) according to the manufacturer's instructions. Using a syringe, the column was equilibrated by washing with coupling buffer (50 mM Tris, 5 mM EDTA, pH 8.5). Mouse macrophage cell-line RAW264.7 plasma membrane fraction was prepared as previously reported (Smart et al., 1995). Plasma membrane was solubilized in coupling buffer containing 0.5% Triton X-100. Samples were then loaded in the coupling buffer and the column was incubated for 1 h at 4°C. Non-bound and excess proteins were removed by washing the column with 3 column volumes of coupling buffer. Elution of bound proteins was carried out using 3 column volumes of coupling buffer containing 1 M mannose and 0.1% Triton X-100. Eluted protein extracts were subjected to 12.5% SDS-PAGE under non-reducing condition. After Coomassie staining, protein bands were excised, destained, and reduced prior to tryptic digestion and peptide mass fingerprinting. MALDI mass spectra were generated using a Voyager DE-STR MALDI-TOF MS system (PerSeptive Biosystems) with delayed extraction in the reflectron mode. Proteins were identified by comparison of peak lists generated from the Data Explorer application (PerSeptive Biosystems) against NCBInr (no redundant) and Swiss-prot databases using the Protein-Prospector V3.4.1 software MS-Fit (http://www.prospector.ucsf.edu).

Moesin-GST Expression and Purification

A pGEX-4T-3 vector (Addgene) carrying Moesin-GST as N-terminal fusion protein was transformed into a bl21de3plysS (Promega, USA) *E. coli* strain. A single colony was picked to inoculate an overnight culture in 100 ml of LB medium supplemented with 100 μg/ml ampicillin at 37°C under shaking at 200 rpm. On the following day the overnight culture was diluted 1:20 in LB supplemented with 100 μg/ml ampicillin and incubated at 37°C at 300 rpm until an OD_{600} of 0.5 was reached. IPTG (Sigma-Aldrich) was added to the final concentration of 1 mM and the culture was incubated for additional 4 h. The bacteria pellet was harvested by centrifugation at 4,000 × g at 4°C for 20 min.

For the purification, bacteria pellet was resuspended in lysis buffer (50 mM Tris, 50 mM NaCl, 5 mM EDTA, 1 μg/ml leupeptin, 1 μg/ml pepstatin, 0.15 mM PMSF, 1 mM DFP, 1 mM 2-ME, pH 8.0) and lysis was completed by sonication. Cell lysate was centrifuged at 48,000 × g for 20 min at 4°C and the clear supernatant loaded on a GSH-agarose affinity column (Thermo Fisher). The column was washed three times to remove unbound material and moesin-GST was eluted with elution buffer (10 mM GSH in 50 mM Tris, 10 mM reduced glutathione, pH 8.0). The eluate was dialyzed against PBS and aliquots were kept at −80°C until use.

For surface plasmon resonance measurements, moesin was released from the moesin-GST fusion protein by thrombin digestion using immobilized thrombin, agarose (Sigma-Aldrich) according to the manufacturer's instruction (Supplementary Figure 1). Briefly, purified moesin was incubated with washed thrombin agarose beads in batch for 2 h at 37°C and the cleaved protein was recovered from the supernatant after centrifugation. Cleaved GST was removed by incubating the product from the thrombin cleavage with GSH-agarose beads in batch for 2 h at RT. Moesin without the GST tag was recovered in the supernatant after centrifugation of the beads at 10,000 × g for 10 min. Purified moesin was dialyzed against PBS and aliquots were frozen until use.

Microarray Binding Assays

GPI microarrays were constructed as previously described (Ratner et al., 2004; Kamena et al., 2008) and covered with a FlexWell-64 (GRACE BIO-LABS, Bend, OR) layer to form a multi-well plate. Wells were then blocked with 5% milk powder in PBS for 1 h at RT followed by three washes with PBS containing 0.05% Tween-20. The wells were incubated with purified moesin-GST in PBS containing 0.05% Tween-20 and 0.5% BSA for 2 h at RT or with FITC-labeled concanavalin A (FITC-ConA) in ConA binding buffer (20 mM Tris; 500 mM NaCl; 1 mM $CaCl_2$; 1 mM $MgCl_2$; pH 7.4). After washing, the slides were incubated with rabbit polyclonal anti-GST antibodies for 1 h at RT. After extensive washing the slides were incubated 1 h at RT with ALEXA-Fluor® 594-labeled anti-rabbit secondary antibody (Invitrogen, Eugene. OR) at 1:1,000 in PBS containing 0.5% BSA and 0.05% Tween-20. The slides were then washed and fluorescence was revealed using an Affymetrix 427 laser scanner (MWG Biotech, Huntsville, AL).

Surface Plasmon Resonance

GPI structure VI (**Figure 1B**) having a free thiol group was covalently attached to a gold surface CM5 chip using a Biacore T100 (GE Healthcare, Uppsala, Sweden). GPI glycan was immobilized on gold chips according to the manufacturer's protocol. Briefly, the carboxymethylated dextran matrix (CM5 chip) was activated at a flow rate of 10 μL/min using an 8 min injection pulse of an aqueous solution containing *N*-hydroxysuccinimide (NHS, 0.05 M) and *N*-ethyl-*N*'-(dimethylaminopropyl) carbodiimide (EDC, 0.2 M). The surface was further activated with a solution of 2-(2-pyridinyldithio) ethanolamine (PDEA, 80 mM in 0.1 M sodium borate; pH 8.5) at the flow rate of 10 μL/min using a 10 min pulse. Next, a solution of synthetic GPI (50 μg/ml) containing 1 mM hexadecyltrimethylammonium chloride was flowed over the activated surface for 10 min at 4 μL/min. Remaining reactive groups on the surface were quenched by injection of a cysteine/NaCl solution (50 mM cysteine and 1 M NaCl in 0.1 M sodium acetate; pH 4.3) for 7.5 min at 10 μL/min. The reference flow cell was activated in parallel and ethanolamine was covalently attached. For K_D determination between immobilized GPI and moesin, HBS-EP buffer (10 mM HEPES, pH 7.4, 150 mM NaCl, 3 mM EDTA, 0.005% v/v surfactant P20) was used as running buffer. Various concentrations of moesin (10, 2, 37.5, 75, 150, and 300 nM) were injected into the flow cell for 10 min each at 20 μL/min at 25°C. After each sample, running buffer flowed over the sensor surface for 10 min to allow dissociation. The chip surface was regenerated for the next sample by injection of the regenerating solution (0.1% SDS, 0.085% H_3PO_4, 1 M NaCl and 0.1% HCl) for 1 min at 80 μL/min flow rate. The responses were calculated as the difference in response unit (RU) between analyte and reference flow cell and monitored as function of time (sensogram). Data processing and kinetic analysis was performed using the BIAevaluation software for T100 (Version 1.1.1) and graphs were plotted using Origin 8.0 (OriginLab, Northampton). Double referenced association and dissociation phase data were globally fitted to a simple 1:1 interaction model ($A + B = AB$).

To calculate the K_D, the signal from the reference flow cell containing ethanolamine was subtracted from each value to correct for the contribution of non-specific interactions and systematic errors.

THP-1 Cells

The human monocytic leukemia cell line THP-1 (ATCC: TIB-202) was a kind gift from Dr. Pedro Moura-Alves (Max Planck Institute for Infection Biology, Berlin, Germany) and was cultured in RPMI 1640 (Gibco, Germany) supplemented with 10% fetal calf serum (FCS; Gibco), 2 mM L-glutamine (Gibco), 100 mM HEPES (Gibco), 1 mM sodium pyruvate (Sigma-Aldrich, Germany), 1% non-essential amino-acids (NEAA) (Gibco) and 55 μM β-mercaptoethanol (Sigma-Aldrich). For differentiation of THP-1 cells into macrophage-like cells, monocytic THP-1 cells were plated at a density of 0.6 × 10 e6 cells/ml in culture medium supplemented with 50–200 nM phorbol 12-myristate 13-acetate (PMA, Sigma-Aldrich) for 72 h (Moura-Alves et al., 2014). Upon transition of THP-1 cells into adherent growth, cells were washed with PBS repeatedly and

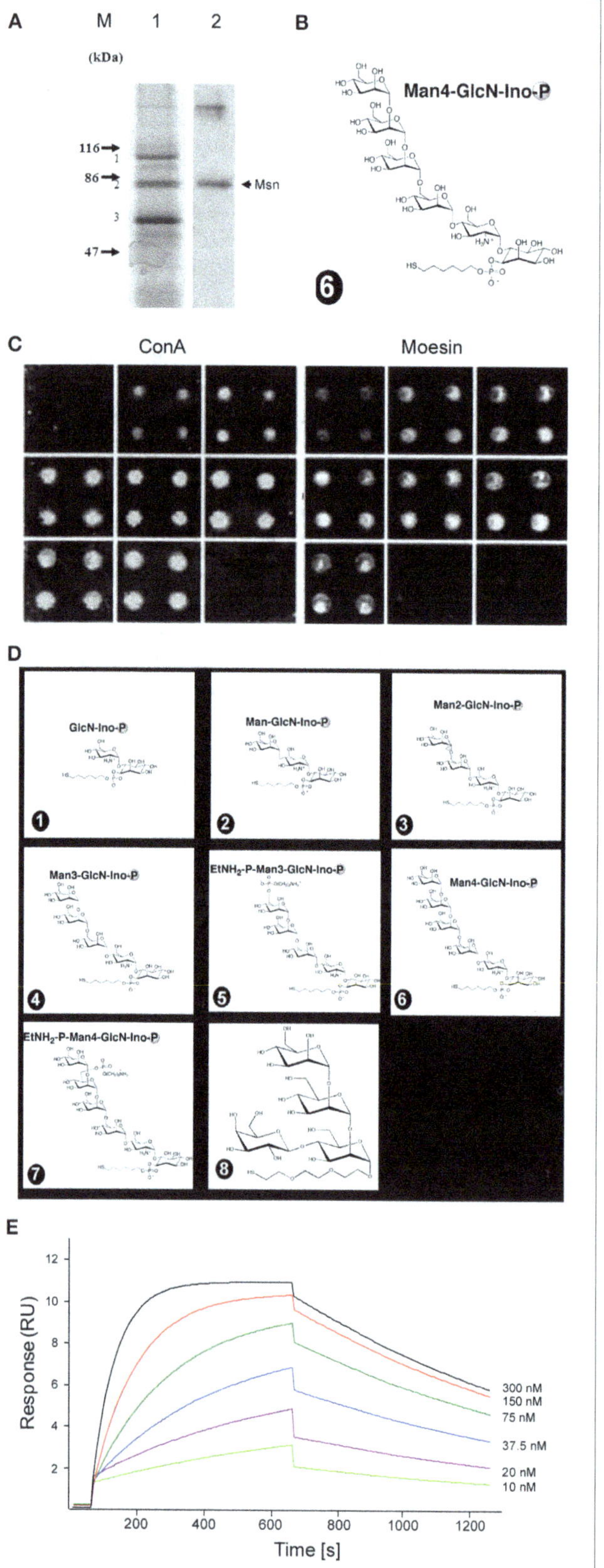

FIGURE 1 | Synthetic *Plasmodium* GPI glycan interacts with moesin. **(A)** GPI-interacting proteins from an affinity chromatography were revealed by Coomassie staining on an SDS-PAGE **(1)** and after identification by mass

(Continued)

FIGURE 1 | Continued

spectrometry moesin was confirmed by western blot using anti-moesin antibody **(2)**. **(B)** The affinity column was generated using the full length glycan moiety of the GPI anchor. **(C,D)** Moesin interacts with GPI on microarray. Seven GPI glycan fragments and a polymannose control structure (depicted in D) were immobilized covalently as quadruplicate on glass slides to generate a microarray. **(C)** The slides were incubated with either FITC-ConA or GST-moesin. After incubation bound proteins were revealed by a fluorescent scanner. **(E)** Surface plasmon resonance measurement of moesin interaction with GPI glycan. Various concentrations of recombinantly expressed moesin (10, 20, 37.5, 75, 150, and 300 nM) were flown through the GPI-coupled gold chip and sensograms recorded and analyzed using the BIAevaluation software (BIAcore Life sciences) and the generated data were exported and graphs plotted using Origin 8.0 (OriginLab, Northampton) to obtain the K_D value. Double referenced association and dissociation phase data were globally fitted to a simple 1:1 interaction model ($A + B = AB$). The GPI glycan immobilized on the sensor chip was the same as that used for the affinity chromatography **(B)**.

rested in culture medium for 24 to 72 h. Successful differentiation was assessed in terms of expression of the cell surface marker CD11b by flow cytometry, since CD11b is not expressed on monocytic THP-1 cells (Schwende et al., 1996).

Bone Marrow-Derived Cells

Bone marrow-derived cells were isolated from C57BL/6 (Charles River Laboratories) or WT and moesin-deficient mice from the Max Planck Institute for Infection Biology breeding facility, according to Gonçalves and Mosser (2015). For the generation of bone marrow-derived macrophages (BMDM), bone marrow-derived cells were cultured in IMDM incomplete (IMDM (Gibco) containing 10% FCS and 2 mM L-glutamine) supplemented with 30% L-929 supernatant and 5% horse serum. Macrophage colony-stimulating factor (M-CSF)-expressing L-929 cells were kindly provided by Soo-Kyung Peuschel (Max Planck Institute for Infection Biology, Berlin, Germany). Medium was added at day 3 after seeding and a third of the volume was replaced at days 6 and 8 of culture. At day 10, differentiation was assessed by flow cytometry in terms of expression of macrophage surface markers CD11b and F4/80 as well as intracellular CD68 (Gonçalves and Mosser, 2015). Cells were re-plated for experiments or preserved in frozen stocks for future use.

For the generation of bone marrow-derived dendritic cells (BMDC), bone marrow-derived cells were further processed according to protocols adapted from Lutz et al. (1999), Brasel et al. (2000), Wells et al. (2005) and Madaan et al. (2014). Briefly, bone marrow-derived cells were resuspended in ACK lysis buffer (pH 7.2) and incubated for 2 min at 37°C for erythrocyte lysis. After washing, cells were cultured in RPMI 1640 supplemented with 10% FCS, 1% NEAA, 2 mM L-glutamine, 100 U/ml penicillin/streptomycin (Gibco), 50 μM β-mercaptoethanol, and 20 ng/ml granulocyte-macrophage colony-stimulating factor (GM-CSF; Miltenyi Biotec, Germany) as well as 20 ng/ml IL-4 (Miltenyi Biotec). After 3 days of culture, fresh medium was added to the cells, and half of the medium was replaced with fresh medium at days 6 and 8. At day 10, loosely adherent cells were collected and re-plated in culture medium without IL-4 and 10 ng/ml GM-CSF for 24 h. Optionally, BMDC were LPS-primed (100 ng/ml) for 24 h to mature. BMDC differentiation was assessed by flow cytometry in terms of expression of DC surface markers CD11b, CD11c, and MHCII, as well as F4/80. Upon successful differentiation, BMDC were re-plated for stimulation experiments.

Cell Stimulation

Cells were stimulated with 10 ng/ml LPS (LPS from *E. coli* 0111:B4, Sigma-Aldrich), 10 ng/ml TNF (Miltenyi Biotec, Germany), *P. falciparum* schizont extract diluted 1:100 in culture medium, *P. berghei* schizont extract diluted 1:1,000 in culture medium, or *P. berghei* schizonts added at a ratio of 1:10, i.e., 10 schizonts per cell. *P. falciparum* schizonts were obtained through a percoll gradient centrifugation of a mixed-stages culture as previously described (Rivadeneira et al., 1983). Purified schizonts were washed in PBS and subsequently sonicated to produce schizont extract. *P. berghei* schizont extract was generated by repeated freeze-thaw cycles and adjusted to contain the extract of 4 × 10 e6 schizonts/μl in PBS.

Schizont Culture

For schizont enrichment, blood of *P. berghei*-infected mice was cultured in RPMI 1640 supplemented with 20% FCS (Gibco) and 15 μg/ml gentamycin (Gibco) with mild shaking for 20–24 h at 37°C and 80% humidity under 5% O_2 and 5% CO_2 (Matz et al., 2015). Schizont development was assessed by Giemsa-stained thin blood smear and schizonts were purified by density gradient centrifugation using 60% Percoll (GE Healthcare, UK) in PBS. Schizonts were collected from the interphase, washed repeatedly and further processed depending on experimental end-point.

Transcript Quantification

RNA was isolated with TRIzol reagent (Ambion, Germany), glycogen (Ambion) and ammoniumacetate (Ambion) according to the manufacturer's instructions. Complementary DNA (cDNA) was synthesized from 1 μg total RNA per sample by reverse transcription using the RETROscript reverse transcription kit (Ambion) according to the manufacturer's instructions. Transcript abundance was determined by qPCR with reactions carried out on a StepOne Plus (Applied Biosystems, Germany) with Power SYBR green master mix (Applied Biosystems) and Quantitect primer assays (Qiagen, Germany) for the following transcripts: *Ppib* (Mm_Ppib_1_SG), *Tnf* (Mm_Tnf_1_SG), *Il1b* (Mm_Il1b_2_SG), *Il12a* (Mm_Il12a_1_SG), *Ifng* (Mm_Ifng_1_SG), as well as with primers Hs_*RPL13A*_fwd 5′-CCTGGAGGAGAAGAGGAAAGAGA-3′, Hs_*RPL13A*_rev 5′-TTGAGGACCTCTGTGTATTTGTCAA-3′ (Rizopoulos et al., 2016), Mm_*Gapdh*_fwd 5′-TGAGGCCGGTGCTGAGTATGTCG-3′, Mm_*Gapdh*_rev 5′-CCACAGTCTTCTGGGTGGCAGTG-3′ (Sato et al., 2014) (synthesized by Eurofins Genomics, Germany). qPCR was performed in technical triplicates with the following cycling conditions: 94°C for 15 min and 40 cycles of 94°C for 15 s, 60°C for 60 s. For determining phagosomal degradation, *P. berghei* 18 s RNA transcripts were amplified as specified in Friesen et al. (2010). Melt curve analysis was included in each run to verify the specificity of each reaction. Relative transcript abundance and fold change were determined using the comparative threshold cycle (C_T) method (Schmittgen and Livak, 2008), while *RPL13A*, *Gapdh*, or *Ppib* served as internal controls.

Western Blot

For the detection of proteins using Western blot, samples were prepared by resuspension in sample buffer (Laemmli 2x concentrate, Sigma-Aldrich), separated by SDS-PAGE, and transferred onto Amersham Hybond P 0.45 PVDF membranes (GE Healthcare). Membranes were incubated with anti-MSN antibody (clone 38/87, Sigma-Aldrich; or clone EP1863Y, Abcam, UK) or anti-GAPDH antibody (clone 71.1, Sigma-Aldrich) as a loading control. Antibodies were detected using corresponding anti-mouse or anti-rabbit antibody coupled to HRP (Jackson Immunoresearch, UK) and ECL Western blotting substrate (Pierce, Germany). PageRuler pre-stained protein ladder (Fermentas) was used to determine the molecular weight of separated proteins.

Quantification of Cytokines and Chemokines

THP-1, BMDM, and BMDC supernatants as well as serum of *P. berghei* ANKA Bergreen-infected mice were assayed for cytokines by human or mouse TNF DuoSet ELISA (R&D systems, USA) in combination with the DuoSet ELISA ancillary reagent kit (R&D systems) or by cytometric bead array for the murine cytokines TNF, IFN-γ, IL-6, IL-10, IL-12p70, and MCP-1/CCL2 by using the CBA mouse inflammation kit (BD Biosciences, Germany). Each kit was used according to the manufacturer's instructions.

Flow Cytometry

Cells were incubated with human or mouse FcR blocking reagent (Miltenyi Biotec) according to the manufacturer's instructions prior to antibody staining. Cells were stained with the following antibodies: anti-human CD11b (ICRF44, eBioscience, Germany), anti-mouse CD11b (M1/70, eBioscience), CD11c (N418, eBioscience), CD68 (FA-11, eBioscience), F4/80 (BM8, eBioscicence), MHCII (M5/114.15.2, eBioscience), anti-Moesin (38/87, Sigma-Aldrich; EP1863Y, Abcam), anti-mouse IgG1 (M1-14D12, eBioscience) or anti-rabbit IgG (poly4064, Biolegend; polyclonal, Invitrogen). Stainings included fixable viability dyes LIVE/DEAD fixable dead cell stain aqua (Invitrogen) or fixable viability dye eFluor780 (eBioscience). Fixable viability dyes and antibodies for cell surface antigens were diluted in PBS and added to cells for 15 min at 4°C. For staining of intracellular proteins, cells were fixed in 2% paraformaldehyde (PFA, Sigma-Aldrich) and permeabilized using Permeabilizing solution 2 (BD Biosciences). Antibodies for intracellular antigens were diluted in PBS and added to cells for 30 min at 4°C. For unconjugated primary antibodies, a further incubation step with a secondary fluorochrome-conjugated antibody was performed (30 min, 4°C). Cells were acquired on a FACSCanto or Fortessa (BD Biosciences) in the flow cytometry core facility of the Deutsches Rheuma-Forschungszentrum and data was analyzed in FlowJo (Treestar, USA). The gating strategy employed excluded doublets and dead cells from the analysis and further gates were set based on fluorescence-minus-one (FMO) and unstained controls.

Phagocytosis Assay

BMDM were incubated with labeled or unlabeled P. *berghei* ANKA Bergreen parasites expressing GFP under the HSP70 promoter (Kooij et al., 2012). Briefly, *P. berghei* ANKA Bergreen schizonts were isolated by density gradient centrifugation and stored in 10% glycerol (Roth) in Alsever's solution (Sigma-Aldrich) at −80°C. Due to freeze-thawing of schizonts, merozoites were released from erythrocytes, subsequently washed with PBS and labeled according to a protocol adapted from Cambos and Scorza (2011). Briefly, merozoites were labeled with 5 μM caroboxyfluorescein diacetate succinimidyl ester (CFDA-SE; Molecular Probes, Germany) or 2.5 μM CellTrace Violet (Molecular Probes) in PBS supplemented with 0.1% FCS for 3 min at room temperature. Residual dye was diluted with 10%FCS in PBS, followed by an additional washing step with 10%FCS in PBS. CFSE- or CellTrace Violet-labeled merozoites were resuspended in BMDM culture medium and added to cells at a ratio of 1:10, i.e., 10 merozoites per one BMDM. Alternatively, *P. berghei* ANKA Bergreen schizonts were isolated and immediately added at a ratio of 1:10 to BMDM without prior labeling. At indicated time points, cells were collected on ice, washed in PBS, and stained for cell surface markers or immediately resuspended in acquisition buffer. Phagocytosis was analyzed by flow cytometry based on detection of CFSE, CellTrace Violet, or GFP for unlabeled schizonts. Gate settings were determined using untreated BMDM.

Ethics Statement

All animal work was conducted in accordance with the German "Tierschutzgesetz in der Fassung vom 22. Juli 2009," which implements Directive 2010/63/EU from the European Parliament and Council (On the Protection of Animals Used for Scientific Purposes). The protocol was approved by the ethics committee of the Berlin state authorities (LaGeSo).

Mice

C57BL/6 and NMRI mice were obtained from Charles River laboratories (Germany). Moesin-deficient (Doi et al., 1999) and corresponding wild type control colonies on a C57BL/6 background were maintained by the Max Planck Institute for Infection Biology breeding facility. SNP genotyping (Taconic, USA) revealed that moesin-deficient mice were backcrossed to the C57BL/6 background for at least six generations. Moesin-deficient mice were identified by PCR using *Taq* DNA polymerase (Fermentas) and standard cycling conditions with primers· *Msn*_fwd1 5′-CTGAAGTCGGACAAAGATTTC CAGG-3′, *Msn*_fwd2 5′-CATCAGTATATGAAACAGCCCCCT G-3′, *Msn*_rev 5′-AGGTGTCTCCCAGAGATACGATTTGG-3′ (synthesized by Eurofins Genomics). Mice were kept under specific pathogen-free conditions with *ad libitum* diet at the Max Planck Institute for Infection Biology animal facility in a 12 h light/12 h dark cycle.

P. berghei ANKA Bergreen *In vivo* Infection

Six to nine week old female *Msn-/-* or WT mice were infected with 10,000 *P. berghei* ANKA Bergreen-infected erythrocytes derived from an NMRI donor mouse by i.v. injection. Parasitemia was determined daily by flow cytometry starting day 3 post-infection. Briefly, blood of infected mice was diluted in Alsever's solution containing Hoechst 33342 (Invitrogen) and acquired on a Fortessa flow cytometer (BD Biosciences). Parasitemia was assessed by determining the fraction of GFP$^+$ Hoechst 33342$^+$ cells in the samples. Blood from a naïve mouse served as control for determination of gate settings. Cells single positive for Hoechst 33342, representing leukocytes, were excluded from the analysis. Additionally, serum was collected by retrobulbar punction at indicated time points. Mice were closely monitored for behavioral symptoms of ECM, such as convulsions, absence of touch escape, and unconsciousness (Lackner et al., 2006), and sacrificed when presenting with severe neurological impairment.

Data Analysis

All data was imported into Prism 7.0 (GraphPad) for statistical analysis. Statistical analyses to determine the *P*-value of each comparison are indicated individually. No statistical analysis was performed on data sets with $n < 3$.

RESULTS

Moesin Interacts with *Pf*GPI

The GPI of *Plasmodium* origin has been widely described to induce pro-inflammatory responses from host immune system via pattern recognition receptors such as TLR2 and TLR4 (Krishnegowda et al., 2005). However, observations that TLR2/4 double knockout mice show no resistance to cerebral malaria (Togbe et al., 2007) prompted the question whether additional receptors might be involved in this process. In order to look for interaction partners of *Pf*GPI, we immobilized chemically synthesized GPI glycan (**Figure 1B**) on an affinity column and performed pull-down experiments using plasma membrane preparation from the mouse macrophage cell line RAW264.7. Proteins bound to synthetic GPI glycan were eluted from the column, subjected to SDS-PAGE and identified after trypsin digestion by peptide mass fingerprinting. The membrane-organizing extension spike protein moesin was identified as one of the most prominent GPI-binding protein, and was confirmed by western blot using anti-moesin antibody (**Figure 1A**). Other proteins were also identified but were mostly very abundant proteins that might easily result from contamination such a keratin, actin, and histones. Additionally, proteins such as CD1b were identified along with moesin as potential binding candidates. However, since moesin showed the highest probability after repeated experiments and given the postulated role in LPS signaling (Tohme et al., 1999; Amar et al., 2001; Iontcheva et al., 2004; Zawawi et al., 2010), moesin was selected for further investigations.

Moesin Binds to *Pf*GPI on Microarray and on Surface Plasmon Resonance (SPR)

In a first attempt to confirm the interaction between moesin and GPI glycans, a carbohydrate microarray containing seven synthetic GPI glycans of different length (**Figure 1D** positions 1 to 7), as well as a cap polysaccharide from *Leishmania* as control (**Figure 1D** position 8) was constructed. Incubation of recombinantly expressed GST-moesin with the carbohydrate array revealed binding of moesin to all GPI fragments but not to the cap polysaccharide. In a control experiment, the mannose-specific lectin concanavalin A bound all mannose-containing GPI fragments as well as the cap polysaccharide, but not the shortest GPI fragment lacking any mannose (**Figure 1C**). Next, we studied the kinetics of the interaction between moesin and *Pf*GPI using surface plasmon resonance (SPR). The full GPI-glycan of *Plasmodium falciparum* (**Figure 1B**) was covalently immobilized on an SPR gold chip. Binding was assessed using various concentrations of purified moesin. The result showed a linear concentration-dependent binding of moesin to GPI-glycan (**Figure 1E**). Strikingly, the binding constant (K_D) for the interaction between moesin and GPI was 9.7×10^{-4} M, which is relatively weak but is in the typical range for carbohydrate interaction with carbohydrate-binding proteins (Goldstein and Poretz, 1986; Lee and Lee, 1995). Taken together these results clearly indicated an interaction between moesin and the carbohydrate moiety of the *Pf*GPI anchor.

Malaria PAMP Do Not Induce Moesin Cell Surface Translocation on Macrophage-Like THP-1 Cells

After clearly establishing the binding of moesin to *Pf*GPI we next sought to determine the physiological relevance of this interaction in the context of malaria. The classification of *Pf*GPI as one of the major malaria toxins is due to its ability to induce the secretion of pro-inflammatory cytokines from host innate immune cells such as macrophages *in vitro* (Schofield and Hackett, 1993; Tachado et al., 1996; Krishnegowda et al., 2005; Zhu et al., 2009). Intriguingly, moesin is primarily described as an intracellular protein (Ponuwei, 2016), yet translocation to the cell surface of e.g., macrophage-like THP-1 cells was reported to be induced by LPS stimulation (Iontcheva et al., 2004). Consequently, it was hypothesized that moesin might acts as a macrophage cell surface receptor for *Plasmodium* GPI. Given that GPI are abundantly present on the parasite surface (Gowda, 2007), preparations of schizont extracts were used as a stimulus containing *Plasmodium* GPI. In order to evaluate the responsiveness of human macrophage-like THP-1 cells to stimulation with LPS or GPI-containing *P. falciparum* schizont extract (*Pf*SE), TNF secretion was determined in cell culture supernatants by ELISA. While macrophage-like THP-1 cells secrete TNF to a great extent when stimulated with LPS, stimulation with *Pf*SE also results in a consistent yet less pronounced induction of TNF secretion from differentiated THP-1 cells (**Figure 2A**). Given the suitability of the stimuli applied to elicit a pro-inflammatory response, next we assessed the cell surface localization of moesin upon stimulation of human macrophage-like THP-1 cells with LPS or *Pf*SE by flow cytometry. Surprisingly, moesin cell surface translocation was not detected on viable differentiated THP-1 cells with anti-moesin antibody 38/87 in either LPS- or *Pf*SE-treated samples at all timepoints tested (**Figure 2B**). This finding was further corroborated by using another anti-moesin antibody clone (EP1863Y) (**Figure 2B**). Moreover, the suitability of the staining protocol was verified by successful intracellular moesin detection with each anti-moesin antibody clone (**Figure 2C**). Taken together, these results indicate that even though macrophage-like THP-1 cells respond to both LPS and *Pf*SE by TNF secretion, this response is not accompanied by recruitment of moesin to the cell surface.

Macrophage Response to Malaria PAMP Is Moesin-Independent

Since *Pf*GPI-induced TNF secretion was reported to be MyD88-dependent (Krishnegowda et al., 2005), another aspect to be investigated by this study was the role of moesin in *Plasmodium* GPI-induced signal transduction leading to the secretion of pro-inflammatory cytokines. In order to address this question *in vitro*, we isolated cells from moesin-deficient mice (Doi et al., 1999). Moesin-deficient mice were identified by PCR (Supplementary Figure 2A) and lack of moesin protein was validated via western blot. Surprisingly, use of anti-moesin antibody 38/87 suggested the presence of moesin in cells isolated from moesin-deficient mice (Supplementary Figure 2B), while anti-moesin antibody EP1863Y confirmed the absence of moesin from moesin-deficient mice (Supplementary Figure 2C). Since anti-moesin antibody 38/87 recognizes a second, slightly heavier protein in human THP-1 cells (Supplementary Figure 2B), and the protein recognized in murine samples corresponds to the size of the upper band detected in human THP-1 cells, it may be concluded that this antibody clone binds unspecifically to a protein other than moesin in murine samples. Consequently, anti-moesin antibody clone EP1863Y was used for subsequent experiments. Next, bone marrow-derived macrophages (BMDM) were generated from both wild type (WT) and moesin-deficient C57BL/6 mice. Successful differentiation was confirmed by flow cytometric analysis of the key mouse macrophage surface markers CD11b and F4/80, as well as intracellular CD68 (Gonçalves and Mosser, 2015). All viable WT and moesin-deficient BMDM expressed both, CD11b and F4/80, and cells were also largely positive for CD68, thus verifying efficient differentiation of bone marrow-derived cells (Supplementary Figure 2D).

Upon confirmation of differentiation of WT and moesin-deficient BMDM, cells were stimulated with LPS, *Pf*SE, *P. berghei* schizont extract (*Pb*SE), and *P. berghei* schizonts (*Pb*S) for 24 h and cell culture supernatants were analyzed for TNF concentrations by ELISA or CBA. Despite previous reports on markedly reduced LPS-induced TNF secretion in the absence of moesin (Iontcheva et al., 2004) or antibody-mediated moesin blocking (Tohme et al., 1999; Amar et al., 2001; Zawawi et al., 2010), TNF concentration in supernatants of LPS-treated moesin-deficient BMDM was similar to WT BMDM in the experimental setting used here (**Figure 3A**). Additionally, the TNF response induced by *Plasmodium*-derived stimuli was not markedly different between WT and moesin-deficient BMDM. Since the TNF response induced by malaria PAMPs was generally low and variable for both WT and moesin-deficient cells, potential differences in TNF secretion may not be detectable in this experimental setting. Therefore, transcript

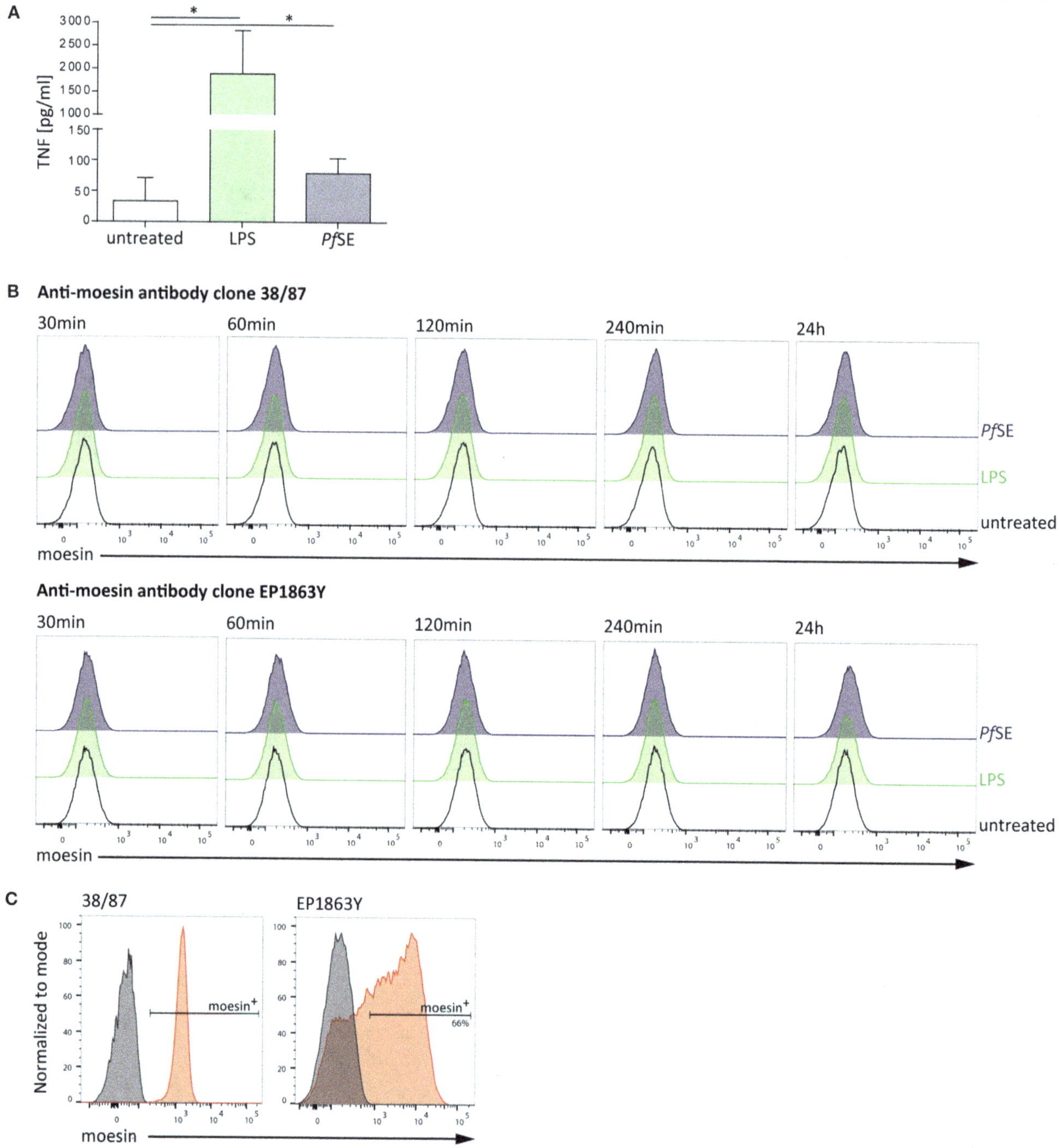

FIGURE 2 | Macrophage-like THP-1 cell response to stimulation is not accompanied by moesin cell surface localization. (A) Macrophage-like THP-1 cell responsiveness to stimulation determined by TNF-ELISA after 24 h treatment; LPS: 10 ng/ml, *P. falciparum* schizont extract (*Pf*SE): 1:100 in medium; $n = 5$, bars indicate mean + SD; One-way ANOVA of paired samples with Dunnett correction revealed $^*P < 0.05$. **(B)** Representative histograms of moesin cell surface staining in macrophage-like THP-1 cells at different time points of stimulation, detected by flow cytometry with time points and treatments indicated, gated on viable CD11b$^+$ cells, detection with anti-moesin antibody clone 38/87, and anti-mouse IgG-FITC [upper panel; cells differentiated with 20 ng/ml PMA for 24 h (Iontcheva et al., 2004)] and with anti-moesin antibody clone EP1863Y and anti-rabbit IgG-PE (lower panel; cells differentiated with 200 nM PMA for 72 h) **(C)** Intracellular staining control for moesin; left: viable undifferentiated THP-1, right: viable differentiated THP-1; gray: secondary antibody staining control, red: moesin$^+$ cells detected with anti-mouse IgG-APC for clone 38/87, and anti-rabbit IgG-PE for clone EP1863Y. Dead cells were excluded from all flow cytometric analyses by using a fixable viability dye.

levels of *Tnf* and *Il1b* were determined by qPCR in both WT and moesin-deficient BMDM after 4 h of stimulation under otherwise unchanged conditions. In good agreement with TNF concentration in BMDM supernatants, induction of TNF transcripts was most pronounced in LPS-treated samples (~100-fold compared to untreated BMDM). Transcription of

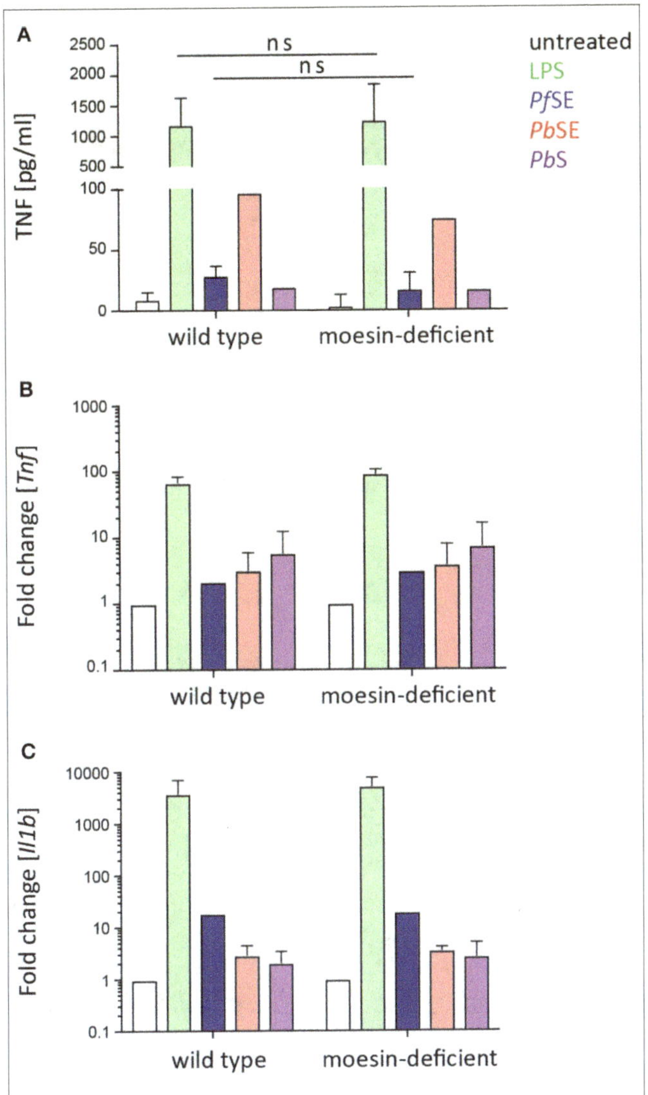

FIGURE 3 | BMDM response to stimulation is moesin-independent. (A) TNF secretion upon BMDM stimulation determined in supernatants after 24 h stimulation by TNF-ELISA and CBA, $n = 4$ for untreated/LPS/*P. falciparum* schizont extract (*Pf*SE), $n = 1$ for *P. berghei* schizont extract (*Pb*SE), and *P. berghei* schizonts (*Pb*S); unpaired *t*-test revealed that differences are not significant (ns); **(B,C)** *Tnf* and *Il1b* expression detected by qPCR, relative expression was calculated with respect to *Gapdh*, relative expression in treated groups was normalized to untreated cells; $n = 2$ for LPS/*Pb*S/*Pb*SE, $n = 1$ for *Pf*SE; LPS: 10 ng/ml, *Pf*SE: 1:100 dilution in medium, *Pb*SE: 1:1,000 dilution in medium, *Pb*S added at a ratio of 1:10. Bars indicate mean + SD.

the *Tnf* gene was also induced by *Plasmodium*-derived stimuli, yet to a much lower extent (~5-fold compared to untreated BMDM) than that initiated by LPS treatment (**Figure 3B**). Nevertheless, induction of TNF transcripts was similar in WT and moesin-deficient BMDM for all conditions tested. Another *Plasmodium* GPI-induced cytokine is IL-1β (Schofield and Hackett, 1993), and LPS-induced secretion of IL-1β has also been demonstrated to be moesin-dependent (Zawawi et al., 2010), thus indicating a role for moesin in signal transduction leading to IL-1β secretion. However, in the present study, induction of *Il1b* gene transcription did not markedly differ in WT and moesin-deficient BMDM for all stimuli applied, including LPS (**Figure 3C**). Taken together, these results demonstrate that the macrophage pro-inflammatory response to malaria PAMPs in terms of TNF secretion as well as *Tnf* and *Il1b* gene transcription is not as pronounced as that elicited by LPS. Furthermore, moesin-deficient and WT BMDM responded similarly to LPS and *Plasmodium*-derived stimuli, suggesting that moesin is not essential in signaling processes leading to TNF secretion and *Il1b* gene transcription in murine BMDM.

Since it cannot be excluded that stimulation-induced cell surface localization of moesin is required for prompting other processes so far not covered in this study, we also investigated the translocation of moesin to the cell surface of macrophages upon stimulation with PAMPs in the murine system. Therefore, WT BMDM were stimulated with LPS, *Pf*SE, and *Pb*SE for different periods of time and analyzed for moesin cell surface expression via flow cytometry. In line with our observations in differentiated human THP-1 cells, localization of moesin to the cell surface of viable WT BMDM was not detected with anti-moesin antibody clone EP1863Y in either LPS-, *Pf*SE-, or *Pb*SE-treated samples at all timepoints tested (**Figure 4A**), while the intracellular staining control demonstrated the suitability of the protocol to detect moesin (**Figure 4B**).

Moesin-Deficient Macrophages Display Unaltered Phagocytic Activity

An alternative site for moesin and *Plasmodium* GPI to interact is at the phagosomal membrane (Desjardins et al., 1994; Defacque et al., 2000) and thus moesin might orchestrate parasite recognition and/or degradation (Defacque et al., 2000; Erwig et al., 2006). Consequently, experiments aimed at investigating whether moesin is critically involved in phagocytic uptake and degradation of *P. berghei* merozoites or schizonts were performed.

In order to determine the impact of moesin-deficiency on *P. berghei* merozoite internalization, CFSE- or CellTrace Violet-labeled *P. berghei* merozoites were added to WT and moesin-deficient BMDM for different periods of time and phagocytosis was analyzed by flow cytometry (**Figures 5A,B**). Since the two approaches revealed comparable phagocytic uptake of *P. berghei* merozoites by WT and moesin-deficient BMDM, unlabeled *P. berghei* schizonts expressing high levels of GFP [ANKA Bergreen; (Kooij et al., 2012)] were used next in order to exclude that excess CFSE or CellTrace Violet dye resulted in BMDM labeling instead of reflecting phagocytosis. Although the three approaches differed in overall detection levels of phagocytic activity, phagocytic uptake of parasites was consistently similar in WT and moesin-deficient BMDM within experiments at all-time points tested (**Figures 5A–C**). Additionally, WT and moesin-deficient BMDM were incubated with *P. berghei* merozoites for 4 and 24 h in order to assess parasite degradation on the RNA level via qPCR. In good agreement with the data obtained by flow cytometry, *P. berghei* rRNA levels were similar in WT and moesin-deficient BMDM after 4 h of incubation (**Figure 5D**), thus confirming that moesin is not essential for phagocytic uptake of *P. berghei* merozoites. Additionally, *P. berghei* rRNA levels were markedly reduced after 24 h of incubation in both WT and moesin-deficient BMDM to a similar extent

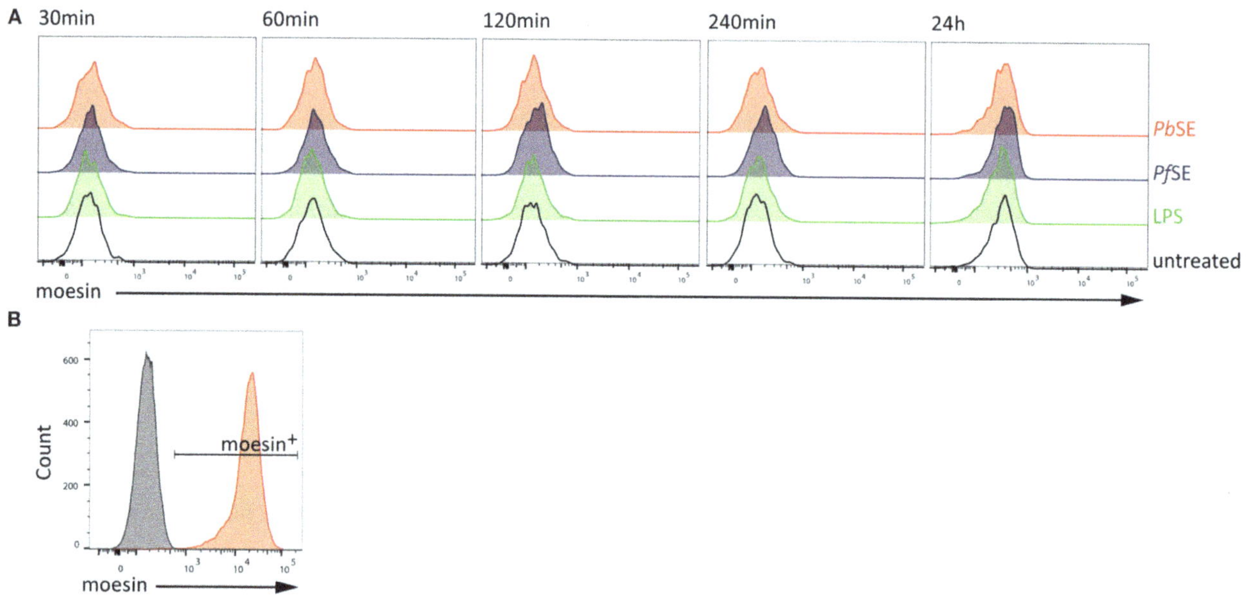

FIGURE 4 | Absence of moesin on BMDM cell surface. (A) Flow cytometric analysis of moesin cell surface localization on viable CD11b+F4/80+ BMDM over time with stimuli indicated; detection of anti-moesin EP1863Y using anti-rabbit-PE; **(B)** Intracellular moesin detection in viable CD11b+ BMDM; gray: secondary antibody control, red: moesin+ cells using anti-moesin antibody EP1863Y and anti-rabbit IgG-AlexaFluor488.

(**Figure 5D**), thereby indicating that lack of moesin does not impair phagosomal degradation of parasite material.

Moesin Deficiency Does Not Affect Dendritic Cell Response to Malaria PAMP

In line with the observations of the present study, Wu et al. (2015) reported that macrophage responsiveness is impaired due to *Plasmodium*-induced phagosomal acidification and that early cytokine responses to *Plasmodium* infection are rather DC-mediated. Given that macrophages and DCs both recognize PAMPs via pattern recognition receptors and are capable of phagocytosis (Gazzinelli et al., 2014), the interaction of moesin and *Plasmodium* GPI may serve a similar function like that proposed for macrophages in DCs. Consequently, bone marrow-derived dendritic cells (BMDC) were generated and successful differentiation was confirmed by flow cytometric analysis of viable WT BMDC which expressed key DC surface markers, i.e., CD11b, CD11c, and MHCII (Lutz et al., 1999), while only few cells expressed the macrophage marker F4/80 (**Figure 6A**). In line with previous reports (Madaan et al., 2014), LPS-priming induced maturation of BMDC, as indicated by a population shift to high level MHCII expression (Villadangos et al., 2005), demonstrating that the cells are properly differentiated.

Next, WT and moesin-deficient BMDC were stimulated with LPS, *PbSE*, and *P. berghei* schizonts and TNF as well as IL-6 concentrations in supernatants were analyzed by CBA. In good agreement with previous observations in BMDM, the LPS- and malaria PAMP-induced response of BMDC revealed subtle and inconsistent differences between WT and moesin-deficient BMDC for all conditions tested (**Figures 6B,C**). Even though the cytokine response to *Plasmodium*-derived stimuli is rather low, these results indicate that the BMDC response to these pathogen-derived stimuli as measured by TNF and IL-6 secretion is independent of the presence of moesin.

Immune Response to *P. berghei* ANKA and Infection Outcome Are Moesin-Independent

While a pivotal role of moesin-*Plasmodium* GPI interaction for macrophage responsiveness or functionality could not be demonstrated with the *in vitro* assays performed in this study, the interaction of moesin with *Plasmodium* GPI may be relevant in other *Plasmodium*-related host responses *in vivo*. Additionally, moesin may be involved in key events leading to the development of malaria pathology independent of its interaction with *Plasmodium* GPI, since moesin was described to be relevant in immunological synapse formation (Itoh et al., 2002; Parameswaran and Gupta, 2013) and in endothelial permeability (Koss et al., 2006; Yao and Tsirka, 2011). Thus, moesin-deficient C57BL/6 mice and the corresponding wild type controls were infected with *P. berghei* ANKA Bergreen blood stage parasites in order to investigate the potential involvement of moesin in the development of ECM. Despite the previously mentioned indications for moesin to play a role during processes leading to ECM, moesin-deficient mice were not protected from development of ECM (**Figure 7A**) concomitant with normal progression of parasite growth (**Figure 7B**). Moreover, lack of moesin did not affect the pro-inflammatory immune response mounted upon *P. berghei* ANKA

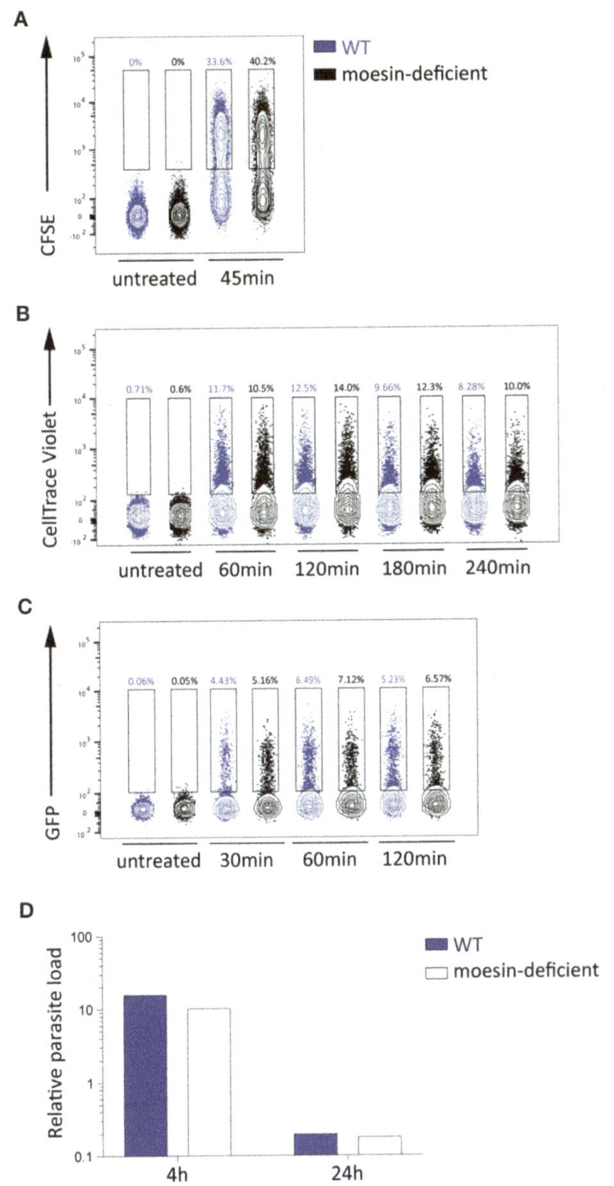

FIGURE 5 | Phagocytosis and phagosomal degration of parasites in BMDM is moesin-independent. (A–C) Flow cytometric analysis of *P. berghei* phagocytosis by WT and moesin-deficient BMDM for the time indicated, numbers represent percentage of BMDM that phagocytosed parasites; $n = 1$ for all sets **(A)** Phagocytosis of CFSE-labeled *P. berghei* ANKA merozoites in viable CD11b$^+$ F4/80$^+$ BMDM; **(B)** Phagocytosis of CellTrace Violet-labeled *P. berghei* ANKA merozoites in BMDM; **(C)** Phagocytosis of unlabeled *P. berghei* ANKA Bergreen (GFP$^+$) schizonts in BMDM; **(D)** Detection of *P. berghei* 18 s rRNA in BMDM by qPCR, expressed as relative parasite load, after 4 and 24 h of incubation with *P. berghei* ANKA merozoites ($n = 1$), reduction in *P. berghei* 18 s rRNA indicates phagosomal degradation.

infection in terms of serum levels of TNF, IL-6 and MCP-1/CCL2 (**Figures 7C,E,F**). Noteworthy, the interferon (IFN)-γ response differed significantly ($p = 0.03$) between WT and moesin-deficient mice at days 3 and 5 post-infection (**Figure 7D**), yet higher serum IFN-γ concentration at day 5 post-infection did not impact the overall course of infection in moesin-deficient mice.

DISCUSSION

In the present study, the ERM protein moesin was found to interact with *Plasmodium* GPI *in vitro* and the relevance of this interaction was further investigated in the context of *Plasmodium*-induced pro-inflammatory responses and pathology. Moesin is a protein of the ERM family, which undergoes conformational change upon phosphatidylinositol-4,5-bisphosphate (PIP_2)-mediated phosphorylation (Neisch and Fehon, 2011) and links actin filaments to transmembrane proteins (Louvet-Vallee, 2000). Thereby, ERM proteins contribute to cytoskeletal rearrangement, cellular migration, and membrane dynamics (Ponuwei, 2016). In addition to ERM proteins interacting with phosphatidylinositide 3-kinase, protein kinase A, or Rho-specific GDP dissociation inhibitors (Ivetic and Ridley, 2004; Niggli and Rossy, 2008; Ponuwei, 2016), it has been suggested that LPS-induced TNF secretion is mediated by moesin signaling through the adapter protein MyD88 (Zawawi et al., 2010).

Moesin is a membrane-associated intracellular protein, which was previously reported to translocate to the cell surface upon LPS stimulation (Iontcheva et al., 2004; Takamatsu et al., 2009) and to be constitutively present on the surface of lymphocyte subsets (Takamatsu et al., 2009). Therefore, it was hypothesized that, upon translocation to the cell surface, moesin might interact with *Plasmodium* GPI. In contrast to previous reports on LPS-induced moesin cell surface translocation (Iontcheva et al., 2004; Takamatsu et al., 2009), we were unable to detect moesin on the cell surface of LPS-stimulated macrophage-like THP-1 cells or BMDM. Since intracellular moesin was detected in THP-1 cells and BMDM, and given that THP-1 cells as well as BMDM and BMDC responded to LPS-stimulation with TNF secretion, we were able to demonstrate that our protocol is generally suitable to detect moesin by flow cytometry and to elicit an LPS-induced pro-inflammatory cytokine response from different cell types. Although transient or nominal cell surface translocation of moesin upon LPS or *Pf*SE/*Pb*SE stimulation may not have been detected with the experimental settings used here, our results indicate permanent absence of moesin from the cell surface of macrophages *in vitro*.

The phagosome may be an alternative site for *Plasmodium* GPI and moesin to interact, since merozoite surface GPI become exposed upon schizont degradation. Moesin was described to be associated with phagosomes in murine J774 and human U937 macrophages (Desjardins et al., 1994; Defacque et al., 2000) and to be involved in phagosomal acidification (Erwig et al., 2006). However, in accordance with a previous study reporting that the rate of phagocytosis of apoptotic cells is moesin-independent (Erwig et al., 2006), moesin-deficiency did not affect non-opsonic uptake of *P. berghei* merozoites or schizonts in three independent experiments. Additionally, the absence of moesin did not have an impact on phagosomal degradation of *P. berghei* 18 s rRNA. Even though degradation of *P. berghei* 18 s rRNA was only analyzed once and at a limited number of time points, markedly reduced 18 s rRNA levels after 24 h of incubation in both wild type and moesin-deficient BMDM indicate that the presence of moesin is not critical for this process. Notably, the degradation of parasite

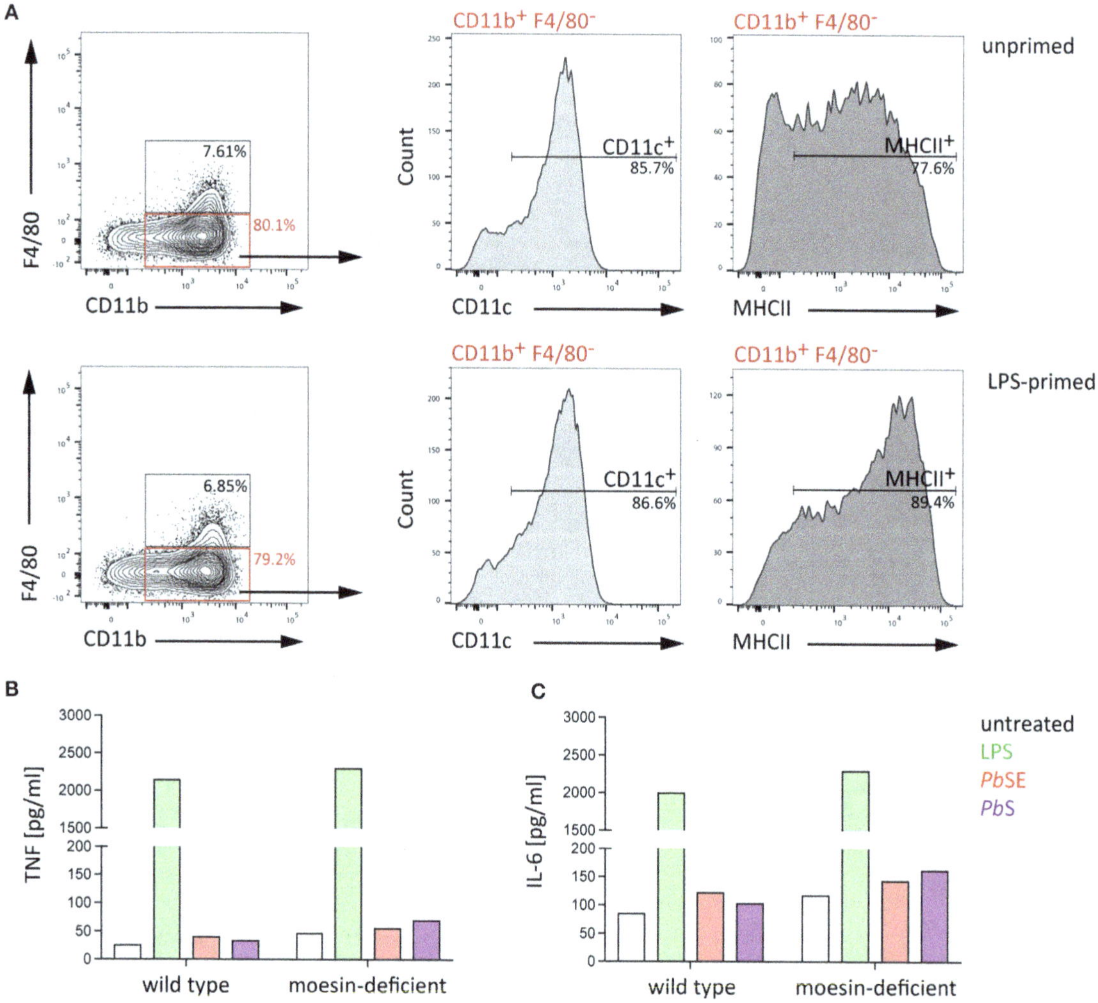

FIGURE 6 | WT and moesin-deficient BMDC respond similarly to stimulation. BMDC were generated from bone marrow-derived cells of C57BL/6 WT mice using GM-CSF and IL-4 **(A)** Representative plots of flow cytometric analysis of BMDC differentiation with and without 24 h LPS priming; F4/80$^+$ cells were excluded and CD11b$^+$ cells analyzed for CD11c and MHCII surface expression, gates were set according to FMO controls and dead cells were excluded from analysis by using a fixable viability dye. **(B,C)** Response of unprimed WT and moesin-deficient BMDC to stimulation with LPS (10 ng/ml), *P. berghei* schizont extract (*Pb*SE, 1:1,000 dilution in medium), and *P. berghei* schizonts (*Pb* schizonts, added at a ratio of 1:10 to BMDC), determined after 24 h incubation by CBA; **(B)** TNF supernatant concentrations of stimulated BMDC, **(C)** IL-6 concentrations in supernatants of BMDC; Due to $n = 1$, no statistical analysis was performed.

components other than 18 s rRNA, e.g., hemozoin, was not quantified. Although Fc receptor-mediated phagocytic uptake of antibody-opsonized *P. berghei* merozoites or schizonts could be affected by moesin-deficiency, previously published data suggest that ERM proteins do not localize to phagosomes containing opsonized cells (Erwig et al., 2006).

Previous studies investigating the pro-inflammatory response to *Plasmodium* GPI demonstrated pronounced TNF secretion from BMDM *in vitro* using purified *Pf*GPI immobilized on gold particles (Krishnegowda et al., 2005; Zhu et al., 2009, 2011). Additionally, purified GPI of other protozoan parasites such as *Toxoplasma gondii* have been described to induce TNF secretion from murine macrophages *in vitro* (Debierre-Grockiego et al., 2003), indicating that protozoan GPI represent conserved PAMP. Although malaria PAMP other than GPI were present in the schizont extracts used here, which could activate pattern recognition receptors independent of moesin, we observed minor cytokine secretion and subtle induction of cytokine transcription in both wild type and moesin-deficient BMDM and BMDC. Thus, it seems unlikely that a potential contribution of moesin to *Plasmodium* GPI-induced signaling has been masked by activation of other pathways leading to cytokine production.

In line with our observation of a subtle induction of pro-inflammatory cytokines upon BMDM stimulation with *P. berghei* schizonts, another recent study reported that the cytokine response of BMDM is impaired upon internalization of *P. falciparum*- or *P. berghei*-infected erythrocytes or merozoites due to pronounced phagosomal acidification and consequential inactivation of endosomal TLR (Wu et al., 2015). Furthermore,

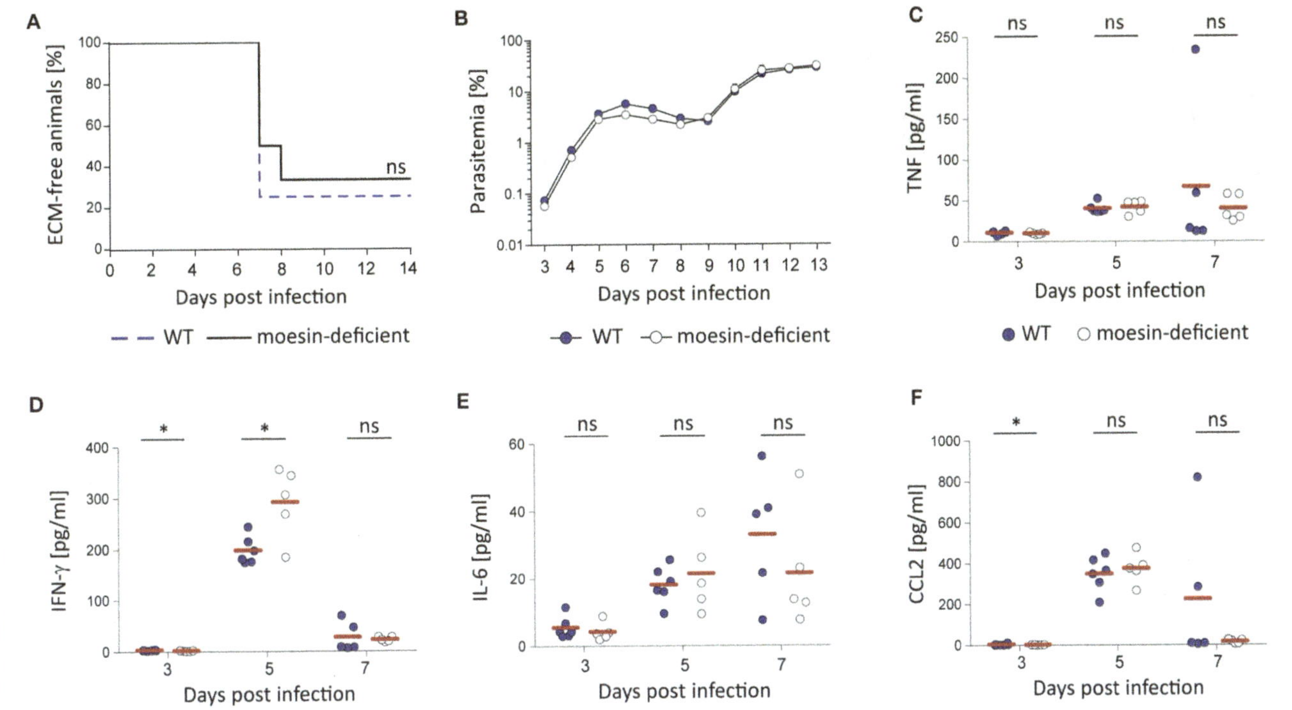

FIGURE 7 | Moesin-deficiency does not protect mice from *P. berghei* ANKA-induced ECM. Moesin-deficient mice and corresponding WT controls were infected by i.v. injection of 10,000 *P. berghei* ANKA Bergreen-infected erythrocytes and the impact of moesin-deficiency on the course of infection and the systemic immune response was analyzed; **(A)** Survival curve indicating development of ECM in both WT and moesin-deficient mice, $n = 12$/genotype; Mantel Cox test revealed that differences are non-significant. **(B)** Representative parasitemia ($n = 6$/genotype) indicating similar progression of parasite growth independent of the host genotype. Parasitemia was determined by flow cytometric analysis of GFP^+ erythrocytes; Dots display mean parasitemia + SD **(C–F)** Serum was collected from infected mice ($n = 6$ for WT, $n = 5$ for $Msn^{-/-}$) at days 3, 5, and 7 post-infection by retrobulbar punction and analyzed for serum concentration of TNF **(C)**, IFN-γ **(D)**, IL-6 **(E)**, and CCL2 **(F)** by CBA. Dots represent individual mice, bars indicate means. Analysis by Mann-Whitney test: $^*P < 0.05$, ns, non-significant.

the majority of splenic macrophages isolated from *P. berghei* ANKA-infected mice did not produce inflammatory cytokines (Wu et al., 2015). Collectively, our data support the notion that macrophages contribute marginally to the pro-inflammatory cytokine response at early stages of infection (Stevenson and Riley, 2004). Interestingly, it was recently demonstrated that *in vitro* stimulation of BMDC with *P. falciparum*-infected erythrocytes or merozoites resulted in cytokine secretion in a dose-dependent manner (Wu et al., 2015). In contrast, the BMDC cytokine responses to *Plasmodium*-derived stimuli observed here were subtle and inconsistent. Since the properties of BMDC generated *in vitro* vary depending on the stimuli used to induce differentiation (Xu et al., 2007), these BMDC may not properly reflect the spectrum of DC subtypes, e.g. monocyte-derived and plasmacytoid DC (Heath and Carbone, 2013), yet cytokine responses to *P. berghei* ANKA infection are DC subtype-dependent *in vivo* (Wu et al., 2015). However, cytokine secretion and transcription were markedly induced by LPS, suggesting that BMDC were generally proficient to respond to TLR ligands. Notably, despite previous reports on considerably reduced LPS-induced TNF secretion from THP-1 cells when moesin was silenced (Iontcheva et al., 2004) or blocked by anti-moesin antibody (Tohme et al., 1999; Amar et al., 2001; Zawawi et al., 2010), the LPS-induced TNF response was not affected by moesin-deficiency when compared to wild type BMDM or BMDC. Consequently, these results indicate that the LPS-induced cytokine response from murine BMDM and BMDC is moesin-independent *in vitro*. Although moesin likely serves similar functions in human and murine cells, further studies are needed to clarify the localization and the role of moesin in the pro-inflammatory immune response to LPS in human cells.

Moesin is the predominantly expressed ERM protein in T-cells (Itoh et al., 2002) and ERM proteins are involved in immunological synapse formation, thereby modulating T and B cell activation (Itoh et al., 2002; Parameswaran and Gupta, 2013). Furthermore, moesin is the predominant ERM protein in endothelial cells (Berryman et al., 1993) and was found to be involved in TNF-induced endothelial cell paracellular gap formation, resulting in increased endothelial permeability *in vitro* (Koss et al., 2006). Nevertheless, moesin-deficiency did not impair pro-inflammatory cytokine responses to *P. berghei* ANKA infection and did not affect ECM-associated mortality *in vivo*. These findings point toward a dispensable role for moesin as well as the interaction of moesin with *Plasmodium* GPI in the immune response to *P. berghei* ANKA infection and in the manifestation of symptoms of ECM.

Collectively, our findings demonstrate that even though *Plasmodium* GPI and moesin interact, the relevance of this interaction in the context of malaria pathology could not be established. Interestingly, although moesin has been described to be the predominantly expressed ERM protein in lymphocytes (Itoh et al., 2002) and endothelial cells (Berryman et al., 1993), it cannot be excluded that moesin-deficiency may be compensated for by other proteins of the ERM family, especially taking partial functional redundancy of ERM proteins into consideration (Niggli and Rossy, 2008). Additionally, given the conflicting *in vitro* data and considering that TLR-deficiency did not protect mice from ECM (Togbe et al., 2007; Lepenies et al., 2008), the precise mechanisms leading to the activation of the innate immune system during *Plasmodium* infection, as well as the relevance of GPI in this process, need to be further investigated to elucidate the underlying mechanisms of malaria pathology.

AUTHOR CONTRIBUTIONS

FK conceived the study. JD, NA, XL, and FK designed and performed the experimental work. JD, NA, PS, and FK analyzed and interpreted data. ST provided moesin-deficient embryos. JD and FK wrote the manuscript. All authors approved the final version of the manuscript.

FUNDING

This work was supported by the German Research Foundation grant to FK (KA 3347/4-1), the German Federal Ministry for Education and Research (BMBF) and the Max Planck Society.

ACKNOWLEDGMENTS

We thank Kai Matuschewski for insightful comments and fruitful discussions. We also thank Toralf Kaiser and Jenny Kirsch of the flow cytometry core facility at the Deutsches Rheuma-Forschungszentrum (Berlin) as well as the Max Planck Institute for Infection Biology breeding facility for technical assistance. We thank Pedro Moura-Alves and Soo-Kyung Peuschel for kindly providing THP-1 and L-929 cells, respectively. Parts of this work have been published previously in a PhD thesis by JD and may therefore present similarities in wording and/or content without constituting plagiarism.

REFERENCES

Amar, S., Oyaisu, K., Li, L., and Van Dyke, T. (2001). Moesin: a potential LPS receptor on human monocytes. *J. Endotoxin Res.* 7, 281–286. doi: 10.1177/09680519010070041001

Berryman, M., Franck, Z., and Bretscher, A. (1993). Ezrin is concentrated in the apical microvilli of a wide variety of epithelial cells whereas moesin is found primarily in endothelial cells. *J. Cell Sci.* 105(Pt 4), 1025–1043.

Boutlis, C. S., Riley, E. M., Anstey, N. M., and De Souza, J. B. (2005). Glycosylphosphatidylinositols in malaria pathogenesis and immunity: potential for therapeutic inhibition and vaccination. *Curr. Top. Microbiol. Immunol.* 297, 145–185. doi: 10.1007/3-540-29967-x_5

Brasel, K., De Smedt, T., Smith, J. L., and Maliszewski, C. R. (2000). Generation of murine dendritic cells from flt3-ligand-supplemented bone marrow cultures. *Blood* 96, 3029–3039. Available online at: http://www.bloodjournal.org/content/96/9/3029

Cambos, M., and Scorza, T. (2011). Robust erythrophagocytosis leads to macrophage apoptosis via a hemin-mediated redox imbalance: role in hemolytic disorders. *J. Leukoc. Biol.* 89, 159–171. doi: 10.1189/jlb.0510249

Cunnington, A. J., Walther, M., and Riley, E. M. (2013). Piecing together the puzzle of severe malaria. *Sci. Transl. Med.* 5, 211ps218. doi: 10.1126/scitranslmed.3007432

Debierre-Grockiego, F., Azzouz, N., Schmidt, J., Dubremetz, J. F., Geyer, H., Geyer, R., et al. (2003). Roles of glycosylphosphatidylinositols of Toxoplasma gondii. Induction of tumor necrosis factor-alpha production in macrophages. *J. Biol. Chem.* 278, 32987–32993. doi: 10.1074/jbc.M304791200

Defacque, H., Egeberg, M., Habermann, A., Diakonova, M., Roy, C., Mangeat, P., et al. (2000). Involvement of ezrin/moesin in de novo actin assembly on phagosomal membranes. *EMBO J.* 19, 199–212. doi: 10.1093/emboj/19.2.199

Desjardins, M., Celis, J. E., Van Meer, G., Dieplinger, H., Jahraus, A., Griffiths, G., et al. (1994). Molecular characterization of phagosomes. *J. Biol. Chem.* 269, 32194–32200.

Doi, Y., Itoh, M., Yonemura, S., Ishihara, S., Takano, H., Noda, T., et al. (1999). Normal development of mice and unimpaired cell adhesion/cell motility/actin-based cytoskeleton without compensatory up-regulation of ezrin or radixin in moesin gene knockout. *J. Biol. Chem.* 274, 2315–2321. doi: 10.1074/jbc.274.4.2315

Erwig, L. P., McPhilips, K. A., Wynes, M. W., Ivetic, A., Ridley, A. J., and Henson, P. M. (2006). Differential regulation of phagosome maturation in macrophages and dendritic cells mediated by Rho GTPases and ezrin-radixin-moesin (ERM) proteins. *Proc. Natl. Acad. Sci. U.S.A.* 103, 12825–12830. doi: 10.1073/pnas.0605331103

Friesen, J., Silvie, O., Putrianti, E. D., Hafalla, J. C., Matuschewski, K., and Borrmann, S. (2010). Natural immunization against malaria: causal prophylaxis with antibiotics. *Sci. Transl. Med.* 2, 40ra49. doi: 10.1126/scitranslmed.3001058

Gazzinelli, R. T., Kalantari, P., Fitzgerald, K. A., and Golenbock, D. T. (2014). Innate sensing of malaria parasites. *Nat. Rev. Immunol.* 14, 744–757. doi: 10.1038/nri3742

Goldstein, I. J., and Poretz, R. D. (1986). "Isolation, physicochemical characterization, and carbohydrate-binding specificity of lectins," in *The Lectins: Properties, Functions, and Applications in Biology and Medicine*, eds I. E. Liener, N. Sharon and I. J. Goldstein (Orlando, FL: Academic Press, Inc.), 33–247.

Gonçalves, R., and Mosser, D. M. (2015). The isolation and characterization of murine macrophages. *Curr. Protoc. Immunol.* 111, 14.01.01–14.01.16. doi: 10.1002/0471142735.im1401s111

Gowda, D. C. (2007). TLR-mediated cell signaling by malaria GPIs. *Trends Parasitol.* 23, 596–604. doi: 10.1016/j.pt.2007.09.003

Heath, W. R., and Carbone, F. R. (2013). The skin-resident and migratory immune system in steady state and memory: innate lymphocytes, dendritic cells and T cells. *Nat. Immunol.* 14, 978–985. doi: 10.1038/ni.2680

Iontcheva, I., Amar, S., Zawawi, K. H., Kantarci, A., and Van Dyke, T. E. (2004). Role for moesin in lipopolysaccharide-stimulated signal transduction. *Infect. Immun.* 72, 2312–2320. doi: 10.1128/IAI.72.4.2312-2320.2004

Itoh, K., Sakakibara, M., Yamasaki, S., Takeuchi, A., Arase, H., Miyazaki, M., et al. (2002). Cutting edge: negative regulation of immune synapse formation by anchoring lipid raft to cytoskeleton through Cbp-EBP50-ERM assembly. *J. Immunol.* 168, 541–544. doi: 10.4049/jimmunol.168.2.541

Ivctic, A., and Ridley, A. J. (2004). Ezrin/radixin/moesin proteins and Rho GTPase signalling in leucocytes. *Immunology* 112, 165–176. doi: 10.1111/j.1365-2567.2004.01882.x

Kamena, F., Tamborrini, M., Liu, X., Kwon, Y. U., Thompson, F., Pluschke, G., et al. (2008). Synthetic GPI array to study antitoxic malaria response. *Nat. Chem. Biol.* 4, 238–240. doi: 10.1038/nchembio.75

Kawai, T., and Akira, S. (2011). Toll-like receptors and their crosstalk with other innate receptors in infection and immunity. *Immunity* 34, 637–650. doi: 10.1016/j.immuni.2011.05.006

Kooij, T. W., Rauch, M. M., and Matuschewski, K. (2012). Expansion of experimental genetics approaches for *Plasmodium berghei* with versatile transfection vectors. *Mol. Biochem. Parasitol.* 185, 19–26. doi: 10.1016/j.molbiopara.2012.06.001

Koss, M., Pfeiffer, G. R. II., Wang, Y., Thomas, S. T., Yerukhimovich, M., Gaarde, W. A., et al. (2006). Ezrin/radixin/moesin proteins are phosphorylated by TNF-α and modulate permeability increases in human pulmonary microvascular endothelial cells. *J. Immunol.* 176, 1218–1227. doi: 10.4049/jimmunol.176.2.1218

Krishnegowda, G., Hajjar, A. M., Zhu, J., Douglass, E. J., Uematsu, S., Akira, S., et al. (2005). Induction of proinflammatory responses in macrophages by the glycosylphosphatidylinositols of *Plasmodium falciparum*: cell signaling receptors, glycosylphosphatidylinositol (GPI) structural requirement, and regulation of GPI activity. *J. Biol. Chem.* 280, 8606–8616. doi: 10.1074/jbc.M413541200

Kwon, Y. U., Soucy, R. L., Snyder, D. A., and Seeberger, P. H. (2005). Assembly of a series of malarial glycosylphosphatidylinositol anchor oligosaccharides. *Chemistry* 11, 2493–2504. doi: 10.1002/chem.200400934

Lackner, P., Beer, R., Heussler, V., Goebel, G., Rudzki, D., Helbok, R., et al. (2006). Behavioural and histopathological alterations in mice with cerebral malaria. *Neuropathol. Appl. Neurobiol.* 32, 177–188. doi: 10.1111/j.1365-2990.2006.00706.x

Langhorne, J., Ndungu, F. M., Sponaas, A. M., and Marsh, K. (2008). Immunity to malaria: more questions than answers. *Nat. Immunol.* 9, 725–732. doi: 10.1038/ni.f.205

Lee, Y. C., and Lee, R. T. (1995). Carbohydrate-protein interactions: basis of glycobiology. *Acc. Chem. Res.* 28, 321–327. doi: 10.1021/ar00056a001

Lepenies, B., Cramer, J. P., Burchard, G. D., Wagner, H., Kirschning, C. J., and Jacobs, T. (2008). Induction of experimental cerebral malaria is independent of TLR2/4/9. *Med. Microbiol. Immunol.* 197, 39–44. doi: 10.1007/s00430-007-0057-y

Liu, X., Kwon, Y. U., and Seeberger, P. H. (2005). Convergent synthesis of a fully lipidated glycosylphosphatidylinositol anchor of *Plasmodium falciparum*. *J. Am. Chem. Soc.* 127, 5004–5005. doi: 10.1021/ja042374o

Louvet-Vallee, S. (2000). ERM proteins: from cellular architecture to cell signaling. *Biol. Cell* 92, 305–316. doi: 10.1016/S0248-4900(00)01078-9

Lutz, M. B., Kukutsch, N., Ogilvie, A. L., Rossner, S., Koch, F., Romani, N., et al. (1999). An advanced culture method for generating large quantities of highly pure dendritic cells from mouse bone marrow. *J. Immunol. Methods* 223, 77–92. doi: 10.1016/S0022-1759(98)00204-X

Madaan, A., Verma, R., Singh, A. T., Jain, S. K., and Jaggi, M. (2014). A stepwise procedure for isolation of murine bone marrow and generation of dendritic cells. *J. Biol. Methods* 1, 1–6. doi: 10.14440/jbm.2014.12

Matz, J. M., Ingmundson, A., Costa Nunes, J., Stenzel, W., Matuschewski, K., and Kooij, T. W. (2015). *In vivo* function of PTEX88 in malaria parasite sequestration and virulence. *Eukaryotic Cell* 14, 528–534. doi: 10.1128/EC.00276-14

Moura-Alves, P., Fae, K., Houthuys, E., Dorhoi, A., Kreuchwig, A., Furkert, J., et al. (2014). AhR sensing of bacterial pigments regulates antibacterial defence. *Nature* 512, 387–392. doi: 10.1038/nature13684

Neisch, A. L., and Fehon, R. G. (2011). Ezrin, Radixin and Moesin: key regulators of membrane-cortex interactions and signaling. *Curr. Opin. Cell Biol.* 23, 377–382. doi: 10.1016/j.ceb.2011.04.011

Niggli, V., and Rossy, J. (2008). Ezrin/radixin/moesin: versatile controllers of signaling molecules and of the cortical cytoskeleton. *Int. J. Biochem. Cell Biol.* 40, 344–349. doi: 10.1016/j.biocel.2007.02.012

Parameswaran, N., and Gupta, N. (2013). Re-defining ERM function in lymphocyte activation and migration. *Immunol. Rev.* 256, 63–79. doi: 10.1111/imr.12104

Ponuwei, G. A. (2016). A glimpse of the ERM proteins. *J. Biomed. Sci.* 23, 35. doi: 10.1186/s12929-016-0246-3

Ratner, D. M., Adams, E. W., Su, J., O'Keefe, B. R., Mrksich, M., and Seeberger, P. H. (2004). Probing protein-carbohydrate interactions with microarrays of synthetic oligosaccharides. *Chembiochem* 5, 379–382. doi: 10.1002/cbic.200300804

Rivadeneira, E. M., Wasserman, M., and Espinal, C. T. (1983). Separation and concentration of schizonts of *Plasmodium falciparum* by Percoll gradients. *J. Protozool.* 30, 367–370. doi: 10.1111/j.1550-7408.1983.tb02932.x

Rizopoulos, Z., Matuschewski, K., and Haussig, J. (2016). Distinct prominent roles for enzymes of plasmodium berghei heme biosynthesis in sporozoite and liver stage maturation. *Infect. Immun.* 84, 3252–3262. doi: 10.1128/IAI.00148-16

Sato, Y., Montagna, G. N., and Matuschewski, K. (2014). Plasmodium berghei sporozoites acquire virulence and immunogenicity during mosquito hemocoel transit. *Infect. Immun.* 82, 1164–1172. doi: 10.1128/IAI.00758-13

Schmittgen, T. D., and Livak, K. J. (2008). Analyzing real-time PCR data by the comparative C(T) method. *Nat. Protoc.* 3, 1101–1108. doi: 10.1038/nprot.2008.73

Schofield, L., and Hackett, F. (1993). Signal transduction in host cells by a glycosylphosphatidylinositol toxin of malaria parasites. *J. Exp. Med.* 177, 145–153. doi: 10.1084/jem.177.1.145

Schofield, L., Hewitt, M. C., Evans, K., Siomos, M. A., and Seeberger, P. H. (2002). Synthetic GPI as a candidate anti-toxic vaccine in a model of malaria. *Nature* 418, 785–789. doi: 10.1038/nature00937

Schwende, H., Fitzke, E., Ambs, P., and Dieter, P. (1996). Differences in the state of differentiation of THP-1 cells induced by phorbol ester and 1,25-dihydroxyvitamin D3. *J. Leukoc. Biol.* 59, 555–561. Available online at: http://www.jleukbio.org/content/59/4/555.long

Smart, E. J., Ying, Y. S., Mineo, C., and Anderson, R. G. (1995). A detergent-free method for purifying caveolae membrane from tissue culture cells. *Proc. Natl. Acad. Sci. U.S.A.* 92, 10104–10108. doi: 10.1073/pnas.92.22.10104

Stevenson, M. M., and Riley, E. M. (2004). Innate immunity to malaria. *Nat. Rev. Immunol.* 4, 169–180. doi: 10.1038/nri1311

Storm, J., and Craig, A. G. (2014). Pathogenesis of cerebral malaria–inflammation and cytoadherence. *Front. Cell. Infect. Microbiol.* 4:100. doi: 10.3389/fcimb.2014.00100

Tachado, S. D., Gerold, P., McConville, M. J., Baldwin, T., Quilici, D., Schwarz, R. T., et al. (1996). Glycosylphosphatidylinositol toxin of Plasmodium induces nitric oxide synthase expression in macrophages and vascular endothelial cells by a protein tyrosine kinase-dependent and protein kinase C-dependent signaling pathway. *J. Immunol.* 156, 1897–1907.

Takamatsu, H., Espinoza, J. L., Lu, X., Qi, Z., Okawa, K., and Nakao, S. (2009). Anti-moesin antibodies in the serum of patients with aplastic anemia stimulate peripheral blood mononuclear cells to secrete TNF-α and IFN-γ. *J. Immunol.* 182, 703–710. doi: 10.4049/jimmunol.182.1.703

Togbe, D., Schofield, L., Grau, G. E., Schnyder, B., Boissay, V., Charron, S., et al. (2007). Murine cerebral malaria development is independent of toll-like receptor signaling. *Am. J. Pathol.* 170, 1640–1648. doi: 10.2353/ajpath.2007.060889

Tohme, Z. N., Amar, S., and Van Dyke, T. E. (1999). Moesin functions as a lipopolysaccharide receptor on human monocytes. *Infect. Immun.* 67, 3215–3220.

Villadangos, J. A., Schnorrer, P., and Wilson, N. S. (2005). Control of MHC class II antigen presentation in dendritic cells: a balance between creative and destructive forces. *Immunol. Rev.* 207, 191–205. doi: 10.1111/j.0105-2896.2005.00317.x

Wells, J. W., Darling, D., Farzaneh, F., and Galea-Lauri, J. (2005). Influence of interleukin-4 on the phenotype and function of bone marrow-derived murine dendritic cells generated under serum-free conditions. *Scand. J. Immunol.* 61, 251–259. doi: 10.1111/j.1365-3083.2005.01556.x

WHO (2016). *World Malaria Report 2016.* Available online at: http://www.who.int/malaria/publications/world-malaria-report-2016/report/en/

Wu, X., Gowda, N. M., and Gowda, D. C. (2015). Phagosomal acidification prevents macrophage inflammatory cytokine production to malaria, and dendritic cells are the major source at the early stages of infection: implication for malaria protective immunity development. *J. Biol. Chem.* 290, 23135–23147. doi: 10.1074/jbc.M115.671065

Xu, Y., Zhan, Y., Lew, A. M., Naik, S. H., and Kershaw, M. H. (2007). Differential development of murine dendritic cells by GM-CSF versus Flt3 ligand has implications for inflammation and trafficking. *J. Immunol.* 179, 7577–7584. doi: 10.4049/jimmunol.179.11.7577

Yao, Y., and Tsirka, S. E. (2011). Truncation of monocyte chemoattractant protein 1 by plasmin promotes blood-brain barrier disruption. *J. Cell Sci.* 124, 1486–1495. doi: 10.1242/jcs.082834

Zawawi, K. H., Kantarci, A., Schulze-Spate, U., Fujita, T., Batista, E. L. Jr., Amar, S., et al. (2010). Moesin-induced signaling in response to lipopolysaccharide in macrophages. *J. Periodont. Res.* 45, 589–601. doi: 10.1111/j.1600-0765.2010.01271.x

Zhu, J., Krishnegowda, G., Li, G., and Gowda, D. C. (2011). Proinflammatory responses by glycosylphosphatidylinositols (GPIs) of *Plasmodium falciparum* are mainly mediated through the recognition of TLR2/TLR1. *Exp. Parasitol.* 128, 205–211. doi: 10.1016/j.exppara.2011.03.010

Zhu, J., Wu, X., Goel, S., Gowda, N. M., Kumar, S., Krishnegowda, G., et al. (2009). MAPK-activated protein kinase 2 differentially regulates *Plasmodium falciparum* glycosylphosphatidylinositol-induced production of tumor necrosis factor-α and interleukin-12 in macrophages. *J. Biol. Chem.* 284, 15750–15761. doi: 10.1074/jbc.M901111200

14

Reciprocal Interactions between Nematodes and their Microbial Environments

Ankur Midha, Josephine Schlosser and Susanne Hartmann *

Department of Veterinary Medicine, Institute of Immunology, Freie Universität Berlin, Berlin, Germany

Edited by:
Lorenza Putignani, Bambino Gesù Ospedale Pediatrico (IRCCS), Italy

Reviewed by:
Mario M. Zaiss, Universitätsklinikum Erlangen, Germany
Chang-Shi Chen, National Cheng Kung University, Taiwan

Correspondence:
Susanne Hartmann
susanne.hartmann@fu-berlin.de

Parasitic nematode infections are widespread in nature, affecting humans as well as wild, companion, and livestock animals. Most parasitic nematodes inhabit the intestines of their hosts living in close contact with the intestinal microbiota. Many species also have tissue migratory life stages in the absence of severe systemic inflammation of the host. Despite the close coexistence of helminths with numerous microbes, little is known concerning these interactions. While the environmental niche is considerably different, the free-living nematode *Caenorhabditis elegans* (*C. elegans*) is also found amongst a diverse microbiota, albeit on decaying organic matter. As a very well characterized model organism that has been intensively studied for several decades, *C. elegans* interactions with bacteria are much more deeply understood than those of their parasitic counterparts. The enormous breadth of understanding achieved by the *C. elegans* research community continues to inform many aspects of nematode parasitology. Here, we summarize what is known regarding parasitic nematode-bacterial interactions while comparing and contrasting this with information from work in *C. elegans*. This review highlights findings concerning responses to bacterial stimuli, antimicrobial peptides, and the reciprocal influences between nematodes and their environmental bacteria. Furthermore, the microbiota of nematodes as well as alterations in the intestinal microbiota of mammalian hosts by helminth infections are discussed.

Keywords: nematode, helminth, microbiota, antimicrobial peptides, antibiotic resistance

INTRODUCTION

Parasitic nematodes are responsible for widespread morbidity in humans and animals. It is estimated that approximately 1.5 billion people are infected with one or more of these organisms (Hotez et al., 2008; World Health Organization, 2017) which also pose a considerable burden for animal production (Eijck and Borgsteede, 2005; Nganga et al., 2008). The extraordinary success of these parasites speaks to their ability to withstand a multitude of stresses such as host immune pressures and infectious challenges from microbes. Most parasitic nematodes inhabit the intestines of their hosts, co-existing with numerous microbial species. In studying these dynamics, researchers have focused extensively on the host-parasite relationship; more recently, the role of the microbiota as a major third party in the relationship is better appreciated due to diverse and far-reaching influences in health and disease (Donaldson et al., 2016). Much attention in these studies is given to host immune mechanisms while the interactions between nematodes and their microbial environments are largely overlooked. Due to many technical and biological challenges associated with studying parasites, these questions can be very difficult to address. The free-living nematode

Caenorhabditis elegans (*C. elegans*) is frequently found in nature amongst a diverse microbiota on decaying organic matter (Frézal and Félix, 2015). *C. elegans* has been very well characterized and its interactions with bacteria studied in considerable detail. As such, these findings might be conveyed to parasitic nematodes and greatly inform our understanding of how parasites interact with the host-microbiota, as many immune-related pathways and responses may be conserved (Tarr, 2012; Rosso et al., 2013). This review will summarize current knowledge regarding how parasitic nematodes and their microbial environments may influence each other, supplemented with insights from work in *C. elegans*.

NEMATODES AND THEIR MICROBIAL ENVIRONMENTS

Studies on intestinal nematodes report a range of alterations to the composition of the microbiota, ranging from increased or decreased diversity, dysbiosis, or in some cases no identifiably significant changes (summarized in **Tables 1, 2**). Responses by *C. elegans* to numerous microbes have also been studied. Accordingly, parasitic helminths illuminate our understanding of how microbial communities can be altered by the presence of nematodes whereas studies of *C. elegans* can explain how microbial populations impact nematode physiology,

TABLE 1 | Effects of helminth infection on host microbiota and metabolism in humans, macaques, and pigs.

Host and helminth(s) species	Microbiota diversity	Microbiota composition	Changes in host metabolism	Sample site(s)	Population details	References
HUMAN						
T. trichiura	→	n.r.	n.r.	Feces	Rural Ecuadorians	Cooper et al., 2013
	↓	*Prevotella* ↑	n.r.	Feces	Rural Malaysians	Ramanan et al., 2016
A. lumbricoides, *T. trichiura* and hookworm (mixed infections)	↓	*Streptococcus* ↑	n.r.	Feces	Rural Ecuadorians *A. lumbricoides* and *T. trichiura*	Cooper et al., 2013
	↑	Prevotellaceae, Mollicutes, Bacteroidales Alphaproteobacteria ↑	Carbohydrate metabolism ↓	Feces	Rural Malaysians *A. lumbricoides*, *T. trichiura*, and hookworm	Lee et al., 2014
N. americanus	→	n.r.	n.r.	Feces	Healthy volunteers (gluten-free diet; 8 wpi)	Cantacessi et al., 2014
	↑	Bacteroidetes and Bacteroidia ↑; *Lachnospira*, *Ruminococcus*, Firmicutes, Tenericutes ↓	Gluten tolerance ↑	Feces	Volunteers with celiac disease (8 wpi), gluten administration in parallel	Giacomin et al., 2015
	n.r.	n.r.	SCFA ↑	Feces	Healthy volunteers (8 wpi)	Zaiss et al., 2015
MACAQUE						
T. trichiura	↑	Cyanobacteria ↓; Tenericutes and Bacteroidetes ↑; bacterial attachment to mucosa ↓	n.r.	Colon	Chronic helminth infection in a colitis model	Broadhurst et al., 2012
PIG						
T. suis	→	*Ruminococcus*, *Oscillibacter* and *Succinivibrio*↓; *Mucispirillum* and *Paraprevotella* ↑	Altered fatty acid metabolism and carbohydrate metabolism, amino acid availability↓	Colon	Larval stage infection (21 dpi)	Li et al., 2012
	n.r.	*Ruminococcus* *Oscillibacter* and *Succinivibrio* ↓; *Campylobacter* ↑	n.r.	Colon	Chronic infection (53 dpi)	Wu et al., 2012
A. suum	↓	*Prevotella* ↑	SCFA ↑	Colon	54 dpi	Paerewijck et al., 2015

→, no change; ↑, increase; ↓, decrease; n.r., not reported; SCFA, short chain fatty acids; dpi, days post-infection; wpi, weeks post-infection; Nod2, nucleotide-binding oligomerization domain-containing protein 2; WT, wild type.

TABLE 2 | Effects of helminth infection on host microbiota and metabolism in mice.

Host and helminth(s) species	Microbiota diversity	Microbiota composition	Changes in host metabolism	Sample site(s)	Infection phase	References
MUS MUSCULUS						
T. muris	↓	Bacteroidetes ↓; *Mucispirillum*, *Bifidobacterium*, Lactobacillaceae, Proteobacteria and Firmicutes ↑	n.r.	Cecum Colon Feces	Chronic infection	Holm et al., 2015
	↓	*Parabaceroides*, *Prevotella* and Bacteroidetes ↓; *Mucispirillum* and Rikenellaceae ↑	weight gain and carbohydrate metabolism ↓	Feces	Chronic infection	Houlden et al., 2015
	↑ *Nod2* deficient mice; ↓ in WT mice	*B. vulgatus*, *Prevotella* and *Bacteroides* ↓; Lachnospiraceae, Lactobacillales and Clostridiales ↑	n.r.	Feces	Acute infection (21 dpi)	Ramanan et al., 2016
H. p. bakeri	n.r.	Lactobacillaceae, Clostridiaceae, Ruminococcaceae and Lachnospiraceae ↑	n.r.	Ileum Cecum	Acute infection (14 dpi)	Walk et al., 2010
	n.r.	*Baceroides*, *Clostridium*, *Lactobacillus* and Enterobacteriaceae ↑	n.r.	Ileum Cecum Colon	Acute infection (14 dpi)	Rausch et al., 2013
	n.r.	Enterobacteriaceae and Lactobacillaceae ↑	n.r.	Duodenum Feces	28 dpi	Reynolds et al., 2014
	n.r.	Clostridiales ↑	SCFA ↑	Cecum	28 - 42 dpi	Zaiss et al., 2015
N. brasiliensis	→	Firmicutes and SFB ↓; Bacteroidetes and Actinobacteria ↑	n.r.	Jejunum Ileum Cecum Colon Feces	11 dpi	Fricke et al., 2015
APODEMUS FLAVICOLLIS						
H. p. bakeri, *Syphacia*. *Hymenolepsis* and *M. muris* (mixed infections)	→	Firmicutes/Bacteroidetes ratio ↑ (with *H. p. bakeri*)	carbohydrate metabolism ↑ (with *H. p. bakeri*)	stomach small intestine cecum colon	Wild caught mice, likely chronic exposure to helminths	Kreisinger et al., 2015

→, no change; ↑, increase; ↓, decrease; n.r., not reported; SCFA, short chain fatty acids; dpi, days post-infection; wpi, weeks post-infection; Nod2, nucleotide-binding oligomerization domain-containing protein 2; WT, wild type; SFB, segmented filamentous bacteria.

reproduction and growth; considered together, one can better understand how these multifactorial biological systems operate. Herein, we focus most of our discussion on selected members of the genera *Trichuris* and *Ascaris*, as well as the rodent parasite *Heligmosomoides polygyrus bakeri* and the free-living *C. elegans*. These organisms have been selected due to their importance to human and animal health along with the abundance of available data in the literature, though additional studies from other helminths are considered where appropriate.

The Nematodes

Trichuris

The whipworms *Trichuris trichiura*, *T. suis*, and *T. muris* infect humans, pigs, and mice respectively. The life cycles of these species are comparable and infection begins with ingestion of developed eggs (Bethony et al., 2006; Klementowicz et al., 2012). Hatching occurs within hours of ingestion, liberating L1 larvae which invade the intestinal wall and undergo successive molts to the L4 stage by 3 weeks post-infection (pi) and finally develop into mature adults by 12 weeks pi (Bethony et al., 2006). Trichurids inhabit the most dense and diverse microbial environments of their hosts: the cecum and colon (Klementowicz et al., 2012). They can survive here for 1–2 years with individual females laying up to 5,000 eggs per day (Bethony et al., 2006).

Ascaris

The roundworms *A. lumbricoides* and the closely related *A. suum* infect humans and pigs respectively. As with Trichuriasis, Ascariasis also spreads via the fecal-oral route in humans as well as in pigs (Dold and Holland, 2011). Within 3 h, ingested eggs containing L3 larvae hatch and by 18 h pi the larvae begin their tissue migratory phase, passing through the liver after invading the cecum and proximal colon (Murrell et al., 1997). The larvae reach the lungs and pharynx by days six to eight pi (Roepstorff et al., 1997), are swallowed and can then be found in the small intestine as L4 stage larvae before further developing into mature adults. Adult Ascarids reside in the small intestine for around 1 year with individual females producing hundreds of thousands of eggs per day (Dold and Holland, 2011).

H. p. bakeri

The trichostrongyloid *H. p. bakeri* is amongst the most common helminth parasites of rodents and a well characterized model for chronic intestinal nematode infection (Wu et al., 2012). Infection is initiated by ingestion of L3 larvae which migrate into the mucosa of the small intestine. By day three pi the larvae develop into L4 within the mucosa before returning to the lumen of the duodenum by day nine pi where they develop into, and remain as, egg-laying adults for approximately 12 weeks in the wood mouse (*Apodemus sylvaticus*) and more than twice as long in BALB/c laboratory mice (Robinson et al., 1989; Gregory et al., 1990; Behnke et al., 2009).

C. elegans

C. elegans is a free-living, bacterivorous nematode found predominantly in humid temperate areas (Félix and Duveau, 2012; Frézal and Félix, 2015). These nematodes can be identified in feeding and reproductive stages in rotting fruit and herbaceous stems. The life cycle is characterized by freshly hatched L1 stage larvae undergoing multiple molts before reaching adulthood in as little as 3 days. Under stressful conditions including crowding, limited food, and heat stress, L1 individuals will pursue an alternate life cycle through a pre-dauer L2 (L2d) stage, followed by a non-feeding, stress-resistant alternate L3 stage called "dauer." Dauer individuals can survive for several months without food before reentering a relatively normal development cycle when conditions are more favorable. In the laboratory, the reference N2 strain is typically cultured on a diet of the rather innocuous *Escherichia coli* OP50. In contrast to controlled laboratory conditions, *C. elegans* shares its natural habitat with a variety of organisms, including bacteria, phages, fungi, isopods, arthropods, and other nematodes (Félix and Duveau, 2012). Additionally, worms can be found in states of starvation or constipation in their natural environments (Barrière and Félix, 2005).

Parasitic Nematodes Influence the Host-Intestinal Microbiota

The mammalian intestine is home to approximately 3.8×10^{13} microbes from all three domains of life, archaea, bacteria, and eukaryotes, collectively referred to as the microbiota (Sender et al., 2016). The different regions of the intestinal tract form divergent habitats, varying in bacterial type and density. In humans, an estimated 10^3–10^4 microbial cells/mL intestinal content reside in the small intestine (Sender et al., 2016). Considerably more bacterial diversity and density is found in the large intestine with as many as 10^{11} cells/mL contents representing thousands of different species (Zoetendal et al., 2008; Sender et al., 2016). Interestingly, microbial density and diversity of intestinal regions are inversely correlated with concentrations of host-derived antimicrobials; specialized secretory Paneth cells are a key source of α-defensins, lysozymes, and C-type lectins and are particularly prominent in the proximal intestine, the intestinal site of lowest microbial richness (Bevins and Salzman, 2011; Donaldson et al., 2016). Additionally, persistence of common gut commensals is partially mediated by resistance to host defense molecules (Cullen et al., 2015). Whether these factors influence helminth niche selection remains to be determined. Various conditions such as age, diet, health status and genetic background can impact the host microbiota composition. Maturation of the gut microbiota is characterized by increasing diversification with age while age-related changes are also due to exposure to a more varied diet (David et al., 2014; Odamaki et al., 2016). Analysis of human fecal samples can detect rapid, diet-mediated changes in microbial composition. For example, consumption of animal products increases the abundance of bile-tolerant species and decreases abundance of species that metabolize plant-derived polysaccharides (David et al., 2014). Dysbiosis, a potentially pathogenic imbalance of microbial communities, can be precipitated by exposure to pharmaceutical substances such as antimicrobials as well as the presence of infectious agents (Donaldson et al., 2016). Acute antibiotic treatment can drastically perturb the gut microbiota, decreasing species diversity (Dethlefsen et al., 2008). Alarmingly, while some changes appear reversible, other alterations can be detected in fecal samples even years after a short course of antibiotic treatment (Jernberg et al., 2007). A major clinical implication of a disturbed gut microbiota is elevated risk of enteric infection, such as with *Clostridium difficile*, which itself is associated with decreased microbial diversity (Milani et al., 2016). Many studies have now shown that intestinal nematodes influence their microbial niches as they establish themselves as part of their wider environment within the host; therefore, the role of helminths in dysbiosis is an area of active investigation (**Figure 1**).

The gut microbiota of humans, pigs, and mice is dominated by two of the 29 known bacterial phyla: Bacteroidetes and Firmicutes, with lower abundance phyla differing between hosts and including Actinobacteria, Deferribacteres, Proteobacteria, Spirochaetes, Tenericutes, and Verrucomicrobia (Leser et al., 2002; Eckburg et al., 2005; Consortium, 2012; Nguyen et al., 2015; Weldon et al., 2015). The diversity of the microbiota is thought to reflect the health of the intestine, with far reaching implications for the overall health of the host; greater species diversity contributes to healthy metabolic and immune functioning. Dysbiosis is associated with a reduction in intestinal biodiversity, predisposing to the outgrowth of particularly harmful bacterial species (Carding et al., 2015). The literature is mixed with respect to whether or not helminths cause dysbiosis, and some reports have indicated beneficial effects in therapeutic settings. The few studies assessing the influence of helminths on intestinal microbial communities are a mix of clinical observations and animal experiments, employing different analytical tools and acquiring microbiota samples from different sources. Hence, it is difficult to draw meaningful and generalizable conclusions from

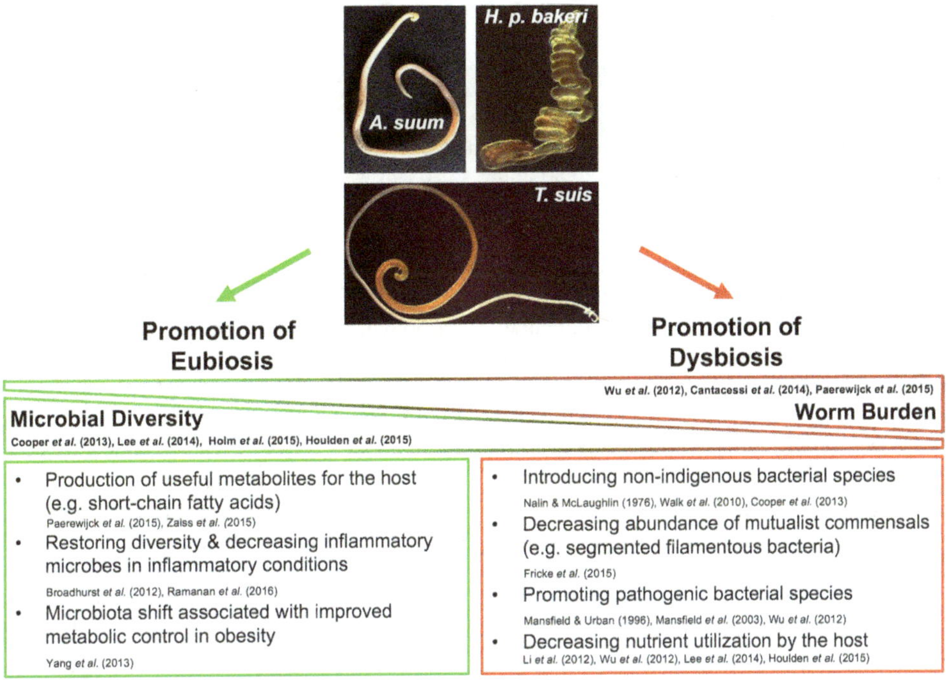

FIGURE 1 | Diverse influences of nematodes on the gut microbiota of their hosts.

the available evidence. Still, through a careful reading of the literature, some common threads emerge.

Analysis of fecal samples from children in rural Ecuador revealed widespread helminth infection (Cooper et al., 2013). Children co-infected with both *T. trichiura* and *A. lumbricoides* appeared to have a decreased microbial diversity compared to uninfected children and children with *T. trichiura* single infections who did not differ from uninfected individuals. Interestingly, in a subset of children with mixed infections the authors also reported a higher abundance of *Streptococcus* spp., not usually dominant in healthy individuals. Taken together, these data suggest dysbiosis in the presence of *A. lumbricoides,* while *T. trichiura* single infections did not result in drastic alterations to the fecal microbiota. Another indication of dysbiosis associated with *Ascaris* infection comes from a study of *A. suum*-infected pigs which showed worm burden-dependent decreased bacterial diversity compared to control animals (Paerewijck et al., 2015). One study in humans found no difference in community structure of fecal samples in healthy volunteers infected with *Necator americanus* (Cantacessi et al., 2014). In contrast, a study of fecal samples from helminth-infected (*T. trichiura, A. lumbricoides,* hookworm) individuals in rural Malaysia found a positive association between helminth-colonization and microbiota diversity (Lee et al., 2014). Burrowed in the epithelia, *T. trichiura* likely interacts with the mucosal microbiota, the composition of which is known to differ considerably from fecal communities (Eckburg et al., 2005). Combined with the obstacles to sampling the small intestine, the site of *A. lumbricoides* and *N. americanus* infections, it is difficult to draw firm conclusions from these human studies regarding beneficial or harmful effects of helminth infections with respect to intestinal microbial composition. Though in the case of *Ascaris,* the local effects seen in the porcine small intestine (Paerewijck et al., 2015) correspond with the distal effects seen in human feces (Cooper et al., 2013).

Animal studies of helminthiases can offer more depth compared to human studies, accounting for the limitations associated with sampling only the fecal microbiota. During the larval stage, *T. suis* appears not to disrupt the porcine colonic microbiota (Li et al., 2012); however, chronic infections in pigs demonstrate worm burden-dependent disruption (Wu et al., 2012). *T. suis* also appears to promote *Campylobacter* infection in pigs, intensifying colitis disease severity (Mansfield and Urban, 1996; Mansfield et al., 2003; Wu et al., 2012). Chronic *T. muris* infections in mice considerably decrease overall microbial diversity, an effect that appears reversible upon worm clearance (Holm et al., 2015; Houlden et al., 2015). In these studies, the murine microbiota also showed a shift away from Bacteroidetes in favor of Firmicutes (Holm et al., 2015; Houlden et al., 2015). A study of wild mice has also observed an increased Firmicutes/Bacteroidetes ratio in helminth-infected individuals (Kreisinger et al., 2015) whereas mice experimentally infected with the small intestinal nematode *Nippostrongylus brasiliensis* showed a decrease of Firmicutes while increasing Bacteroidetes (Fricke et al., 2015). Though *N. brasiliensis* decreases the Firmicutes/Bacteroidetes ratio, it also promotes the reduction of segmented filamentous bacteria (SFB) which are thought to prevent colonization by bacterial pathogens, as it was shown in SFB-colonized mice with enhanced resistance to the pathogenic *Citrobacter rodentium* (Ivanov et al., 2009; Fricke et al., 2015). Mice with chronic *T. muris* infections (Holm et al., 2015; Houlden et al., 2015) as well as those with acute *H. p. bakeri* infections (Rausch et al., 2013) have higher abundance of Enterobacteriaceae, a family shown to overgrow during intestinal inflammation (Lupp et al., 2007) and strongly correlated with Crohn's disease (Gevers et al., 2014) and *C. difficile* infection (Milani et al., 2016) in humans. These data indicate a propensity for helminths to associate with a simplified microbiota; however, whether these observations are generalizable across helminth infections in diverse mammalian hosts remains to be determined; nonetheless, these animal experiments are suggestive of helminths promoting dysbiosis in their hosts.

Despite the evidence for dysbiosis, a fairly consistent finding across various helminth infections is an increased abundance of Lactobacillaceae (Walk et al., 2010; Rausch et al., 2013; Reynolds et al., 2014; Fricke et al., 2015; Holm et al., 2015; Houlden et al., 2015; Ramanan et al., 2016), a family composed primarily of *Lactobacillus* spp., currently under intense investigation for use as probiotics (Walter, 2008; Salvetti et al., 2012). Additionally, studies employing intestinal nematodes as therapeutic interventions to treat intestinal inflammatory conditions have shown beneficial outcomes (Broadhurst et al., 2012; Giacomin et al., 2015; Ramanan et al., 2016). Macaques with idiopathic chronic diarrhea show signs characteristic of dysbiosis such as decreased diversity, increased bacterial attachment to the intestinal mucosa, and increased abundance of Enterobacteriaceae (Broadhurst et al., 2012). Bacterial attachment and abundance of Enterobacteriaceae were effectively decreased by *T. trichiura* infection, while bacterial diversity was restored, indicating a protective effect of helminth infection in this setting. Similarly, mice deficient in *Nod2* are susceptible to Crohn's disease and can be colonized by inflammatory *Bacteroides* spp., while *T. muris* infection protects against pathogenic colonization (Ramanan et al., 2016). In patients with celiac disease, low-level infection with *N. americanus* increases gluten tolerance (Croese et al., 2015), while also increasing microbial richness when combined with gluten consumption (Giacomin et al., 2015). Taken together, these findings indicate that intestinal nematodes possess great therapeutic potential and may promote microbial restoration in conditions of pre-existing dysbiosis.

From taxonomic data referring to the microbiota composition alone it is challenging to conclude whether intestinal nematodes contribute to or ameliorate dysbiosis. As such, the influence of helminths on gut metabolic profiles may offer more clues. Methodological and technological advances allow for metabolic profiling of gut microbiota, along with identification and quantification of metabolites of interest (Vernocchi et al., 2016). Such experiments can be quite informative, though they are currently far less abundant than those reporting taxonomic changes. Metabolomic analysis of the colonic microbiota of pigs infected with *T. suis* demonstrated reduced capacity to metabolize and utilize carbohydrates relative to control animals, an effect seen in acute and chronic infections (Li et al., 2012; Wu et al., 2012). Interestingly, *T. suis*-infected pigs also showed signs of altered fatty acid metabolism, including higher levels of oleic acid relative to control pigs (Li et al., 2012). Notably, oleic acid possesses antibacterial activity (Dilika et al., 2000) and may therefore influence microbial composition during *Trichuris* infection. Mice chronically infected with *T. muris* also showed signs of reduced carbohydrate and amino acid metabolism and nutrient uptake compared to naïve animals, features which likely contribute to decreased weight gain during helminth infection (Houlden et al., 2015). Observational analysis of helminth-infected humans has attributed decreased carbohydrate metabolism to *Ascaris* infection (Lee et al., 2014). In contrast, wild mice infected with helminths showed mixed effects with respect to metabolomic shifts (Kreisinger et al., 2015). Notably, wild mice with *H. p. bakeri* appeared to have an increased capacity to metabolize carbohydrates; however, metabolites were not measured and mouse weights were not reported. Together, these observations suggest helminth-mediated microbiota changes tend to reduce metabolic capability in the gut, ultimately manifesting as nutritional deficiencies.

While dietary carbohydrate utilization may be impaired by intestinal nematodes, other experiments demonstrate potential benefits of helminth infection such as increased abundance of intestinal short-chain fatty acids (SCFAs), typically produced from microbial processing of indigestible oligosaccharides (Paerewijck et al., 2015; Zaiss et al., 2015; Vernocchi et al., 2016). SCFAs can serve as energy sources and anti-inflammatory compounds and are therefore under investigation for their therapeutic potential (Vernocchi et al., 2016). Increased SCFAs have been detected during infection with *H. p. bakeri* in mice, *A. suum* in pigs, and *N. americanus* in humans (Paerewijck et al., 2015; Zaiss et al., 2015). Furthermore, *H. p. bakeri* and *A. suum* can produce SCFAs directly (Tielens et al., 2010; Zaiss et al., 2015). Reduced weight gain associated with helminth infection may also prove to be therapeutic in different circumstances, as illustrated by Yang et al. in a study of obese mice and mice fed obesity-inducing diets (Yang et al., 2013). In agreement with other observations, *N. brasiliensis* infection attenuated weight gain. Importantly, helminth infection decreased adiposity and hepatic lipid storage while improving glycemic control, implying a reversal of metabolic disease. These studies indicate that microbiota alterations and metabolomic changes associated with intestinal nematodes may offer certain benefits.

The mixed observations described herein highlight the difficulties of generalizing findings from these studies, simultaneously hinting at the massive potential to apply these insights in diverse therapeutic settings. Animal studies designed to induce strong immune responses are typically a result of a high infection dose and thus high worm burdens and may not reflect average worm burdens seen in nature. Indeed, some of the aforementioned animal experiments demonstrate microbiota changes suggestive of dysbiosis (Li et al., 2012; Wu et al., 2012; Holm et al., 2015; Houlden et al., 2015). In contrast, observations from natural settings or studies inducing low-level helminth infections suggest less dramatic changes (Cantacessi et al., 2014; Kreisinger et al., 2015). Additionally, when intestinal nematodes are introduced into individuals with intestinal inflammation or metabolic abnormalities, they appear beneficial (Broadhurst et al., 2012; Yang et al., 2013; Giacomin et al., 2015). Taken together, these data emphasize co-evolution of helminths, gut microbiota, and mammalian hosts, such that helminths can be considered less strictly as intruders but rather members of the gut macrobiota (Gause and Maizels, 2016). In order to establish themselves in the mammalian intestine, rather than being solely beneficial or causing outright harm, nematodes must shape the niche such that a new ecological balance is found. This task is aided by some microbes and challenged by others, and the insights gained from understanding these dynamics can provide opportunities to better understand and perhaps manipulate incredibly complex biological systems. It should be noted that many potential mechanisms have been identified which act in concert to shape the intestinal microbiota. Immune mechanisms such as modifying the balance between Th1/Th17 vs. Th2 responses as well as the induction of regulatory T cells have been characterized and discussed elsewhere (Reynolds et al., 2015; Gause and Maizels, 2016; Zaiss and Harris, 2016). Furthermore, the bulk of work done thus far has focused primarily on bacteria and far less is known about the archaeal and fungal components of intestinal microbial communities. In addition to metabolomic factors touched upon here, important considerations which are relatively under-studied and not frequently discussed are the direct signals between helminths and microbes. These reciprocal interactions are considered below.

Environmental Microbes Impact *C. elegans* Physiology

The study of intestinal parasites is particularly amenable to understanding alterations to microbial communities of the gut, though the microbial influence on helminths is relatively difficult to assess in these systems. As a model organism with many available genetic tools, *C. elegans* can bridge some of the knowledge gaps encountered when studying parasitic nematodes. When recovered from compost or isopods, which worms may use as vectors to shuttle between food sources, *C. elegans* is frequently found in the dauer stage (Félix and Duveau, 2012). In contrast, proliferating populations of nematodes can be found in microbe-dense environments, particularly rotting fruits or vegetation. A study by Samuel et al. characterized the natural bacterial microenvironment of *C. elegans* (Samuel et al., 2016). The most prevalent bacterial phyla in decaying apples were Proteobacteria, Bacteroidetes, Firmicutes, and Actinobacteria. The Enterobacteriaceae family within Proteobacteria encompassed the most abundant genera detected, while *Lactococcus, Lactobacillus, Acetobacter, Gluconobacter,* and *Gluconoacetobacter* were also quite prevalent. In some samples, *Escherichia* spp. were also identified, though they were not particularly abundant. Considering the immensity of bacterial diversity coming from 29 extant phyla (Yarza et al., 2014), there is considerable overlap in the microbial environments of parasitic and free-living nematodes. Experiments assessing the effect of *C. elegans* on an experimental microbiota could be designed, whereby the nematodes are introduced into a defined microbial environment and followed over time to assess changes to bacterial constituents. Such studies would be analogous, albeit profoundly simplified, to studies assessing gut microbial changes in helminth infections and could shed light on the underlying mechanisms contributing to compositional alterations. Akin to some reports of parasitic nematodes, observations from rotting fruit suggest that growth of *C. elegans* is enhanced amongst a simpler microbiota (Samuel et al., 2016).

Many studies have demonstrated the susceptibility of the *C. elegans* intestine to a multitude of pathogens (Couillault and Ewbank, 2002), including *Salmonella enterica* serovar Typhimurium (*S. typhimurium*) (Lee et al., 2015), *Enterococcus faecalis* (Sim and Hibberd, 2016), *Burkholderia* spp. (Lee et al., 2013), *Staphylococcus aureus* (JebaMercy and Balamurugan, 2012), *Proteus mirabilis* (JebaMercy and Balamurugan, 2012), and *Pseudomonas aeruginosa* (Dai et al., 2015). Beyond posing a threat to the nematode intestine, bacteria may also damage and infect the nematode surface. In experimental settings, *Yersinia* spp. can form biofilms that block the oral cavity of the worms, resulting in starvation and death (Tan and Darby, 2004). Wild nematodes are subject to cuticular infection by *Microbacterium nematophilum* (O'Rourke et al., 2006) and the fungal pathogen *Drechmeria coniospora* (Engelmann et al., 2011). Additionally, *Elizabethkingia* are capable of digesting the nematode cuticle components keratin and collagen (Riffel et al., 2003; Félix and Duveau, 2012). *C. elegans* is also infected by intracellular pathogens such as the microsporidian parasite *Nematocida parisii* (Troemel et al., 2008) and the Orsay virus (Félix et al., 2011). Though studies have demonstrated the ability of bacteria to colonize parasitic nematodes, no information is available concerning which microbes might be beneficial or harmful for them. In contrast, numerous studies in *C. elegans* have shown beneficial and harmful effects of specific bacterial strains. Alphaproteobacteria and *Lactococcus* spp. tend to be beneficial and promote *C. elegans* proliferation while Bacteroidetes and Gammaproteobacteria seem to impair nematode physiology and induce stress/immune responses (Samuel et al., 2016). It stands to reason that similar interactions exist between bacteria and parasitic nematodes and that the composition of the host microbiota would then influence the health of parasitic nematodes in the gut. Interestingly, nematode fecundity is subject to various stresses; the host immune response can decrease helminth fecundity, exemplified by reduced egg production by *H. p. bakeri* during a type 2 helper T cell-mediated immune response (Strandmark et al., 2016). As bacteria influence *C. elegans* fecundity (Szewczyk et al., 2006), it is possible that communities within the microbiota may also influence the reproductive capacity of parasites. Larger populations of proliferating *C. elegans* are found in more highly degraded apples containing larger microbial populations, thereby providing more nutritional sources for the nematodes. Also, apples with higher populations of worms had microbiota which were more similar to each other than apples with lower/no worms. Apples containing proliferating populations of *C. elegans* also had significantly fewer bacterial species and diversity than apples with non-proliferating populations. Most importantly, proliferation was associated with Alphaproteobacteria and the absence of potential pathogens from Gammaproteobacteria and Bacteroidetes. Perhaps there is a general preference by nematodes for decreased abundance of several Bacteroidetes organisms, given the observations in parasite-host microbiota studies discussed previously. As Lactobacillaceae are more predictive of successful *H. p. bakeri* establishment in mice (Reynolds et al., 2014), Enterobacteriaceae and Acetobacteraceae are predictive for larger proliferating *C. elegans* populations in rotting apples, while Gammaproteobacteria show an inverse relationship (Samuel et al., 2016). It is not fully understood how intestinal nematodes establish in specific habitats such as the cecum and colon in the case of Trichurids, or the small intestine in the case of Ascarids and *H. p. bakeri*; however, some speculate the choice is based on the abundance of nutrients or the relative lack of harmful stimuli (Davey, 1964; Bansemir and Sukhdeo, 1994, 2001). While determining the nature of habitat selection in these settings may prove experimentally elusive, the available data suggest that parasitic nematodes, as with their free-living counterparts such as *C. elegans*, have advantageous associations with some microbial species and detrimental interactions with others.

Colonization of Nematodes by Microbes

All animals, including nematodes, live in association with a multitude of other species. The host-microbe relationship has gained a lot of attention in recent studies, with various reciprocal interactions ranging from parasitism, to commensalism and mutualism, seen as potent forces guiding the co-evolution of species. In addition to influencing the rich and diverse microbial environments that they inhabit, nematodes inevitably also harbor their own microbiota that is likely essential for normal development and physiology, as is the case for other organisms. Though the data are limited, studies have documented the ability of bacteria to colonize *Ascaris, H. p. bakeri,* as well as *C. elegans.*

Earlier studies demonstrated nematode-associated bacterial communities in *A. suum* (Hsu et al., 1986; Shahkolahi and Donahue, 1993). One study aimed at identifying the source of serotonin present in nematodes, which generally lack the enzymes necessary for *de novo* synthesis of serotonin from tryptophan, revealed 4×10^9 bacteria per gram of nematode intestine (Hsu et al., 1986). In addition to *E. coli, Enterobacter, Klebsiella, Acinetobacter, Citrobacter, Pseudomonas, Aeromonas,* and *Shigella* were identified among gram-negatives while *Staphylococcus, Streptococcus, Corynebacterium,* and *Bacillus* were identified amongst gram-positive organisms. The species identified suggest that the nematode's intestinal microbiota may have been derived from that of the host. Another study demonstrated that antibiotic treatment of *ex vivo* cultured *A. suum* reduced, but did not eliminate, the bacterial load carried by the worms and determined that the posterior portion of the intestine harbored the highest number of culturable bacteria (Shahkolahi and Donahue, 1993). Studies that employ more modern methods while sampling site-specific host- and parasite-associated microbial communities could greatly enhance our understanding of the selectivity and development of an *Ascaris*-specific microbiota.

Another study showed that *A. lumbricoides* nematodes isolated from cholera patients were colonized by *Vibrio cholerae* (Nalin and McLaughlin, 1976). Worms were retrieved from patients after being spontaneously passed or after de-worming and a majority of worms were colonized by *V. cholerae* of the same serotypes found in stool samples of cholera patients. Serial sectioning of the worms revealed colonization along the entire length of the intestine, from oral cavity to anus. The bacteria were recovered and viable even after worms were in culture in saline for 6 days. The authors reported retrieval of one hookworm which also revealed two colonies of bacteria which were not *V. cholerae.* The authors reasoned that pathogenic bacteria may survive inside parasites when parasites are passed in the stool, as happens commonly during a cholera infection, thereby contributing to environmental spread of microbial pathogens. Further, the authors discussed the possibility of pathogenic microbes reaching the reproductive tract of female nematodes during copulation and adhering to egg shells which may also serve as a vehicle for transmission. There was no indication in this study that *V. cholerae* are pathogenic to Ascarids and further study in this area could reveal interesting associations between different enteric infections. Taken together, these findings highlight the clinical relevance of understanding interactions between intestinal nematodes and environmental microbes.

Walk et al. provided evidence for a *H. p. bakeri*-associated microbiota when they sampled L3 and adult nematodes (Walk et al., 2010), finding only 28 16S sequences obtained from larvae, concluding that they are associated with few bacteria; however, the L3-associated microbiota was completely unique and consisted of 6 bacterial families, unlike the adult-associated microbiota which was very similar to the ileum of the murine host. As *H. p. bakeri* hatch outside of the host, they likely enter their hosts with a distinct microbiota which changes over time in the new environment. This L3-specific microbiota may also serve as a source of non-indigenous microbes for the mammalian host.

A special microbe-helminth relationship is also well documented for filarial nematodes in which the gram-negative intracellular bacterium *Wolbachia* is obligatory for normal larval growth and development, embryogenesis, and survival of adult worms (Taylor et al., 2005). Such endosymbiotic relationships probably emerged from ancestral infections of the host nematode by free-living bacteria, concomitant with gene losses and genome rearrangements on both sides during coevolution (Masson et al., 2016). So far, such an endosymbiotic relationship has not been detected in other parasitic nematode species, but parallels to other microbe-nematode partnerships may be drawn. For example, *Ascaris* requires and absorbs Vitamin B12 from microbial sources (Zam and Martin, 1969). *Wolbachia* displays cell tropism and is restricted to somatic tissues in adult male worms, whereas females also harbor bacteria in the germline (Kozek, 1977; Taylor et al., 1999). The level of infection varies substantially during filarial development, where shortly after transmission to the mammalian host a dramatic increase in the bacterial population occurs (McGarry et al., 2004). As bacterial loads within individual worms differ, Taylor et al. hypothesized that higher levels of *Wolbachia* infection within a worm may potentially confer selective advantages in terms of filarial development or fecundity (Taylor et al., 2013). Transcriptomic analysis of the *Wolbachia* genome of *Onchocerca ochengi* indicated that *Wolbachia* may have a mitochondrion-like function in the soma, generating ATP for the nematode host (Darby et al., 2012). Hence, recent trials aim at utilizing antibiotics such as tetracycline (Hoerauf et al., 1999), and other chemotherapeutics targeting *Wolbachia* as a novel tool for the treatment of filarial infection and disease, reviewed in Taylor et al. (2014).

C. elegans nematodes isolated from the wild are observed to harbor live bacteria in their intestine which may exist as commensals or which may proliferate and cause obstruction and pathology of the worm gut (Félix and Duveau, 2012). Worms isolated from the wild also carry a distinct and diverse microbiota when compared to other nematode species in the same environment (Dirksen et al., 2016). Dirksen et al. reported a microbiota rich in unclassified Proteobacteria from the family Enterobacteriaceae, as well as members of the genera *Pseudomonas, Stenotrophomonas, Ochrobactrum,* and *Sphingomonas.* When isolated worms were enriched on plates of *E. coli* OP50, their microbiota maintained considerable similarity to freshly isolated samples despite 3 weeks in culture on *E. coli* plates, suggestive of a *C. elegans*-specific microbiota and closely developed microbial-host community. This study did not mention any changes in overall microbial population sizes over time. In the same study, a subset of 14 bacterial isolates were chosen in order to cultivate nematodes on an experimental microbiota with bacterial frequencies mirroring the nematode-associated microbiota of worms isolated from the wild. Three genotypes of *C. elegans,* including two natural isolates (MY316 and MY379) and the laboratory N2 strain, were cultured from hatched sterilized eggs through to adulthood. The investigators found significant influences of genotype and life stage on the microbial composition of the nematodes. Interestingly, certain bacteria including *Ochrobactrum* MYb71 and *Stenotrophomonas* MYb57 were enriched in the nematode samples relative to the agar plates. The effect was quite pronounced in the case of *Ochrobactrum* which was present in only trace amounts in the agar plates but represented as much as 20% of the nematode-associated bacterial community. *Ochrobactrum* was also able to persist in the intestine even under starvation conditions without being used as a food source or eliminated during the ensuing stress response, which can include upregulation of antimicrobial effectors such as lysozymes (Uno et al., 2013). This bacterial strain may be a prominent symbiont for *C. elegans* as it seems to use the nematode as an environmental niche in the absence of apparent fitness costs to the worm. The experimental microbiota was also shown to enhance growth and nematode population size relative to worms cultured on *E. coli.* While detailed analysis of this sort is absent for parasitic nematodes, the ability of microbes to colonize these worms supports the idea of worm-associated microbial communities, providing benefits similar to those seen in *C. elegans* and other organisms, such as supplying nutrients and providing protection from pathogens (Cabreiro and Gems, 2013; Watson et al., 2014; Lee et al., 2015; Dirksen et al., 2016).

THE INFLUENCE OF BACTERIA ON PARASITIC NEMATODES

Living in intimate association with microbes, nematodes are subject to diverse microbial influences. Beneficial effects of microbes on nematodes may include nutrition, promotion of longevity, protection from infection by other microbes, and contributions to a hospitable environment (Cabreiro and Gems, 2013; MacNeil and Walhout, 2013). From the perspective of mammalian hosts, the question arises whether a specific microbial environment might significantly influence susceptibility to helminth infection. Further, microbes might also be a source of competition, stress, and disease for nematodes.

The microbial environment can profoundly impact establishment and propagation of parasitic nematode infections by influencing egg hatching and reproductive success. *T. muris* eggs may require the presence of selected bacterial species to induce hatching, as demonstrated using murine cecal explants as well as *E. coli, S. typhimurium, S. aureus,* and *P. aeruginosa* (Hayes et al., 2010). Live bacteria appear to be necessary for these effects as heat inactivation prevented hatching, while bacteriostatic gentamycin treatment did not. It was proposed that physical contact between the bacteria and eggs is required as Type 1 fimbriae facilitate *E. coli*-induced hatching, though additional mechanisms likely exist. The authors also reported that mice pre-treated with antibiotics had significantly lower worm burdens at day 21 pi compared to untreated animals, indicating a significant role for bacterial communities in parasitic nematode establishment. Interestingly, bacteria-induced *T. muris* egg hatching seems to occur efficiently with members of Proteobacteria (*E. coli*) and Firmicutes (*Enterococcus caccae, Streptococcus hyointestinalis, Lactobacillus reuteri,* and *Lactobacillus amylovorus*). It is possible that many different bacterial species contribute via different mechanisms for optimal *T. muris* egg hatching (Vejzagić et al., 2015).

Lactobacillaceae abundance in the duodenum positively correlates with susceptibility to *H. p. bakeri* infection (Reynolds et al., 2014). Low-level vancomycin treatment prior to nematode infection did not significantly reduce total bacteria but elevated abundance of Lactobacillaceae and Enterobacteriaceae while reducing *Eubacterium*/*Clostridium* species in the fecal microbiota. This was associated with *H. p. bakeri* persistence in the host. *H. p. bakeri* infection also elevated duodenal Lactobacillaceae and Enterobacteriaceae. Administration of *Lactobacillus taiwanensis* enhanced susceptibility to *H. p. bakeri* infection and worm fecundity, thought to be due to the induction of immunosuppressive regulatory T cells. This study demonstrated a reciprocal interaction whereby *Lactobacillus* spp. promote nematode establishment which then promote growth of *Lactobacilli.* Similar to *T. muris* infections discussed above, studies in germfree mice revealed higher *H. p. bakeri* worm burdens in conventionally raised mice, implicating the host microbiota as a key part of the parasite's environmental niche (Wescott, 1968). Bacterial populations also influence the host's immune status which can have a profound influence on the intestinal environment for parasite establishment, though specific immune variables and bacterial species are still being identified (Cattadori et al., 2016). These data suggest not only that the microbiota is essential for parasite development, but also that particular bacteria facilitate helminth establishment.

While *C. elegans* and other free-living nematodes are known to subsist on microbes, the food sources of intestinal nematodes are less well established. The digested remains of yeasts can be found in the intestines of *C. elegans* isolated from the wild, demonstrating the capability of these nematodes to use eukaryotic cells as a food source in addition to bacteria (Félix and Duveau, 2012). There is corresponding evidence suggestive of consumption of intestinal epithelia by *A. suum* in pigs as well as *H. p. bakeri* in mice (Davey, 1964; Bansemir and Sukhdeo, 1994). Freshly isolated *Ascaris* nematodes were found to accumulate eukaryotic cellular material in their buccal cavities, thought to be of host origin (Davey, 1964). Labeling studies sought to determine whether *H. p. bakeri* accumulates ingesta, host blood, or host tissue material and found an accumulation of host tissue components rather than blood or ingesta (Bansemir and Sukhdeo, 1994). These studies did not assess the intestinal contents of the worms and these data do not preclude the ability of intestinal nematodes to digest bacterial cells, especially considering bacteria are counted amongst the intestinal contents of *A. suum* and *A. lumbricoides* as discussed previously. Further insights using modern methods could be provided by studies designed to specifically assess uptake and digestion of microbes by intestinal nematodes.

Bacteria can promote or hinder nematode proliferation by various means. From serving as direct food sources or by producing essential nutrients, microbes are required for nematode growth. Furthermore, specific species are well documented to promote helminth establishment while themselves being reinforced by nematodes, as discussed. One could imagine that intentional manipulation of microbial variables could influence parasite establishment and might possibly impact how parasitic diseases are treated in the future. In the case of *C. elegans*, characterizing its interactions with microbes beyond *E. coli* OP50 serves to improve this powerful model and enhances its utility to investigators with diverse objectives. Together, these diverse systems complement each other in elucidating the varied interactions between nematodes and microbes, thereby setting a stable foundation upon which future research can build.

SENSING THE MICROBIAL ENVIRONMENT

Nematodes are confronted with a tremendous and highly diverse microbial environment, presenting many infectious challenges. Alterations in the intestinal microbiota during helminth infection, coupled with studies demonstrating distinctly beneficial or harmful outcomes to *C. elegans* physiology in response to various bacteria, illustrate the ability of nematodes to sense their microbial environments and possibly discriminate between microbial species. Parasitic nematodes must have evolved particular strategies to overcome colonization by microbes, likely employing selected antibacterial defense mechanisms to coexist with the host microbiota. *C. elegans* has become an important model organism for the study of innate immune defense against pathogenic bacteria (Schulenburg et al., 2004; Irazoqui et al., 2010). The *C. elegans* immune system is seemingly of ancient origin, and there exist homologs of nearly all of its components in other organisms, including humans (Schulenburg et al., 2008). Consequently, sensing of the microbial environment might follow conserved or comparable mechanisms in parasitic nematodes as well.

C. elegans uses different protective mechanisms when confronted with potential pathogens, such as avoidance behavior (Meisel and Kim, 2014) and activation of stress and immune responses (Samuel et al., 2016) leading to the production and release of defense molecules with antimicrobial activities (Mallo et al., 2002). Identification of microbe-associated molecular patterns is followed by signal transduction via several signaling cascades, culminating in transcriptional alterations, reviewed in Rosso et al. (2013) and Kim and Ewbank (2015). While the pathogen-recognition receptors responsible for initiating immune responses are not entirely known, candidates include F-box proteins, lectins, follicle stimulating hormone receptor homolog-1, scavenger receptors, and the Toll-like receptor TOL-1 (Kim and Ewbank, 2015). Stress and immune responses illustrate an overlap between microbial and abiotic stresses; the main responses involved include: autophagy, insulin-like receptor (DAF-2), mitogen-activated protein kinases (MAPK), transforming growth factor-β-like (DBL-1), programmed cell death pathways, and unfolded protein responses (UPR) (Kim and Ewbank, 2015). Perhaps surprisingly, *C. elegans* lacks a homolog of NF-κB, an essential transcription factor in the innate immune response of many invertebrate and vertebrate species (Vallabhapurapu and Karin, 2009). Other proteins regulating transcription of infection and stress-modulated genes have been identified, including cyclic AMP-dependent transcription factor-7 (ATF-7), forkhead box O (FOXO) ortholog DAF-16, GATA transcription factors (ELT-2, ELT-3), helix loop helix-30 (HLH-30), heat-shock factor-1 (HSF-1), NF-E2-related factor SKN-1, signal transducer and activator of transcription STA-2, X-box binding protein-1 (XBP-1), and basic leucine zipper domain transcription factor ZIP-2 (Kim and Ewbank, 2015). As indicated, the intricacies of these responses have been reviewed elsewhere; as such, only examples of particular interest are highlighted here.

Pathogen Recognition

Infectious risks could be mitigated and resources preserved if pathogens were simply not encountered. Avoidance behavior is facilitated by the sole *C. elegans* toll-like receptor, TOL-1 (Pujol et al., 2001), and is characterized by the detection of specific microbial products, such as serrawettin W2 produced by *Serratia marcescens*, resulting in worms migrating away from the offending agents (Pradel et al., 2007). Unlike other organisms, *C. elegans* may not rely heavily on toll-like signaling for immune defense, though reports on this are conflicting (Pujol et al., 2001; Couillault et al., 2004; Tenor and Aballay, 2008). Other mechanisms such as aerotaxis also contribute to pathogen avoidance, as demonstrated by *C. elegans* avoidance of *P. aeruginosa* (Reddy et al., 2009). Lectins, carbohydrate-binding proteins implicated in multiple facets of immunity in a diverse range of species, may sense or neutralize microbes (Zelensky and Gready, 2005). Finally, there is evidence for an important role for scavenger receptors such as cell death abnormal-1 (CED-1) and scavenger (SCAV) proteins in pathogen recognition and resistance (Nicholas and Hodgkin, 2004; Means et al., 2009). Comparable studies of differential activation of recognition receptors in parasites by microbial communities from different intestinal regions might provide insights into how parasitic nematodes recognize threats and whether or not activation of such pathways impacts their niche selection.

Surveillance Immunity

In addition to sensing microbes and their toxins, organisms induce immunity-related genes due to disruptions of core physiologic processes by pathogens. *C. elegans* employs this surveillance immunity in response to inhibited translation, cellular damage, and mitochondrial stress, all of which can result from infection and exposure to microbial toxins (Pukkila-Worley, 2016). Transcriptional responses to these stresses include activation of immune signaling and xenobiotic metabolic pathways (Pukkila-Worley, 2016).

Toxins produced by several microbes, including diphtheria toxin from *Corynebacterium diphtheria* (Collier, 2001), cholix toxin from *Vibrio cholerae* (Jørgensen et al., 2008), and exotoxin A (ToxA) from *P. aeruginosa* (Dunbar et al., 2012), interfere with protein translation. When non-pathogenic *E. coli* engineered to express ToxA are fed to *C. elegans*, immune pathways required for resistance to the toxin, especially MAPK pathways, are upregulated by the worms (McEwan et al., 2012). Also, the aminoglycoside antibiotic hygromycin B blocks elongation of the amino acid chain during protein translation like ToxA (McEwan et al., 2012). Taken together, *C. elegans* likely responds to translation inhibition by ToxA rather than to the protein itself. An RNAi screen showed that disrupting core processes, including translation, activatesbasic leucine zipper domain transcription factor ZIP-2-dependent immune signaling, similar to responses seen during *P. aeruginosa* infection of *C. elegans* and following exposure to ToxA (Dunbar et al., 2012). More recently, another transcription factor called CCAAT-enhancer-binding-protein-2 (CEBP-2) was identified to act in concert with ZIP-2 to promote defense by *C. elegans* against *P. aeruginosa,* ToxA, and in response to inhibition of translation and other core processes (Reddy et al., 2016).

In addition to surveillance of disrupted physiologic processes, *C. elegans* also induces immune responses after injury of its epidermis by microbial infection and sterile wounding (Pujol et al., 2008a). During infection with *D. coniospora,* a fungal pathogen which damages the nematode cuticle, 4-hydoxyphenyllactic acid (HPLA) acts as a damage-associated molecular pattern recognized by the G protein-coupled receptor DCAR-1 which is required for AMP expression during fungal infection (Zugasti et al., 2014). Another study showed that epidermal damage liberates the STAT-like transcription factor STA-2, triggering AMP production (Zhang et al., 2015). These findings exemplify the ability of epithelial barriers to surveil physical damage and respond by activating innate immune pathways.

Microbial infection can often lead to mitochondrial stress; a survey of *C. elegans* responses to bacteria isolated from the nematode's natural environment found that 101 strains of the >550 isolates tested induced the mitochondrial stress reporter promoter *hsp-6::GFP* (Samuel et al., 2016). Interestingly, mitochondrial disruption also induces drug-detoxification enzymes belonging to the cytochrome P450 superfamily (CYPs) and enzymes involved in glucuronidation (Liu et al., 2014) as well as infection response gene-1 (*irg-1*) which is also induced during *P. aerugionsa* infection in a ZIP-2-dependent manner (Estes et al., 2010; Dunbar et al., 2012). Another toxin of *P. aeruginosa,* pyoverdin, disrupts the mitochondria of *C. elegans.* The nematodes respond by a specialized form of autophagy called mitophagy, whereby damaged mitochondria are degraded to resist *P. aeruginosa*-mediated killing (Kirienko et al., 2015).

By sensing various forms of cellular stress and damage, *C. elegans* is able to launch an integrated response which promotes survival and longevity (Pukkila-Worley, 2016). These responses can be induced by microbes and xenobiotics, activating immune and detoxification pathways (Melo and Ruvkun, 2012; Pukkila-Worley et al., 2014; Pukkila-Worley, 2016). As helminths may employ similar strategies to deal with microbial and xenobiotic stresses, the overlap between immune and drug detoxification responses is of particular interest. Various contributing factors have been identified for the development of anthelmintic resistance, including resistance alleles in detoxification genes, parasites not exposed to treatments, and underdosing (Vercruysse et al., 2011). The concept of surveillance immunity raises the notion that elements within the host microbiota prime helminths to resist anthelmintic treatments. Whether certain microbial species of the host intestine can promote drug resistance by activating xenobiotic detoxification within intestinal nematodes has not yet been studied.

Signal Transduction Pathways and Transcriptional Responses

As illustrated by many studies, MAPK pathways have a fundamental function in *C. elegans* stress and immune responses, including the p38 PMK-1 and extracellular signal-regulated kinase (ERK) pathways. Mutations at multiple levels of the NSY-1-SEK-1-PMK-1 pathway increase susceptibility to *P. aeruginosa* without impacting growth on *E. coli* OP50 (Kim et al., 2002). PMK-1 is activated by the toll-interleukin-1 receptor domain adaptor protein TIR-1 which is required for resisting killing by numerous microbial pathogens (Couillault et al., 2004). Phosphorylation of the ATF-7 transcription factor by PMK-1 activates transcription of lectins and candidate antimicrobial peptides (AMPs), conferring intestinal resistance to various species, including *P. aeruginosa, S. marcescens,* and *E. faecalis* (Shivers et al., 2010). Small molecule-mediated stimulation of the PMK-1 pathway and subsequent activation of ATF-7 can also increase lifespan in the presence of *E. faecalis* (Pukkila-Worley et al., 2012). Growth of *C. elegans* on soil-derived non-pathogenic bacteria, *Bacillus megaterium* and *Pseudomonas mendocina* also enhanced resistance to *P. aeruginosa* in a PMK-1 dependent fashion (Montalvo-Katz et al., 2013). Additionally, the PMK-1 pathway is active in epidermal infections as shown by induced expression of AMPs in response to *D. coniospora* as well in response to epidermal injury (Pujol et al., 2008a,b). Another MAPK pathway involving ERK signaling has been shown to be protective against rectal infection by *M. nematophilum*, (Gravato-Nobre et al., 2005). Based on these observations, one could speculate that MAPK pathways are also essential for helminth survival amongst numerous microbes.

Insulin-like signaling via DAF-2 highlights the intersection between immunity and metabolism. DAF-2 signaling inhibits DAF-16 activation by preventing its localization to the nucleus. Loss of function mutations of *daf-2* confer pathogen resistance and longevity by allowing activation of the DAF-16 transcription factor (Kenyon et al., 1993; Garsin et al., 2003). DAF-16 activation also increases resistance to non-microbial insults, such as heat stress and oxidative stress (Barsyte et al., 2001). Intriguingly, *C. elegans* can be primed to withstand pathogens and heat stress when exposed to pathogens during development, increasing the worm's lifespan (Leroy et al., 2012). DAF-16 activation appears to increase antimicrobial gene transcription as well as stress and detoxification genes, placing this transcription factor at the nexus of stress and immune signaling (McElwee et al., 2003). Autophagy, a lysosomal degradation pathway, is also implicated in longevity and its inhibition increases intracellular replication of *S. typhimurium* in *C. elegans* intestinal epithelia (Jia et al., 2009).

As intestinal nematodes are typically much larger than *C. elegans*, with female *Ascaris* worms growing up to 35 cm in length (Dold and Holland, 2011), the surface area available for attachment and infection by microbes is extensive. Furthermore, these nematodes are much longer-lived than *C. elegans*. Stress responses, especially autophagy, may be of particular importance in these organisms, though this area remains virtually unexplored. An intriguing study by Voronin *et al.* identified autophagy as a bactericidal mode of action in filarial worms targeting the bacterium *Wolbachia* (Voronin et al., 2012). The activation of autophagy coincided with the onset of rapid bacterial growth and expansion, showing that in spite of their mutualistic association, the nematode may recognize *Wolbachia* as a stressor and respond to regulate bacterial abundance (Taylor et al., 2013). Further studies assessing antibacterial responses by intestinal nematodes are largely lacking; however, two reports have shed some light on the issue. Adult female *A. suum* nematodes challenged with heat-inactivated *E. coli* respond by increasing transcription of two AMP families, the *Ascaris suum* antibacterial factors (ASABF) and the Cecropins (Pillai et al., 2003, 2005). Worms were challenged by injection of heat-killed bacteria into the pseudocoelom and appeared to demonstrate tissue-specific responses. While these data suggest an inducible defense system in *A. suum*, it would be relevant to study tissue-specific AMP expression using live bacterial cultures introduced externally, without wounding the worms, coupled with modern transcriptomic methods. Such an experiment would preserve pathogen-associated molecular patterns without invoking pathogen-independent, epithelial-damage responses, thereby allowing identification of transcriptional changes induced specifically by infection.

EFFECTORS OF INNATE IMMUNE SIGNALING IN NEMATODES

After sensing microbes, typical responses by nematodes include the production and release of factors possessing antimicrobial activity (**Table 3**). Among the different effectors of innate immunity, AMPs constitute the most ancient gene-encoded antimicrobial tools of eukaryotes (Zasloff, 2002). Nematodes produce different families of AMPs, many of which have been well characterized in *C. elegans*, while some have also been identified in parasitic nematodes. Antimicrobial activity has been experimentally demonstrated for many of these factors. AMPs can be classified based on their amino acid constituents and structural characteristics: α-helices, β–sheets, extended, and

TABLE 3 | Selected antimicrobial molecules of nematodes.

	Parasites			Free-living	
	***Ascaris* spp.**	***Trichuris* spp.**	***H. p. bakeri***	***C. elegans***	**References**
Antibacterial factors	Yes	–	–	Yes	Kato et al., 2002; Andersson et al., 2003; Pillai et al., 2003
Cecropins	Yes	–	–	–	Andersson et al., 2003; Pillai et al., 2005
Lectins	Yes*	–	Yes	Yes*	Cuperlović et al., 1987; Mallo et al., 2002; Harcus et al., 2009; Engelmann et al., 2011; Wang et al., 2013; Miltsch et al., 2014
Lysozymes	Yes	–	Yes	Yes	Mallo et al., 2002; O'Rourke et al., 2006; Schulenburg and Boehnisch, 2008; Hewitson et al., 2011; Tarr, 2012; Wang et al., 2013; Gravato-Nobre et al., 2016
Nemapores	Yes	Yes	–	Yes	Bányai and Patthy, 1998; Coolon et al., 2009; Roeder et al., 2010; Tarr, 2012
Nematode products	Tissue extracts, pseudocoelomic fluid	ESP	–	–	Wardlaw et al., 1994; Kato, 1995; Abner et al., 2001

*Yes, detected; -, not detected; *, lectin-like activity detected; gray shading, demonstrated bactericidal activity.*

looped (Melo et al., 2009). Many of the best-characterized AMPs tend to be small, cationic, amphipathic molecules thought to act by membrane disruption. While many candidate immune effectors have been proposed in the literature for *C. elegans*, reviewed in Kim and Ewbank (2015), here we focus on effectors with corresponding data from parasitic nematodes. AMPs such as antibacterial factors and cecropins are discussed along with larger proteins involved in the immune response including lectins, nemapores, and lysozymes. We will then conclude this section by discussing antimicrobial activities of helminth-derived products.

Antibacterial Factors

First identified in *A. suum*, ABFs are present in at least 25 nematode species, including seven ASABFs produced by *Ascaris* and six ABFs produced by *C. elegans* (Tarr, 2012). Sequence analysis reported by Tarr shows that other parasitic nematode species expressing ABFs include the human hookworm *N. americanus*, the ruminant nematode *Haemonchus contortus*, and the rodent model parasite *N. brasiliensis* (Tarr, 2012). Body fluid isolated from the pseudocoelem of *A. suum* demonstrated bactericidal activity, particularly against gram positive organisms (Wardlaw et al., 1994; Kato, 1995). Kato *et al.* isolated ASABF-α (Kato and Komatsu, 1996) and subsequently demonstrated broad-spectrum antibacterial and weak antifungal activity of a recombinant form of the peptide (Zhang et al., 2000). The observed activity was rapid, killing *S. aureus* in under 1 min, and could be inhibited by increasing salt concentrations (Zhang et al., 2000). Andersson *et al.* isolated ASABF-β and γ from *A. lumbricoides* which also showed antimicrobial activity, especially against gram positives (Andersson et al., 2003). ABFs were the first AMPs described in *C. elegans*, based on sequence similarity to their Ascarid counterparts and also demonstrated antimicrobial activity (Kato et al., 2002). ABFs belong to the cysteine-stabilized-αβ (CS-αβ) group of AMPs, are cationic, and contain a cysteine-stabilized α-helix and two β-sheets (Kato and Komatsu, 1996; Tarr, 2012). Transcripts for ASABFs have been detected in all tissues of *A. suum*, with some members upregulated in the body wall, intestine, and ovaries after bacterial challenge (Pillai et al., 2003). Expression patterns and anatomical localization of ABFs in *C. elegans* are indicative of roles in defense and digestion (Kato et al., 2002). For example, ABF-1 and 2 are detected in the pharynx, and ABF-1 and 3 in the intestine of *C. elegans*. The expression of some ABFs is inducible by different pathogens: ABF-2 by *S. typhimurium* (Alegado and Tan, 2008), ABF-1 and 2 by *Cryptococcus neoformans*, and ABF-3 by *S. aureus* (Alper et al., 2007).

Cecropins

In contrast to ABFs which seem to be widely distributed amongst nematodes, the cecropin family of AMPs has only been found in three Ascarids: *A. suum, A. lumbricoides*, and *Toxocara canis* (Pillai et al., 2005; Tarr, 2012). The first described nematode cecropin, Cecropin P1, was originally thought to be of porcine origin due to its isolation from pig intestine (Lee et al., 1989). Subsequently, its production was correctly attributed to *A. suum* (Andersson et al., 2003). Andersson et al. also isolated Cecropin P1 from *A. lumbricoides* and demonstrated antibacterial activity against gram negative organisms (Andersson et al., 2003). Pillai et al. demonstrated broad-spectrum antimicrobial activity of all four *Ascaris* cecropins as well as bacterial inducibility as detected for ASABFs (Pillai et al., 2005). Cecropins are typically 31–39 amino acids in length, strongly basic, cationic, α-helical peptides which are thought to disrupt microbial membranes by first laying on the membrane surface before reorientation and insertion into the membrane leading to disrupted lipid packing and subsequent membrane disintegration (Sipos et al., 1992; Gazit et al., 1995).

Lectins

Proteins containing lectin domains are conserved across Metazoans, including nematodes (Zelensky and Gready, 2005). Harcus et al. isolated one C-type lectin (CTL) from *H. p. bakeri* and two from *N. brasiliensis* (Harcus et al., 2009). Moreover, lectin-like carbohydrate-binding activity has previously been reported in the intestine of *A. suum* (Cuperlović et al., 1987) and lectins have been identified in excreted and secreted products (ESPs) of *A. suum* larvae (Wang et al., 2013). In general, CTLs are capable of binding carbohydrates and function in pathogen recognition and neutralization (Zelensky and Gready, 2005). CTLs from *H. p. bakeri* and *N. brasiliensis* are predominantly expressed by gut-dwelling adults rather than larvae; while Harcus et al. made a compelling case for host-immunomodulation by their reported CTLs, a dual role in pathogen neutralization or recognition is worth testing for parasite-derived lectins (Harcus et al., 2009). Parasite-derived CTL molecules localize in the nematode cuticle but could also be found in ESPs (Page et al., 1992). The CTLs detected in parasitic nematodes were most similar to the *C. elegans*-CTLs *clec-48, -49*, and -50. *Clec-50* is expressed in the *C. elegans* intestine and upregulated in response to the bacterium *S. marcescens* (Mallo et al., 2002). Though Harcus et al. did not report antimicrobial activity for the parasite-derived molecules, studies in *C. elegans* suggest they may have a role in defense. In addition to *clec-50, clec-49* is also upregulated in response to *S. marcescens* (Engelmann et al., 2011) and mutants deficient in this protein and another CTL, *clec-39*, have increased susceptibility to, and reduced survival and fecundity during, *S. marcescens* infection compared to wild-type worms (Miltsch et al., 2014). Furthermore, recombinant *clec-39* and *clec-49* bind *S. marcescens* in the absence of bactericidal activity (Miltsch et al., 2014). Additionally, in response to *M. nematophilum*, CTLs were found to be the most up-regulated protein class in *C. elegans* (O'Rourke et al., 2006). While nematode-derived lectins have not yet been shown to possess bactericidal activity, the mammalian lectin RegIIIγ is antibacterial and promotes commensalism by maintaining segregation between the microbiota and the host epithelium in mice (Vaishnava et al., 2011). Though many questions remain, the limited evidence available is suggestive of a role for lectins during infectious challenges and it is possible that parasite-derived lectins may confer resistance to different bacteria as has been demonstrated for *C. elegans*.

Lysozymes

Lysozymes are polysaccharide hydrolases, targeting bacterial peptidoglycan leading to cell lysis (Ellison and Giehl, 1991; Monzingo et al., 1996), and have been widely found in different nematode species. Lysozymes are encoded in the genomes of Ascarids, *N. americanus, H. contortus, N. brasiliensis, Brugia malayi,* and *Wuchereria bancrofti*, though missing from the Trichurids included in the sequence analysis by Tarr (2012). Lysozymes were also detected in the ESPs of *A. suum* (Wang et al., 2013) and *H. p. bakeri* (Hewitson et al., 2011), though further study is required to determine antibacterial activities of these helminth-lysozymes. 15 lysozymes were detected in *C. elegans*, divided into 10 protist-type (*lys-1–lys-10*) and five invertebrate-type (*ilys-1–ilys-5*), so named for sequence similarities to other organisms (Schulenburg and Boehnisch, 2008). Some lysozymes are markedly upregulated by *C. elegans* in response to bacterial infection (Mallo et al., 2002; O'Rourke et al., 2006; Gravato-Nobre et al., 2016). Lysozymes expressed in the *C. elegans* intestine (Schulenburg and Boehnisch, 2008) have been proposed to act in concert with caenopores (discussed in the next section)

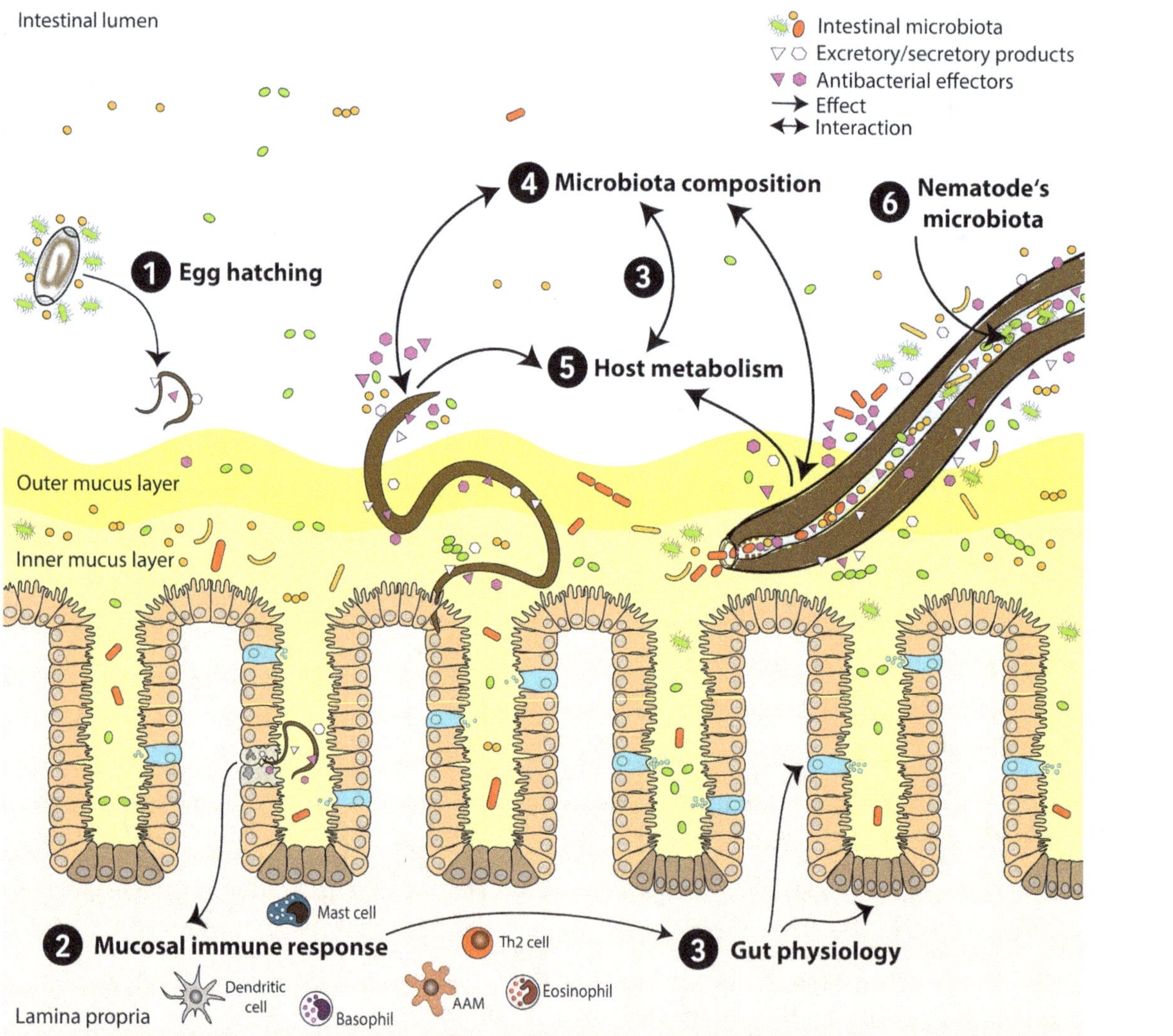

FIGURE 2 | Mutual influences of intestinal nematodes and host-gut bacteria. Establishment and persistence of intestinal nematodes in the host's gut are affected by bacterial communities and lead to substantial changes of the gut microbiota. Here, nematode-microbiota interactions and their impact on the host immune response and physiology are exemplified. (1) Egg hatching: Interaction of eggs with the intestinal microbiota is needed for some species, enabling larvae to hatch. (2) Mucosal immune response: Attachment to the epithelium and tissue migratory phase might lead to bacterial translocation and manipulation of immune responses. The anti-helminth immune response is predominantly a T helper type 2 response. (3) Gut physiology: Immune responses induce changes in gut physiology via induction of goblet cell hyperplasia, mucus production, and epithelial turnover, leading to changes in the host microbiota and its metabolome. Specific subsets of bacteria directly influence host physiology through their metabolic activities (e.g., short chain fatty acids-producing bacteria). (4) Microbiota composition: Intestinal nematodes modify intestinal microbial communities via different mechanisms: a) directly via secretion of antibacterial molecules and/or excretory/secretory products, b) indirectly by metabolic and physiologic shifts influencing the gut milieu. Chronic infections often lead to reduction in bacterial diversity and outgrowth of specific bacterial species beneficial for parasite survival. **(5) Host metabolism:** Intestinal nematodes modify host metabolism and nutrient uptake, e.g., alter amino acid, fatty acid, and carbohydrate metabolism, with subsequent influence on gut physiology, immune reactivity, and intestinal microbiota composition. (6) Nematode's microbiota: Nematode-associated bacterial communities might reflect the host microbiota and may also serve as transmission vehicles for pathogenic bacteria. Th2 cell, T helper type 2 cell; AAM, alternatively activated macrophage.

in digestion and immunity (Bányai and Patthy, 1998). For example, the *C. elegans* invertebrate lysozyme ILYS-3 is needed for physiological pharyngeal grinder function and for defense against bacterial pathogens (Gravato-Nobre et al., 2016). It was also shown that ILYS-3 is induced by danger signals generated both by bacterial pathogens and starvation (Gravato-Nobre et al., 2016). In healthy *C. elegans*, intestinal *ilys-3* expression undergoes a post-developmental regulatory oscillation: levels increase after L1 hatching, decline after the L2 transition, and increase again after L4 transition becoming abundantly expressed in the intestine of adult worms (Gravato-Nobre et al., 2016). Notably, coelomocytes of *C. elegans* also express *ilys-3* (Gravato-Nobre et al., 2016) and are scavenger cells that endocytose fluid from the pseudocoelom (Fares and Greenwald, 2001). The role of coelomocytes in parasitic nematodes is not well understood and they have not been studied in immunity. Given the demonstrated importance of lysozymes for *C. elegans* and the wide distribution of this protein family across species, it is expected that they support helminth survival amongst the host-microbiota.

Nemapores

Known as caenopores in *C. elegans*, nemapores contain a saposin domain and share similarity with protozoan amoebapores and mammalian NK-lysin and granulysin (Leippe, 1995; Roeder et al., 2010). As with ABFs, nemapores are also cysteine-rich, but contain multiple α-helices (Mysliwy et al., 2010). Nemapores are widely distributed and in addition to *C. elegans*, have been found in 46 nematode species including Ascarids, Trichurids, and the human filarial worms *B. malayi* and *W. bancrofti* (Tarr, 2012). Only caenopores have been studied experimentally, with caenopore-1 and 5 demonstrating antimicrobial activity (Bányai and Patthy, 1998; Roeder et al., 2010). Caenopore-5 is constitutively expressed in the intestine, while caenopore-3 is induced by starvation as well as the bacterial strains *B. megaterium* and *Micrococcus luteus*, suggesting functions in nutrition and immune defense (Roeder et al., 2010). Interestingly, the free-living soil bacteria *B. megaterium* and *M. luteus* are both frequently found with Rhabditid nematodes (Coolon et al., 2009) and may be present in the environment of *C. elegans*. As with lysozymes, experimental evidence of nemapore function in parasitic nematodes is currently lacking.

Antimicrobial Activities of Helminth-Derived Products

In addition to studies demonstrating antimicrobial activities of specific helminth-derived molecules described here, activity can also be detected from the ESPs of parasites. In one study, ESPs from the filarial worm *O. ochengi* were analyzed revealing 36 candidate AMPs (Eberle et al., 2015). Of the 36 candidates, the investigators were able to unambiguously attribute bactericidal activity against *E. coli* to three peptides while the other 33 peptides had been assessed as part of peptide mixtures. Antibacterial activity has also been shown for ESPs from adult *T. suis* worms (Abner et al., 2001). Different bacterial strains were tested, including *S. aureus*, *E. coli*, and *C. jejuni*. The observed activity was shown to be due to small (<10 kDa), boiling-resistant molecules, indicative of AMPs. Interestingly, pore-forming proteins have also been isolated from *T. trichiura* and *T. muris*, indicating that antimicrobial activity of nematode ESPs is likely due to multiple components of varying sizes and mechanisms (Drake et al., 1994). As nematodes produce a variety of antimicrobial factors, innate immune responses to microbes by helminths likely offer protection using several different strategies.

CONCLUSIONS AND PERSPECTIVES

Antibiotic resistance is a rapidly escalating problem with devastating consequences for human and animal health. Drug resistance mechanisms described for microbes and helminths foreshadow the emergence of immense clinical and economic challenges associated with previously treatable infectious diseases. Meanwhile, inflammatory and metabolic diseases also inflict great suffering and are a source of considerable strain on healthcare systems; therefore, novel solutions are sought after to combat these difficulties. As nematodes have evolved over millions of years in a diverse microbial environment, a better understanding of how nematodes interact with microbial populations may offer innovative strategies for treating human and animal diseases. Given the importance of the microbiota and the ability of helminths to influence microbial communities in the gut (**Figure 2**), helminth infections and helminth products are being studied for their role in dysbiosis. Preliminary data suggest potential benefits of helminths in inflammatory diseases and in individuals with metabolic abnormalities. An additional application of the impact of nematodes on microbes is the development of new antimicrobials. AMPs are under investigation for their therapeutic potential and an understanding of how antimicrobial effectors are used by organisms living amongst diverse microbial populations can guide development efforts. In elucidating the impacts of different bacteria on nematodes, one can anticipate the discovery of novel anthelmintic targets. Moreover, these studies also provide insights into conserved innate immune mechanisms. The divergent environments and experimental systems of parasitic and free-living nematodes offer unique tools to investigators, the combination of which enhance our comprehension of nematode biology and evolutionary ecology.

AUTHOR CONTRIBUTIONS

All authors listed have made substantial contributions to the planning and writing of this work. All authors have approved this work for publication.

FUNDING

The work was supported by the German Research Foundation: GRK 2046 (AM and SH) and HA2542/3-2 (SH).

REFERENCES

Abner, S. R., Parthasarathy, G., Hill, D. E., and Mansfield, L. S. (2001). Trichuris suis: detection of antibacterial activity in excretory-secretory products from adults. *Exp. Parasitol.* 99, 26–36. doi: 10.1006/expr.2001.4643

Alegado, R. A., and Tan, M.-W. (2008). Resistance to antimicrobial peptides contributes to persistence of salmonella typhimurium in the *C. Elegans* INTESTINE. *Cell. Microbiol.* 10, 1259–1273. doi: 10.1111/j.1462-5822.2008.01124.x

Alper, S., McBride, S. J., Lackford, B., Freedman, J. H., and Schwartz, D. A. (2007). Specificity and complexity of the *Caenorhabditis elegans* innate immune response. *Mol. Cell. Biol.* 27, 5544–5553. doi: 10.1128/MCB.02070-06

Andersson, M., Boman, A., and Boman, H. H. (2003). *Ascaris* nematodes from pig and human make three antibacterial peptides: isolation of cecropin P1 and two ASABF peptides. *Cell. Mol. Life Sci.* 60, 599–606. doi: 10.1007/s000180300051

Bansemir, A. D., and Sukhdeo, M. V. (1994). The food resource of adult *Heligmosomoides Polygyrus* in the small intestine. *J. Parasitol.* 80, 24–28. doi: 10.2307/3283340

Bansemir, A. D., and Sukhdeo, M. V. (2001). Intestinal distribution of worms and host ingesta in *Nippostrongylus brasiliensis*. *J. Parasitol.* 87, 1470–1472. doi: 10.1645/0022-3395(2001)087[1470:IDOWAH]2.0.CO;2

Bányai, L., and Patthy, L. (1998). Amoebapore homologs of *Caenorhabditis elegans*. *Biochim. Biophys. Acta* 1429, 259–264. doi: 10.1016/S0167-4838(98)00237-4

Barrière, A., and Félix, M. (2005). High local genetic diversity and low outcrossing rate in *Caenorhabditis elegans* natural populations. *Curr. Biol.* 15, 1176–1184. doi: 10.1016/j.cub.2005.06.022

Barsyte, D., Lovejoy, D. A., and Lithgow, G. J. (2001). Longevity and heavy metal resistance in Daf-2 and age-1 long-lived mutants of *Caenorhabditis elegans*. *FASEB J.* 15, 627–634. doi: 10.1096/fj.99-0966com

Behnke, J. M., Menge, D. M., and Noyes, H. (2009). Heligmosomoides bakeri: a model for exploring the biology and genetics of resistance to chronic gastrointestinal nematode infections. *Parasitology* 136, 1565–1580. doi: 10.1017/S0031182009006003

Bethony, J., Brooker, S., Albonico, M., Geiger, S. M., Loukas, A., Diemert, D., et al. (2006). Soil-transmitted helminth infections: ascariasis, trichuriasis, and hookworm. *Lancet* 367, 1521–1532. doi: 10.1016/S0140-6736(06)68653-4

Bevins, C. L., and Salzman, N. H. (2011). Paneth cells, antimicrobial peptides and maintenance of intestinal homeostasis. *Nat. Rev. Microbiol.* 9, 356–368. doi: 10.1038/nrmicro2546

Broadhurst, M. J., Ardeshir, A., Kanwar, B., Mirpuri, J., Gundra, U. M., Leung, J. M., et al. (2012). Therapeutic helminth infection of macaques with idiopathic chronic diarrhea alters the inflammatory signature and mucosal microbiota of the colon. *PLoS Pathog.* 8:e1003000. doi: 10.1371/journal.ppat.1003000

Cabreiro, F., and Gems, D. (2013). Worms need microbes too: microbiota, health and aging in *Caenorhabditis elegans*. *EMBO Mol. Med.* 5, 1300–1310. doi: 10.1002/emmm.201100972

Cantacessi, C., Giacomin, P., Croese, J., Zakrzewski, M., Sotillo, J., McCann, L., et al. (2014). Impact of experimental hookworm infection on the human gut microbiota. *J. Infect. Dis.* 210, 1431–1434. doi: 10.1093/infdis/jiu256

Carding, S., Verbeke, K., Vipond, D. T., Corfe, B. M., and Owen, L. J. (2015). Dysbiosis of the gut microbiota in disease. *Microb. Ecol. Health Dis.* 26:26191. doi: 10.3402/mehd.v26.26191

Cattadori, I. M., Sebastian, A., Hao, H., Katani, R., Albert, I., Eilertson, K. E., et al. (2016). Impact of helminth infections and nutritional constraints on the small intestine microbiota. *PLoS ONE* 11:e0159770. doi: 10.1371/journal.pone.0159770

Collier, R. J. (2001). Understanding the mode of action of diphtheria toxin: a perspective on progress during the 20th century. *Toxicon* 39, 1793–1803. doi: 10.1016/S0041-0101(01)00165-9

Consortium, T. H. M. P. (2012). Structure, function and diversity of the healthy human microbiome. *Nature* 486, 207–214. doi: 10.1038/nature11234

Coolon, J. D., Jones, K. L., Todd, T. C., Carr, B. C., and Herman, M. A. (2009). *Caenorhabditis elegans* genomic response to soil bacteria predicts environment-specific genetic effects on life history traits. *PLoS Genet.* 5:e1000503. doi: 10.1371/journal.pgen.1000503

Cooper, P., Walker, A. W., Reyes, J., Chico, M., Salter, S. J., Vaca, M., et al. (2013). Patent human infections with the whipworm, *Trichuris trichiura*, are not associated with alterations in the faecal microbiota. *PLoS ONE* 8:e76573. doi: 10.1371/journal.pone.0076573

Couillault, C., and Ewbank, J. J. (2002). Diverse bacteria are pathogens of *Caenorhabditis elegans* infect. *Immun.* 70, 4705–4707. doi: 10.1128/IAI.70.8.4705-4707.2002

Couillault, C., Pujol, N., Reboul, J., Sabatier, L., Guichou, J.-F., Kohara, Y., et al. (2004). TLR-independent control of innate immunity in *Caenorhabditis elegans* by the TIR domain adaptor protein TIR-1, an ortholog of human SARM. *Nat. Immunol.* 5, 488–494. doi: 10.1038/ni1060

Croese, J., Giacomin, P., Navarro, S., Clouston, A., McCann, L., Dougall, A., et al. (2015). Experimental hookworm infection and gluten microchallenge promote tolerance in celiac disease. *J. Allergy Clin. Immunol.* 135, 508–516. doi: 10.1016/j.jaci.2014.07.022

Cullen, T. W., Schofield, W. B., Barry, N. A., Putnam, E. E., Rundell, E. A., Trent, M. S., et al. (2015). Antimicrobial peptide resistance mediates resilience of prominent gut commensals during inflammation. *Science* 347, 170–175. doi: 10.1126/science.1260580

Cuperlović, M., Movsesijan, M., and Hajduković, L. (1987). *Ascaris* lumbricoides: lectin activity in the gastrointestinal system. *Exp. Parasitol.* 63, 237–239. doi: 10.1016/0014-4894(87)90167-6

Dai, L.-L., Gao, J.-X., Zou, C.-G., Ma, Y.-C., and Zhang, K.-Q. (2015). mir-233 modulates the unfolded protein response in *C. elegans* during *Pseudomonas aeruginosa* infection. *PLoS Pathog.* 11:e1004606. doi: 10.1371/journal.ppat.1004606

Darby, A. C., Armstrong, S. D., Bah, G. S., Kaur, G., Hughes, M. A., Kay, S. M., et al. (2012). Analysis of gene expression from the *Wolbachia* genome of a filarial nematode supports both metabolic and defensive roles within the symbiosis. *Genome Res.* 22, 2467–2477. doi: 10.1101/gr.138420.112

Davey, K. G. (1964). The food of *Ascaris*. *Can. J. Zool.* 42, 1160–1161. doi: 10.1139/z64-115

David, L. A., Maurice, C. F., Carmody, R. N., Gootenberg, D. B., Button, J. E., Wolfe, B. E., et al. (2014). Diet rapidly and reproducibly alters the human gut microbiome. *Nature* 505, 559–563. doi: 10.1038/nature12820

Dethlefsen, L., Huse, S., Sogin, M. L., and Relman, D. A. (2008). The pervasive effects of an antibiotic on the human gut microbiota, as revealed by deep 16S rRNA sequencing. *PLoS Biol.* 6:e280. doi: 10.1371/journal.pbio.0060280

Dilika, F., Bremner, P. D., and Meyer, J. J. (2000). Antibacterial activity of linoleic and oleic acids isolated from Helichrysum pedunculatum: a plant used during circumcision rites. *Fitoterapia* 71, 450–452. doi: 10.1016/S0367-326X(00)00150-7

Dirksen, P., Marsh, S. A., Braker, I., Heitland, N., Wagner, S., Nakad, R., et al. (2016). The native microbiome of the nematode *Caenorhabditis elegans*: gateway to a new host-microbiome model. *BMC Biol.* 14:38. doi: 10.1186/s12915-016-0258-1

Dold, C., and Holland, C. V. (2011). Ascaris and ascariasis. *Microbes Infect.* 13, 632–637. doi: 10.1016/j.micinf.2010.09.012

Donaldson, G. P., Lee, S. M., and Mazmanian, S. K. (2016). Gut biogeography of the bacterial microbiota. *Nat. Rev. Microbiol.* 14, 20–32. doi: 10.1038/nrmicro3552

Drake, L., Korchev, Y., Bashford, L., Djamgoz, M., Wakelin, D., Ashall, F., et al. (1994). The major secreted product of the whipworm, Trichuris, is a pore-forming protein. *Proc. Biol. Sci.* 257, 255–261. doi: 10.1098/rspb.1994.0123

Dunbar, T. L., Yan, Z., Balla, K. M., Smelkinson, M. G., and Troemel, E. R. (2012). *C. elegans* detects pathogen-induced translational inhibition to activate immune signaling. *Cell Host Microbe* 11, 375–386. doi: 10.1016/j.chom.2012.02.008

Eberle, R., Brattig, N. W., Trusch, M., Schlüter, H., Achukwi, M. D., Eisenbarth, A., et al. (2015). Isolation, identification and functional profile of excretory-secretory peptides from Onchocerca ochengi. *Acta Trop.* 142, 156–166. doi: 10.1016/j.actatropica.2014.11.015

Eckburg, P. B., Bik, E. M., Bernstein, C. N., Purdom, E., Dethlefsen, L., Sargent, M., et al. (2005). Diversity of the human intestinal microbial flora. *Science* 308, 1635–1638. doi: 10.1126/science.1110591

Eijck, I. A. and Borgsteede, F. H. (2005). A survey of gastrointestinal pig parasites on free-range, organic and conventional pig farms in The Netherlands. *Vet. Res. Commun.* 29, 407–414. doi: 10.1007/s11259-005-1201-z

Ellison, R. T., and Giehl, T. J. (1991). Killing of gram-negative bacteria by lactoferrin and lysozyme. *J. Clin. Invest.* 88, 1080–1091. doi: 10.1172/JCI115407

Engelmann, I., Griffon, A., Tichit, L., Montañana-Sanchis, F., Wang, G., Reinke, V., et al. (2011). A comprehensive analysis of gene expression changes provoked by bacterial and fungal infection in *C. elegans*. *PLoS ONE* 6:e19055. doi: 10.1371/journal.pone.0019055

Estes, K. A., Dunbar, T. L., Powell, J. R., Ausubel, F. M., and Troemel, E. R. (2010). bZIP transcription factor zip-2 mediates an early response to *Pseudomonas aeruginosa* infection in *Caenorhabditis elegans*. *Proc. Natl. Acad. Sci. U.S.A.* 107, 2153–2158. doi: 10.1073/pnas.0914643107

Fares, H., and Greenwald, I. (2001). Genetic analysis of endocytosis in *Caenorhabditis elegans*: coelomocyte uptake defective mutants. *Genetics* 159, 133–145.

Félix, M.-A., Ashe, A., Piffaretti, J., Wu, G., Nuez, I., Bélicard, T., et al. (2011). Natural and experimental infection of Caenorhabditis nematodes by novel viruses related to nodaviruses. *PLoS Biol.* 9:e1000586. doi: 10.1371/journal.pbio.1000586

Félix, M.-A., and Duveau, F. (2012). Population dynamics and habitat sharing of natural populations of *Caenorhabditis elegans* and C. briggsae. *BMC Biol.* 10:59. doi: 10.1186/1741-7007-10-59

Frézal, L., and Félix, M.-A. (2015). *C. elegans* outside the Petri dish. *Elife* 4:e05849. doi: 10.7554/eLife.05849

Fricke, W. F., Song, Y., Wang, A.-J., Smith, A., Grinchuk, V., Mongodin, E., et al. (2015). Type 2 immunity-dependent reduction of segmented filamentous bacteria in mice infected with the helminthic parasite *Nippostrongylus brasiliensis*. *Microbiome* 3:40. doi: 10.1186/s40168-015-0103-8

Garsin, D. A., Villanueva, J. M., Begun, J., Kim, D. H., Sifri, C. D., Calderwood, S. B., et al. (2003). Long-lived *C. elegans* daf-2 mutants are resistant to bacterial pathogens. *Science* 300:1921. doi: 10.1126/science.1080147

Gause, W. C., and Maizels, R. M. (2016). Macrobiota - helminths as active participants and partners of the microbiota in host intestinal homeostasis. *Curr. Opin. Microbiol.* 32, 14–18. doi: 10.1016/j.mib.2016.04.004

Gazit, E., Boman, A., Boman, H. G., and Shai, Y. (1995). Interaction of the mammalian antibacterial peptide cecropin P1 with phospholipid vesicles. *Biochemistry (Mosc.)* 34, 11479–11488. doi: 10.1021/bi00036a021

Gevers, D., Kugathasan, S., Denson, L. A., Vázquez-Baeza, Y., Van Treuren, W., Ren, B., et al. (2014). The treatment-naive microbiome in new-onset Crohn's disease. *Cell Host Microbe* 15, 382–392. doi: 10.1016/j.chom.2014.02.005

Giacomin, P., Zakrzewski, M., Croese, J., Su, X., Sotillo, J., McCann, L., et al. (2015). Experimental hookworm infection and escalating gluten challenges are associated with increased microbial richness in celiac subjects. *Sci. Rep.* 5:13797. doi: 10.1038/srep13797

Gravato-Nobre, M. J., Nicholas, H. R., Nijland, R., O'Rourke, D., Whittington, D. E., Yook, K. J., et al. (2005). Multiple genes affect sensitivity of *Caenorhabditis elegans* to the bacterial pathogen *Microbacterium nematophilum*. *Genetics* 171, 1033–1045. doi: 10.1534/genetics.105.045716

Gravato-Nobre, M. J., Vaz, F., Filipe, S., Chalmers, R., and Hodgkin, J. (2016). The invertebrate lysozyme effector ILYS-3 is systemically activated in response to danger signals and confers antimicrobial protection in *C. elegans*. *PLoS Pathog.* 12:e1005826. doi: 10.1371/journal.ppat.1005826

Gregory, R. D., Keymer, A. E., and Clarke, J. R. (1990). Genetics, sex and exposure: the ecology of *Heligmosomoides polygyrus* (Nematoda) in the wood mouse. *J. Anim. Ecol.* 59, 363–378. doi: 10.2307/5178

Harcus, Y., Nicoll, G., Murray, J., Filbey, K., Gomez-Escobar, N., and Maizels, R. M. (2009). C-type lectins from the nematode parasites *Heligmosomoides polygyrus* and *Nippostrongylus brasiliensis*. *Parasitol. Int.* 58, 461–470. doi: 10.1016/j.parint.2009.08.011

Hayes, K. S., Bancroft, A. J., Goldrick, M., Portsmouth, C., Roberts, I. S., and Grencis, R. K. (2010). Exploitation of the intestinal microflora by the parasitic nematode Trichuris muris. *Science* 328, 1391–1394. doi: 10.1126/science.1187703

Hewitson, J. P., Harcus, Y., Murray, J., van Agtmaal, M., Filbey, K. J., Grainger, J. R., et al. (2011). Proteomic analysis of secretory products from the model gastrointestinal nematode *Heligmosomoides polygyrus* reveals dominance of Venom Allergen-Like (VAL) proteins. *J. Proteomics* 74, 1573–1594. doi: 10.1016/j.jprot.2011.06.002

Hoerauf, A., Nissen-Pähle, K., Schmetz, C., Henkle-Dührsen, K., Blaxter, M. L., Büttner, D. W., et al. (1999). Tetracycline therapy targets intracellular bacteria in the filarial nematode Litomosoides sigmodontis and results in filarial infertility. *J. Clin. Invest.* 103, 11–18. doi: 10.1172/JCI4768

Holm, J. B., Sorobetea, D., Kiilerich, P., Ramayo-Caldas, Y., Estellé, J., Ma, T., et al. (2015). Chronic Trichuris muris infection decreases diversity of the intestinal microbiota and concomitantly increases the abundance of *Lactobacilli*. *PLoS ONE* 10:e0125495. doi: 10.1371/journal.pone.0125495

Hotez, P. J., Brindley, P. J., Bethony, J. M., King, C. H., Pearce, E. J., and Jacobson, J. (2008). Helminth infections: the great neglected tropical diseases. *J. Clin. Invest.* 118, 1311–1321. doi: 10.1172/JCI34261

Houlden, A., Hayes, K. S., Bancroft, A. J., Worthington, J. J., Wang, P., Grencis, R. K., et al. (2015). Chronic Trichuris muris Infection in C57BL/6 mice causes significant changes in host microbiota and metabolome: effects reversed by pathogen clearance. *PLoS ONE* 10:e0125945. doi: 10.1371/journal.pone.0125945

Hsu, S. C., Johansson, K. R., and Donahue, M. J. (1986). The bacterial flora of the intestine of Ascaris suum and 5-hydroxytryptamine production. *J. Parasitol.* 72, 545–549. doi: 10.2307/3281505

Irazoqui, J. E., Urbach, J. M., and Ausubel, F. M. (2010). Evolution of host innate defence: insights from *C. elegans* and primitive invertebrates. *Nat. Rev. Immunol.* 10, 47–58. doi: 10.1038/nri2689

Ivanov, I. I., Atarashi, K., Manel, N., Brodie, E. L., Shima, T., Karaoz, U., et al. (2009). Induction of intestinal Th17 cells by segmented filamentous bacteria. *Cell* 139, 485–498. doi: 10.1016/j.cell.2009.09.033

JebaMercy, G., and Balamurugan, K. (2012). Effects of sequential infections of *Caenorhabditis elegans* with *Staphylococcus aureus* and *Proteus mirabilis*. Microbiol. *Immunol.* 56, 825–835. doi: 10.1111/j.1348-0421.2012.00509.x

Jernberg, C., Löfmark, S., Edlund, C., and Jansson, J. K. (2007). Long-term ecological impacts of antibiotic administration on the human intestinal microbiota. *ISME J.* 1, 56–66. doi: 10.1038/ismej.2007.3

Jia, K., Thomas, C., Akbar, M., Sun, Q., Adams-Huet, B., Gilpin, C., et al. (2009). Autophagy genes protect against Salmonella typhimurium infection and mediate insulin signaling-regulated pathogen resistance. *Proc. Natl. Acad. Sci. U.S.A.* 106, 14564–14569. doi: 10.1073/pnas.0813319106

Jørgensen, R., Purdy, A. E., Fieldhouse, R. J., Kimber, M. S., Bartlett, D. H., and Merrill, A. R. (2008). Cholix Toxin, a novel ADP-ribosylating factor from *Vibrio cholerae*. *J. Biol. Chem.* 283, 10671–10678. doi: 10.1074/jbc.M710008200

Kato, Y. (1995). Humoral defense of the nematode Ascaris suum: antibacterial, bacteriolytic and agglutinating activities in the body fluid. *Zoolog. Sci.* 12, 225–230. doi: 10.2108/zsj.12.225

Kato, Y., Aizawa, T., Hoshino, H., Kawano, K., Nitta, K., and Zhang, H. (2002). abf-1 and abf-2, ASABF-type antimicrobial peptide genes in *Caenorhabditis elegans*. *Biochem. J.* 361, 221–230. doi: 10.1042/bj3610221

Kato, Y., and Komatsu, S. (1996). ASABF, a novel cysteine-rich antibacterial peptide isolated from the nematode Ascaris suum. Purification, primary structure, and molecular cloning of cDNA. *J. Biol. Chem.* 271, 30493–30498. doi: 10.1074/jbc.271.48.30493

Kenyon, C., Chang, J., Gensch, E., Rudner, A., and Tabtiang, R. (1993). A *C. elegans* mutant that lives twice as long as wild type. *Nature* 366, 461–464. doi: 10.1038/366461a0

Kim, D. H., and Ewbank, J. J. (2015). Signaling in the innate immune response. *WormBook* doi: 10.1895/wormbook.1.83.2. [Epub ahead of print].

Kim, D. H., Feinbaum, R., Alloing, G., Emerson, F. E., Garsin, D. A., Inoue, H., et al. (2002). A conserved p38 MAP kinase pathway in *Caenorhabditis elegans* innate immunity. *Science* 297, 623–626. doi: 10.1126/science.1073759

Kirienko, N. V., Ausubel, F. M., and Ruvkun, G. (2015). Mitophagy confers resistance to siderophore-mediated killing by *Pseudomonas aeruginosa*. *Proc. Natl. Acad. Sci. U.S.A.* 112, 1821–1826. doi: 10.1073/pnas.1424954112

Klementowicz, J. E., Travis, M. A., and Grencis, R. K. (2012). Trichuris muris: a model of gastrointestinal parasite infection. *Semin. Immunopathol.* 34, 815–828. doi: 10.1007/s00281-012-0348-2

Kozek, W. J. (1977). Transovarially-transmitted intracellular microorganisms in adult and larval stages of *Brugia malayi*. *J. Parasitol.* 63, 992–1000. doi: 10.2307/3279832

Kreisinger, J., Bastien, G., Hauffe, H. C., Marchesi, J., and Perkins, S. E. (2015). Interactions between multiple helminths and the gut microbiota in wild rodents. *Philos. Trans. R. Soc. Lond. B. Biol. Sci.* 370:20140295. doi: 10.1098/rstb.2014.0295

Lee, J., Choe, J., Kim, J., Oh, S., Park, S., Kim, S., et al. (2015). Heat-killed Lactobacillus spp. cells enhance survivals of *Caenorhabditis elegans* against Salmonella and Yersinia infections. *Lett. Appl. Microbiol.* 61, 523–530. doi: 10.1111/lam.12478

Lee, J. Y., Boman, A., Sun, C. X., Andersson, M., Jörnvall, H., Mutt, V., et al. (1989). Antibacterial peptides from pig intestine: isolation of a mammalian cecropin. *Proc. Natl. Acad. Sci. U.S.A.* 86, 9159–9162. doi: 10.1073/pnas.86.23.9159

Lee, S. C., Tang, M. S., Lim, Y. A. L., Choy, S. H., Kurtz, Z. D., Cox, L. M., et al. (2014). Helminth colonization is associated with increased diversity of the gut microbiota. *PLoS Negl. Trop. Dis.* 8:e2880. doi: 10.1371/journal.pntd.0002880

Lee, S.-H., Wong, R.-R., Chin, C.-Y., Lim, T.-Y., Eng, S.-A., Kong, C., et al. (2013). *Burkholderia* pseudomallei suppresses *Caenorhabditis elegans* immunity by specific degradation of a GATA transcription factor. *Proc. Natl. Acad. Sci. U.S.A.* 110, 15067–15072. doi: 10.1073/pnas.1311725110

Leippe, M. (1995). Ancient weapons: NK-lysin, is a mammalian homolog to pore-forming peptides of a protozoan parasite. *Cell* 83, 17–18. doi: 10.1016/0092-8674(95)90229-5

Leroy, M., Mosser, T., Manière, X., Alvarez, D. F., and Matic, I. (2012). Pathogen-induced *Caenorhabditis elegans* developmental plasticity has a hormetic effect on the resistance to biotic and abiotic stresses. *BMC Evol. Biol.* 12:187. doi: 10.1186/1471-2148-12-187

Leser, T. D., Amenuvor, J. Z., Jensen, T. K., Lindecrona, R. H., Boye, M., and Møller, K. (2002). Culture-independent analysis of gut bacteria: the pig gastrointestinal tract microbiota revisited. *Appl. Environ. Microbiol.* 68, 673–690. doi: 10.1128/AEM.68.2.673-690.2002

Li, R. W., Wu, S., Li, W., Navarro, K., Couch, R. D., Hill, D., et al. (2012). Alterations in the porcine colon microbiota induced by the gastrointestinal nematode Trichuris suis. *Infect. Immun.* 80, 2150–2157. doi: 10.1128/IAI.00141-12

Liu, Y., Samuel, B. S., Breen, P. C., and Ruvkun, G. (2014). *Caenorhabditis elegans* pathways that surveil and defend mitochondria. *Nature* 508, 406–410. doi: 10.1038/nature13204

Lupp, C., Robertson, M. L., Wickham, M. E., Sekirov, I., Champion, O. L., Gaynor, E. C., et al. (2007). Host-mediated inflammation disrupts the intestinal microbiota and promotes the overgrowth of Enterobacteriaceae. *Cell Host Microbe* 2, 119–129. doi: 10.1016/j.chom.2007.06.010

MacNeil, L. T., and Walhout, A. J. (2013). Food, pathogen, signal. *Worm* 2:e26454. doi: 10.4161/worm.26454

Mallo, G. V., Kurz, C. L., Couillault, C., Pujol, N., Granjeaud, S., Kohara, Y., et al. (2002). Inducible antibacterial defense system in *C. elegans*. *Curr. Biol. CB* 12, 1209–1214. doi: 10.1016/S0960-9822(02)00928-4

Mansfield, L., Gauthier, D. T., Abner, S. R., Jones, K. M., Wilder, S. R., and Urban, J. F. (2003). Enhancement of disease and pathology by synergy of Trichuris suis and Campylobacter jejuni in the colon of immunologically naive swine. *Am. J. Trop. Med. Hyg.* 68, 70–80. doi: 10.4269/ajtmh.2003.68.70

Mansfield, L. S., and Urban, J. F. (1996). The pathogenesis of necrotic proliferative colitis in swine is linked to whipworm induced suppression of mucosal immunity to resident bacteria. *Vet. Immunol. Immunopathol.* 50, 1–17. doi: 10.1016/0165-2427(95)05482-0

Masson, F., Zaidman-Rémy, A., and Heddi, A. (2016). Antimicrobial peptides and cell processes tracking endosymbiont dynamics. *Philos. Trans. R. Soc. B* 371:20150298. doi: 10.1098/rstb.2015.0298

McElwee, J., Bubb, K., and Thomas, J. H. (2003). Transcriptional outputs of the *Caenorhabditis elegans* forkhead protein DAF-16. *Aging Cell* 2, 111–121. doi: 10.1046/j.1474-9728.2003.00043.x

McEwan, D. L., Kirienko, N. V., and Ausubel, F. M. (2012). Host translational inhibition by *Pseudomonas aeruginosa* exotoxin a triggers an immune response in *Caenorhabditis elegans*. *Cell Host Microbe* 11, 364–374. doi: 10.1016/j.chom.2012.02.007

McGarry, H. F., Egerton, G. L., and Taylor, M. J. (2004). Population dynamics of *Wolbachia* bacterial endosymbionts in *Brugia malayi*. *Mol. Biochem. Parasitol.* 135, 57–67. doi: 10.1016/j.molbiopara.2004.01.006

Means, T. K., Mylonakis, E., Tampakakis, E., Colvin, R. A., Seung, E., Puckett, L., et al. (2009). Evolutionarily conserved recognition and innate immunity to fungal pathogens by the scavenger receptors SCARF1 and CD36. *J. Exp. Med.* 206, 637–653. doi: 10.1084/jem.20082109

Meisel, J. D., and Kim, D. H. (2014). Behavioral avoidance of pathogenic bacteria by *Caenorhabditis elegans*. *Trends Immunol.* 35, 465–470. doi: 10.1016/j.it.2014.08.008

Melo, J. A., and Ruvkun, G. (2012). Inactivation of conserved *C. elegans* genes engages pathogen- and xenobiotic-associated defenses. *Cell* 149, 452–466. doi: 10.1016/j.cell.2012.02.050

Melo, M. N., Ferre, R., and Castanho, M. A. R. B. (2009). Antimicrobial peptides: linking partition, activity and high membrane-bound concentrations. *Nat. Rev. Microbiol.* 7, 245–250. doi: 10.1038/nrmicro2095

Milani, C., Ticinesi, A., Gerritsen, J., Nouvenne, A., Lugli, G. A., Mancabelli, L., et al. (2016). Gut microbiota composition and *Clostridium difficile* infection in hospitalized elderly individuals: a metagenomic study. *Sci. Rep.* 6:25945. doi: 10.1038/srep25945

Miltsch, S. M., Seeberger, P. H., and Lepenies, B. (2014). The C-type lectin-like domain containing proteins Clec-39 and Clec-49 are crucial for *Caenorhabditis elegans* immunity against *Serratia marcescens* infection. *Dev. Comp. Immunol.* 45, 67–73. doi: 10.1016/j.dci.2014.02.002

Montalvo-Katz, S., Huang, H., Appel, M. D., Berg, M., and Shapira, M. (2013). Association with soil bacteria enhances p38-dependent infection resistance in *Caenorhabditis elegans*. *Infect. Immun.* 81, 514–520. doi: 10.1128/IAI.00653-12

Monzingo, A. F., Marcotte, E. M., Hart, P. J., and Robertas, J. D. (1996). Chitinases, chitosanases, and lysozymes can be divided into procaryotic and eucaryotic families sharing a conserved core. *Nat. Struct. Mol. Biol.* 3, 133–140. doi: 10.1038/nsb0296-133

Murrell, K. D., Eriksen, L., Nansen, P., Slotved, H. C., and Rasmussen, T. (1997). Ascaris suum: a revision of its early migratory path and implications for human ascariasis. *J. Parasitol.* 83, 255–260. doi: 10.2307/3284450

Mysliwy, J., Dingley, A. J., Stanisak, M., Jung, S., Lorenzen, I., Roeder, T., et al. (2010). Caenopore-5: the three-dimensional structure of an antimicrobial protein from *Caenorhabditis elegans*. *Dev. Comp. Immunol.* 34, 323–330. doi: 10.1016/j.dci.2009.11.003

Nalin, D. R., and McLaughlin, J. (1976). Colonization of ascaris lumbricoides by *V. cholerae*. *J. Parasitol.* 62, 839–841. doi: 10.2307/3278979

Nganga, C. J., Karanja, D. N., and Mutune, M. N. (2008). The prevalence of gastrointestinal helminth infections in pigs in Kenya. *Trop. Anim. Health Prod.* 40, 331–334. doi: 10.1007/s11250-007-9112-3

Nguyen, T. L. A., Vieira-Silva, S., Liston, A., and Raes, J. (2015). How informative is the mouse for human gut microbiota research? *Dis. Model. Mech.* 8, 1–16. doi: 10.1242/dmm.017400

Nicholas, H. R., and Hodgkin, J. (2004). Responses to infection and possible recognition strategies in the innate immune system of *Caenorhabditis elegans*. *Mol. Immunol.* 41, 479–493. doi: 10.1016/j.molimm.2004.03.037

O'Rourke, D., Baban, D., Demidova, M., Mott, R., and Hodgkin, J. (2006). Genomic clusters, putative pathogen recognition molecules, and antimicrobial genes are induced by infection of *C. elegans* with M. nematophilum. *Genome Res.* 16, 1005–1016. doi: 10.1101/gr.50823006

Odamaki, T., Kato, K., Sugahara, H., Hashikura, N., Takahashi, S., Xiao, J.-Z., et al. (2016). Age-related changes in gut microbiota composition from newborn to centenarian: a cross-sectional study. *BMC Microbiol.* 16:90. doi: 10.1186/s12866-016-0708-5

Paerewijck, O., Vlaminck, J., Li, R. W., Urban, J., Zaiss, M. M., Harris, N. L., et al. (2015). *The Influence of an Infection with Ascaris Suum on the Intestinal Microbiota of the Host.* IPVS Belgian Branch Studiedag, Abstracts. International Pig Veterinary Society (IPVS). Belgian Branch. Abstract retrieved from Ghent University Academic Bibliography. Available online at: http://hdl.handle.net/1854/LU-7277973

Page, A. P., Hamilton, A. J., and Maizels, R. M. (1992). Toxocara canis: monoclonal antibodies to carbohydrate epitopes of secreted (TES) antigens localize to different secretion-related structures in infective larvae. *Exp. Parasitol.* 75, 56–71. doi: 10.1016/0014-4894(92)90122-Q

Pillai, A., Ueno, S., Zhang, H., and Kato, Y. (2003). Induction of ASABF (Ascaris suum antibacterial factor)-type antimicrobial peptides by bacterial injection: novel members of ASABF in the nematode Ascaris suum. *Biochem. J.* 371, 663–668. doi: 10.1042/bj20021948

Pillai, A., Ueno, S., Zhang, H., Lee, J. M., and Kato, Y. (2005). Cecropin P1 and novel nematode cecropins: a bacteria-inducible antimicrobial peptide family in the nematode Ascaris suum. *Biochem. J.* 390, 207–214. doi: 10.1042/BJ20050218

Pradel, E., Zhang, Y., Pujol, N., Matsuyama, T., Bargmann, C. I., and Ewbank, J. J. (2007). Detection and avoidance of a natural product from the pathogenic bacterium *Serratia marcescens* by *Caenorhabditis elegans*. *Proc. Natl. Acad. Sci. U.S.A.* 104, 2295–2300. doi: 10.1073/pnas.0610281104

Pujol, N., Cypowyj, S., Ziegler, K., Millet, A., Astrain, A., Goncharov, A., et al. (2008a). Distinct innate immune responses to infection and wounding in the *C. elegans* epidermis. *Curr. Biol. CB* 18, 481–489. doi: 10.1016/j.cub.2008.02.079

Pujol, N., Link, E. M., Liu, L. X., Kurz, C. L., Alloing, G., Tan, M. W., et al. (2001). A reverse genetic analysis of components of the Toll signaling pathway in *Caenorhabditis elegans*. *Curr. Biol. CB* 11, 809–821. doi: 10.1016/S0960-9822(01)00241-X

Pujol, N., Zugasti, O., Wong, D., Couillault, C., Kurz, C. L., Schulenburg, H., et al. (2008b). Anti-fungal innate immunity in *C. elegans* is enhanced by evolutionary diversification of antimicrobial peptides. *PLoS Pathog.* 4:e1000105. doi: 10.1371/journal.ppat.1000105

Pukkila-Worley, R. (2016). Surveillance immunity: an emerging paradigm of innate defense activation in *Caenorhabditis elegans*. *PLoS Pathog.* 12:e1005795. doi: 10.1371/journal.ppat.1005795

Pukkila-Worley, R., Feinbaum, R., Kirienko, N. V., Larkins-Ford, J., Conery, A. L., and Ausubel, F. M. (2012). Stimulation of host immune defenses by a small molecule protects C. elegans from bacterial infection. *PLoS Genet.* 8:e1002733. doi: 10.1371/journal.pgen.1002733

Pukkila-Worley, R., Feinbaum, R. L., McEwan, D. L., Conery, A. L., and Ausubel, F. M. (2014). The evolutionarily conserved mediator subunit MDT-15/MED15 links protective innate immune responses and xenobiotic detoxification. *PLoS Pathog.* 10:e1004143. doi: 10.1371/journal.ppat.1004143

Ramanan, D., Bowcutt, R., Lee, S. C., Tang, M. S., Kurtz, Z. D., Ding, Y., et al. (2016). Helminth infection promotes colonization resistance via type 2 immunity. *Science* 352, 608–612. doi: 10.1126/science.aaf3229

Rausch, S., Held, J., Fischer, A., Heimesaat, M. M., Kühl, A. A., Bereswill, S., et al. (2013). Small intestinal nematode infection of mice is associated with increased enterobacterial loads alongside the intestinal tract. *PLoS ONE* 8:e74026. doi: 10.1371/journal.pone.0074026

Reddy, K. C., Andersen, E. C., Kruglyak, L., and Kim, D. H. (2009). A Polymorphism in npr-1 Is a behavioral determinant of pathogen susceptibility in *C. elegans*. *Science* 323, 382–384. doi: 10.1126/science.1166527

Reddy, K. C., Dunbar, T. L., Nargund, A. M., Haynes, C. M., and Troemel, E. R. (2016). The *C. elegans* CCAAT-enhancer-binding protein gamma is required for surveillance immunity. *Cell Rep.* 14, 1581–1589. doi: 10.1016/j.celrep.2016.01.055

Reynolds, L. A., Finlay, B. B., and Maizels, R. M. (2015). Cohabitation in the intestine: interactions among helminth parasites, bacterial microbiota, and host immunity. *J. Immunol.* 195, 4059–4066. doi: 10.4049/jimmunol.1501432

Reynolds, L. A., Smith, K. A., Filbey, K. J., Harcus, Y., Hewitson, J. P., Redpath, S. A., et al. (2014). Commensal-pathogen interactions in the intestinal tract: *Lactobacilli* promote infection with, and are promoted by, helminth parasites. *Gut Microbes* 5, 522–532. doi: 10.4161/gmic.32155

Riffel, A., Lucas, F., Heeb, P., and Brandelli, A. (2003). Characterization of a new keratinolytic bacterium that completely degrades native feather keratin. *Arch. Microbiol.* 179, 258–265. doi: 10.1007/s00203-003-0525-8

Robinson, M., Wahid, F., Behnke, J. M., and Gilbert, F. S. (1989). Immunological relationships during primary infection with *Heligmosomoides polygyrus, Nematospiroides dubius*): dose-dependent expulsion of adult worms. *Parasitology* 98, 115–124. doi: 10.1017/S0031182000059758

Roeder, T., Stanisak, M., Gelhaus, C., Bruchhaus, I., Grötzinger, J., and Leippe, M. (2010). Caenopores are antimicrobial peptides in the nematode *Caenorhabditis elegans* instrumental in nutrition and immunity. *Dev. Comp. Immunol.* 34, 203–209. doi: 10.1016/j.dci.2009.09.010

Roepstorff, A., Eriksen, L., Slotved, H. C., and Nansen, P. (1997). Experimental Ascaris suum infection in the pig: worm population kinetics following single inoculations with three doses of infective eggs. *Parasitology* 115, 443–452. doi: 10.1017/S0031182097001480

Rosso, M. N., Pujol, N., and Ewbank, J. J. (2013). "Innate immunity in *Caenorhabditis elegans* and other nematodes," in *Parasitic Nematodes: Molecular Biology, Biochemistry and Immunology*, eds M. W. Kennedy and W. Harnett (Wallingford: CABI), 42–66.

Salvetti, E., Torriani, S., and Felis, G. E. (2012). The genus lactobacillus. probiotics antimicrob. *Proteins* 4, 217–226. doi: 10.1007/s12602-012-9117-8

Samuel, B. S., Rowedder, H., Braendle, C., Félix, M.-A., and Ruvkun, G. (2016). *Caenorhabditis elegans* responses to bacteria from its natural habitats. *Proc. Natl. Acad. Sci. U.S.A.* 113, E3941–E3949. doi: 10.1073/pnas.1607183113

Schulenburg, H., and Boehnisch, C. (2008). Diversification and adaptive sequence evolution of Caenorhabditis lysozymes (Nematoda: Rhabditidae). *BMC Evol. Biol.* 8:114. doi: 10.1186/1471-2148-8-114

Schulenburg, H., Hoeppner, M. P., Weiner, J. III., and Bornberg-Bauer, E. (2008). Specificity of the innate immune system and diversity of C-type lectin domain (CTLD) proteins in the nematode *Caenorhabditis elegans*. *Immunobiology* 213, 237–250. doi: 10.1016/j.imbio.2007.12.004

Schulenburg, H., Kurz, C. L., and Ewbank, J. J. (2004). Evolution of the innate immune system: the worm perspective. *Immunol. Rev.* 198, 36–58. doi: 10.1111/j.0105-2896.2004.0125.x

Sender, R., Fuchs, S., and Milo, R. (2016). Revised estimates for the number of human and bacteria cells in the body. *PLoS Biol.* 14:e1002533. doi: 10.1371/journal.pbio.1002533

Shahkolahi, A. M., and Donahue, M. J. (1993). Bacterial flora, a possible source of serotonin in the intestine of adult female Ascaris suum. *J. Parasitol.* 79, 17–22. doi: 10.2307/3283271

Shivers, R. P., Pagano, D. J., Kooistra, T., Richardson, C. E., Reddy, K. C., Whitney, J. K., et al. (2010). Phosphorylation of the conserved transcription factor ATF-7 by PMK-1 p38 MAPK regulates innate immunity in *Caenorhabditis elegans*. *PLoS Genet.* 6:e1000892. doi: 10.1371/journal.pgen.1000892

Sim, S., and Hibberd, M. L. (2016). *Caenorhabditis elegans* susceptibility to gut *Enterococcus faecalis* infection is associated with fat metabolism and epithelial junction integrity. *BMC Microbiol.* 16:6. doi: 10.1186/s12866-016-0624-8

Sipos, D., Andersson, M., and Ehrenberg, A. (1992). The structure of the mammalian antibacterial peptide cecropin P1 in solution, determined by proton-NMR. *Eur. J. Biochem.* 209, 163–169. doi: 10.1111/j.1432-1033.1992.tb17273.x

Strandmark, J., Steinfelder, S., Berek, C., Kühl, A. A., Rausch, S., and Hartmann, S. (2016). Eosinophils are required to suppress Th2 responses in Peyer's patches during intestinal infection by nematodes. *Mucosal Immunol.* doi: 10.1038/mi.2016.93. [Epub ahead of print].

Szewczyk, N. J., Udranszky, I. A., Kozak, E., Sunga, J., Kim, S. K., Jacobson, L. A., et al. (2006). Delayed development and lifespan extension as features of metabolic lifestyle alteration in *C. elegans* under dietary restriction. *J. Exp. Biol.* 209, 4129–4139. doi: 10.1242/jeb.02492

Tan, L., and Darby, C. (2004). A movable surface: formation of yersinia sp. biofilms on motile *Caenorhabditis elegans*. *J. Bacteriol.* 186, 5087–5092. doi: 10.1128/JB.186.15.5087-5092.2004

Tarr, D. E. K. (2012). Distribution and characteristics of ABFs, cecropins, nemapores, and lysozymes in nematodes. *Dev. Comp. Immunol.* 36, 502–520. doi: 10.1016/j.dci.2011.09.007

Taylor, M. J., Bandi, C., and Hoerauf, A. (2005). *Wolbachia* bacterial endosymbionts of filarial nematodes. *Adv. Parasitol.* 60, 245–284. doi: 10.1016/S0065-308X(05)60004-8

Taylor, M. J., Bilo, K., Cross, H. F., Archer, J. P., and Underwood, A. P. (1999). 16S rDNA phylogeny and ultrastructural characterization of *Wolbachia* intracellular bacteria of the filarial nematodes *Brugia malayi*, B. pahangi, and Wuchereria bancrofti. *Exp. Parasitol.* 91, 356–361. doi: 10.1006/expr.1998.4383

Taylor, M. J., Hoerauf, A., Townson, S., Slatko, B. E., and Ward, S. A. (2014). Anti-*Wolbachia* drug discovery and development: safe macrofilaricides for onchocerciasis and lymphatic filariasis. *Parasitology* 141, 119–127. doi: 10.1017/S0031182013001108

Taylor, M. J., Voronin, D., Johnston, K. L., and Ford, L. (2013). *Wolbachia* filarial interactions. *Cell. Microbiol.* 15, 520–526. doi: 10.1111/cmi.12084

Tenor, J. L., and Aballay, A. (2008). A conserved Toll-like receptor is required for *Caenorhabditis elegans* innate immunity. *EMBO Rep.* 9, 103–109. doi: 10.1038/sj.embor.7401104

Tielens, A. G. M., van Grinsven, K. W. A., Henze, K., van Hellemond, J. J., and Martin, W. (2010). Acetate formation in the energy metabolism of parasitic helminths and protists. *Int. J. Parasitol.* 40, 387–397. doi: 10.1016/j.ijpara.2009.12.006

Troemel, E. R., Félix, M.-A., Whiteman, N. K., Barrière, A., and Ausubel, F. M. (2008). Microsporidia are natural intracellular parasites of the nematode *Caenorhabditis elegans*. *PLoS Biol.* 6:e309. doi: 10.1371/journal.pbio.0060309

Uno, M., Honjoh, S., Matsuda, M., Hoshikawa, H., Kishimoto, S., Yamamoto, T., et al. (2013). A fasting-responsive signaling pathway that extends life span in *C. elegans*. *Cell Rep.* 3, 79–91. doi: 10.1016/j.celrep.2012.12.018

Vaishnava, S., Yamamoto, M., Severson, K. M., Ruhn, K. A., Yu, X., Koren, O., et al. (2011). The antibacterial lectin RegIIIgamma promotes the spatial segregation of microbiota and host in the intestine. *Science* 334, 255–258. doi: 10.1126/science.1209791

Vallabhapurapu, S., and Karin, M. (2009). Regulation and function of NF-κB transcription factors in the immune system. *Annu. Rev. Immunol.* 27, 693–733. doi: 10.1146/annurev.immunol.021908.132641

Vejzagić, N., Adelfio, R., Keiser, J., Kringel, H., Thamsborg, S. M., and Kapel, C. M. O. (2015). Bacteria-induced egg hatching differs for Trichuris muris and Trichuris suis. Parasit. *Vectors* 8:371. doi: 10.1007/s00436-015-4476-1

Vercruysse, J., Albonico, M., Behnke, J. M., Kotze, A. C., Prichard, R. K., McCarthy, J. S., et al. (2011). Is anthelmintic resistance a concern for the control of human soil-transmitted helminths? Int. *J. Parasitol. Drugs Drug Resist.* 1, 14–27. doi: 10.1016/j.ijpddr.2011.09.002

Vernocchi, P., Del Chierico, F., and Putignani, L. (2016). Gut Microbiota profiling: metabolomics based approach to unravel compounds affecting human health. *Front. Microbiol.* 7:1144. doi: 10.3389/fmicb.2016.01144

Voronin, D., Cook, D. A. N., Steven, A., and Taylor, M. J. (2012). Autophagy regulates *Wolbachia* populations across diverse symbiotic associations. *Proc. Natl. Acad. Sci. U.S.A.* 109, E1638–E1646. doi: 10.1073/pnas.1203519109

Walk, S. T., Blum, A. M., Ewing, S. A.-S., Weinstock, J. V., and Young, V. B. (2010). Alteration of the murine gut microbiota during infection with the parasitic helminth *Heligmosomoides polygyrus* inflamm. *Bowel Dis.* 16, 1841–1849. doi: 10.1002/ibd.21299

Walter, J. (2008). Ecological role of *Lactobacilli* in the gastrointestinal tract: implications for fundamental and biomedical research. *Appl. Environ. Microbiol.* 74, 4985–4996. doi: 10.1128/AEM.00753-08

Wang, T., Van Steendam, K., Dhaenens, M., Vlaminck, J., Deforce, D., Jex, A. R., et al. (2013). Proteomic analysis of the excretory-secretory products from larval stages of Ascaris suum reveals high abundance of glycosyl hydrolases. *PLoS Negl. Trop. Dis.* 7:e2467. doi: 10.1371/journal.pntd.0002467

Wardlaw, A. C., Forsyth, L. M., Crompton, D. W. (1994). Bactericidal activity in the pig roundworm Ascaris suum. *J. Appl. Bacteriol.* 76, 36–41. doi: 10.1111/j.1365-2672.1994.tb04412.x

Watson, E., MacNeil, L. T., Ritter, A. D., Yilmaz, L. S., Rosebrock, A. P., Caudy, A. A., et al. (2014). Interspecies systems biology uncovers metabolites affecting *C. elegans* gene expression and life history traits. *Cell* 156, 759–770. doi: 10.1016/j.cell.2014.01.047

Weldon, L., Abolins, S., Lenzi, L., Bourne, C., Riley, E. M., and Viney, M. (2015). The gut microbiota of wild mice. *PLoS ONE* 10:e0134643. doi: 10.1371/journal.pone.0134643

Wescott, R. B. (1968). Experimental Nematospiroides dubius infection in germfree and conventional mice. *Exp. Parasitol.* 22, 245–249. doi: 10.1016/0014-4894(68)90099-4

World Health Organization (2017). *Fact Sheet: Soil-Transmitted Helminth Infections [WWW Document]*. WHO. Available online at: http://www.who.int/mediacentre/factsheets/fs366/en/ (accessed 3.27.17).

Wu, S., Li, R. W., Li, W., Beshah, E., Dawson, H. D., and Urban, J. F. (2012). Worm burden-dependent disruption of the porcine colon microbiota by Trichuris suis infection. *PLoS ONE* 7:e35470. doi: 10.1371/journal.pone.0035470

Yang, Z., Grinchuk, V., Smith, A., Qin, B., Bohl, J. A., Sun, R., et al. (2013). Parasitic nematode-induced modulation of body weight and associated metabolic dysfunction in mouse models of obesity. *Infect. Immun.* 81, 1905–1914. doi: 10.1128/IAI.00053-13

Yarza, P., Yilmaz, P., Pruesse, E., Glöckner, F. O., Ludwig, W., Schleifer, K.-H., et al. (2014). Uniting the classification of cultured and uncultured bacteria and archaea using 16S rRNA gene sequences. *Nat. Rev. Microbiol.* 12, 635–645. doi: 10.1038/nrmicro3330

Zaiss, M. M., and Harris, N. L. (2016). Interactions between the intestinal microbiome and helminth parasites. *Parasite Immunol.* 38, 5–11. doi: 10.1111/pim.12274

Zaiss, M. M., Rapin, A., Lebon, L., Dubey, L. K., Mosconi, I., Sarter, K., et al. (2015). The intestinal microbiota contributes to the ability of helminths to modulate allergic inflammation. *Immunity* 43, 998–1010. doi: 10.1016/j.immuni.2015.09.012

Zam, S. G., and Martin, W. E. (1969). Binding of 60Co-vitamin B12 by Ascaris suum intestine. *J. Parasitol.* 55, 480–485. doi: 10.2307/3277283

Zasloff, M. (2002). Antimicrobial peptides of multicellular organisms. *Nature* 415, 389–395. doi: 10.1038/415389a

Zelensky, A. N., and Gready, J. E. (2005). The C-type lectin-like domain superfamily. *FEBS J.* 272, 6179–6217. doi: 10.1111/j.1742-4658.2005.05031.x

Zhang, H., Yoshida, S., Aizawa, T., Murakami, R., Suzuki, M., Koganezawa, N., et al. (2000). *In vitro* antimicrobial properties of recombinant ASABF, an antimicrobial peptide isolated from the nematode Ascaris suum. *Antimicrob. Agents Chemother.* 44, 2701–2705. doi: 10.1128/AAC.44.10.2701-2705.2000

Zhang, Y., Li, W., Li, L., Li, Y., Fu, R., Zhu, Y., et al. (2015). Structural damage in the *C. elegans* epidermis causes release of STA-2 and induction of an innate immune response. *Immunity* 42, 309–320. doi: 10.1016/j.immuni.2015.01.014

Zoetendal, E. G., Rajilic-Stojanovic, M., and de Vos, W. M. (2008). High-throughput diversity and functionality analysis of the gastrointestinal tract microbiota. *Gut* 57, 1605–1615. doi: 10.1136/gut.2007.133603

Zugasti, O., Bose, N., Squiban, B., Belougne, J., Kurz, C. L., Schroeder, F. C., et al. (2014). Activation of a G protein-coupled receptor by its endogenous ligand triggers the innate immune response of *Caenorhabditis elegans*. *Nat. Immunol.* 15, 833–838. doi: 10.1038/ni.2957

15

The Intestinal Eukaryotic and Bacterial Biome of Spotted Hyenas: The Impact of Social Status and Age on Diversity and Composition

Emanuel Heitlinger[1,2*†], *Susana C. M. Ferreira*[3†], *Dagmar Thierer*[3], *Heribert Hofer*[3] *and Marion L. East*[3]

[1] Research Group Ecology and Evolution of Molecular Parasite Host Interactions, Leibniz Institute for Zoo and Wildlife Research, Berlin, Germany, [2] Institute for Biology, Molecular Parasitology, Humboldt University, Berlin, Germany, [3] Department of Evolutionary Ecology, Leibniz Institute for Zoo and Wildlife Research, Berlin, Germany

Edited by:
Susanne Hartmann,
Freie Universität Berlin, Germany

Reviewed by:
Anastasios D. Tsaousis,
University of Kent, United Kingdom
Jingwen Wang,
Yale University, United States

***Correspondence:**
Emanuel Heitlinger
heitlinger@izw-berlin.de;
emanuel.heitlinger@hu-berlin.de

† Shared first author.

In mammals, two factors likely to affect the diversity and composition of intestinal bacteria (bacterial microbiome) and eukaryotes (eukaryome) are social status and age. In species in which social status determines access to resources, socially dominant animals maintain better immune processes and health status than subordinates. As high species diversity is an index of ecosystem health, the intestinal biome of healthier, socially dominant animals should be more diverse than those of subordinates. Gradual colonization of the juvenile intestine after birth predicts lower intestinal biome diversity in juveniles than adults. We tested these predictions on the effect of: (1) age (juvenile/adult) and (2) social status (low/high) on bacterial microbiome and eukaryome diversity and composition in the spotted hyena (*Crocuta crocuta*), a highly social, female-dominated carnivore in which social status determines access to resources. We comprehensively screened feces from 35 individually known adult females and 7 juveniles in the Serengeti ecosystem for bacteria and eukaryotes, using a set of 48 different amplicons (4 for bacterial 16S, 44 for eukaryote 18S) in a multi-amplicon sequencing approach. We compared sequence abundances to classical coprological egg or oocyst counts. For all parasite taxa detected in more than six samples, the number of sequence reads significantly predicted the number of eggs or oocysts counted, underscoring the value of an amplicon sequencing approach for quantitative measurements of parasite load. In line with our predictions, our results revealed a significantly less diverse microbiome in juveniles than adults and a significantly higher diversity of eukaryotes in high-ranking than low-ranking animals. We propose that free-ranging wildlife can provide an intriguing model system to assess the adaptive value of intestinal biome diversity for both bacteria and eukaryotes.

Keywords: eukaryotome, eukaryome, parasites, amplicon sequencing, spotted hyena, social status, bacterial microbiome, age classes

INTRODUCTION

Mammalian hosts have a long evolutionary history with the diverse communities of prokaryotes (Dethlefsen et al., 2007; Ley et al., 2008; Douglas and Werren, 2016) and eukaryotes (Hafner and Nadler, 1988; Glendinning et al., 2014), here designated as the intestinal biome, present in their gastrointestinal tract. Although the intestinal biome was traditionally viewed as a rather inert species assembly, recent insights have revealed that its composition is influenced by many host traits and that it in turn can have a considerable impact on its host (Turnbaugh et al., 2007; Graham, 2008; Costello et al., 2012; Wegner Parfrey et al., 2014; Kreisinger et al., 2015). Recently, interest in the community of bacteria in the intestine (often called the microbiome, even though bacteria do not comprise all microscopic organisms in the intestines) has grown (Round and Mazmanian, 2009; Turnbaugh et al., 2009; Lozupone et al., 2012), whereas the communities of unicellular (Wegner Parfrey et al., 2014) and especially multicellular eukaryotes in the gastrointestinal tract (eukaryome or eukaryotome) have received less attention.

Following birth, the mammalian gastrointestinal tract is gradually colonized by prokaryotes and eukaryotes (Palmer et al., 2007; Koenig et al., 2011; Lozupone et al., 2012; Yatsunenko et al., 2012). Throughout an individual's lifespan, the composition of the intestinal biome can be altered by various factors, including diet (Turnbaugh et al., 2009; Amato et al., 2013), as exemplified by the transition from the consumption of milk during infancy (Pond, 1977) to an "adult" diet when weaned. Composition and diversity is also influenced by interactions between species within the intestinal biome (Ezenwa, 2004; Benson et al., 2010; Glendinning et al., 2014; Lee et al., 2014; Kreisinger et al., 2015), developmental changes in immune function (Dowling and Levy, 2014) and age related changes in exposure to prokaryotes and eukaryotes in the environment, food and conspecifics (Palmer et al., 2007; Koenig et al., 2011; Lozupone et al., 2012). Despite these factors that induce variation in the intestinal biome among individuals within a species, there is evidence of species-specific bacterial microbiome signatures in mammals (Ley et al., 2008; Ochman et al., 2010; Yildirim et al., 2010; Degnan et al., 2012; Menke et al., 2014).

While the majority of studies on the diversity and composition of bacterial microbiomes are based on partial sequencing of 16S ribosomal RNA genes, the application of metagenomics (the sequencing of the complete genetic repertoire of the host's intestinal microbiome) has revealed links between the bacterial microbiome of the intestine and the host's metabolism (Gill et al., 2006; The Human Microbiome Consortium, 2012). The bacterial microbiome influences host nutrition, fat storage and the metabolism of vitamins and minerals (Turnbaugh et al., 2009; Tremaroli and Bäckhed, 2012; Leone et al., 2015). Experimental studies with germ-free mice also show that the bacterial microbiome of the intestine can affect postnatal development of the hypothalamic-pituitary-adrenal axis (Sudo et al., 2004). Furthermore, bacterially derived fermentation products from the intestinal microbiome help regulate the maturation of microglia which contribute to an active immune defense of the central nervous system (Erny et al., 2015) and there is now general agreement that the bacterial microbiome influences the host immune system (Round and Mazmanian, 2009; Hooper et al., 2012; Sivan et al., 2015).

The impact of intestinal eukaryotes on their hosts has mostly been studied in relation to the pathologies caused by specific helminths and protozoans (Wegener Parfrey et al., 2011; Andersen et al., 2013; Rajilić-Stojanović and de Vos, 2014). We are not aware of any studies on intestinal biomes comprehensively screening for eukaryotes, including multicellular species. This is surprising, as it has been argued that eukaryotes may have an important ecological function in intestinal ecosystems similar to that of keystone species in terrestrial or aquatic ecosystems (Lukeš et al., 2015). By extension this should particularly apply to large multicellular eukaryotes. Currently, most research on the intestinal biomes of mammals has focused on the bacterial microbiome of humans, wild and captive non-human primates, laboratory mice and zoo animals; hence knowledge on the intestinal biomes of free-ranging wild mammals is limited.

In social mammals, social status often determines access to resources (Clutton-Brock and Huchard, 2013) thereby affecting health status (Sapolsky, 2005), wound healing (Archie et al., 2012), immune gene expression (Tung et al., 2012), immune defenses (Flies et al., 2016; Snyder-Mackler et al., 2016) and the likelihood and impact of pathogen infection (East et al., 2001, 2015; Höner et al., 2012). Social status is also likely to affect the species composition and abundance of bacteria and eukaryotes in the gastrointestinal tract.

We present, to our knowledge, the first study to simultaneously investigate both the bacterial microbiome and eukaryome of a wild mammalian species. We applied a multi-amplicon sequencing approach for bacteria and eukaryotes (metabarcoding) to fresh feces to investigate the effect of social status and age on the (distal) intestinal bacterial microbiome and eukaryome of individually known spotted hyenas (*Crocuta crocuta*) in the Serengeti National Park (NP) in northwestern Tanzania. This highly social carnivore lives in fission-fusion groups termed clans, in which natal females and their offspring are socially dominant over immigrant males (Kruuk, 1972). Migratory movements of ungulates cause large fluctuations in the abundance of food resources in clan territories (Hofer and East, 1993a,b), which profoundly affect the foraging behavior of clan members (Hofer and East, 1993a,b). When migratory ungulates are absent, clan members undertake regular long-distance (approximately 80–140 km) foraging trips (termed commuting trips) to areas containing abundant migratory prey (Hofer and East, 1993b). As access to food within a clan's territory is determined by social status, high-ranking females commute far less often than low-ranking females (Hofer and East, 2003) and their reduced foraging effort is reflected in their lower fecal glucocorticoid metabolite (fGCM) concentrations (Goymann et al., 2001b).

High-ranking females are more often exposed to infectious pathogens than low-ranking females because of their more frequent social interactions with clan members (East et al., 2001). Even so, high-ranking females have lower intestinal parasite burdens than low-ranking females, probably because they can allocate more resources to immune processes than low-ranking females (East et al., 2015). Hence, we expect the bacterial microbiome and the eukaryome of high-ranking animals to be more diverse than those of low-ranking animals, because high species diversity is generally considered an index of ecosystem health (Cardinale et al., 2006; Costello et al., 2012; Reich et al., 2012). In contrast, we expect the intestinal biome of low-ranking animals to be less diverse than those of high-ranking animals.

As in all mammals, the intestinal bacterial microbiome and the eukaryome of juvenile spotted hyenas develops after birth. In our study population, juveniles are more often infected with specific pathogens than adults (Goller et al., 2013; Nikolin et al., 2017), including the eukaryote *Dipylidium* sp. (East et al., 2013). Moreover, juveniles have lower protection from antibodies (East et al., 2001) and their diet includes maternal milk until 12–18 months of age (Hofer and East, 1995). For these reasons we expect the bacterial microbiome and eukaryome of juveniles to be less diverse than that of adults.

We tested our predictions concerning the effects of age and social status by assessing sequence read counts of taxonomically annotated ribosomal sequence variants (RSV) and hence the composition and abundance of genera in the bacterial microbiome and the eukaryome of individually known hosts. We also compared these results with those generated by the classical coprological method of parasite egg or oocyst counts as applied, for instance, by East et al. (2015) to assess whether the results of these methods were strongly correlated.

METHODS

Study Population

The spotted hyena (hereafter hyena) study population included three closely monitored clans that are part of an ongoing long-term research program in the center of Serengeti NP, northwest Tanzania. Individuals were recognized by their spot patterns, ear notches, scars and bald patches (Frank, 1986; Hofer and East, 1993a) and sexed using the dimorphic shape of the phallic gland (Frank et al., 1990). Age was determined from the observed date of birth or based on observations of pelage, position of the ears, level of coordination when walking and body size, with an accuracy of ±7 days as previously described (East et al., 2003). Animals were categorized as juveniles when <24 months of age, and adult when ≥24 months of age. Females were allocated a social rank within the dominance hierarchy using submissive responses in dyadic interactions (East et al., 2003). To compare rank positions across clans, individuals were assigned a standardized rank within a dominance hierarchy by distributing ranks evenly between the highest rank (standardized rank +1) and the lowest rank (standardized rank −1), with the median rank being scored as 0 (Goymann et al., 2001a). Females holding standardized ranks with 0 or above 0 were categorized as high-ranking, those holding a standardized rank of less than 0 as low ranking.

Sampling

Forty-two fecal samples (35 adult females and 7 juveniles) were collected immediately after defecation from individually known animals between 2009 and 2012. Samples were thoroughly mixed and aliquots were stored in formalin (4%) for parasite egg counts and preserved in RNAlater (Sigma–Aldrich, St Louis, MO, USA) for molecular genetic analyses. Samples in RNAlater were initially stored frozen at −10°C, transported frozen and then stored at −80°C for genetic analysis (East et al., 2013). DNA was extracted using the Macherey-Nagel Nucleo-spin soil DNA extraction kit (Macherey-Nagel, Düren, Germany) following the manufacturer's recommendations and using the Peqlab Precellys 24 homogenisator (VWR International Group, Erlangen, Germany). We assume that fecal biomes are representative of intestinal biomes, since a strong relationship between the two was demonstrated for freshly collected (Menke et al., 2015) and properly stored samples (Menke et al., 2017).

Parasite Egg Counts

Parasite egg or oocyst counts were conducted on aliquots of a subset of 32 fecal samples (27 adult females and 5 juveniles, 20 high-ranking and 12 low-ranking individuals) that were suitable for this procedure using a modification of the McMaster flotation technique (Gordon and Whitlock, 1939). To enhance the detectability of eggs, a solution of potassium iodide (KI) was used with a specific weight of 1.5 g ml^{-1} (Meyer-Lucht and Sommer, 2005; Schwensow et al., 2007). Four McMaster chambers were counted for each sample with a dilution factor of 1:15. After combining the feces with the KI solution, it was vortexed for 3 min and then sieved in order to remove bigger debris. Parasite eggs or oocysts were identified according to their morphology and counted using a light microscope, 1 h after preparing the fecal suspension, with a magnification of 100x (10x eyepiece lens × 10x objective lens). Pictures were captured using the software ProgRes CapturePro version 2.5, 2007 (Jenoptik, Jena, Germany). During fecal egg or oocyst counts, eukaryote parasites were identified at the genus or family level on the basis of their morphology and size, with the exception of oocysts from the order Coccidia because they are very similar in terms of their morphological appearance. For *Ancylostoma*, the Taeniidae and the Coccidia two morphological types based on two size classes of eggs or oocysts were distinguished. For the nematode *Ancylostoma*, the two identified size classes for eggs were <80 µm and ≥80 µm, for the cestodes from Taeniidae, the two size classes were < 45 µm and ≥45 µm, and for the Coccidia oocysts, the two size classes were <20 µm and ≥20 µm, respectively. The results are expressed as fecal egg counts per g feces (FEC) or fecal oocyst counts per g feces (FOC). All egg and oocyst counts were done blind with respect to the life history stages and characteristics (age, social status) of the individual hyenas from which the fecal sample was taken and analyzed.

Multi-Amplicon PCRs and Sequencing

The Fluidigm Access Array integrated fluidic circuit (Fluidigm, San Francisco, California, USA) was used to run 48 × 48 PCR reactions in 2,306 compartments of a microfluidics device. Target specific PCR primers (Supplementary File 1) for 18S and 16S small ribosomal subunits (SSU) were used in a "four primer" PCR approach, following the manual provided by Fluidigm. Briefly, target specific primer pairs were combined with "CS1" and "CS2" adapters at their 5′ and 3′ ends, respectively, on the microfluidics device. These target specific primer pairs were used to prime 48 target specific reactions for each of 48 samples, using default cycling parameters. After harvesting all products from the separate samples into a 96 well microliter plate, a second PCR was performed on a 10-fold dilution, by introducing Illumina sequencing oligonucleotides "PE5" at the "CS1" adapter and "PE7" at the "CS2" adapter as well as a sample identifier sequence between "CS2" and "PE7" based on the Access Array Barcode Library (Fluidigm, San Francisco, California, USA) for Illumina Sequencers (384 single direction). Samples were pooled and selected by size using Agencourt AMPure XP Reagent beads (Beckman Coulter Life Sciences, Krefeld, Germany). For further cleanup, PCR fragments between 400 and 1,000 bp were purified by PippinPrep using the 1.5% agarose DNA gel cassettes (Sage Science Inc., Beverly, Massachusetts, USA). Suitability of PCR products for sequencing (e.g., by checking for an absence of primer multi-meres) was confirmed using the Agilent 2200 Tape Station with D1000 ScreenTapes and D1000 Reagents (Agilent Technologies, Santa Clara, California, USA). Sequences were generated at the Berlin Center for Genomics in Biodiversity Research (BeGenDiv) on the Illumina MiSeq machine (Illumina, San Diego, California, USA) using version 3 chemistry and 600 cycles of (paired-end) sequencing. The sequencing data can be accessed through the accession number PRJNA386767 at NCBI Short Read Archive (SRA).

Bioinformatic Analyses

Sorting of sequencing reads in different samples was performed using the bcl2fastq utility version 2.17.1.14 (Illumina, San Diego, California, USA) based on the sample identifier oligos. All subsequent bioinformatic, taxonomic and statistical analyses were performed in R version 3.3.2 (R Development Core Team, 2016); below we cite the R packages used for specific steps in the analysis.

Sequences were quality trimmed and screened for erroneous reads using the fastqPairedFilter function of package dada2 version 1.2.1 (Callahan et al., 2016) with parameter settings of truncLen=c(170,170), maxN=0, maxEE=2, truncQ=2. Further stratification of the full "samples by amplicon" matrix was performed using package MultiAmplicon version 0.1 (Heitlinger, 2017): primer sequences were trimmed in read pairs matching with zero mismatches starting at position one in both forward and reverse reads. Sequencing reads were sorted into an amplicon when they contained the sequences of a specific pair of primers. The MultiAmplicon package was also used as a wrapper to process identified amplicons with the dada2 workflow. Briefly, sequences were dereplicated, RSVs were inferred using the function dadaMulti (with options err=NULL, selfConsist=TRUE), forward and reverse reads were concatenated (using function mergeMulti, option justConcatenate=TRUE), a table of RSV occurrence was collated for each sample and sequences likely to be chimeric and introduced during PCR were screened and discarded.

Technical replicates for which PCRs failed were identified by hierarchical clustering of primer-stratified read numbers, with water as negative controls, and marked for exclusion. For each sample, RSV counts were obtained as the sum of the remaining technical replicates and normalized for sequencing depth using a simple scaling by the median of the per sample RSV counts. All taxonomic assignments were done blind with respect to the life history stages and characteristics (age, social status) of the individual hyenas from which the fecal sample was taken and analyzed.

Taxonomic and Statistical Analyses

Taxonomy was inferred for RSVs using a ribosomal database project naïve Bayesian classifier (Wang et al., 2007) through dada2's "assignTaxonomy" function. As a training data set for the classifier, the SILVA_123 database (Quast et al., 2013) was expanded with highest scoring unique BLAST hits (blastn; Altschul et al., 1997) of our RSVs in the NCBI nt database. This training dataset was thus curated with a focus on eukaryotic 18S sequences in our study system and then used in an assignment of the taxonomy levels "phylum," "class," "order," "family," and "genus" to each of our RSVs. Problems arose for annotation of putative *Eimeria* reads (among others) because of an incongruence between the taxonomic systems of SILVA and NCBI, so two separate sets of results will be described for this genus.

RSV counts, annotation with taxonomy information and hyena specific sample data were combined into a single R object for all amplicons using the package phyloseq version 1.18.0 (McMurdie and Holmes, 2013). Data were merged across different amplicons via their taxonomic annotation at the genus level using the function "tax_glom" with the parameter "NArm=TRUE." This excludes genera not annotated at the genus level (or annotated with uninformative terms such as "undefined"). We also excluded genera annotated as the only genus in their respective phylum and genera with an "undefined" phylum annotation. We report estimates of RSV diversity derived from different amplicons with caution, as we recognize that many raw RSVs prior to taxonomic annotation represent different parts of the same marker genes and hence our diversity estimates are inflated for this measure. Even so, they can be used to compare the diversity between individuals, because all samples were processed using the same amplification and bioinformatics workflow.

We used the strength of association between "sequence abundance" (number of ribosomal sequence reads annotated for specific genera or higher level taxa) and FEC or FOC to screen for the most likely sequenced taxon in samples for which we had morphological evidence from the egg or oocyst counts. Because the larger size class of *Ancylostoma* occurred in only two samples, FEC for both size classes were added together for the correlation of egg counts with sequence abundance data. Spearman rank correlation coefficients were calculated in R base and recorded not only for "target taxa" within the taxonomic scope of morphological discrimination but in a "blinded" approach for the comprehensive set of all sequence counts at all levels of taxonomy. The strongest correlations were then screened for taxonomic agreement with FEC and FOC. The four highest positive correlations always contained the target taxa as defined by the observed morphology. In the results (below) we report

p-values to test for significant association between the number of ribosomal sequence reads and FEC or FOC for the highest or second highest Spearman correlation coefficients. We also constructed linear models using (1+$\log_{10}$) transformed data to visualize the linearity of the association and report the regression equations as a predictive tool.

Richness—the number of taxa (RSVs or genera) present —, evenness—the evenness in the distribution of sequencing read numbers for different taxa—and diversity—an index that takes into account both richness and evenness—(see Legendre and Legendre, 2012) were calculated after the random selection of a data subset (rarefaction) from all sample counts at the sequencing depth of the library sequenced to the lowest depth. We used rarefaction instead of normalization for diversity estimates to avoid problems of overestimating presence in more deeply sequenced samples. We used the package phyloseq with its function estimate_diversity to estimate measures of diversity and species richness with the help of package vegan version 2.4-1. We calculated the number of genera as "observed richness," the Chao1 index of diversity (Chao, 1984) as a measure of species diversity and Pielou's J as a measure of evenness (Pielou, 1975). Number of genera, Chao1 index and Pielou's J were compared between juveniles and adults or high-ranking and low-ranking hyenas using the exact version of the Mann-Whitney U test in the package coin version 1.1-2 (Hothorn et al., 2006) to obtain appropriate p-values for small sample sizes and in the presence of ties.

In order to compare the composition of the bacterial microbiome and the eukaryome between individuals, life history stages and social status categories, the diversity of the bacterial microbiomes and eukaryomes and its underlying variation across individuals was efficiently summarized by multidimensional scaling (MDS), a non-parametric ordination technique. This technique has previously been highly successful in summarizing similarly complex data sets (e.g., Burgener et al., 2009), along new dimensions called here MDS axes. MDS uses pairwise Bray-Curtis dissimilarities (Bray and Curtis, 1957) on (1+$\log_{10}$) transformed data of sequence abundances per genus. On the same transformed data partial least squares (PLS) models (Hastie et al., 2013), as calculated by package caret version 6.0-73, were used as a supervised machine learning technique (Wold et al., 1984) to predict age and rank category for the individual from which the sample was collected. PLS models also produce a set of axes or "directions" (Hastie et al., 2013) called here PLS axes. The optimal number of PLS axes retained in the final model was determined using leave-one-out cross-validation. Each sample received a PLS score on each PLS axis, which documents how well sample categories can be differentiated on that axis, and each taxonomic unit as a "predictor" received a PLS "loading" on each axis which documents to what extent the taxonomic unit contributed to the PLS axis. We subsequently used Fisher's exact test from R base to test for overrepresentation or underrepresentation of phyla visually identified to be abundant at the extremes of the distribution of loadings. We tested highest and lowest quartile of loadings on the single PLS axis of the model addressing rank category differences in the eukaryome. As the PLS model for differences of the microbiome in age categories contained more than one axis, the PLS loadings of the first two axes separating the samples were combined by multiplication before this procedure.

Package DESeq2 version 1.14.0 (Love et al., 2014) (function "DESeq") was used to test for differences in the abundance of individual genera between age and rank categories. In contrast to normalization or rarefaction used in other analyses the function estimated "size factors" to address differences in sequencing depth between different samples. These factors were then used as offset when a mean abundance was fitted for each taxon in generalized linear models (glm) using a negative binomial distribution and a dispersion parameter specific to that taxon. Maximum likelihood estimates for glm coefficients were obtained and likelihood ratio tests were conducted by subtracting the log-likelihood of the full model including different estimates for a focal contrast (age or rank category) from a reduced model without this difference. The resulting likelihood-ratio was compared then to a χ^2-distribution. Resulting p-values were corrected for multiple testing using the Benjamini and Hochberg method (Benjamini and Hochberg, 1995) and expressed as false discovery rates, with the significance threshold set to 0.05.

RESULTS

High throughput sequencing of multiple amplicons provided a comprehensive survey of the intestinal biome of hyenas, comprising 986 genera, most of which belonged to the eukaryotic biome, as described in detail below.

Sequencing Based Assessment

We obtained a total of 3,195,831 sequencing read-pairs from amplicon sequencing for 18S small ribosomal subunits of eukaryotes and 16S ribosomal subunits of bacteria. Variant inference on a single base resolution level for these sequences revealed a total of 24,604 RSVs, which were summarized via shared taxonomic assignments at the genus level.

Taxonomic Diversity of Hyena Intestinal Biomes

We identified 201 genera (3,725 RSVs) of bacteria as constituents of the bacterial microbiome of the hyena. We also identified 656 genera (20,879 RSVs) of eukaryotes in the same fecal samples. The number of genera annotated varied greatly between phyla of both bacteria and eukaryotes (**Figure 1A**, **Table 1**). High genus level diversity was observed in the bacterial phylum Firmicutes and in the eukaryote phyla Ascomycota, Chlorophyta and Basidiomycota. The classic phyla of intestinal parasites—Nematoda, Apicomplexa and Platyhelminthes—showed an intermediate number of genera but a high number of sequencing reads. Phylum Chordata was represented with few genera and a large number of sequencing reads (**Figure 1A**, **Table 1**).

The eukaryote sequences derived from 18S amplification did not solely originate from organisms in the eukaryome but also included organisms that were part of the hyena's diet or those that were accidentally ingested. Taxonomic annotation of eukaryote derived DNA can help to assess these potential sources. For some taxa a role as intestinal inhabitants or food items can safely be assigned. We therefore categorized eukaryote phyla in

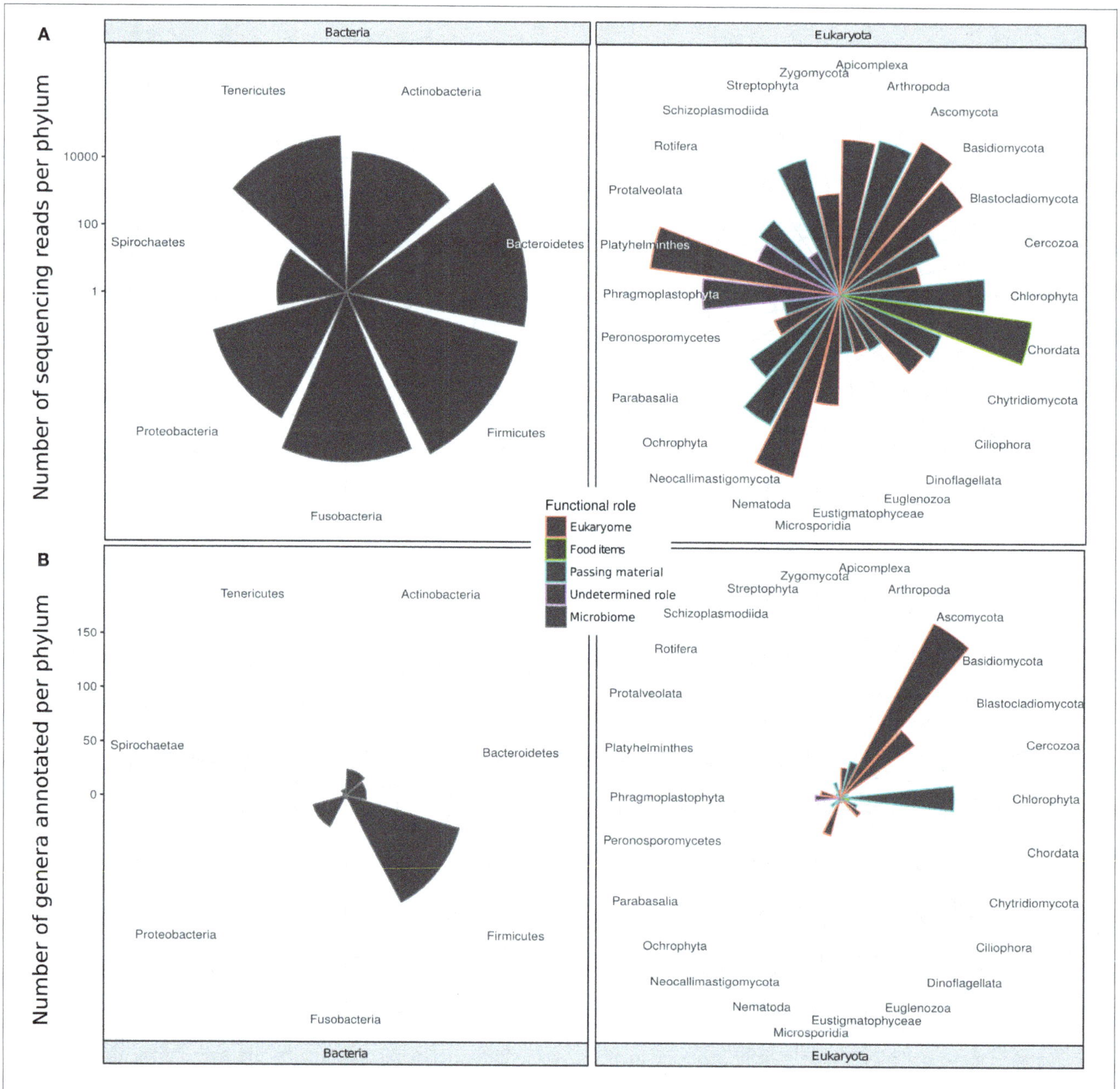

FIGURE 1 | Taxonomic diversity of the intestinal bacterial microbiome and eukaryome of the spotted hyena in terms of **(A)** number of genera and **(B)** number of sequence reads inferred for different phyla of bacteria and eukaryotes from taxonomically annotated multi-amplicon sequencing reads. Bars are colored according to the likely predominant interaction with their host conventionally assumed for these taxa (see main text).

our taxonomic annotation in categories of likely (1) eukaryome (including parasites, commensals and mutualists), (2) food items, (3) passing material, and (4) undetermined role (**Table 1**). We consider for example Nematoda, Platyhelminthes, Apicomplexa and Microsporidia as classical eukaryotic parasites and hence members of the eukaryome. Other organisms not conventionally considered to be parasites but rather commensals or with an unknown effect on their host comprised most phyla of fungi. DNA sequences from the phylum Chordata were most likely originating from hyena food items (**Table 1**).

Sequence Based Abundance Counts Correlate with Fecal Egg or Oocyst Counts but Are More Sensitive

Eukaryote parasites were identified at a genus level for the genus *Ancylostoma* (detected in 25 of 32 samples), more conservatively at the family level for cestodes in families Diphyllobothriidae (detected in 26 of 32 samples) and Taeniidae (detected in 6 of 32 samples) and protists only at the level of order for Coccidia (detected in 17 of 32 samples). We also detected in one or two

TABLE 1 | The diversity of genera and phyla of bacteria and eukaryotes recorded from the intestinal biome of the spotted hyena as extracted by amplicon sequencing of fecal samples.

Taxon	Functional role	Ribosomal sequencing variants (RSV)	Identified genera	Number of sequencing reads
Bacteria	**Microbiome**	**3,559/*3,725**	**201/*202**	**768,581/*807,654**
Actinobacteria	Microbiome	184	24	14,690
Bacteroidetes	Microbiome	787	20	328,848
Firmicutes	Microbiome	2,073	112	259,513
Fusobacteria	Microbiome	183	3	105,138
Proteobacteria	Microbiome	248	33	16,881
Spirochaetes	Microbiome	13	3	140
Tenericutes	Microbiome	71	6	43,371
Undetermined**	Microbiome	166	1**	38,928
Eukaryotes	**Multiple**	**18,202/*20,879**	**656/*784**	**2,129,418/*2,388,177**
Apicomplexa	Eukaryome (parasites)	1,074	28	39,899
Arthropoda	Food items	600	35	53,075
Ascomycota	Eukaryome	4,841	184	146,864
Basidiomycota	Eukaryome	1,675	85	36,241
Blastocladiomycota	Passing material	126	7	1,676
Cercozoa	Eukaryome	47	4	288
Chlorophyta	Passing material	1,131	107	25,680
Chordata	Food items	1,743	8	782,156
Chytridiomycota	Passing material	144	17	1,944
Ciliophora	Eukaryome	254	32	1,264
Dinoflagellata	Passing material	30	4	74
Euglenozoa	Eukaryome	13	4	61
Eustigmatophyceae	Passing material	6	3	53
Microsporidia	Eukaryome (parasites)	39	4	1,869
Nematoda	Eukaryome (parasites)	1,431	36	380,347
Neocallimastigomycota	Passing material	337	6	25,520
Ochrophyta	Passing material	184	11	2,008
Parabasalia	Eukaryome	29	3	131
Peronosporomycetes	Passing material	11	3	52
Phragmoplastophyta	Undetermined role	420	24	13,602
Platyhelminthes	Eukaryome (parasites)	1,195	19	600,119
Protalveolata	Undetermined role	85	3	478
Rotifera	Passing material	100	5	930
Schizoplasmodiida	Undetermined role	11	2	28
Streptophyta	Passing material	107	15	14,066
Zygomycota	Eukaryome	98	7	993
Undetermined**	Undetermined role	2,471	128**	216,753

The first number is for the annotated dataset analyzed for genera; the second number is the full dataset analyzed for RSVs.

***Number of genera not considered correctly annotated based on phylum level abundance (see methods) or annotated as "undefined" at the phylum level.*

samples species from Spirurida, *Trichuris* spp. and *Dipylidium* spp. (**Table 2**).

The amplicon sequencing based abundance estimates correlated significantly and positively with egg or oocyst counts, as detailed below, for those species for which we had more than six positive FEC or FOC samples. These correlations also helped to assign plausible taxonomic status to taxa with morphologically indistinguishable eggs or oocysts. *Ancylostoma* FEC correlated best with the sequence counts for the genus *Ancylostoma* among all reported genera (Spearman's rho, $\rho = 0.54$, $n = 32$, $p = 0.002$). There was a slightly better positive correlation with counts summarized for the order Rhabditida, to which *Ancylostoma* belongs ($\rho = 0.58$, $n = 32$, $p < 0.001$): seven samples with relatively high sequencing counts (range 84–4,035) and zero FECs were recovered and all samples reporting FEC in Rhabditida had at least 407 sequences counted for *Ancylostoma*. Within this order, annotations for 23 other genera were reported. The genus *Ancylostoma* contributed most (59%) sequencing reads annotated within the order. The genera *Ostertagia* (20%) and *Haemonchus* (12%) also contributed substantial numbers of sequencing reads annotated as Rhabditida. Adding together reads annotated as *Ancylostoma* and *Haemonchus* resulted in

TABLE 2 | The intensity of infection in terms of parasite egg or oocyst counts per g feces from fecal samples ($n = 32$) of spotted hyenas.

Taxon	Taxon level	Phylum	Prevalence	Intensity of infection					
			%	Mean	Confidence intervals		Median	Confidence intervals	
					Low	High		Low	High
Diphyllobothriidae	family	Platyhelminthes	81.2	21,461	1,137	41,784	3,650	850	6,850
Ancylostoma total	genus	Nematoda	78.1	802	320	1,284	275	100	773
Ancylostoma < 80 μm	spp.	Nematoda	78.1	786	308	1,264	275	100	773
Ancylostoma ≥ 80 μm	spp.	Nematoda	6.2	200	0 [−94]	494	200	NA	NA
Coccidia total	order	Apicomplexa	53.2	2,171	0 [−664]	5,007	50	25	75
Coccidia < 20 μm	spp.	Apicomplexa	12.5	8,800	0 [−1504]	19,104	6,588	NA	NA
Coccidia ≥ 20 μm	spp.	Apicomplexa	53.1	101	29	173	50	25	50
Taeniidae total	family	Platyhelminthes	18.8	89	15	164	62	25	75
Taeniidae < 45 μm	spp.	Platyhelminthes	3.1	85	10	161	50	25	75
Taeniidae ≥ 45 μm	spp.	Platyhelminthes	18.8	25	NA	NA	25	NA	NA
Spirurida	order	Nematoda	6.2	412	0 [−249]	1,074	412	NA	NA
Trichuris	genus	Nematoda	3.1	50	NA	NA	50	NA	NA
Dipylidium	genus	Platyhelminthes	3.1	50	NA	NA	50	NA	NA

Indicated are identified taxa, their prevalence in %, the mean and median with respective 95% confidence intervals. Table was sorted by prevalence. "spp.": an unknown number of species which may or may not belong to more than one genus.

a correlation slightly stronger ($\rho = 0.59$, $n = 32$, $p < 0.001$) than that observed for the whole order Rhabditida. When reads classified as *Ostertagia* were added to the reads annotated as *Ancylostoma*, the correlation with *Ancylostoma* spp. in the FEC became slightly weaker ($\rho = 0.54$, $n = 32$, $p = 0.002$) (**Figure 2A**).

Similarly, FEC for taxa identified as originating from one or several species in the family Diphyllobothriidae correlated best with annotated RSV counts for the family Diphyllobothriidae ($\rho = 0.69$, $n = 32$, $p < 0.001$). The genus *Diphyllobothrium* provided the vast majority (98%) of counts annotated in the family Diphyllobothriidae and reads for the genus *Spirometra* provided the remaining (2%) of counts in this family. The correlation of FEC with annotated RSV counts for *Spirometra* alone was slightly weaker ($\rho = 0.67$, $n = 32$, $p < 0.001$) than for the entire family. The FEC results for four samples contained no *Diphyllobothrium* eggs but produced positive *Diphyllobothrium* sequence results, with annotated RSV counts ranging from 9 to 39,699; all samples with FEC above zero produced annotated RSV counts in the range of 79–44,993 for Diphyllobothriidae. **Figure 2B** visualizes this relationship.

When annotated RSV counts for the genera *Besnoitia*, *Toxoplasma*, *Isospora*, and *Eimeria* were added together, their total number correlated best ($\rho = 0.79$, $n = 32$, $p < 0.001$) with FOC for the small size class (<20 μm) of Coccidia oocysts. This comparison produced a linear model on log transformed data with an excellent fit ($r^2 = 0.92$; **Figure 2C**). FOC were zero for three samples with sequencing counts ranging from four to five for these genera. The number of RSV counts annotated as *Eimeria* correlated best ($\rho = 0.60$, $n = 32$, $p < 0.001$) with the large size class (≥20 μm) of Coccidia oocyst counts (**Figure 2D**). This relationship did not follow the pattern reported for other correlations, since substantial numbers of FOC were reported for samples with zero abundance in terms of annotated RSV reads.

Adult Female Hyenas Have a Bacterial Microbiome Which Is More Diverse Than and Differs in Composition from That of Juveniles

Consistent with our prediction, the bacterial microbiome of juvenile hyenas contained a significantly lower number of genera (lower richness; Mann-Whitney U-test, $U = 184.5$, $n = 42$, $p = 0.012$), had a lower diversity ($U = 174.5$, $n = 42$, $p = 0.034$) and showed a trend toward lower evenness ($U = 168$, $n = 42$, $p = 0.063$) than that of adults (**Figure 3A**). The bacterial microbiome of adult hyenas contained a median of 49 bacterial genera whereas those of juveniles hosted a median of 41 genera.

A more detailed analysis for each bacterial phylum revealed that the higher richness and diversity of genera in adults than juveniles predominantly occurred in the phyla Tenericutes ($U = 203$, $n = 42$, $p < 0.001$) and Bacteroidetes ($U = 173$, $n = 42$, $p = 0.037$). Microbiomes of adults had a significantly lower diversity for Actinobacteria than those of juveniles ($U = 53$, $n = 42$, $p = 0.021$). The differences in composition between the bacterial microbiomes of juveniles and adults were confirmed using multidimensional scaling ordination, which showed that juvenile microbiomes are less uniform in composition between individuals than those of adults (**Figure 3B**).

The distinct composition of adult and juvenile bacterial microbiomes was underlined by the results of a PLS regression which correctly assigned samples to age categories with an accuracy of 93% in leave-one-out cross evaluations. The optimal model retained three PLS axes, the first two of which are plotted with PLS scores of samples and loadings of bacteria phyla in **Figure 3C**, illustrating how well age categories were separated by their PLS scores. A more detailed analysis demonstrated that genera in the phyla Tenericutes tended to be (odds ratio = 4.83, Fisher test, $p = 0.069$)

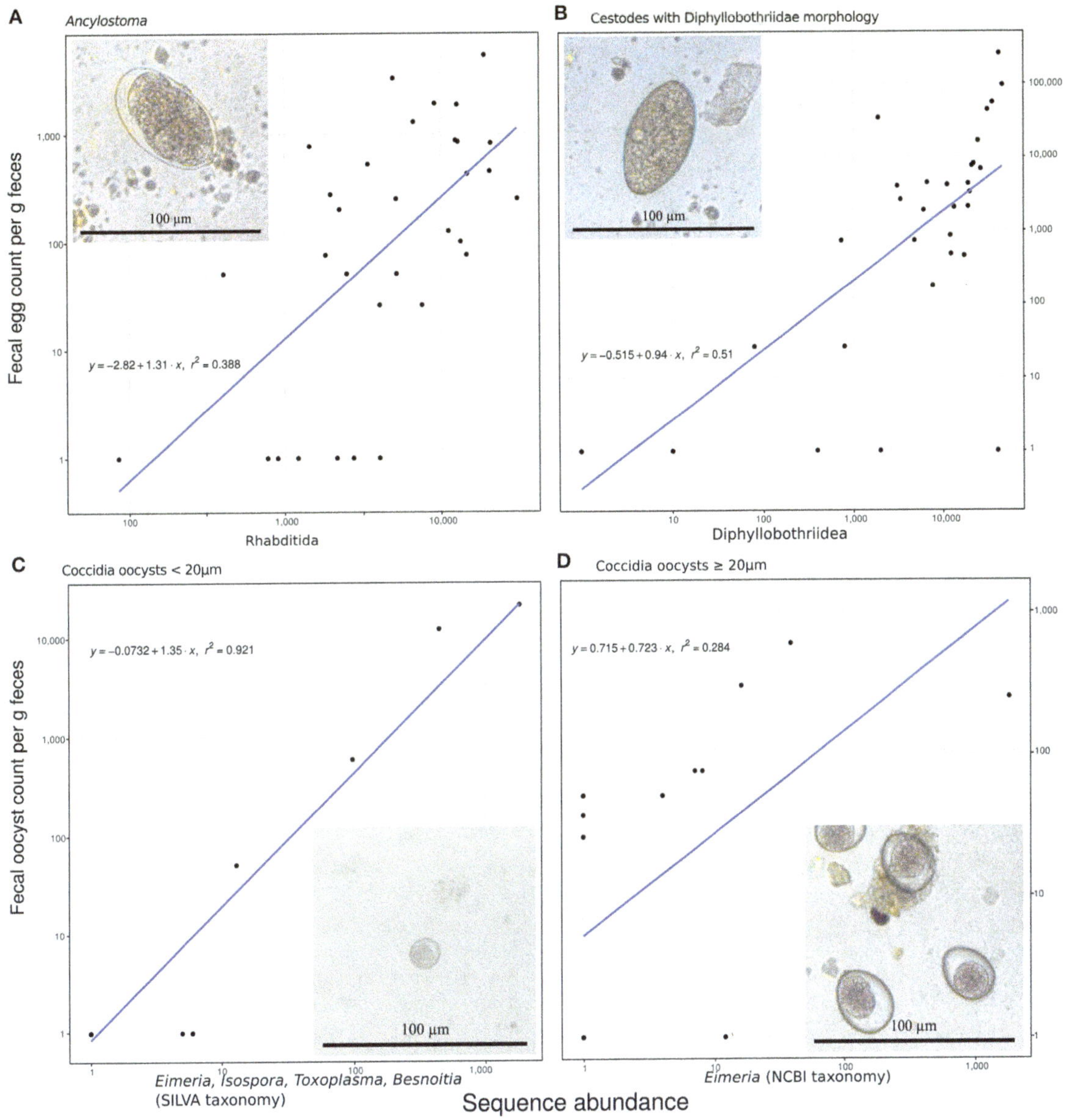

FIGURE 2 | Predicting fecal egg or oocyst counts per g feces from the number of annotated ribosomal sequence variants reads. **(A)** *Ancylostoma* FEC vs. sequence counts for the order Rhabditida. **(B)** Diphyllobothriidae FEC vs. sequence counts for the same family. **(C)** A small size class of oocyst counts vs. added sequence counts for *Eimeria*, *Isospora*, *Besnoitia*, and *Toxoplasma*. **(D)** A large size class of coccidian oocysts vs. *Eimeria* sequences. All panels contain the formula for the specific linear model on (1+$\log_{10}$) transformed data, R^2 as a measure of goodness of fit, and a line representing the predicted relationship. The panels additionally include a representative micrograph depicting the egg or oocyst counted.

and Bacteroidetes were (odds ratio = 5.42, Fisher test, $p < 0.001$) characteristic for adult microbiomes, Actinobacteria for juvenile microbiomes (odds ratio = 2.93, Fisher test, $p = 0.009$). Testing individual genera of bacteria for differences in abundance between age categories resulted in six genera with significant false discovery rates of <0.05, with three more abundant in juveniles and three more abundant in adults (**Figure 3D**).

In contrast to the bacterial microbiome, we detected no significant differences in eukaryome richness ($U = 106$, $n = 42$, $p = 0.75$), diversity ($U = 96$, $n = 42$, $p = 0.50$), evenness ($U = 128$, $n = 42$, $p = 0.68$) or genus abundance between hyena age categories (false discovery rate for all single genera glms >0.05).

A More Diverse Eukaryome in High-Ranking Than Low-Ranking Hyenas

Estimates of observed richness ($U = 293$, $n = 42$, $p = 0.004$) and diversity ($U = 288$, $n = 42$, $p = 0.007$) in terms of RSVs in the eukaryome were significantly higher in high-ranking than low-ranking hyenas (**Figure 4A**). The same was true for inferred genera (richness, $U = 299$, $n = 42$, $p = 0.002$; diversity,

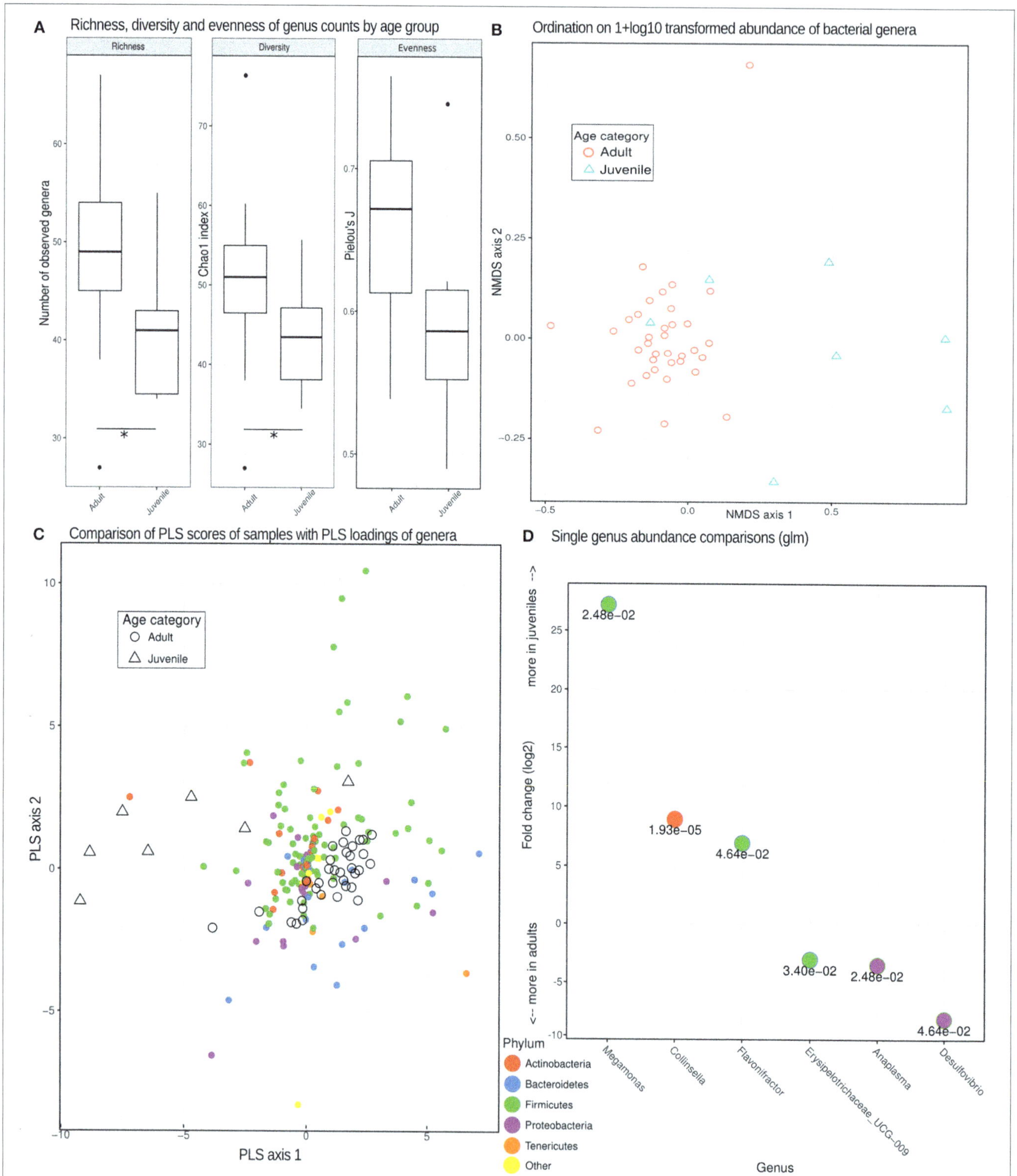

FIGURE 3 | Bacterial genera richness, diversity and microbiome composition in different age categories. **(A)** Box plots depicting distributions of richness (observed counts of genera richness per phylum), diversity (Chao1 index) and evenness (Pielou's *J*) estimates on rarefied (see methods) genera counts for juveniles and adults. *Significant differences ($p < 0.05$) based on exact Mann-Whitney U tests. **(B)** Non-metric multidimensional scaling (MDS) ordination based on pairwise Bray-Curtis dissimilarities partially separated juvenile from adult samples based on different compositions of taxonomic units. **(C)** A comparison of PLS scores (for samples) and PLS loadings (for genera) from the first two PLS axes of an optimized partial least squares model, demonstrating a clear separation of adult and juvenile samples. Genera colored by phylum can be used to assess the taxa contributing (PLS loading) to the differences underlying this distinction. **(D)** Log2-fold change inferred by generalized linear models testing for differences between adults and juveniles for each genus with a false discovery rate (adjusted p-value) of < 0.05. The numerical value of the false discovery rate is given below the dot for each genus color-coded for its respective phylum.

$U = 299.5$, $n = 42$, $p = 0.002$; **Figure 4B**). Social status had no significant effect on eukaryome evenness. A significantly higher number of genera (richness) occurred in high-ranking than low-ranking individuals for the phyla Basidiomycota ($U = 275$, $n = 42$, $p = 0.021$), Ascomycota ($U = 272.5$, $n = 42$, $p = 0.025$) and Blastocladiomycota ($U = 250$, $n = 42$, $p = 0.049$). There was a trend toward higher diversity in high-ranking than low-ranking hyenas for Apicomplexa ($U = 254.5$, $n = 42$, $p = 0.079$).

It was not possible to determine compositional differences between eukaryomes of high-ranking and low-ranking animals in our dataset using unsupervised ordination techniques. PLS regression models, however, were able to assign animals to social status categories with 71% accuracy in leave-one-out cross evaluations. Most high-ranking individuals were clearly separated from low-ranking individuals by the single PLS axis retained in the model, the overlap with low-ranking individuals being confined to a minority of high-ranking individuals (**Figure 4C**). The loading of several genera belonging to the phylum Basidiomycota tended to increase the PLS scores for high-ranking individuals (odds ratio = 1.55, Fisher test, $p = 0.074$). There was also a trend that genera in the Apicomplexa through their loadings increased the PLS scores for low-ranking individuals (odds ratio = 2.01, Fisher test, $p = 0.057$). Both trends contributed to the separation of high-ranking and low-ranking individuals. Interestingly, different genera in the Apicomplexa were drivers in terms of their PLS loadings on the single PLS axis for the classification of samples as belonging to both high-ranking and low-ranking individuals (odds ratio = 3.17, $p = 0.011$; testing the combined upper and lower quartiles of loadings).

In contrast to the eukaryome, we detected no significant differences in bacterial microbiome richness ($U = 184.5$ $n = 42$, $p = 0.84$), diversity ($U = 182.5$, $n = 42$, $p = 0.80$), evenness ($U = 184$, $n = 42$, $p = 0.84$) or genus abundance between high-ranking and low-ranking animals (false discovery rate for all individual genera glms >0.05).

DISCUSSION

Amplicon sequencing (metabarcoding) revealed that spotted hyenas in the Serengeti NP had a diverse intestinal biome, with at least 201 identified genera of bacteria and 656 identified genera of eukaryotes (**Table 1**, **Figure 1A**). The bacterial phylum with the highest diversity of identified genera was the Firmicutes, as were the Ascomycota, Chlorophyta and Basidiomycota among the eukaryotes (**Figure 1B**). Positive, significant correlations between amplicon sequence abundance estimates and FEC or FOC (**Figure 2**) suggest that results from amplicon sequencing are quantitatively valid and highly sensitive measures, and also can aid the differentiation of taxa with similar egg and oocyst morphologies. Consistent with our predictions, adult females had a significantly more diverse intestinal bacterial microbiome than juveniles (**Figure 3**) and the diversity of eukaryotes was significantly greater in high-ranking than low-ranking animals (**Figure 4**). However, contrary to our prediction, there was no effect of social status on the diversity of the bacterial microbiome and also no difference between the diversity of eukaryotes in adult and juvenile intestinal biomes.

Studies of the intestinal bacterial microbiome in humans report an increase in the number of taxa and taxonomic diversity of bacteria with age (Palmer et al., 2007; Tannock, 2007; Koenig et al., 2011). Our results were similar in that the distal intestinal bacterial microbiome of adult hyenas was significantly more diverse and differed in composition from that in juvenile hyenas. Probably both social and physiological factors contributed to these age related differences. During approximately the first 12 months of life, juveniles remain at the clan's communal den (Hofer and East, 1993c) and for most daylight hours they rest together in underground burrows where conditions are probably conducive to the spread of bacteria among resting juveniles (Höner et al., 2012). Dens also function as important social centers where clan members meet and interact, thereby enhancing the transmission of hyena-associated pathogens between clan members (East et al., 2013; Olarte-Castillo et al., 2016). Greeting ceremonies (East et al., 1993), in which participants stand head-to-tail and sniff and lick each other's anogenital area, are probably important for the spread of bacteria and their inclusion in the intestinal biome by the fecal-oral route. Since juveniles frequently participate in greeting ceremonies (East et al., 1993), greetings probably aid the colonization of the juvenile intestinal biome by both bacteria and eukaryotes. In line with this idea there is growing evidence that socially mediated transmission contributes to the maintenance of a diverse bacterial microbiome in a taxonomically broad range of species, including chimpanzees (*Pan troglodytes*), in which social processes help maintain a diversity rich in commensals and mutualists (Moeller et al., 2016), and social insects where social transmission of bacteria provides protection against virulent pathogens (Koch and Schmid-Hempel, 2011). Throughout the long period in which they are nursed, juvenile hyenas receive bacteria from their mother, and the nutritional and immunological components of milk (Hofer et al., 2016) may also affect the composition of the intestinal bacterial microbiome of juvenile hyenas.

As high-ranking individuals are highly sought after social partners, we predicted a socially mediated spread of a more diverse bacterial microbiome in high-ranking than low-ranking individuals but our results did not show this. One possible explanation is that our resolution, to the level of RSVs and genera, was insufficient. Our approach might have failed to distinguish functional differences in the relationship (e.g., mutualistic vs. pathogenic) of variants of the same species with their hosts, as in the case of distinct variants of *Escherichia coli* (von Mentzer et al., 2014). Hence our taxonomic resolution—even at the RSV level—was possibly insufficient for a fine-grained analysis of the diversity of the bacterial microbiome and the functional relationships of variants to their host. An alternative interpretation of our results is that high rates of contact between adult female clan members homogenize their intestinal bacterial biomes, as proposed by ecological network theory (Wilson, 1992).

In contrast to the bacterial microbiome, intestinal eukaryotes are—with the exception of some fungi—traditionally considered parasites and thus detrimental to their host. However, extending

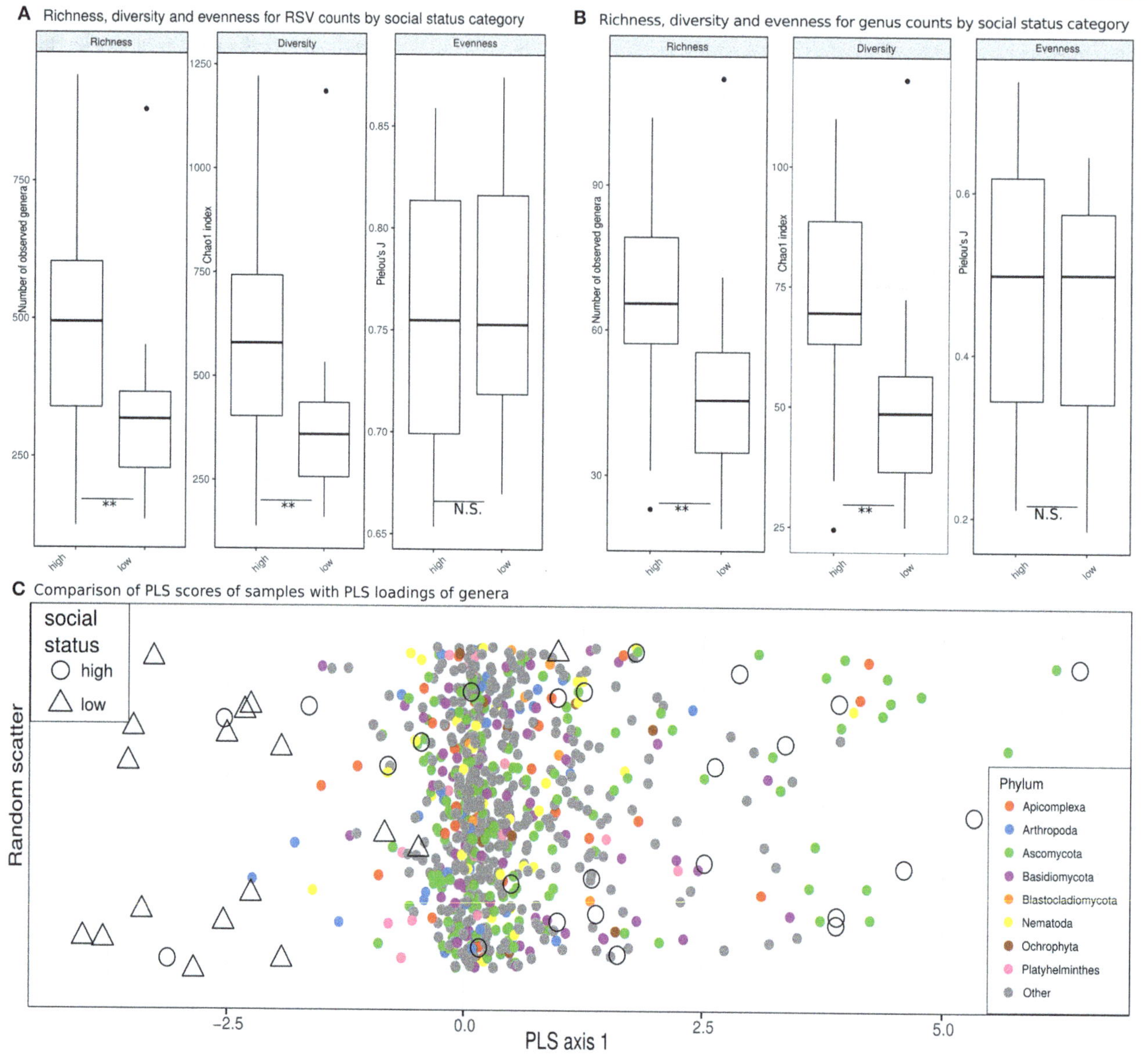

FIGURE 4 | Eukaryome diversity and composition in high ranking vs. low ranking hyenas. **(A)** Estimates of richness (observed counts of genera richness per phylum), diversity (Chao1 index) and evenness (Pielou's *J*) on rarefied (see methods) ribosomal sequence variant (RSV) counts for high-ranking and low-ranking individuals. **(B)** Counts for annotated RSV per genus are compared in box plots for high and low ranking hyenas. **Significant differences ($p < 0.01$) based on exact Mann-Whitney U tests. **(C)** A comparison of PLS scores (for samples) and PLS loadings (for genera) are visualized on the single PLS axis of an optimized partial least squares model, demonstrating a separation of the majority of samples from high-ranking individuals from samples from low-ranking animals. On the y-axis random scatter is introduced for visualization. The underlying genera are color-coded for their respective phylum.

the findings made on bacteria in the last decades it seems likely that the mammalian intestinal biome also includes diverse commensals and mutualists (Wegner Parfrey et al., 2014; Lukeš et al., 2015). In microbial communities at least, an increase in species richness increases the potential for metabolic interactions and dependencies between community members, resulting in more stable communities because they become more independent from the environment (Zelezniak et al., 2015). More stable communities are less likely to suffer perturbations in their composition (dysbiosis) as reported for many diseases. To what extent this also applies to intestinal eukaryotic communities is unclear at present. We found that high-ranking animals had a significantly more diverse eukaryome than low-ranking animals and we interpret this result to indicate a healthier intestinal ecosystem in high-ranking animals. Previously we have shown that female social status determines access to food resources within the clan territory and foraging effort (Hofer and East, 1993b). As a result, low-ranking females have higher foraging costs and higher fGCM concentrations (Goymann et al., 2001b) indicative of an elevated allostatic load. Low-ranking adult females more often resort to resource allocation trade-offs that reduce allocation of resources to immune processes, which therefore resulted in higher burdens of the intestinal helminth *Ancylostoma* spp., especially during lactation (East et al., 2015). A greater allocation of resources by high-ranking females to immune processes might contribute to maintaining mutualistic microorganisms whilst keeping pathogens in check (Hooper et al., 2012). It seems likely that the immune system of high-ranking females better limits parasitic infections than those of low-ranking females. Their higher contact rate with other clan members (East et al., 2001) and monopolization of parasite-infected social resting sites and parts of carcasses (on which they feed) can then enable high-ranking females to absorb, establish and maintain a more diverse eukaryome.

To alleviate primer bias and handling problems arising from primers targeting mainly food items we used a multi-amplicon sequencing approach (Heitlinger, 2017). To assess to what extent these methods provide a quantitative estimate of the abundance at a particular level of resolution achieved between taxa, we correlated FEC or FOC with sequence reads. Our results indicate that sequencing based estimates were more sensitive both in the detection and the identification of parasite taxa than morphologically based FEC or FOC. We also found that the number of sequence reads was moderately to strongly positively correlated with FEC or FOC counts (**Figure 2**), which generally indicates that a degree of quantification was possible using amplicon sequencing, as reported by previous studies (Kartzinel et al., 2015; Pornon et al., 2016). For analyses of this kind, it is important to take into account the fact that taxa vary in the amount of DNA present in traditionally counted entities such as eggs, oocysts or whole individuals as this will influence the number of sequencing reads obtained (Blanckenhorn et al., 2016). The stronger correlations between the number of annotated sequence reads and coccidian FOC counts than between annotated sequence reads and helminth FEC may be due to the different life cycles of these parasites. Coccidian parasites live in the cells of the epithelial lining, thus contribute DNA via oocytes shed into the lumen of the intestines whereas adult helminths reside in the lumen of the intestines, thus potentially can contributed DNA both in the eggs they shed and from adult worms. The extent of discrepancies introduced by adult worm DNA would then depend on the relationship between egg numbers and helminth tissue in the DNA preparation. For some helminth parasites, this relationship may also depend on adult female/male ratios and other biological processes such as density-dependent effects on worm fecundity, which introduce biases in the estimate of hookworm burdens (Anderson and Schad, 1985).

Cestodes in the family Diphyllobothriidae produce eggs with a very similar morphology, thus reliable identification of *Spirometra* spp. and *Diphyllobothrium* spp. based on egg morphology is challenging (Thanchomnang et al., 2016). Our sequencing based taxonomic assignments suggest that eggs from both *Spirometra* spp. and *Diphyllobothrium* spp. were included in these egg counts. Similarly, *Ancylostoma* spp. have a typical strongyle egg type, hence differentiation between *Ancylostoma* spp. eggs and those of species such as *Haemonchus* spp. is difficult. Although *Haemonchus* spp. are parasites of ungulates, they might be detected in hyena feces by both amplicon sequencing and FEC after ingestion if hyenas fed on the viscera of an infected ungulate prey. The detection of *Haemonchus* spp. eggs in the feces of hyena does not indicate to us at present that these parasite species are members of the hyena's eukaryome. Our sequencing results revealed that our FOC counts for the order Coccidia (phylum Apicomplexa) likely comprised oocysts from species in three genera. We thus conclude that our amplicon sequencing approach offered an improved resolution and sensitivity over traditional egg or oocyst identification techniques and that combining the results from both approaches can provide complementary information.

Currently, little is known about the gastrointestinal biome of most wildlife species in "natural" ecosystems. Nevertheless, components of Darwinian fitness correlated with intestinal biome features can provide insight into the function of associated organisms for their host. At a more basic level, research on a broad range of wild mammals is required to permit the correct functional role (parasite, commensal or mutualist) to be assigned to individual taxa present in intestinal biomes, and in the case of predatory species to correctly differentiate passaging material such as parasites of prey from true host gastrointestinal biome constituents. For the latter, high resolution amplicon markers (e.g., COI; Hebert et al., 2003) and analysis of correlations of the composition of the apparent intestinal biome and ingested food items might offer solutions. Annotation of taxa with functional roles additionally requires databases collating such information (Poelen et al., 2014). Whereas studies on humans and laboratory animals have revealed the importance of the bacterial microbiome in host nutrition, physiology and immune processes, little is known about the impact of intestinal eukaryote diversity and composition on any host. We propose that the assessment of intestinal biomes in free-ranging wildlife in the context of host fitness in terms of survival or reproductive success can help to identify beneficial and adverse community compositions for different demographic or social categories of host populations and distinguish those from dysbiosis. The hologenome concept of evolution proposes that evolution in complex organisms should, in addition to considering interactions between an individual's genome and its environment, also consider its interactions with the products and physiological processes arising from the combined genomes of the microorganisms it hosts (Zilber-Rosenberg and Rosenberg, 2008; but see Douglas and Werren, 2016). This has led some to suggest that, during the current period of rapid environmental change, the plasticity of the gastrointestinal microbiome may help some vertebrate populations adjust in an appropriate manner (Alberdi et al., 2016). We suggest that research on the roles of intestinal biomes for humans and wildlife should in addition encompass both unicellular and multicellular eukaryotes, including those traditionally thought of as parasites and the vast majority of organism so far unknown for their impact on hosts, before we can arrive at a balanced view of and the vast majority of organism so far unknown for their impact on hosts, before we can arrive at a balanced view of the benefits and costs of different community compositions of intestinal biomes.

DATA DEPOSITION

Raw data has been deposited under accession number PRJNA386767 at NCBI Short Read Archive (SRA).

ETHICS STATEMENT

All protocols were non-invasive and adhered to the laws and guidelines of Tanzania. Permission to conduct research in Tanzania was granted to HH, ME, and SF by the Tanzania Commission for Science and Technology. Permission to undertake research within the Serengeti National Park was granted by the Tanzanian National Parks Authority, and the research was approved by the Tanzanian Wildlife Research Institute. The research was also approved by the Committee for Ethics and Animal Welfare of the Leibniz Institute for Zoo and Wildlife Research under the approval number 2008-11-02.

AUTHOR CONTRIBUTIONS

EH, SF, HH, and ME designed the study, EH, SF, DT, HH, and ME collected the data, EH and SF analyzed the data, EH, SF, HH, and ME wrote the manuscript. All authors approved the final version of the manuscript.

FUNDING

The study was funded by the Leibniz Institute for Zoo and Wildlife Research and the DFG Research Training Group 2046 "Parasite Infections: From Experimental Models to Natural Systems" (SF).

ACKNOWLEDGMENTS

We thank Sarah Benhaiem, Nelly Boyer, Annie Francis, Katja Goller, Janine Helms, Thomas Shabani for their assistance, Luis Santos for his contribution to PCR primer selection, Ines Lesniak for help with preparing the Fluidigm Access Array PCR chips and two reviewers for their constructive comments on the manuscript.

REFERENCES

Alberdi, A., Aizpurua, O., Bohmann, K., Zepeda-Mendoza, M. L., and Gilbert, M. T. P. (2016). Do vertebrate gut metagenomes confer rapid ecological adaptation? *Trends Ecol. Evol. (Amst).* 31, 689–699. doi: 10.1016/j.tree.2016.06.008

Altschul, S. F., Madden, T. L., Schaffer, A. A., Zhang, J. H., Zhang, Z., Miller, W., et al. (1997). Gapped BLAST and PSI-BLAST: a new generation of protein database search programs. *Nucleic Acids Res.* 25, 3389–3402. doi: 10.1093/nar/25.17.3389

Amato, K. R., Yeoman, C. J., Kent, A., Righini, N., Carbonero, F., Estrada, A., et al. (2013). Habitat degradation impacts black howler monkey (*Alouatta pigra*) gastrointestinal microbiomes. *ISME J.* 7, 1344–1353. doi: 10.1038/ismej.2013.16

Andersen, L. O., Vedel Nielsen, H., and Stensvold, C. R. (2013). Waiting for the human intestinal Eukaryotome. *ISME J.* 7, 1253–1255. doi: 10.1038/ismej.2013.21

Anderson, R. M., and Schad, G. A. (1985). Hookworm burdens and faecal egg counts: an analysis of the biological basis of variation. *Trans. R. Soc. Trop. Med. Hyg.* 79, 812–825. doi: 10.1016/0035-9203(85)90128-2

Archie, E. A., Altmann, J., and Alberts, S. C. (2012). Social status predicts wound healing in wild baboons. *Proc. Natl. Acad. Sci. U.S.A.* 109, 9017–9022. doi: 10.1073/pnas.1206391109

Benjamini, Y., and Hochberg, Y. (1995). Controlling the false discovery rate: a practical and powerful approach to multiple testing. *J. R. Stat. Soc. Ser. B* 57, 289–300.

Benson, A. K., Kelly, S. A., Legge, R., Ma, F., Low, S. J., Kim, J., et al. (2010). Individuality in gut microbiota composition is a complex polygenic trait shaped by multiple environmental and host genetic factors. *Proc. Natl. Acad. Sci. U.S.A.* 107, 18933–18938. doi: 10.1073/pnas.1007028107

Blanckenhorn, W. U., Rohner, P. T., Bernasconi, M. V., Haugstetter, J., and Buser, A. (2016). Is qualitative and quantitative metabarcoding of dung fauna biodiversity feasible? *Environ. Toxicol. Chem.* 35, 1970–1977. doi: 10.1002/etc.3275

Bray, J. R., and Curtis, J. T. (1957). An ordination of the upland forest communities of southern Wisconsin. *Ecol. Monogr.* 27, 325–349. doi: 10.2307/1942268

Burgener, N., East, M. L., Hofer, H., and Dehnhard, M. (2009). Does anal scent signal identity in the spotted hyena? *Anim. Behav.* 77, 707–715. doi: 10.1016/j.anbehav.2008.11.022

Callahan, B. J., McMurdie, P. J., Rosen, M. J., Han, A. W., Johnson, A. J. A., and Holmes, S. P. (2016). DADA2: high resolution sample inference from Illumina amplicon data. *Nat. Methods* 13, 581–583. doi: 10.1038/nmeth.3869

Cardinale, B. J., Srivastava, D. S., Emmett Duffy, J., Wright, J. P., Downing, A. L., Sankaran, M., et al. (2006). Effects of biodiversity on the functioning of trophic groups and ecosystems. *Nature* 443, 989–992. doi: 10.1038/nature05202

Chao, A. (1984). Nonparametric estimation of the number of classes in a population. *Scand. J. Stat.* 11, 265–270.

Clutton-Brock, T. H., and Huchard, E. (2013). Social competition and its consequences in female mammals. *J. Zool.* 289, 151–171. doi: 10.1111/jzo.12023

Costello, E. K., Stagaman, K., Dethlefsen, L., Bohannan, B. J. M., and Relman, D. A. (2012). The application of ecological theory towards an understanding of the human microbiome. *Science* 336, 1255–1262. doi: 10.1126/science.1224203

Degnan, P. H., Pusey, A. E., Lonsdorf, E. V., Goodall, J., Wroblewski, E. E., Wilson, M. L., et al. (2012). Factors associated with the diversification of the gut microbial communities within chimpanzees from Gombe National Park. *Proc. Natl. Acad. Sci. U.S.A.* 109, 13034–13039. doi: 10.1073/pnas.1110994109

Dethlefsen, L., McFall-Ngai, M., and Relman, D. A. (2007). An ecological and evolutionary perspective on human-microbe mutualism and disease. *Nature* 449, 811–818. doi: 10.1038/nature06245

Douglas, A. E., and Werren, J. H. (2016). Holes in the Hologenome: why host-microbe symbioses are not holobionts. *MBio* 7:e02099-15. doi: 10.1128/mBio.02099-15

Dowling, D. J., and Levy, O. (2014). Ontogeny of early life immunity. *Trends Immunol.* 35, 299–310. doi: 10.1016/j.it.2014.04.007

East, M. L., Burke, T., Wilhelm, K., Greig, C., and Hofer, H. (2003). Sexual conflict in spotted hyenas: male and female mating tactics and their reproductive outcome with respect to age, social status and tenure. *Proc. R. Soc. Lond.* B270, 1247–1254. doi: 10.1098/rspb.2003.2363

East, M. L., Hofer, H., Cox, J. H., Wulle, U., Wiik, H., and Pitra, C. (2001). Regular exposure to rabies virus and lack of symptomatic disease in Serengeti spotted hyenas. *Proc. Natl. Acad. Sci. U.S.A.* 98, 15026–15031. doi: 10.1073/pnas.261411898

East, M. L., Hofer, H., and Wickler, W. (1993). The erect 'penis' as a flag of submission in a female-dominated society: greetings in Serengeti spotted hyenas. *Behav. Ecol. Sociobiol.* 33, 355–370. doi: 10.1007/BF00170251

East, M. L., Kurze, C., Wilhelm, K., Benhaiem, S., and Hofer, H. (2013). Factors influencing *Dipylidium* sp. infection in a free-ranging social carnivore, the spotted hyaena *(Crocuta crocuta)*. *Int. J. Parasitol. Parasites Wildl.* 2, 257–265. doi: 10.1016/j.ijppaw.2013.09.003

East, M. L., Otto, E., Helms, J., Thierer, D., Cable, J., and Hofer, H. (2015). Does lactation lead to resource allocation trade-offs in the spotted hyaena? *Behav. Ecol. Sociobiol.* 69, 805–814. doi: 10.1007/s00265-015-1897-x

Erny, D., Hrabě de Angelis, A. L., Jaitin, D., Wieghofer, P., Staszewski, O., David, E., et al. (2015). Host microbiota constantly control maturation and function of microglia in the CNS. *Nat. Neurosci.* 18, 965–977. doi: 10.1038/nn.4030

Ezenwa, V. O. (2004). Interactions among host diet, nutritional status and gastrointestinal parasite infection in wild bovids. *Int. J. Parasitol.* 34, 535–542. doi: 10.1016/j.ijpara.2003.11.012

Flies, A. S., Mansfield, L. S., Flies, E. J., Grant, C. K., and Holekamp, K. E. (2016). Socioecological predictors of immune defences in wild spotted hyenas. *Funct. Ecol.* 30, 1549–1557. doi: 10.1111/1365-2435.12638

Frank, L. G. (1986). Social organization of the spotted hyaena *Crocuta crocuta*. II. Dominance and reproduction. *Anim. Behav.* 34, 1510–1527. doi: 10.1016/S0003-3472(86)80221-4

Frank, L. G., Glickman, S. E., and Powch, I. (1990). Sexual dimorphism in the spotted hyaena (*Crocuta crocuta*). *J. Zool. Lond.* 221, 308–313. doi: 10.1111/j.1469-7998.1990.tb04001.x

Gill, S. R., Pop, M., DeBoy, R. T., Eckburg, P. B., Turnbaugh, P. J., Samuel, B. S., et al. (2006). Metagenomic analysis of the human distal gut microbiome. *Science* 312, 1355–1359. doi: 10.1126/science.1124234

Glendinning, L., Nausch, N., Free, A., Taylor, D. W., and Mutapi, F. (2014). The microbiota and helminths: sharing the same niche in the human host. *Parasitology* 141, 1255–1271. doi: 10.1017/S0031182014000699

Goller, K. V., Fickel, J., Hofer, H., Beier, S., and East, M. L. (2013). Coronavirus genotype diversity and prevalence of infection in wild carnivores in the Serengeti National Park, Tanzania. *Arch. Virol.* 158, 729–734. doi: 10.1007/s00705-012-1562-x

Gordon, H. M., and Whitlock, H. (1939). A new technique for counting nematode eggs in sheep faeces. *J. Counc. Sci. Ind. Res.* 12, 50–52.

Goymann, W., East, M. L., and Hofer, H. (2001a). Androgens and the role of female "hyperaggressiveness" in spotted hyenas (*Crocuta crocuta*). *Horm. Behav.* 39, 83–92. doi: 10.1006/hbeh.2000.1634

Goymann, W., East, M. L., Wachter, B., Höner, O., Möstl, E., Van't Hof, T. J., et al. (2001b). Social, state-dependent and environmental modulation of faecal corticosteroid levels in free-ranging female spotted hyaenas. *Proc. R. Soc. Lond.* B268, 2453–2459. doi: 10.1098/rspb.2001.1828

Graham, A. L. (2008). Ecological rules governing helminth–microparasite coinfection. *Proc. Natl. Acad. Sci. U.S.A.* 105, 566–570. doi: 10.1073/pnas.0707221105

Hafner, M. S., and Nadler, S. A. (1988). Phylogenetic trees support the coevolution of parasites and their hosts. *Nature* 332, 258–259. doi: 10.1038/332258a0

Hastie, T., Tibshirani, R., and Friedman, J. (2013). *The Elements of Statistical Learning: Data Mining, Inference, and Prediction, 2nd Edn.* Berlin: Springer Verlag.

Hebert, P. D. N., Cywinska, A., Ball, S. L., and de Waard, J. R. (2003). Biological identifications through DNA barcodes. *Proc. R. Soc. Lond.* B270, 313–321. doi: 10.1098/rspb.2002.2218

Heitlinger, E. (2017). *Derele/MultiAmplicon version 0.01 [R - package]*. Zenodo.

Hofer, H., Benhaiem, S., Golla, W., and East, M. L. (2016). Trade-offs in lactation and milk intake by competing siblings in a fluctuating environment. *Behav. Ecol.* 27, 1567–1578. doi: 10.1093/beheco/arw078

Hofer, H., and East, M. (1995). "Population dynamics, population size, and the commuting system of Serengeti spotted hyenas," in *Serengeti II: Dynamics, Management, and Conservation of an Ecosystem*, eds A. R. E. Sinclair and P. Arcese (Chicago, IL: University of Chicago Press), 332–363.

Hofer, H., and East, M. L. (1993a). The commuting system of Serengeti spotted hyaenas: how a predator copes with migratory prey. I. Social organization. *Anim. Behav.* 46, 547–557. doi: 10.1006/anbe.1993.1222

Hofer, H., and East, M. L. (1993b). The commuting system of Serengeti spotted hyaenas: how a predator copes with migratory prey. II. Intrusion pressure and commuters' space use. *Anim. Behav.* 46, 559–574. doi: 10.1006/anbe.1993.1223

Hofer, H., and East, M. L. (1993c). The commuting system of Serengeti spotted hyaenas: how a predator copes with migratory prey. III. Attendance and maternal care. *Anim. Behav.* 46, 575–589. doi: 10.1006/anbe.1993.1224

Hofer, H., and East, M. L. (2003). Behavioural processes and costs of co-existence in female spotted hyenas: a life history perspective. *Evol. Ecol.* 17, 315–331. doi: 10.1023/A:1027352517231

Höner, O. P., Wachter, B., Goller, K. V., Hofer, H., Runyoro, V., Thierer, D., et al. (2012). The impact of a pathogenic bacterium on a social carnivore population. *J. Anim. Ecol.* 81, 36–46. doi: 10.1111/j.1365-2656.2011.01873.x

Hooper, L. V., Littman, D. R., and Macpherson, A. J. (2012). Interactions between the microbiota and the immune system. *Science* 336, 1268–1273. doi: 10.1126/science.1223490

Hothorn, T., Hornik, K., van de Weil, M. A., and Zeileis, A. (2006). A Lego system for conditional inference. *Am. Statist.* 60, 257–263. doi: 10.1198/000313006X118430

Kartzinel, T. R., Chen, P. A., Coverdale, T. C., Erickson, D. L., Kress, W. J., Kuzmina, M. L., et al. (2015). DNA metabarcoding illuminates dietary niche partitioning by African large herbivores. *Proc. Natl. Acad. Sci. U.S.A* 112, 8019–8024. doi: 10.1073/pnas.1503283112

Koch, H., and Schmid-Hempel, P. (2011). Socially transmitted gut microbiota protect bumble bees against an intestinal parasite. *Proc. Natl. Acad. Sci. U.S.A.* 108, 19288–19292. doi: 10.1073/pnas.1110474108

Koenig, J. E., Spor, A., Scalfone, N., Fricker, A. D., Stombaugh, J., Knight, R., et al. (2011). Succession of microbial consortia in the developing infant gut microbiome. *Proc. Natl. Acad. Sci. U.S.A.* 108(Suppl. 1), 4578–4585. doi: 10.1073/pnas.1000081107

Kreisinger, J., Bastien, G., Hauffe, H. C., Marchesi, J., and Perkins, S. E. (2015). Interactions between multiple helminths and the gut microbiota in wild rodents. *Phil. Trans. R. Soc. Lond.* B370:20140295. doi: 10.1098/rstb.2014.0295

Kruuk, H. (1972). *The Spotted Hyena: A Study of Predation and Social Behavior.* Chicago, IL: University of Chicago Press.

Lee, S. C., Tang, M. S., Lim, Y. A. L., Choy, S. H., Kurtz, Z. D., Cox, L. M., et al. (2014). Helminth colonization is associated with increased diversity of the gut microbiota. *PLoS Negl. Trop. Dis.* 8:e2880. doi: 10.1371/journal.pntd.0002880

Legendre, P., and Legendre, L. F. J. (2012). *Numerical Ecology, 3rd Edn.* Amsterdam: Elsevier.

Leone, V., Gibbons, S. M., Gilbert, J. A., Chang, E. B., Leone, V., Gibbons, S. M., et al. (2015). Effects of diurnal variation of gut microbes and high-fat feeding on host circadian clock function and metabolism. *Cell Host Microbe* 17, 681–689. doi: 10.1016/j.chom.2015.03.006

Ley, R. E., Hamady, M., Lozupone, C., Turnbaugh, P., Ramey, R. R., Bircher, J. S., et al. (2008). Evolution of mammals and their gut microbes. *Science* 320, 1647–1651. doi: 10.1126/science.1155725

Love, M. I., Huber, W., and Anders, S. (2014). Moderated estimation of fold change and dispersion for RNA-seq data with DESeq2. *Genome Biol.* 15:550. doi: 10.1186/s13059-014-0550-8

Lozupone, C. A., Stombaugh, J. I., Gordon, J. I., Jansson, J. K., and Knight, R. (2012). Diversity, stability and resilience of the human gut microbiota. *Nature* 489, 220–230. doi: 10.1038/nature11550

Lukeš, J., Stensvold, C. R., Jirku-Pomajbíková, K., and Wegener Parfrey, L. (2015). Are human intestinal eukaryotes beneficial or commensals? *PLoS Pathog.* 11:e1005039. doi: 10.1371/journal.ppat.1005039

McMurdie, P. J., and Holmes, S. (2013). phyloseq: an R package for reproducible interactive analysis and graphics of microbiome census data. *PLoS ONE* 8:e61217. doi: 10.1371/journal.pone.0061217

Menke, S., Gillingham, M. A. F., Wilhelm, K., and Sommer, S. (2017). Home-made cost effective preservation buffer is a better alternative to commercial preservation methods for microbiome research. *Front. Microbiol.* 8:102. doi: 10.3389/fmicb.2017.00102

Menke, S., Meier, M., and Sommer, S. (2015). Shifts in the gut microbiome observed in wildlife faecal samples exposed to natural weather conditions: lessons from time-series analyses using next-generation sequencing for application in field studies. *Meth. Ecol. Evol.* 6, 1080–1087. doi: 10.1111/2041-210X.12394

Menke, S., Wasimuddin, Meier, M., Melzheimer, J., Mfune, J. K. E., Heinrich, S., et al. (2014). Oligotyping reveals differences between gut microbiomes of free-ranging sympatric Namibian carnivores (*Acinonyx jubatus, Canis mesomelas*) on a bacterial species-like level. *Front. Microbiol.* 5:526. doi: 10.3389/fmicb.2014.00526

Meyer-Lucht, Y., and Sommer, S. (2005). MHC diversity and the association to nematode parasitism in the yellow-necked mouse (*Apodemus flavicollis*). *Mol. Ecol.* 14, 2233–2243. doi: 10.1111/j.1365-294X.2005.02557.x

Moeller, A. H., Foerster, S., Wilson, M. L., Pusey, A. E., Hahn, B. H., and Ochman, H. (2016). Social behavior shapes the chimpanzee pan-microbiome. *Sci. Adv.* 2:e1500997. doi: 10.1126/sciadv.1500997

Nikolin, V. N., Olarte-Castillo, X. A., Osterrieder, N., Hofer, H., Dubovi, E., Mazzoni, C. J., et al. (2017). Canine distemper virus in the Serengeti ecosystem: molecular adaptation to different carnivore species. *Mol. Ecol.* 26, 2111–2130. doi: 10.1111/mec.13902

Ochman, H., Worobey, M., Kuo, C.-H., Ndjango, J.-B. N., Peeters, M., Hahn, B. H., et al. (2010). Evolutionary relationships of wild hominids recapitulated by gut microbial communities. *PLoS Biol.* 8:e1000546. doi: 10.1371/journal.pbio.1000546

Olarte-Castillo, X. A., Hofer, H., Goller, K. J., Martella, V., Moehlman, P. D., and East, M. L. (2016). Divergent sapovirus strains and infection prevalence in wild carnivores in the Serengeti ecosystem: a long-term study. *PLoS ONE* 11:e0163548. doi: 10.1371/journal.pone.0163548

Palmer, C., Bik, E. M., DiGiulio, D. B., Relman, D. A., and Brown, P. O. (2007). Development of the human infant intestinal microbiota. *PLoS Biol.* 5:e177. doi: 10.1371/journal.pbio.0050177

Pielou, E. C. (1975). *Ecological Diversity*. New York, NY: John Wiley.

Poelen, J. H., Simons, J. D., and Mungall, C. J. (2014). Global biotic interactions: an open infrastructure to share and analyze species-interaction datasets. *Ecol. Inform.* 24, 148–159. doi: 10.1016/j.ecoinf.2014.08.005

Pond, C. M. (1977). The significance of lactation in the evolution of mammals. *Evolution* 31, 177–199. doi: 10.1111/j.1558-5646.1977.tb00995.x

Pornon, A., Escaravage, N., Burrus, M., Holota, H., Khimoun, A., Mariette, J., et al. (2016). Using metabarcoding to reveal and quantify plant-pollinator interactions. *Sci. Rep.* 6:27282. doi: 10.1038/srep27282

Quast, C., Pruesse, E., Yilmaz, P., Gerken, J., Schweer, T., Yarza, P., et al. (2013). The SILVA ribosomal RNA gene database project: improved data processing and web-based tools. *Nucleic Acids Res.* 41, D590–D596. doi: 10.1093/nar/gks1219

Rajilić-Stojanović, M., and de Vos, W. M. (2014). The first 1000 cultured species of the human gastrointestinal microbiota. *FEMS Microbiol. Rev.* 38, 996–1047. doi: 10.1111/1574-6976.12075

R Development Core Team (2016). *R: A Language and Environment for Statistical Computing*. Vienna: R Foundation for Statistical Computing. Available online at: http://www.R-project.org

Reich, P. B., Tilman, D., Isbell, F., Mueller, K., Hobbie, S. E., Flynn, D. F. B., et al. (2012). Impacts of biodiversity loss escalate through time as redundancy fades. *Science* 336, 589–592. doi: 10.1126/science.1217909

Round, J. L., and Mazmanian, S. K. (2009). The gut microbiota shapes intestinal immune responses during health and disease. *Nat. Rev. Immunol.* 9, 313–323. doi: 10.1038/nri2515

Sapolsky, R. M. (2005). The influence of social hierarchy on primate health. *Science* 308, 648–652. doi: 10.1126/science.1106477

Schwensow, N., Fietz, J., Dausmann, K. H., and Sommer, S. (2007). Neutral versus adaptive genetic variation in parasite resistance: importance of major histocompatibility complex supertypes in a free-ranging primate. *Heredity* 99, 265–277. doi: 10.1038/sj.hdy.6800993

Sivan, A., Corrales, L., Hubert, N., Williams, J. B., Aquino-michaels, K., Earley, Z. M., et al. (2015). Commensal Bifidobacterium promotes antitumor immunity and facilitates anti−PD-L1 efficacy. *Science* 350, 1084–1089. doi: 10.1126/science.aac4255

Snyder-Mackler, N., Sanz, J., Kohn, J. N., Brinkworth, J. F., Morrow, S., Shaver, A. O., et al. (2016). Social status alters immune regulation and response to infection in macaques. *Science* 354, 1041–1045. doi: 10.1126/science.aah3580

Sudo, N., Chida, Y., Aiba, Y., Sonoda, J., Oyama, N., Yu, X.-N., et al. (2004). Postnatal microbial colonization programs the hypothalamic–pituitary–adrenal system for stress response in mice. *J. Physiol.* 558, 263–275. doi: 10.1113/jphysiol.2004.063388

Tannock, G. W. (2007). What immunologists should know about bacterial communities of the human bowel. *Semin. Immunol.* 19, 94–105. doi: 10.1016/j.smim.2006.09.001

Thanchomnang, T., Tantrawatpan, C., Intapan, P. M., Sanpool, O., Lulitanond, V., Tourtip, S., et al. (2016). Rapid identification of nine species of diphyllobothriidean tapeworms by pyrosequencing. *Sci. Rep.* 6:37228. doi: 10.1038/srep37228

The Human Microbiome Consortium (2012). Structure, function and diversity of the healthy human microbiome. *Nature* 486, 207–214. doi: 10.1038/nature11234

Tremaroli, V., and Bäckhed, F. (2012). Functional interactions between the gut microbiota and host metabolism. *Nature* 489, 242–249. doi: 10.1038/nature11552

Tung, J., Barreiro, L. B., Johnson, Z. P., Hansen, K. D., Michopoulos, V., Toufexis, D., et al. (2012). Social environment is associated with gene regulatory variation in the rhesus macaque immune system. *Proc. Natl. Acad. Sci. U.S.A.* 109, 6490–6495. doi: 10.1073/pnas.1202734109

Turnbaugh, P. J., Hamady, M., Yatsunenko, T., Cantarel, B. L., Duncan, A., Ley, R. E., et al. (2009). A core gut microbiome in obese and lean twins. *Nature* 457, 480–484. doi: 10.1038/nature07540

Turnbaugh, P. J., Ley, R. E., Hamady, M., Fraser-Liggett, C., Knight, R., and Gordon, J. I. (2007). The human microbiome project: exploring the microbial part of ourselves in a changing world. *Nature* 449, 804–810. doi: 10.1038/nature06244

von Mentzer, A., Connor, T. R., Wieler, L. H., Semmler, T., Iguchi, A., Thomson, N. R., et al. (2014). Identification of enterotoxigenic *Escherichia coli* (ETEC) clades with long-term global distribution. *Nat. Genet.* 46, 1321–1326. doi: 10.1038/ng.3145

Wang, Q., Garrity, G. M., Tiedje, J. M., and Cole, J. R. (2007). Naïve Bayesian classifier for rapid assignment of rRNA sequences into the new bacterial taxonomy. *Appl. Environ. Microbiol.* 73, 5261–5267. doi: 10.1128/AEM.00062-07

Wegener Parfrey, L., Walters, W. A., and Knight, R. (2011). Microbial eukaryotes in the human microbiome: ecology, evolution, and future directions. *Front. Microbiol.* 2:153. doi: 10.3389/fmicb.2011.00153

Wegner Parfrey, L., Walters, W. A., Lauber, C. L., Clements, J. C., Berg-Lyons, D., Teiling, C., et al. (2014). Communities of microbial eukaryotes in the mammalian gut within the context of environmental eukaryotic diversity. *Front. Microbiol.* 5:298. doi: 10.3389/fmicb.2014.00298

Wilson, D. S. (1992). Complex interactions in metacommunities, with implications for biodiversity and higher levels of selection. *Ecology* 73, 1984–2000. doi: 10.2307/1941449

Wold, S., Ruhe, A., Wold, H., and Dunn, I., W. (1984). The collinearity problem in linear regression. The partial least squares (PLS) approach to generalized inverses. *SIAM J. Sci. Stat. Comput.* 5, 735–743. doi: 10.1137/0905052

Yatsunenko, T., Rey, F. E., Manary, M. J., Trehan, I., Dominguez-Bello, M. G., Contreras, M., et al. (2012). Human gut microbiome viewed across age and geography. *Nature* 486, 222–227. doi: 10.1038/nature11053

Yildirim, S., Yeoman, C. J., Sipos, M., Torralba, M., Wilson, B. A., Goldberg, T. L., et al. (2010). Characterization of the fecal microbiome from non-human wild primates reveals species specific microbial communities. *PLoS ONE* 5:e13963. doi: 10.1371/journal.pone.0013963

Zelezniak, A., Andrejev, S., Ponomarova, O., Mende, D. R., Bork, P., and Patil, K. R. (2015). Metabolic dependencies drive species co-occurrence in diverse microbial communities. *Proc. Natl. Acad. Sci. U.S.A.* 112, 6449–6454. doi: 10.1073/pnas.1421834112

Zilber-Rosenberg, I., and Rosenberg, E. (2008). Role of microorganisms in the evolution of animals and plants: the hologenome theory of evolution. *FEMS Microbiol. Rev.* 32, 723–735. doi: 10.1111/j.1574-6976.2008.00123.x

16

Cytokines and Chemokines in Cerebral Malaria Pathogenesis

Josefine Dunst[1,2,3]*, *Faustin Kamena*[1,2,3] *and Kai Matuschewski*[1,2]

[1] Parasitology Unit, Max Planck Institute for Infection Biology, Berlin, Germany, [2] Institute of Chemistry and Biochemistry, Free University, Berlin, Germany, [3] Molecular Parasitology, Institute of Biology, Humboldt University, Berlin, Germany

Edited by:
Slobodan Paessler,
University of Texas Medical Branch,
United States

Reviewed by:
Tracey Lamb,
University of Utah, United States
Teresa Carvalho,
La Trobe University, Australia

***Correspondence:**
Josefine Dunst
dunstj@zedat.fu-berlin.de

Cerebral malaria is among the major causes of malaria-associated mortality and effective adjunctive therapeutic strategies are currently lacking. Central pathophysiological processes involved in the development of cerebral malaria include an imbalance of pro- and anti-inflammatory responses to *Plasmodium* infection, endothelial cell activation, and loss of blood-brain barrier integrity. However, the sequence of events, which initiates these pathophysiological processes as well as the contribution of their complex interplay to the development of cerebral malaria remain incompletely understood. Several cytokines and chemokines have repeatedly been associated with cerebral malaria severity. Increased levels of these inflammatory mediators could account for the sequestration of leukocytes in the cerebral microvasculature present during cerebral malaria, thereby contributing to an amplification of local inflammation and promoting cerebral malaria pathogenesis. Herein, we highlight the current knowledge on the contribution of cytokines and chemokines to the pathogenesis of cerebral malaria with particular emphasis on their roles in endothelial activation and leukocyte recruitment, as well as their implication in the progression to blood-brain barrier permeability and neuroinflammation, in both human cerebral malaria and in the murine experimental cerebral malaria model. A better molecular understanding of these processes could provide the basis for evidence-based development of adjunct therapies and the definition of diagnostic markers of disease progression.

Keywords: malaria, *Plasmodium*, cerebral malaria, cytokines, chemokines, endothelial activation, blood-brain barrier, neuroinflammation

INTRODUCTION

Malaria is one of the most prevalent infectious diseases worldwide and contributes considerably to the global disease burden. With ~200 million new cases and an estimated 430,000 deaths annually (WHO, 2016), malaria remains the most important vector-borne infectious disease. The human-adapted *Plasmodium* species *P. falciparum* and *P. vivax* account for the majority of malaria cases and are transmitted by the bite of an infective *Anopheles* mosquito. Despite considerable progress in malaria eradication over the past 15 years (WHO, 2016),

Abbreviations: CD, cluster of differentiation; CM, cerebral malaria; CSF, cerebrospinal fluid; DAMP, danger-associated molecular patterns; DC, dendritic cell; ECM, experimental cerebral malaria; EPCR, endothelial protein C receptor; GPI, glycosylphosphatidylinositol; ICAM, intercellular adhesion molecule; IFN, interferon; IL, interleukin; IP-10, IFN-γ-inducible protein 10; KC, keratinocyte chemoattractant; LPS, lipopolysaccharide; LT, lymphotoxin; MCP-1, monocyte chemoattractant protein 1; MIG, monokine induced by IFN-γ; MIP, macrophage inflammatory protein; NK, natural killer; NLR, NOD-like receptors, PAMP, pathogen-associated molecular pattern; PF4, platelet factor 4; *Pf*EMP1, *Plasmodium falciparum* erythrocyte membrane protein 1; PRR, pattern recognition receptor; TLR, Toll-like receptor; TNF, tumor necrosis factor; VCAM, vascular cell adhesion molecule; ZO-1, zonula occludens 1.

efforts are hampered by emerging *Plasmodium* resistance to commonly used anti-malaria drugs (Cui et al., 2015) and limited efficacy of the currently most advanced vaccine candidate (White et al., 2015; Olotu et al., 2016).

Among infections by human host-adapted *Plasmodium* species, *P. falciparum* infections are most likely to progress to organ-related pathology and severe malaria, and thereby account for the vast majority of malaria-associated fatalities. Along with severe anemia and respiratory distress, cerebral malaria (CM) is one of the major manifestations of severe malaria (Haldar et al., 2007). CM manifests with impaired consciousness and coma in both children and adults (Idro et al., 2010), while other clinical features differ. In addition to the characteristic diffuse encephalopathy, retinal abnormalities are frequent in children and less common in adults with CM (Beare et al., 2006; Idro et al., 2010). In contrast, CM in adults is accompanied by multi-organ disorder including renal failure and pulmonary edema, which are less frequently observed in children suffering from CM (Idro et al., 2010). Although anti-malaria treatment using artesunate was reported to improve CM outcome in children and adults (Dondorp et al., 2005, 2010), the case-fatality rate of pediatric CM is approximately 20% (Haldar et al., 2007) and sustained cognitive and/or neurological impairment may occur (John et al., 2008a). Consequently, treatment strategies, which not only target the parasite but also other mechanisms underlying CM pathogenesis, need to be developed. Since the pathogenesis of CM is still incompletely understood, further investigations are an important medical research priority, especially in the context of adjunctive therapies. Since accumulating evidence indicates that an imbalance in pro- and anti-inflammatory immune responses partially contributes to CM pathogenesis, such therapeutic approaches could target cytokines and chemokines associated with CM severity. Cytokines are polypeptides, which mediate and generate inflammatory responses. Along with their contribution to disease pathogenesis in general, cytokines also exert physiological roles at lower concentrations (Clark and Vissel, 2017). Chemokines are chemotactic cytokines, which recruit lymphocytes and monocytes to the site of pathogen encounter by binding to their respective chemokine receptor (Griffith et al., 2014). Given that leukocytes were found to sequester in the microvasculature of the brain in human CM and murine ECM (Hunt and Grau, 2003), local chemokine gradients may mediate leukocyte recruitment and thus promote CM pathogenesis. Chemokines exert their function through binding to their respective G protein-coupled chemokine receptors (**Table 1**), which induces activation of phosphatidylinositol 3-kinase (PI3K) and Rho GTPase signaling pathways, thus leading to F-actin polymerization and migration (Viola and Luster, 2008).

In this review, we highlight findings from both experimental murine models and natural human infections, and assess the current knowledge on the role of host cytokine and chemokine responses in the severe malaria complication of cerebral malaria. We also emphasize the potential inflammatory cascade resulting from *Plasmodium* life cycle progression after sporozoite inoculation and ultimately culminating in cerebral malaria pathology (**Figure 1**).

CURRENT CONCEPTS IN CEREBRAL MALARIA PATHOGENESIS

Two central concepts to explain CM pathogenesis have evolved and they are likely mutually dependent- the vascular occlusion hypothesis and the inflammation hypothesis (Storm and Craig, 2014).

The concept of vascular occlusion leading to CM is based on the ability of mature *P. falciparum*-infected erythrocytes to sequester in the microvasculature through binding of *P. falciparum* erythrocyte membrane protein 1 (*Pf*EMP1) present on the erythrocyte surface to endothelial cell surface proteins, such as intercellular adhesion molecule 1 (ICAM-1), vascular cell adhesion molecule 1 (VCAM-1), cluster of differentiation 36 (CD36), or endothelial protein C receptor (EPCR) (Pasloske and Howard, 1994; Chen et al., 2000; Rowe et al., 2009; Smith et al., 2013; Turner et al., 2013; Lennartz et al., 2017). Sequestration occurs in various organs and, along with increased rigidity of erythrocytes, is believed to cause vascular occlusion (Dondorp et al., 2004). Additionally, microvascular obstruction during *P. falciparum* infection may be worsened by the formation of rosettes and clumps (Chen et al., 2000; Rowe et al., 2009; Adams et al., 2014), i.e., the binding of uninfected erythrocytes by infected erythrocytes (Handunnetti et al., 1989), and aggregation of infected erythrocytes and platelets (Pain et al., 2001), respectively. These events may cause a reduction in microvascular blood flow, ischemia, and tissue hypoxia (Medana and Turner, 2006), thereby accounting for cerebral pathology. Reduced vessel perfusion and occlusion was indeed observed by fluorescein angiography of the retina in pediatric CM cases (Beare et al., 2009) and by *in vivo* imaging of the microcirculation in adult patients with CM or other manifestations of severe malaria (Dondorp et al., 2008), although further studies are needed to determine the underlying cause of these observations. Additionally, sequestration of *P. falciparum*-infected erythrocytes was observed in the cerebral microvasculature of CM patients in *post mortem* brain histology studies (Ponsford et al., 2012; Milner et al., 2014, 2015).

Despite accumulating evidence, the relevance of sequestration in the development of CM is still incompletely understood, since the degree of sequestration in brains of non-fatal CM cases cannot be investigated non-invasively and is, thus, unspecified (Miller et al., 2002). Occasionally, fatal CM cases present little sequestration and vessel occlusion similar to non-CM severe malaria cases (Ponsford et al., 2012). Moreover, isolated CM cases were reported in children and adults with confirmed *P. vivax* mono-infections in India (Kochar et al., 2009), although *P. vivax* is unlikely to sequester in the microvasculature since late-stage *P. vivax*-infected erythrocytes are present in peripheral blood (Anstey et al., 2009). Together, cerebral malaria occasionally develops in a few *P. vivax* infections without obvious signs of sequestration *in vivo* or microvascular obstruction.

Given the unresolved role of sequestration in the pathogenesis of CM, additional factors may determine disease severity. Notably, other infectious diseases that result in systemic inflammation and fever also progress to severe forms,

TABLE 1 | Selected human and murine chemokines and their receptors[a].

Chemokine	Other names	Gene		Receptors	Key function
		Human	Mouse		
CCL2	MCP-1 JE (mouse)	*CCL2*	*Ccl2*	CCR2	Inflammatory monocyte trafficking
CCL3 CCL4 CCL5	MIP-1α MIP-1β RANTES	*CCL3* *CCL4* *CCL5*	*Ccl3* *Ccl4* *Ccl5*	CCR1, CCR5 CCR5 CCR1, CCR3, CCR5	Macrophage and NK cell migration, T cell-DC interactions
CCL11	Eotaxin	*CCL11*	*Ccl11*	CCR3, CCR5	Eosinophil and basophil migration
CCL20	MIP-3α	*CCL20*	*Ccl20*	CCR6	Th17 responses, B cell and DC homing
CXCL1 CXCL3	GROα Gm1960 (mouse) GROγ KC (mouse)	*CXCL1* *CXCL3*	*Cxcl3* *Cxcl1*	CXCR2 CXCR2	Neutrophil trafficking
CXCL4 CXCL4L1	PF4 PF4V1	*PF4* *PF4V1*	– *Pf4*	CXCR3-B CXCR3-B	Procoagulant
CXCL8	IL-8	*IL-8*	–	CXCR1, CXCR2	Neutrophil trafficking
CXCL9 CXCL10	MIG IP-10	*CXCL9* *CXCL10*	*Cxcl9* *Cxcl10*	CXCR3 CXCR3	T cell and NK cell trafficking

[a]*Modified from Zlotnik and Yoshie (2012) and Griffith et al. (2014).*

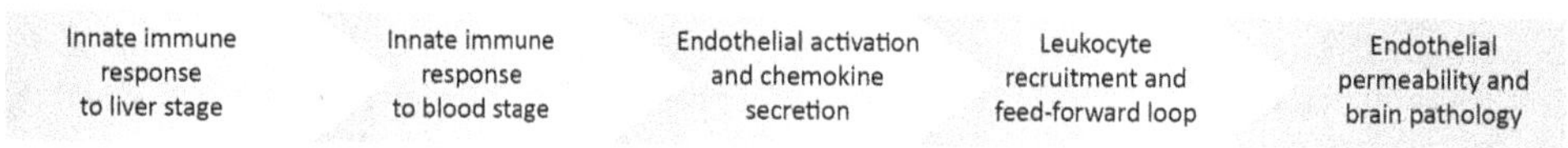

FIGURE 1 | Overview of a potential inflammatory cascade culminating in cerebral malaria pathology. Five consecutive events shape the outcome of a *Plasmodium* infection and contribute to cerebral malaria. During *Plasmodium* infection of the mammalian host, two consecutive parasite replication phases in the liver and red blood cells lead to distinct innate responses, which modulate downstream parasite/host cell interactions. Upon parasite accumulation in the microvasculature, endothelial cells become activated, leading to enhanced chemokine secretion, which in turn enhances leukocyte recruitment. Acute pathology is caused by permeabilization of the endothelial barrier. See **Figures 2–6** for the central roles of chemokines and cytokines in the individual events.

including neurological complications such as sepsis-associated encephalopathy (De Backer et al., 2002; Clark et al., 2004). Strikingly, systemic cytokine levels have been described to correlate with disease severity in malaria as well as sepsis (Prakash et al., 2006; Bozza et al., 2007). These findings corroborate an earlier proposal that an imbalance in pro- and anti-inflammatory immune responses triggers immune-induced pathology and might be a leading cause of CM pathogenesis, which may be further amplified by sequestration (Clark and Rockett, 1994). In addition to inflammation and sequestration, CM is associated with endothelial activation and increased blood-brain barrier permeability, and these processes might act reciprocally and have synergistic effects (van der Heyde et al., 2006). In line with this notion, certain *Pf*EMP1 variants, which are associated with CM, were described to compete with activated protein C in binding to EPCR (Turner et al., 2013; Bernabeu et al., 2016). Therefore, the anti-coagulant, anti-inflammatory, cytoprotective properties, which are induced upon interaction of protein C with EPCR, might be impeded by *Pf*EMP1-EPCR interaction and consequently, disease mechanisms may be further exacerbated (Bernabeu and Smith, 2017; Wassmer and Grau, 2017). However, the impact of the interaction between *Pf*EMP1 and EPCR on inflammation and coagulation remains to be demonstrated.

Insights into the mechanisms underlying CM in humans are limited and mostly based on *post mortem* histopathology or correlations of serum parameters with disease outcome (Hunt and Grau, 2003). Despite potential differences in human and murine CM pathogenesis (Riley et al., 2010; Craig et al., 2012), *P. berghei* (strain ANKA) infection reliably causes signature symptoms of CM in susceptible C57BL/6 mice (de Souza and Riley, 2002; Hunt and Grau, 2003). This host-parasite combination is a widely used and well-established murine model for CM, termed experimental cerebral malaria (ECM), which permits mechanistic studies (Craig et al., 2012). Consequently, studies highlighted in this review include reports on human cerebral malaria cases combined with mechanistic insights based on the murine ECM model and *in vitro* studies.

INNATE IMMUNE ACTIVATION DURING LIVER STAGE DEVELOPMENT

Upon transmission by the bite of an infective *Anopheles* mosquito, *Plasmodium* sporozoites rapidly migrate to the liver, invade hepatocytes and develop into thousands of merozoites. Since this developmental stage of *Plasmodium* parasites is clinically silent, the immune response mounted by the host in order to limit parasite expansion during liver stage development remains largely unexplored (Hafalla et al., 2011). However, it seems likely that sporozoite and liver stage recognition primes the innate immune system locally and well below the pyrogenic threshold. In fact, innate immune cells have occasionally been observed to surround *P. berghei*-infected hepatocytes, indicating that *Plasmodium* does not remain undetected during liver stage development (Liehl and Mota, 2012). Additionally, a type I interferon (IFN) response is induced in livers of mice infected with *P. yoelii* or *P. berghei* (Liehl et al., 2014; Miller et al., 2014). Such an initial type I IFN response might induce chemokines, including IFN-γ-inducible protein 10 (IP-10)/CXCL10, which in turn could recruit cells expressing the corresponding chemokine receptor CXCR3, such as T, natural killer (NK), and NKT cells, to the site of infection, which might contribute to the local immune response by IFN-γ secretion (**Figure 2**; Liehl et al., 2014; Miller et al., 2014). In good agreement, an increase in IFN-γ plasma concentration prior to onset of detectable blood-stage infection was reported in controlled human *P. falciparum* infection (Hermsen et al., 2003). Clearly, the initial cytokine response fails to arrest liver stage development and, thus, does not curtail the proceeding to erythrocyte infection. Interestingly, *P. berghei* sporozoite and blood stage infections result in ECM symptoms in a similar time frame (Kordes et al., 2011), suggesting that immune responses against liver stages might not modulate CM pathogenesis. Whether this first immune response reduces the initial parasite number released into the blood stream and thereby influences the magnitude of early blood stage-induced immune responses remains to be tested.

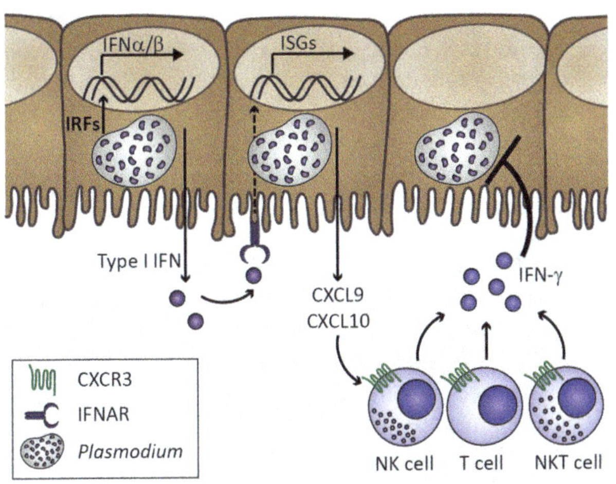

FIGURE 2 | Innate immune response to *Plasmodium* liver stage infection. *Plasmodium* infection of hepatocytes activates interferon regulatory factors (IRF), which induce transcription of type I interferons (IFN) IFNα and IFNβ. Secretion of type I IFNs activates IFNα/β receptor IFNAR in an autocrine or paracrine manner. IFNAR signaling results in transcription of IFN-stimulated genes (ISGs), which includes chemokines, such as CXCL9 and CXCL10. Upon secretion from hepatocytes, these chemokines might recruit cells expressing the corresponding chemokine receptor CXCR3, including natural killer (NK), T, and NKT cells. Upon activation by type I IFN at the site of infection, these cell types could contribute to limiting *Plasmodium* liver stage expansion by IFN-γ secretion. Based on Liehl et al. (2014) and Miller et al. (2014).

BLOOD STAGE-INDUCED INNATE IMMUNE RESPONSES

Concomitant with the release of merozoites into the bloodstream and infection of erythrocytes, a *Plasmodium* infection progresses from the clinically silent liver stage to the symptomatic blood stage. Merozoites are only very briefly (~60 s) exposed to the immune system before they rapidly enter new erythrocytes (Gilson and Crabb, 2009; Beeson et al., 2016), and blood stage infection is the exclusive cause of malaria symptoms, which is associated with systemic inflammation and fever. Fever is a common and effective host defense against microbial pathogens and swiftly initiated upon the first host-pathogen interaction. The febrile response is likely triggered through a universal mechanism, in which pyrogens, such as the pro-inflammatory cytokines interleukin 1α (IL-1α), IL-1β, IL-6, or tumor necrosis factor (TNF), are secreted by innate immune cells upon recognition of pathogen-associated molecular patterns (PAMPs) or host-derived danger-associated molecular patterns (DAMPs) by pattern recognition receptors (PRRs) (Evans et al., 2015). In *Plasmodium* infection, the characteristic recurrent fever coincides with synchronized rupture of infected erythrocytes in the schizont stage (Oakley et al., 2011). Release of parasite- and host-derived molecules due to erythrocyte rupture was described to induce TNF *in vitro* (Kwiatkowski et al., 1989; Bate and Kwiatkowski, 1994), and peaks in TNF serum concentration were found to coincide with elevated body temperature during *P. vivax* infection (Karunaweera et al., 1992), indicating that malaria fever is elicited by repeated release of PAMPs and DAMPs. Although an increase in core body temperature is associated with resolution of infection (Oakley et al., 2011), such a pro-inflammatory immune response needs to be counterbalanced by anti-inflammatory mechanisms in order to avoid a dysregulated immune response, which might lead to complications such as cerebral malaria.

The innate immune system represents the first line of defense against pathogens and mediates recognition and clearance of *Plasmodium* parasites (**Figure 3**). Cells of the innate immune system such as macrophages and dendritic cells (DCs) as well as non-professional immune cells such as endothelial cells and fibroblasts express PRR. These include Toll-like receptors (TLR), C-type lectin receptors (CLR), Retinoic acid-inducible gene (RIG)-I-like receptors, and NOD-like receptors (NLR), which recognize PAMPs and host-derived DAMPs (Takeuchi and Akira, 2010). Most malaria PAMPs and DAMPs known so far are apparently recognized by TLR. Activation of TLR initiates a signaling cascade including the adaptor protein MyD88 and the transcription factors NF-κB, AP-1, and interferon regulatory factor (IRF). As a consequence, expression of genes encoding pro-inflammatory cytokines such as type I IFN, IFN-γ, IL-6, IL-12, and TNF, is induced (Eriksson et al., 2013; Gazzinelli et al., 2014).

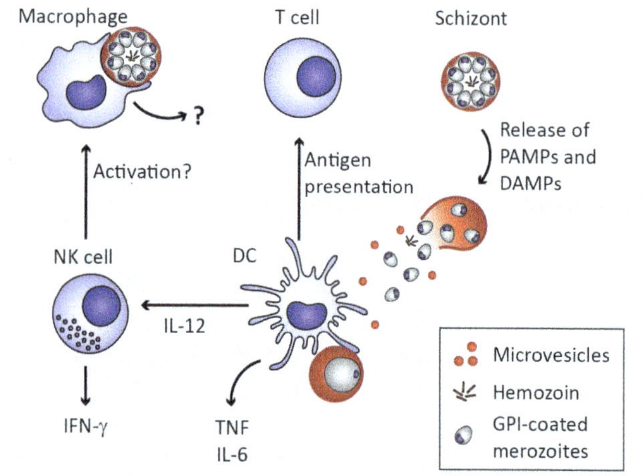

FIGURE 3 | Innate immune response to *Plasmodium* blood stage infection in the spleen. Macrophages as well as dendritic cells (DC) remove infected erythrocytes from the circulation by phagocytosis. In macrophages, uptake of infected erythrocytes might not lead to secretion of pro-inflammatory cytokines due to phagosomal acidification (Wu et al., 2015). Upon rupture of infected erythrocytes, pathogen-associated molecular patterns (PAMPs) and danger-associated molecular patterns (DAMPs) are released, including microvesicles, hemozoin, and glycosylphosphatidylinositols (GPI). These potential PAMPs and DAMPs might be recognized by DC through pattern recognition receptors, resulting in the secretion of interleukin 12 (IL-12), tumor necrosis factor (TNF), and IL-6 (Wu et al., 2015). DC-derived IL-12 might activate natural killer (NK) cells, which in turn secrete interferon γ (IFN-γ) and could thereby activate macrophages (Stevenson and Riley, 2004).

Several *Plasmodium*-derived molecules have been recognized as malaria PAMPs based on their ability to induce cytokine responses *in vitro* (**Figure 3**). One of the candidate malaria PAMPs are glycosylphosphatidylinositols (GPI). Although GPI are present in all eukaryotic cells where they serve as membrane anchors for certain cell surface proteins, *Plasmodium* GPI are structurally distinct from human GPI (Gowda, 2007). Consequently, *Plasmodium* GPI moieties may be recognized by the host immune system. Indeed, *P. falciparum* GPI were reported to induce the pro-inflammatory cytokines TNF and IL-1β in murine macrophages *in vitro* (Schofield and Hackett, 1993; Tachado et al., 1996). Moreover, purified GPI immobilized on gold particles elicited pronounced TNF responses from murine macrophages *in vitro* (Krishnegowda et al., 2005; Zhu et al., 2009, 2011), which was attributed to recognition of *P. falciparum* GPI through TLR2 or heterodimers of TLR2/1 and TLR2/6 (Krishnegowda et al., 2005; Zhu et al., 2011). However, given that TLR-deficiency did not impair immune responses elicited by *P. berghei* ANKA *in vivo* and did not protect mice from ECM (Togbe et al., 2007; Lepenies et al., 2008), the mechanism of GPI-induced innate immune activation *in vivo* remains to be determined.

Another potential malaria PAMP is hemozoin, an insoluble polymer formed inside the digestive vacuole to detoxify heme and its conjugated redox-active iron, which is released during hemoglobin proteolysis (Francis et al., 1997; Sigala and Goldberg, 2014). Hemozoin becomes accessible during erythrocyte rupture and upon phagocytosis of infected erythrocytes, and has been described to induce expression of pro-inflammatory cytokines, such as TNF and IL-1β, as well as chemokines from human monocytes, murine macrophages (Olivier et al., 2014), and human monocyte-derived DCs (Bujila et al., 2016). Hemozoin or hemozoin-bound nucleic acids are recognized by endosomal TLR9 (Coban et al., 2005; Parroche et al., 2007), cytoplasmic inflammasomes, or cytoplasmic sensors (Kalantari et al., 2014). However, it remains unresolved whether hemozoin itself or molecules bound to hemozoin, such as DNA, activate TLR9 (Liehl and Mota, 2012). In fact, the AT-rich *Plasmodium* genomic DNA, a feature shared by many pathogens including *Schistosoma*, was described to be immunomodulatory *in vitro*, but this response is apparently TLR9-independent (McCutchan et al., 1984; Sharma et al., 2011).

In addition to inducing pro-inflammatory responses, recognition of parasites and *Plasmodium*-infected erythrocytes is crucial for the phagocytic uptake and thus removal of parasites from the circulation by macrophages and DCs (McGilvray et al., 2000; Stevenson and Riley, 2004; **Figure 3**). Interestingly, although macrophages and DCs may both contribute to early pro-inflammatory cytokine responses *via* activation of PRR-mediated signaling, a recent study suggests that macrophage responsiveness is strongly compromised upon phagocytosis of *P. falciparum*- or *P. berghei*-infected erythrocytes or free merozoites due to pronounced phagosomal acidification (Wu et al., 2015). Instead, DCs contribute to increased serum levels of pro-inflammatory cytokines early during *P. berghei* infection, including IL-6, IL-12p40, and TNF (Wu et al., 2015).

Apart from parasite-derived stimuli, host-derived DAMPs such as urate crystals, heme, and microvesicles released from damaged host cells may activate the innate immune system, although so far this has only been demonstrated for microvesicles (Gazzinelli et al., 2014). *Plasmodium falciparum*-infected erythrocyte-derived microvesicles have been reported to induce TNF and IL-10 from monocyte-derived human macrophages *in vitro*, potentially through phagocytic uptake of microvesicles (Mantel et al., 2013). In line with this observation, plasma microparticles derived from *P. berghei* -infected mice stimulated bone marrow-derived macrophages to secrete TNF *in vitro*, and TNF induction was reported to be TLR4-dependent (Couper et al., 2010). In humans, increased numbers of plasma microparticles have been detected during *P. falciparum* and *P. vivax* infection, and microparticle numbers were higher in severe malaria cases, including CM, than in uncomplicated *P. falciparum* infections (Campos et al., 2010; Nantakomol et al., 2011; Sahu et al., 2013). Furthermore, two studies point toward infection-induced alterations in the microvesicle cargo, suggesting that not only microvesicle frequency but also content are relevant in inducing pro-inflammatory responses (Couper et al., 2010; Tiberti et al., 2016). Together, these studies indicate that microvesicles might contribute to CM pathogenesis and to other manifestations of severe malaria, and the association with pro-inflammatory immune responses warrants further investigations.

Although parasite-derived stimuli have been repeatedly reported to induce pro-inflammatory responses, the real qualitative and quantitative nature of the stimuli remains inadequately understood and may point toward a complex synergistic effect of multiple stimuli. Pro-inflammatory cytokines such as TNF, IL-1α (Kwiatkowski et al., 1990; Tchinda et al., 2007), IFN-γ and IL-12p40 (Hermsen et al., 2003), as well as chemokines, including IL-8/CXCL8 (Hermsen et al., 2003), platelet factor 4 (PF4)/CXCL4, and IP-10/CXCL10 (Wilson et al., 2011), are clearly elevated during *P. falciparum* infection. Several cytokines and chemokines, including TNF and CXCL10, have been found to be associated with CM severity (Kwiatkowski et al., 1990; Wilson et al., 2011), while a more recent study reported that neither plasma nor cerebrospinal fluid (CSF) TNF concentration were indicative of CM-associated mortality, yet elevated levels of TNF in CSF of pediatric CM cases were associated with long-term neurologic and cognitive deficits (Shabani et al., 2017). Consequently, it remains to be conclusively determined which cytokines and/or chemokines present suitable prognostic signatures of disease progression.

While many early studies focused on the identification of single inflammatory cytokines critically involved in malaria pathology, it is likely that numerous immune players are modulated during the course of a *Plasmodium* infection - sequentially and/or simultaneously. Accordingly, it is conceivable that a complex interplay of immune mediators contributes to the development of severe malaria in general, and to CM pathogenesis in particular. Several studies have addressed this issue by systematically analyzing pro- and anti-inflammatory markers. Since these studies included patients from different study sites of varying age and at various time points of infection, the cytokines identified to be associated with disease severity varied substantially, and the combination of selected analytes was heterogenous between studies (Prakash et al., 2006; Jain et al., 2008; Thuma et al., 2011). An early study reported two clusters of cytokines associated with mild and cerebral malaria, respectively, in *P. falciparum*-infected adults (Prakash et al., 2006). According to this study, IFN-γ, IL-2, IL-5, IL-6 and IL-12 were increased in mild malaria whereas TGF-β, TNF, IL-10 and IL-1β were particularly elevated in CM. In a study cohort of *P. falciparum*-infected children and adults, serum TNF levels did not correlate with disease severity, and instead IP-10/CXCL10, sTNF-R2, and sFas were proposed as biomarkers of CM severity and mortality (Jain et al., 2008). Additional cytokines were elevated in malaria cases compared to healthy controls and included IL-1ra, IL-10, IL-8/CXCL8, and macrophage inflammatory protein 1β (MIP-1β)/CCL4 (Jain et al., 2008). In two cohorts of *P. falciparum*-infected children, TNF concentration was slightly, albeit non-significantly, elevated in CM compared to severe anemia cases (Thuma et al., 2011; Mandala et al., 2017). In the study by Thuma et al. (2011) conducted in Zambia, IL-10, IL-1α, IL-6, and IP-10/CXCL10 plasma levels were higher in children suffering from CM than in children with severe anemia (Thuma et al., 2011). In line with these findings, Mandala et al. (2017) found higher IL-10 and IL-6 serum levels in Malawian children suffering from CM compared to those with severe anemia, while IFN-γ and IL-8/CXCL-8 were also elevated in pediatric CM cases.

In summary, cytokine profiling continues to aid in identifying distinct patterns of pro- and anti-inflammatory cytokines and chemokines in CM patients. Although a common cytokine/chemokine signature associated with CM severity has not yet been identified, which is in part due to the fact that the combination of markers investigated varies among studies, collectively, these studies point toward important roles for certain immunoregulatory molecules in modulating CM severity. In order to describe how inflammatory mediators associated with *Plasmodium* infection may contribute to CM pathogenesis, we will highlight their roles in endothelial activation, blood-brain barrier permeability, and neuroinflammation, by drawing on findings obtained from *in vitro* studies and the murine ECM model.

INFLAMMATION AND ENDOTHELIAL ACTIVATION

Functions of healthy endothelium include anti-coagulant properties through inhibiting platelet adhesion and aggregation, regulation of blood flow by releasing nitric oxide, controlling endothelial permeability, preventing extravasation of plasma proteins to tissue, and preventing leukocyte adhesion through suppressing adhesion molecule expression and sequestering chemokines within Weibel-Palade-bodies (Pober and Sessa, 2007). Under inflammatory conditions such as systemic inflammation during *Plasmodium* infection, endothelial activation may seriously impair endothelial function (**Figure 4**). A hallmark of endothelial activation is the expression of adhesion molecules such as VCAM-1 and ICAM-1 on the endothelial cell surface. Systemic endothelial activation was reported in *P. falciparum*-infected and in sepsis patients based on plasma levels of soluble adhesion molecules (Turner et al., 1998). Moreover, immunohistochemical analysis of fatal *P. falciparum* -infected CM cases revealed that expression of ICAM-1 was

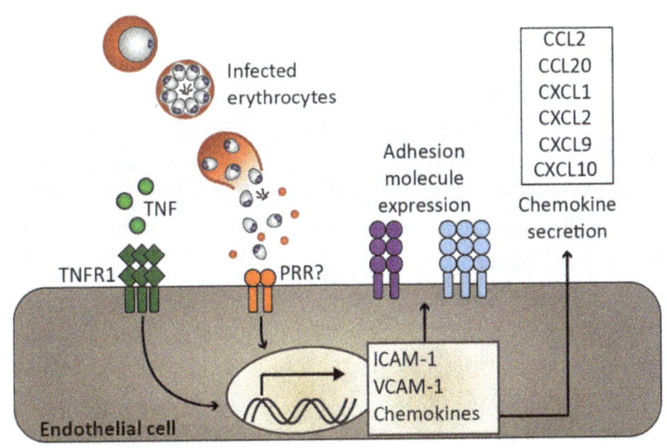

FIGURE 4 | Endothelial activation and chemokine secretion. A characteristic feature of *Plasmodium* infection is endothelial activation, which is likely induced by elevated serum tumor necrosis factor (TNF) levels. Binding of TNF to its receptor (TNFR1) induces transcription of adhesion molecules, including ICAM-1 and VCAM-1, as well as chemokines (Pober and Sessa, 2007). Endothelial activation might be directly induced by infected erythrocytes, possibly through activation of pattern recognition receptors (PRR), resulting in elevated expression of ICAM-1 and chemokine secretion (Viebig et al., 2005; Tripathi et al., 2006, 2009; Chakravorty et al., 2007).

most pronounced in the brain microvasculature compared to other organs and biopsies from non-malaria cases (Turner et al., 1994). In good agreement, ICAM-1 staining was described to be more pronounced on brain endothelial cells from *P. berghei* (strain ANKA)-infected mice during ECM than in those isolated from *P. yoelii*-infected (non-ECM) mice (Grau et al., 1991). Accordingly, *Icam1*-deficiency protected mice from *P. berghei*-induced ECM (Favre et al., 1999). Considering that adhesion molecules are thought to promote binding of infected erythrocytes and leukocytes to endothelial cells, and that human as well as murine CM is associated with intravascular accumulation of leukocytes in the brain (Hunt and Grau, 2003), these findings signify a critical role for endothelial activation in CM pathogenesis.

Among other factors, endothelial activation may be induced by inflammatory cytokines. TNF and lymphotoxin α (LTα) activate human endothelial cells *in vitro* (Cavender et al., 1989; Pober and Cotran, 1990). Similarly, IFN-γ, IL-1α, and IL-1β function in endothelial activation (Pober and Cotran, 1990; Bauer et al., 2002). These pro-inflammatory cytokines have been found to be elevated in serum or plasma of *P. falciparum*-infected patients and TNF as well as IL-1α and IL-1β were described to be associated with CM severity (Prakash et al., 2006; Thuma et al., 2011). Consequently, endothelial activation observed in *P. falciparum* infection might in part be mediated by these cytokines. In accordance with a proposed role for endothelial activation in CM, the pathology observed in murine ECM is associated with a T helper 1 (Th 1) immune response, and cytokines, such as IFN-γ, TNF, and LTα, and immune cells, e.g., $CD4^+$ and $CD8^+$ T cells together with NK cells are involved in ECM (Yanez et al., 1996; Lucas et al., 1997; Engwerda et al., 2002; Hunt and Grau, 2003; Schofield and Grau, 2005; Langhorne et al., 2008). Of note, despite an association of TNF with disease severity in CM, *Tnf*-deficient mice were not protected from ECM (Engwerda et al., 2002), and blocking of TNF by anti-TNF antibodies or pentoxifylline did not improve survival in human CM (Di Perri et al., 1995; van Hensbroek et al., 1996). Consequently, blocking TNF was demonstrated to be insufficient to prevent fatal CM, and, therefore, additional mechanisms are likely to critically contribute to CM pathogenesis. Moreover, these early therapeutic interventions highlight the complexity of this malaria syndrome, indicating that single serum cytokines associated with CM severity do not necessarily translate into therapeutic approaches. Notably, elevated serum TNF in particular may represent a secondary immune response, which might further amplify severity while not being critical in initiating CM pathogenesis.

Apart from the induction of endothelial activation by pro-inflammatory cytokines, endothelial cells are an important part of the innate immune response since they recognize PAMPs through expression of PRR such as TLR and NLR. Endothelial cells were found to secrete pro-inflammatory cytokines, including IL-1α, IL-1β, or IL-6, as well as immunomodulatory cytokines, namely IL-10 and TGF-β, and chemokines, e.g., monocyte chemoattractant protein 1 (MCP-1)/CCL2, RANTES/CCL5, and IL-8/CXCL8, upon stimulation by pro-inflammatory cytokines or lipopolysaccharide (LPS) *in vitro* (Mai et al., 2013). Notably, microvascular endothelial cells derived from subcutaneous adipose tissue of patients with uncomplicated malaria and fatal CM were demonstrated to differ in their endothelial inflammatory response to TNF stimulation *ex vivo* in that MCP-1/CCL2 and IL-6 were induced to a larger extent in endothelial cells derived from CM patients. Consequently, it was proposed that inter-individual differences in the endothelial response to inflammation might account for CM severity (Wassmer et al., 2011). These results support the notion that the pro-inflammatory microvascular environment during *P. falciparum* infection might be enhanced by endothelial cells. Interestingly, human brain microvascular endothelial cells have been described to phagocytose *P. berghei* merozoites *in vitro* (Howland et al., 2015b). Furthermore, upon co-culture with *P. falciparum*-infected erythrocytes, human endothelial cell lines were reported to upregulate ICAM-1 expression (Viebig et al., 2005; Tripathi et al., 2006), to increase transcription of *CCL20*, *CXCL1*, *CXCL2*, *CXCL8*, and *IL6* (Tripathi et al., 2009), and to secrete MCP-1/CCL2, MIP-3α/CCL20, and IL-8/CXCL8 (Viebig et al., 2005; Chakravorty et al., 2007) (**Figure 4**). Together, these *in vitro* observations suggest that endothelial cells are potentially directly involved in the immune response to *Plasmodium* infection. Since leukocyte sequestration in the microvasculature of the brain was described in human CM and murine ECM (Hunt and Grau, 2003), local chemokine gradients originating from brain endothelial cells might orchestrate leukocyte migration and thus promote local inflammation, thereby contributing to the development of CM.

Although the extent of the contribution of endothelial cell-derived chemokines in the process of leukocyte accumulation in brains of patients suffering from CM and of ECM mice remains to be established, a number of clinical studies reported that several chemokines are elevated in serum and CSF of CM patients, thereby providing a potential link between serum or CSF chemokine levels and progression from mild malaria to CM. Chemokines that were elevated in human CM cases included MCP-1/CCL2, MIP-1β/CCL4, PF4/CXCL4, IL-8/CXCL8, and IP-10/CXCL10 (Jain et al., 2008; Wilson et al., 2011). Particularly, MCP-1/CCL2, Eotaxin/CCL11, and IP-10/CXLC10 were reported to be indicative of disease severity (Armah et al., 2007; Jain et al., 2008; Thuma et al., 2011; Wilson et al., 2011). Moreover, *post mortem* MIP-1β/CCL4, IL-8/CXCL8, and IP-10/CXCL10 levels were significantly elevated in cerebrospinal fluid (CSF) of fatal *P. falciparum*-induced CM cases when compared to fatal severe malarial anemia cases and non-malaria deaths (Armah et al., 2007). In another study, IL-8/CXCL8 was elevated in CSF of non-fatal CM cases of *P. falciparum*-infected children (John et al., 2008b), while MCP-1/CCL2, MIP-1α/CCL3, MIP-1β/CCL4, and RANTES/CCL5 levels were comparable to malaria-free controls. The relevance of certain chemokines in cerebral malaria pathogenesis was demonstrated in the murine ECM model, in which *Cxcl4*-, *Cxcl9*-, or *Cxcl10*-deficiency resulted in reduced ECM-associated mortality (Campanella et al., 2008; Srivastava et al., 2008; Nie et al., 2009). Notably, PF4/CXCL4 was elevated in plasma of *P. berghei* ANKA-infected mice and demonstrated to induce TNF secretion from peritoneal macrophages and T cells *in vitro*, and *Cxcl4*-deficiency resulted in reduced serum TNF and IFN-γ levels during *P. berghei* ANKA-infection (Srivastava et al., 2008), indicating that PF4/CXCL4 contributes to establishing a pro-inflammatory environment, which might amplify further immune responses and could thereby promote CM pathogenesis. Furthermore, protection from ECM in *Cxcl10*-deficient mice was associated with a decrease in leukocyte sequestration in brains of *P. berghei* ANKA-infected mice, while parasite-specific $CXCR3^+$ T cells were increased in spleens of *Cxcl10*-deficient compared to WT mice (Nie et al., 2009), suggesting that IP-10/CXCL10-mediated recruitment of $CXCR3^+$ T cells to the brain might contribute to the development of ECM. A similar phenomenon might account for a decrease in ECM-associated mortality described for *Cxcl9*-deficient mice (Campanella et al., 2008), since recruitment of CXCR3-expressing cells can also be initiated by monokine induced by IFN-γ (MIG)/CXCL9. However, the precise mechanism by which MIG/CXCL9 contributes to ECM pathogenesis is yet to be determined. Apart from studies using specific gene deletions, chemokine transcripts were found to be induced to a higher extent in brains of ECM- compared to non-ECM mice. These transcripts included *Ccl2, Ccl3, Ccl4, Ccl5, Cxcl1, Cxcl9,* and *Cxcl10* (Miu et al., 2008; Van den Steen et al., 2008), supporting the finding that apart from NK and T cells, monocytes and neutrophils also sequester in the microvasculature (Renia et al., 2012), e.g., through recruitment by MCP-1/CCL2 and keratinocyte chemoattractant (KC)/*Cxcl1*, respectively. Nevertheless, studies to identify the cell types producing these chemokines in the brain are very limited. For instance, CXCL9 was demonstrated to be expressed by endothelial cells, while the source(s) of CXCL10 in the brain during *P. berghei* infection remain to be conclusively determined, and could include neurons, astrocytes, or endothelial cells (Campanella et al., 2008; Miu et al., 2008) as well as recruited monocytes (Ioannidis et al., 2016).

Together, activated endothelial cells likely contribute to local inflammation by secreting cytokines and chemokines, thereby recruiting leukocytes, including monocytes, macrophages, neutrophils and T cells, which accumulate in brains of mice and humans during ECM and CM, respectively (Renia et al., 2012; Storm and Craig, 2014). Since these cell types might secrete cytokines and chemokines themselves, local inflammation and endothelial activation could be further exacerbated (**Figure 5**). For instance, potential endothelial cell-induced recruitment of neutrophils and monocytes expressing IP-10/CXCL10 may promote further recruitment of $CXCR3^+$ cells such as NK and T cells to the brain (Ioannidis et al., 2016).

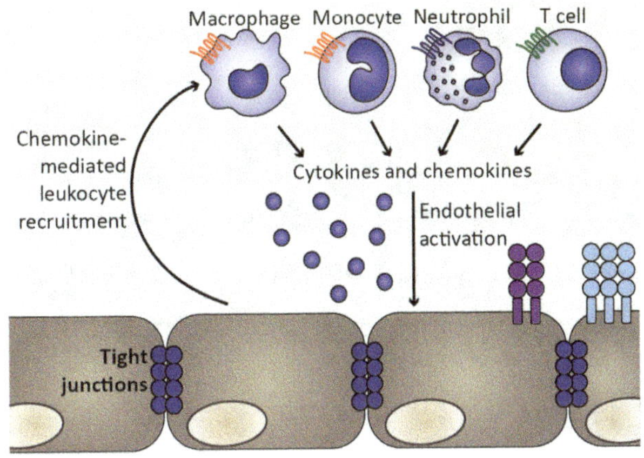

FIGURE 5 | Chemokine-mediated leukocyte recruitment and progression of local inflammation. As a consequence of endothelial activation by pro-inflammatory cytokines, such as TNF, and infected erythrocytes, chemokines are secreted from endothelial cells, which initiate recruitment of leukocytes expressing the respective chemokine receptors, including macrophages, monocytes, neutrophils, and T cell. These cell types were also found to sequester in the microvasculature during human CM as well as murine ECM (Hunt and Grau, 2003; Renia et al., 2012). Upon arrival at the site of the inflammatory insult, these leukocyte subsets may in turn secrete cytokines as well as chemokines, thereby further promoting endothelial activation and leukocyte recruitment. Thus, a feed-forward loop is initiated which exacerbates local inflammation in the brain.

ENDOTHELIAL ACTIVATION AND BLOOD-BRAIN BARRIER INTEGRITY

The blood-brain barrier is comprised of endothelial cells forming a continuous barrier through tight junctions, a basement membrane and astrocytes, which are in direct contact with neurons and microglia. This composition is critical to minimize local inflammation and neuronal damage (Obermeier et al., 2013). In the course of *Plasmodium* infection, endothelial activation may progress to vascular permeability and loss of blood-brain barrier integrity, as indicated by hemorrhages in brains of CM patients and extravasation of dyes or antibodies into the brain parenchyma in ECM (Renia et al., 2012). Although the extent of pathological events related to blood-brain barrier function in human CM is variable, dysfunction of the blood-brain barrier appears to be associated with progression of cerebral disease (Medana and Turner, 2006). Histology of brain sections from fatal human CM cases revealed a redistribution of the tight junction proteins occludin, vinculin, and zonula occludens 1 (ZO-1), which are central to blood-brain barrier integrity (Brown et al., 1999). Moreover, immunohistochemistry of brain sections derived from pediatric fatal CM cases indicated blood-brain barrier impairment in areas containing sequestered *P. falciparum*-infected erythrocytes, where they were associated with focal loss of endothelial intercellular junctions (Brown et al., 2001). Additionally, *in vitro* studies have demonstrated a decrease in endothelial resistance upon addition of *P. falciparum*-infected erythrocytes to endothelial cells (Tripathi et al., 2007; Jambou et al., 2010). This model, however, only partially reflects the response at the blood-brain barrier due to lack of barrier components such as astrocytes and pericytes (Medana and Turner, 2007).

Interestingly, MCP-1/CCL2 induces redistribution of tight junction proteins and increases endothelial permeability *in vitro* (Stamatovic et al., 2003; Song and Pachter, 2004; Yao and Tsirka, 2011). Thus, chemokines may contribute to organ-specific inflammation by inducing signals that promote endothelial permeability (**Figure 6**). The roles of the respective chemokine receptors are less clear in this context. This is exemplified in the

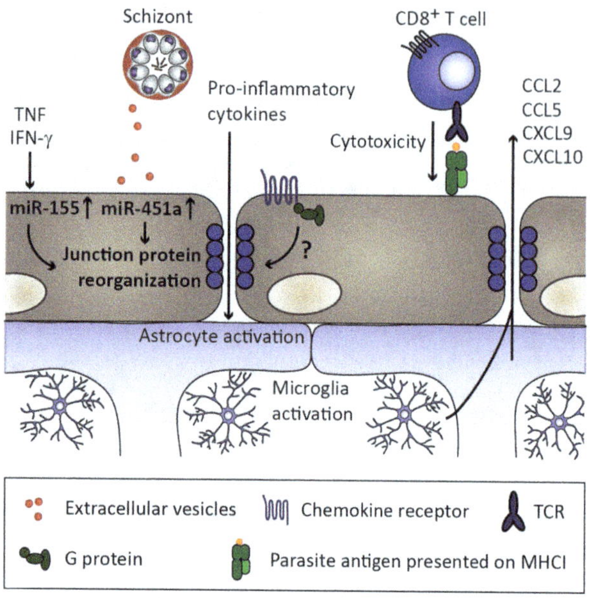

FIGURE 6 | Endothelial permeability and neuroinflammation. Through continued inflammatory insults toward endothelial cells by, for instance, circulating tumor necrosis factor (TNF) and interferon γ (IFN-γ), miR-155 might be upregulated in endothelial cells. Along with uptake of miR-451a from *P. falciparum*-infected erythrocyte-derived extracellular vesicles, reorganization of tight junction proteins such as zonula occludens 1 (ZO-1) is induced and could contribute to endothelial permeability during cerebral malaria (Lopez-Ramirez et al., 2014; Mantel et al., 2016). Additionally, chemokine receptors might induce redistribution of tight junction proteins in a G protein-dependent manner (Stamatovic et al., 2003; Song and Pachter, 2004; Yao and Tsirka, 2011), while the contribution of chemokine-induced opening of tight junctions is less clear in the context of cerebral malaria. CD8$^+$ T cell-mediated cytotoxity toward endothelial cells through recognition of parasite antigen presented on MHC class I molecules on endothelial cells likely contributes substantially to blood-brain barrier permeability during cerebral malaria (Howland et al., 2015a,b). Consequently, pro-inflammatory cytokines enter the brain parenchyma and could thereby activate astrocytes and microglia, which in turn could secrete chemokines (Capuccini et al., 2016) and thus promote leukocyte recruitment and local inflammation.

MCP-1/CCL2 receptor CCR2. *Ccr2*-deficiency abrogated CCL2-induced endothelial permeability *in vitro* (Stamatovic et al., 2003), but did not protect against ECM (Belnoue et al., 2003), indicating that other chemokines and/or additional mechanisms induce blood-brain barrier permeability.

Along with the observed redistribution of endothelial tight junction proteins and loss of intercellular junctions, growing evidence from the murine ECM model suggests that CD8$^+$ T cells are primary mediators in CM disease pathogenesis by contributing considerably to the loss of blood-brain barrier integrity (Howland et al., 2015a). Indeed, the accumulation of CD8$^+$ T cells in brains of *P. berghei* ANKA-infected mice appears to be critical for the development of ECM (Villegas-Mendez et al., 2012), and blood-brain barrier disruption was proposed to be a consequence of CD8$^+$ T cell-mediated cytotoxicity toward endothelial cells cross-presenting parasite antigen (Howland et al., 2015b) (**Figure 6**). Recruitment of CD8$^+$ T cells to the brain of infected mice has been described to be partly mediated by expression of the chemokine receptor CXCR3 and its IFN-γ-inducible ligands MIG/CXCL9 as well as IP-10/CXCL10 (Hansen et al., 2007; Villegas-Mendez et al., 2012). Indeed, NK cell-derived IFN-γ has been demonstrated to be crucial for the induction of CXCR3 expression on T cells and subsequent T-cell migration to the brain of *P. berghei* ANKA-infected mice (Hansen et al., 2007). In line with these findings, brain transcripts of *Cxcr3* were reduced in mice deficient for IFN-γR1 in comparison to wild type mice infected with *P. berghei* ANKA. Additionally, while expression of MIG/CXCL9 and IP-10/CXCL10 is induced in brains of *P. berghei* ANKA-infected wild type mice, expression levels of these chemokines in *Ifngr1*-deficient mice were similar to those of uninfected mice (Palomo et al., 2013). Collectively, these findings suggest that IFN-γ-induced signaling is crucial for chemokine-mediated leukocyte recruitment to the brain during ECM, while it remains to be established to which extent activated endothelium might contribute to this chemokine response.

Importantly, *Cxcr3*-deficient mice were less likely to succumb to ECM (Campanella et al., 2008; Miu et al., 2008), and numbers of CD4$^+$ and CD8$^+$ T cells in brains of *Cxcr3*-deficient mice were reported to be reduced compared to wild type mice during *P. berghei* ANKA infection. However, the extent of CD8$^+$ T cell recruitment was similar in *Cxcr3*-deficient mice which were either resistant or susceptible to ECM (Miu et al., 2008). These results indicate that the quantity of CD8$^+$ T cells in brains of *P. berghei* ANKA-infected mice is not critical for the development of ECM. Rather, additional aspects such as CD8$^+$ T-cell specificity toward parasite antigen presented on endothelium, expression levels of key cytotoxic effector molecules perforin and granzyme B by CD8$^+$ T cells, and localization of these CD8$^+$ T cells within the brain might play a substantial role in the development of ECM (Miu et al., 2008; Haque et al., 2011; Howland et al., 2015b; Huggins et al., 2017). Nevertheless, it remains to be determined why susceptibility to ECM among *Cxcr3*-deficient mice is variable. Moreover, these findings indicate that additional mechanisms other than CD8$^+$ T cell-mediated cytotoxicity might be involved in the loss of blood-brain barrier integrity.

In fact, in addition to CD8$^+$ T cells and chemokines, extracellular vesicles derived from *P. falciparum*-infected erythrocytes were recently implicated in blood-brain barrier permeability *in vitro* (Mantel et al., 2016; **Figure 6**). These extracellular vesicles contained miRNA miR-451a, which, upon endocytosis by endothelial cells, correlated with reduced endothelial caveolin-1 expression. Interestingly, MCP-1/CCL2-induced redistribution of tight junction proteins and concomitant endothelial permeability (Stamatovic et al., 2003) was also accompanied by a decrease in caveolin-1 protein (Song and Pachter, 2004), thus pointing toward a common underlying mechanism in the induction of endothelial permeability by CCL2 and extracellular vesicles derived from *P. falciparum*-infected erythrocytes. Since sequestration of infected erythrocytes in the microvasculature is likely promoted by expression of adhesion molecules upon endothelial activation, locally increased release of *P. falciparum*-infected erythrocyte-derived extracellular vesicles carrying miRNA miR-451a might be an additional mechanism involved in blood-brain barrier permeability in CM.

In addition to miR-451a, another miRNA, miR-155, was implicated in inflammation-associated blood-brain barrier permeability. Upon stimulation of human brain endothelial cells with pro-inflammatory cytokines TNF and IFN-γ *in vitro*, miR-155 was found to be upregulated. The tight junction protein claudin-1 was reported to be among the candidate targets of miR-155, and cytokine stimulation or miR-155 overexpression resulted in reorganization of the tight junction protein ZO-1 along with increased endothelial permeability (Lopez-Ramirez et al., 2014), indicating that cytokines such as TNF and IFN-γ might directly contribute to blood-brain barrier permeability through induction of regulatory miRNAs. Interestingly, levels of miR-155 were recently reported to be elevated in extracellular vesicles in the circulation of *P. berghei* ANKA-infected mice, and *miR-155*-deficiency resulted in preservation of blood-brain barrier integrity and reduced ECM-associated mortality (Barker et al., 2017). Notably, plasma concentrations of IL-6, IFN-γ, and MCP-1/CCL2 were significantly elevated in *P. berghei* ANKA-infected *miR-155*-deficient compared to wild type mice in this study, suggesting that miR-155 might have additional targets other than tight junction proteins. Importantly, whether miR-155-carrying extracellular vesicles are derived from activated endothelium, and their impact on tight junction reorganization in the context of ECM, remain to be determined. Nevertheless, inhibition of the function of miR-155 might present a useful target for therapeutic approaches (Barker et al., 2017). These processes of chemokine induction, microvascular sequestration of infected erythrocytes and leukocytes, and release of extracellular vesicles carrying regulatory miRNAs are most likely not exclusive to the brain. However, endothelial permeability is likely more detrimental in the brain than in other organs and, hence, cerebral malaria may be the most severe manifestation of these processes. Additionally, brain endothelial cells have been described to express comparably low levels of thrombin-binding thrombomodulin, and excess of unbound thrombin may further promote local endothelial activation by inducing further expression of adhesion molecules (Clark et al., 2006).

Together, cytokine- or *Plasmodium*-induced endothelial activation may lead to chemokine induction and leukocyte recruitment as well as sequestration of infected erythrocytes, which may act synergistically in promoting endothelial permeability. Nevertheless, the precise molecular mechanisms that trigger loss of blood-brain barrier integrity in CM are incompletely understood and need to be further investigated.

NEUROINFLAMMATION

Upon disruption of the blood-brain barrier, cytokines, chemokines, and soluble parasite products might enter the brain parenchyma and, thereby, activate astrocytes and microglia, and result in symptoms of neuroinflammation in the absence of extravasation of infected erythrocytes or leukocytes into the brain parenchyma (Combes et al., 2010). Indeed, activation of microglia and astrocytes has been observed in murine and human CM (Hunt et al., 2006; Combes et al., 2010). For instance, transcriptome analysis of microglia isolated from *P. berghei*-infected mice revealed that several chemokines as well as transcripts related to type I IFN signaling were differentially upregulated (Capuccini et al., 2016). This finding was confirmed *in vitro* by stimulation of a murine microglia cell line with IFN-β, which resulted in secretion of MCP-1/CCL2, RANTES/CCL5, MIG/CXCL9, and IP-10/CXCL10. Moreover, stimulation of human primary astrocytes with a combination of IFN-γ and LTα synergistically induced IP-10/CXCL10 secretion *in vitro* (Bakmiwewa et al., 2016). Additionally, co-culture of *P. berghei*-infected erythrocytes with a mixed astrocyte-microglia culture resulted in phagocytic uptake of infected erythrocytes and of parasitized erythrocyte-derived microvesicles by microglia and astrocytes, respectively, which in turn was associated with an induction in IP-10/CXCL10 secretion (Shrivastava et al., 2017). Furthermore, astrocytes and microglia may secrete various cytokines and chemokines upon activation (Dong and Benveniste, 2001; Medana et al., 2001). Consequently, loss of blood-brain barrier integrity and subsequent activation of microglia and astrocytes might result in further chemokine-mediated recruitment of leukocytes to the brain and subsequent amplification of inflammation (**Figure 6**). Additionally, activation of microglia might induce expression of FasL, which, upon binding to Fas expressed on astrocytes, could induce astrocyte damage (Hunt et al., 2006). However, to our knowledge, this has so far not been demonstrated in the context of CM. Since astrocytes are critically involved in maintaining blood-brain barrier properties and survival of neurons (Combes et al., 2010), their functional impairment might disrupt neuronal activity and could thereby account for the neurological impairment observed in some CM cases (Hunt et al., 2006).

SUMMARY AND PERSPECTIVES

The human and murine immune system are in part strikingly different (Stevenson and Riley, 2004). For instance, IL-8/CXCL8 was reported to be associated with cerebral malaria (Armah et al., 2007; John et al., 2008b), while this chemokine is not expressed in mice (Viola and Luster, 2008). However, KC/*Cxcl1* is considered a functional homolog of IL-8/CXCL8 in mice (Hol et al., 2010), which mediates neutrophil recruitment, and *Cxcl1* transcripts were reported to be elevated in brains of ECM compared to non-ECM mice (Miu et al., 2008), suggesting that KC/*Cxcl1* might be similarly involved in ECM pathogenesis. Yet, the precise contribution of IL-8/CXCL8 and KC/*Cxcl1* to human CM and murine ECM, respectively, needs to be further investigated. Moreover, the murine ECM model shares several features with human CM, including aspects of histopathology and inflammatory responses. Importantly, mechanistic insights can only be gained from the murine ECM model, and many observations are in remarkably good agreement with clinical data obtained from *P. falciparum*-induced CM. Although a comprehensive representation of the events leading to CM pathogenesis remains elusive, a working model of an inflammatory cascade leading to CM is conceivable (**Figure 1**).

Upon establishing liver stage infection, a first type I IFN response is mounted by hepatocytes, leading to a primary activation of IFN-γ-producing NK cells (Liehl et al., 2014; Miller et al., 2014; **Figure 2**) and, consequently, induction of MIG/CXCL9 and IP-10/CXCL10 secretion, potentially from endothelial cells (Campanella et al., 2008; Miu et al., 2008). Upon progression of the *Plasmodium* infection to the blood stages, infected erythrocytes are recognized by DCs and induce the secretion of IL-12 and TNF (Wu et al., 2015; **Figure 3**). IL-12 contributes to further activation of NK and differentiation of Th1 cells (Stevenson and Riley, 2004), while TNF and IFN-γ activate chemokine transcription and adhesion molecule expression on endothelial cells (Pober and Sessa, 2007; Miu et al., 2008; Griffith et al., 2014). As the infection progresses further, *Plasmodium*-infected erythrocytes are recognized by endothelial cells and induce expression of chemokines, such as MCP-1/CCL2 and IL-8/CXCL8 (Viebig et al., 2005; Chakravorty et al., 2007; Tripathi et al., 2009; **Figure 4**). As a result, leukocytes are recruited, including monocytes, macrophages, neutrophils, as well as T cells, and initiate a local inflammatory response (Renia et al., 2012; Storm and Craig, 2014; **Figure 5**). These cell types secrete chemokines, thereby amplifying the response leading to further leukocyte recruitment and intensifying local inflammation. Additionally, endothelial cells phagocytose merozoites and parasite material released during schizont rupture and present parasite antigens to CD8$^+$ T cells (Howland et al., 2015b; **Figure 6**), which may result in targeted elimination of antigen-presenting endothelial cells and, thus, cause damages to the endothelial lining of the blood-brain barrier. This process can be further exacerbated by openings of tight junctions mediated by chemokines and extracellular vesicle-derived miRNAs (Song and Pachter, 2004; Mantel et al., 2016). As a result, small molecules can enter the brain parenchyma and potentially activate brain-resident microglia and astrocytes, further amplifying local inflammation through cytokine secretion and leukocyte recruitment and impairing neuronal functionality (Hunt et al., 2006; Combes et al., 2010).

Even though the febrile response elicited during *Plasmodium* blood stage infection together with the concomitant inflammatory cytokine responses limit parasite growth and mediate the resolution of infection, imbalances in pro-inflammatory and anti-inflammatory cytokines cause progression of malaria disease to manifestations of severe malaria, such as CM, and death. Adjunctive therapies that prevent adverse effects of the immune response to *Plasmodium* infection are therefore urgently needed. Although immunomodulation is a promising approach to alleviate immune-mediated pathology, such therapies need to be designed carefully in order to maintain efficient control of parasite growth. Notably, adjunct therapies modulating chemokine responses may have fewer side-effects compared to therapies based on neutralizing cytokines (Ioannidis et al., 2014). Indeed, antibody-mediated targeting of IP-10/CXCL10 was demonstrated to result in reduced ECM-induced mortality and parasite burden in mice, which was likely mediated by retention and expansion of parasite-specific T cells in the spleen (Nie et al., 2009). Such treatments may be relevant in other contexts as well: murine *Toxoplasma* encephalitis has been described to be associated with constant expression of *Ccl2*, *Ccl3*, *Ccl4*, *Ccl5*, and *Cxcl10* in brains of infected mice concomitant with continuous recruitment of CD4$^+$ and CD8$^+$ T cells, which was not the case for mice in which the infection developed into chronic latency (Strack et al., 2002). Furthermore, targeted neutralization of single chemokines, including MCP-1/CCL2, MIP-1α/CCL3, RANTES/CCL5, or IP-10/CXCL10, resulted in protection of mice from experimental autoimmune encephalomyelitis, a murine model for multiple sclerosis (Karin and Wildbaum, 2015). These findings from other neuroinflammatory diseases highlight that chemokines might present a valuable target for intervention strategies in several diseases. However, efforts to design chemokine-based therapies are challenged by the complexity of the chemokine system as well as properties such as redundancy, pleiotropy, and speciation (Viola and Luster, 2008). In fact, most cell populations express several different chemokine receptors and thus single chemokine or chemokine receptor blockade may not affect disease outcome in certain pathological conditions.

Together, reliable biomarkers which predict disease outcome and allow for potential prophylactic measures are yet to be identified. Several clinical studies have reported potential diagnostic and prognostic biomarkers for CM, which apart from chemokines such as IP-10/CXCL10 and PF4/CXCL4 also include *P. falciparum* histidine-rich protein 2 (*Pf*HRP2), a protein which correlates with parasite biomass, as well as regulators of endothelial activation angiopoietin-1 and -2 (summarized in Sahu et al., 2015). Still, comprehensive studies with defined clinical parameters and systematic assessment of plasma levels of multiple inflammatory mediators need to be performed to determine whether distinct clusters of markers can be associated with disease severity in order to identify patients at risk of developing CM early during infection. Such studies will inform future investigations into mechanisms underlying disease pathogenesis in order to develop novel evidence-based malaria intervention strategies.

AUTHOR CONTRIBUTIONS

All authors listed have made a substantial, direct and intellectual contribution to the work, and approved it for publication.

ACKNOWLEDGMENTS

Work on chemokines and cytokines in murine malaria models is funded by the Deutsche Forschungsgemeinschaft (KA 3347/4-1) and partly by the Max Planck Society.

REFERENCES

Adams, Y., Kuhnrae, P., Higgins, M. K., Ghumra, A., and Rowe, J. A. (2014). Rosetting *Plasmodium falciparum*-infected erythrocytes bind to human brain microvascular endothelial cells *in vitro*, demonstrating a dual adhesion phenotype mediated by distinct *P. falciparum* erythrocyte membrane protein 1 domains. *Infect. Immun.* 82, 949–959. doi: 10.1128/IAI.01233-13

Anstey, N. M., Russell, B., Yeo, T. W., and Price, R. N. (2009). The pathophysiology of *vivax* malaria. *Trends Parasitol.* 25, 220–227. doi: 10.1016/j.pt.2009.02.003

Armah, H. B., Wilson, N. O., Sarfo, B. Y., Powell, M. D., Bond, V. C., Anderson, W., et al. (2007). Cerebrospinal fluid and serum biomarkers of cerebral malaria mortality in Ghanaian children. *Malar. J.* 6:147. doi: 10.1186/1475-2875-6-147

Bakmiwewa, S. M., Weiser, S., Grey, M., Heng, B., Guillemin, G. J., Ball, H. J., et al. (2016). Synergistic induction of CXCL10 by interferon-gamma and lymphotoxin-alpha in astrocytes: possible role in cerebral malaria. *Cytokine* 78, 79–86. doi: 10.1016/j.cyto.2015.11.024

Barker, K. R., Lu, Z., Kim, H., Zheng, Y., Chen, J., Conroy, A. L., et al. (2017). miR-155 modifies inflammation, endothelial activation and blood-brain barrier dysfunction in cerebral malaria. *Mol. Med.* 23, 24–33. doi: 10.2119/molmed.2016.00139

Bate, C. A., and Kwiatkowski, D. P. (1994). Stimulators of tumour necrosis factor production released by damaged erythrocytes. *Immunology* 83, 256–261.

Bauer, P. R., Van Der Heyde, H. C., Sun, G., Specian, R. D., and Granger, D. N. (2002). Regulation of endothelial cell adhesion molecule expression in an experimental model of cerebral malaria. *Microcirculation* 9, 463–470. doi: 10.1038/sj.mn.7800159

Beare, N. A., Harding, S. P., Taylor, T. E., Lewallen, S., and Molyneux, M. E. (2009). Perfusion abnormalities in children with cerebral malaria and malarial retinopathy. *J. Infect. Dis.* 199, 263–271. doi: 10.1086/595735

Beare, N. A., Taylor, T. E., Harding, S. P., Lewallen, S., and Molyneux, M. E. (2006). Malarial retinopathy: a newly established diagnostic sign in severe malaria. *Am. J. Trop. Med. Hyg.* 75, 790–797. doi: 10.4269/ajtmh.2006.75.790

Beeson, J. G., Drew, D. R., Boyle, M. J., Feng, G., Fowkes, F. J., and Richards, J. S. (2016). Merozoite surface proteins in red blood cell invasion, immunity and vaccines against malaria. *FEMS Microbiol. Rev.* 40, 343–372. doi: 10.1093/femsre/fuw001

Belnoue, E., Costa, F. T., Vigario, A. M., Voza, T., Gonnet, F., Landau, I., et al. (2003). Chemokine receptor CCR2 is not essential for the development of experimental cerebral malaria. *Infect. Immun.* 71, 3648–3651. doi: 10.1128/IAI.71.6.3648-3651.2003

Bernabeu, M., Danziger, S. A., Avril, M., Vaz, M., Babar, P. H., Brazier, A. J., et al. (2016). Severe adult malaria is associated with specific PfEMP1 adhesion types and high parasite biomass. *Proc. Natl. Acad. Sci. U.S.A.* 113, E3270–E3279. doi: 10.1073/pnas.1524294113

Bernabeu, M., and Smith, J.D. (2017). EPCR and malaria severity: the center of a perfect storm. *Trends Parasitol.* 33, 295–308. doi: 10.1016/j.pt.2016.11.004

Bozza, F. A., Salluh, J. I., Japiassu, A. M., Soares, M., Assis, E. F., Gomes, R. N., et al. (2007). Cytokine profiles as markers of disease severity in sepsis: a multiplex analysis. *Crit. Care* 11, R49. doi: 10.1186/cc5783

Brown, H., Hien, T. T., Day, N., Mai, N. T., Chuong, L. V., Chau, T. T., et al. (1999). Evidence of blood-brain barrier dysfunction in human cerebral malaria. *Neuropathol. Appl. Neurobiol.* 25, 331–340. doi: 10.1046/j.1365-2990.1999.00188.x

Brown, H., Rogerson, S., Taylor, T., Tembo, M., Mwenechanya, J., Molyneux, M., et al. (2001). Blood-brain barrier function in cerebral malaria in Malawian children. *Am. J. Trop. Med. Hyg.* 64, 207–213. doi: 10.4269/ajtmh.2001.64.207

Bujila, I., Schwarzer, E., Skorokhod, O., Weidner, J. M., Troye-Blomberg, M., and Ostlund Farrants, A. K. (2016). Malaria-derived hemozoin exerts early modulatory effects on the phenotype and maturation of human dendritic cells. *Cell. Microbiol.* 18, 413–423. doi: 10.1111/cmi.12521

Campanella, G. S., Tager, A. M., El Khoury, J. K., Thomas, S. Y., Abrazinski, T. A., Manice, L. A., et al. (2008). Chemokine receptor CXCR3 and its ligands CXCL9 and CXCL10 are required for the development of murine cerebral malaria. *Proc. Natl. Acad. Sci. U.S.A.* 105, 4814–4819. doi: 10.1073/pnas.0801544105

Campos, F. M., Franklin, B. S., Teixeira-Carvalho, A., Filho, A. L., De Paula, S. C., Fontes, C. J., et al. (2010). Augmented plasma microparticles during acute *Plasmodium vivax* infection. *Malar. J.* 9:327. doi: 10.1186/1475-2875-9-327

Capuccini, B., Lin, J., Talavera-Lopez, C., Khan, S. M., Sodenkamp, J., Spaccapelo, R., et al. (2016). Transcriptomic profiling of microglia reveals signatures of cell activation and immune response, during experimental cerebral malaria. *Sci. Rep.* 6:39258. doi: 10.1038/srep39258

Cavender, D. E., Edelbaum, D., and Ziff, M. (1989). Endothelial cell activation induced by tumor necrosis factor and lymphotoxin. *Am. J. Pathol.* 134, 551–560.

Chakravorty, S. J., Carret, C., Nash, G. B., Ivens, A., Szestak, T., and Craig, A. G. (2007). Altered phenotype and gene transcription in endothelial cells, induced by *Plasmodium falciparum*-infected red blood cells: pathogenic or protective? *Int. J. Parasitol.* 37, 975–987. doi: 10.1016/j.ijpara.2007.02.006

Chen, Q., Schlichtherle, M., and Wahlgren, M. (2000). Molecular aspects of severe malaria. *Clin. Microbiol. Rev.* 13, 439–450. doi: 10.1128/CMR.13.3.439-450.2000

Clark, I. A., Alleva, L. M., Mills, A. C., and Cowden, W. B. (2004). Pathogenesis of malaria and clinically similar conditions. *Clin. Microbiol. Rev.* 17, 509–539. doi: 10.1128/CMR.17.3.509-539.2004

Clark, I. A., Budd, A. C., Alleva, L. M., and Cowden, W. B. (2006). Human malarial disease: a consequence of inflammatory cytokine release. *Malar. J.* 5:85. doi: 10.1186/1475-2875-5-85

Clark, I. A., and Rockett, K. A. (1994). The cytokine theory of human cerebral malaria. *Parasitol. Today* 10, 410–412. doi: 10.1016/0169-4758(94)90237-2

Clark, I.A., and Vissel, B. (2017). The meteorology of cytokine storms, and the clinical usefulness of this knowledge. *Semin. Immunopathol.* 39, 505–516. doi: 10.1007/s00281-017-0628-y

Coban, C., Ishii, K. J., Kawai, T., Hemmi, H., Sato, S., Uematsu, S., et al. (2005). Toll-like receptor 9 mediates innate immune activation by the malaria pigment hemozoin. *J. Exp. Med.* 201, 19–25. doi: 10.1084/jem.20041836

Combes, V., El-Assaad, F., Faille, D., Jambou, R., Hunt, N. H., and Grau, G. E. (2010). Microvesiculation and cell interactions at the brain-endothelial interface in cerebral malaria pathogenesis. *Prog. Neurobiol.* 91, 140–151. doi: 10.1016/j.pneurobio.2010.01.007

Couper, K. N., Barnes, T., Hafalla, J. C., Combes, V., Ryffel, B., Secher, T., et al. (2010). Parasite-derived plasma microparticles contribute significantly to malaria infection-induced inflammation through potent macrophage stimulation. *PLoS Pathog.* 6:e1000744. doi: 10.1371/journal.ppat.1000744

Craig, A. G., Grau, G. E., Janse, C., Kazura, J. W., Milner, D., Barnwell, J. W., et al. (2012). The role of animal models for research on severe malaria. *PLoS Pathog.* 8:e1002401. doi: 10.1371/journal.ppat.1002401

Cui, L., Mharakurwa, S., Ndiaye, D., Rathod, P. K., and Rosenthal, P. J. (2015). Antimalarial drug resistance: literature review and activities and findings of the ICEMR network. *Am. J. Trop. Med. Hyg.* 93, 57–68. doi: 10.4269/ajtmh.15-0007

De Backer, D., Creteur, J., Preiser, J. C., Dubois, M. J., and Vincent, J. L. (2002). Microvascular blood flow is altered in patients with sepsis. *Am. J. Respir. Crit. Care Med.* 166, 98–104. doi: 10.1164/rccm.200109-016OC

de Souza, J. B., and Riley, E. M. (2002). Cerebral malaria: the contribution of studies in animal models to our understanding of immunopathogenesis. *Microbes Infect.* 4, 291–300. doi: 10.1016/S1286-4579(02)01541-1

Di Perri, G., Di Perri, I. G., Monteiro, G. B., Bonora, S., Hennig, C., Cassatella, M., et al. (1995). Pentoxifylline as a supportive agent in the treatment of cerebral malaria in children. *J. Infect. Dis.* 171, 1317–1322. doi: 10.1093/infdis/171.5.1317

Dondorp, A. M., Fanello, C. I., Hendriksen, I. C., Gomes, E., Seni, A., Chhaganlal, K. D., et al. (2010). Artesunate versus quinine in the treatment of severe *falciparum* malaria in African children (AQUAMAT): an open-label, randomised trial. *Lancet* 376, 1647–1657. doi: 10.1016/S0140-6736(10)61924-1

Dondorp, A. M., Ince, C., Charunwatthana, P., Hanson, J., Van Kuijen, A., Faiz, M. A., et al. (2008). Direct *in vivo* assessment of microcirculatory dysfunction in severe *falciparum* malaria. *J. Infect. Dis.* 197, 79–84. doi: 10.1086/523762

Dondorp, A. M., Pongponratn, E., and White, N. J. (2004). Reduced microcirculatory flow in severe *falciparum* malaria: pathophysiology and electron-microscopic pathology. *Acta Trop.* 89, 309–317. doi: 10.1016/j.actatropica.2003.10.004

Dondorp, A., Nosten, F., Stepniewska, K., Day, N., White, N., and South East Asian Quinine Artesunate Malaria Trial, G. (2005). Artesunate versus quinine for treatment of severe *falciparum* malaria: a randomised trial. *Lancet* 366, 717–725. doi: 10.1016/S0140-6736(05)67176-0

Dong, Y., and Benveniste, E. N. (2001). Immune function of astrocytes. *Glia* 36, 180–190. doi: 10.1002/glia.1107

Engwerda, C. R., Mynott, T. L., Sawhney, S., De Souza, J. B., Bickle, Q. D., and Kaye, P. M. (2002). Locally up-regulated lymphotoxin alpha, not systemic tumor necrosis factor alpha, is the principle mediator of murine cerebral malaria. *J. Exp. Med.* 195, 1371–1377. doi: 10.1084/jem.20020128

Eriksson, E. M., Sampaio, N. G., and Schofield, L. (2013). Toll-like Receptors and malaria: sensing and susceptibility. *J. Trop. Dis.* 2:126. doi: 10.4172/2329-891X.1000126

Evans, S. S., Repasky, E. A., and Fisher, D. T. (2015). Fever and the thermal regulation of immunity: the immune system feels the heat. *Nat. Rev. Immunol.* 15, 335–349. doi: 10.1038/nri3843

Favre, N., Da Laperousaz, C., Ryffel, B., Weiss, N. A., Imhof, B. A., Rudin, W., et al. (1999). Role of ICAM-1 (CD54) in the development of murine cerebral malaria. *Microbes Infect.* 1, 961–968. doi: 10.1016/S1286-4579(99)80513-9

Francis, S. E., Sullivan, D. J. Jr., and Goldberg, D.E. (1997). Hemoglobin metabolism in the malaria parasite *Plasmodium falciparum*. *Annu. Rev. Microbiol.* 51, 97–123. doi: 10.1146/annurev.micro.51.1.97

Gazzinelli, R. T., Kalantari, P., Fitzgerald, K. A., and Golenbock, D. T. (2014). Innate sensing of malaria parasites. *Nat. Rev. Immunol.* 14, 744–757. doi: 10.1038/nri3742

Gilson, P. R., and Crabb, B. S. (2009). Morphology and kinetics of the three distinct phases of red blood cell invasion by *Plasmodium falciparum* merozoites. *Int. J. Parasitol.* 39, 91–96. doi: 10.1016/j.ijpara.2008.09.007

Gowda, D. C. (2007). TLR-mediated cell signaling by malaria GPIs. *Trends Parasitol.* 23, 596–604. doi: 10.1016/j.pt.2007.09.003

Grau, G. E., Pointaire, P., Piguet, P. F., Vesin, C., Rosen, H., Stamenkovic, I., et al. (1991). Late administration of monoclonal antibody to leukocyte function-antigen 1 abrogates incipient murine cerebral malaria. *Eur. J. Immunol.* 21, 2265–2267. doi: 10.1002/eji.1830210939

Griffith, J. W., Sokol, C. L., and Luster, A. D. (2014). Chemokines and chemokine receptors: positioning cells for host defense and immunity. *Annu. Rev. Immunol.* 32, 659–702. doi: 10.1146/annurev-immunol-032713-120145

Hafalla, J. C., Silvie, O., and Matuschewski, K. (2011). Cell biology and immunology of malaria. *Immunol. Rev.* 240, 297–316. doi: 10.1111/j.1600-065X.2010.00988.x

Haldar, K., Murphy, S. C., Milner, D. A., and Taylor, T. E. (2007). Malaria: mechanisms of erythrocytic infection and pathological correlates of severe disease. *Annu. Rev. Pathol.* 2, 217–249. doi: 10.1146/annurev.pathol.2.010506.091913

Handunnetti, S. M., David, P. H., Perera, K. L., and Mendis, K. N. (1989). Uninfected erythrocytes form "rosettes" around *Plasmodium falciparum* infected erythrocytes. *Am. J. Trop. Med. Hyg.* 40, 115–118. doi: 10.4269/ajtmh.1989.40.115

Hansen, D. S., Bernard, N. J., Nie, C. Q., and Schofield, L. (2007). NK cells stimulate recruitment of CXCR3+ T cells to the brain during *Plasmodium berghei*-mediated cerebral malaria. *J. Immunol.* 178, 5779–5788. doi: 10.4049/jimmunol.178.9.5779

Haque, A., Best, S. E., Unosson, K., Amante, F. H., De Labastida, F., Anstey, N. M., et al. (2011). Granzyme B expression by CD8+ T cells is required for the development of experimental cerebral malaria. *J. Immunol.* 186, 6148–6156. doi: 10.4049/jimmunol.1003955

Hermsen, C. C., Konijnenberg, Y., Mulder, L., Loe, C., Van Deuren, M., Van Der Meer, J. W., et al. (2003). Circulating concentrations of soluble granzyme A and B increase during natural and experimental *Plasmodium falciparum* infections. *Clin. Exp. Immunol.* 132, 467–472. doi: 10.1046/j.1365-2249.2003.02 160.x

Hol, J., Wilhelmsen, L., and Haraldsen, G. (2010). The murine IL-8 homologues KC, MIP-2, and LIX are found in endothelial cytoplasmic granules but not in Weibel-Palade bodies. *J. Leukoc. Biol.* 87, 501–508. doi: 10.1189/jlb .0809532

Howland, S. W., Claser, C., Poh, C. M., Gun, S. Y., and Renia, L. (2015a). Pathogenic CD8+ T cells in experimental cerebral malaria. *Semin. Immunopathol.* 37, 221–231. doi: 10.1007/s00281-015-0476-6

Howland, S. W., Poh, C. M., and Renia, L. (2015b). Activated brain endothelial cells cross-present malaria antigen. *PLoS Pathog.* 11:e1004963. doi: 10.1371/journal.ppat.1004963

Huggins, M. A., Johnson, H. L., Jin, F., N'Songo A., Hanson, L. M., Lafrance, S. J., et al. (2017). Perforin expression by CD8 T cells Is sufficient to cause fatal brain edema during experimental cerebral malaria. *Infect. Immun.* 85, e00985–e00916. doi: 10.1128/IAI.00985-16

Hunt, N. H., Golenser, J., Chan-Ling, T., Parekh, S., Rae, C., Potter, S., et al. (2006). Immunopathogenesis of cerebral malaria. *Int. J. Parasitol.* 36, 569–582. doi: 10.1016/j.ijpara.2006.02.016

Hunt, N. H., and Grau, G. E. (2003). Cytokines: accelerators and brakes in the pathogenesis of cerebral malaria. *Trends Immunol.* 24, 491–499. doi: 10.1016/S1471-4906(03)00229-1

Idro, R., Marsh, K., John, C. C., and Newton, C. R. (2010). Cerebral malaria: mechanisms of brain injury and strategies for improved neurocognitive outcome. *Pediatr. Res.* 68, 267–274. doi: 10.1203/PDR.0b013e3181eee738

Ioannidis, L. J., Nie, C. Q., and Hansen, D. S. (2014). The role of chemokines in severe malaria: more than meets the eye. *Parasitology* 141, 602–613. doi: 10.1017/S0031182013001984

Ioannidis, L. J., Nie, C. Q., Ly, A., Ryg-Cornejo, V., Chiu, C. Y., and Hansen, D. S. (2016). Monocyte- and neutrophil-derived CXCL10 impairs efficient control of blood-stage malaria infection and promotes severe disease. *J. Immunol.* 196, 1227–1238. doi: 10.4049/jimmunol.1501562

Jain, V., Armah, H. B., Tongren, J. E., Ned, R. M., Wilson, N. O., Crawford, S., et al. (2008). Plasma IP-10, apoptotic and angiogenic factors associated with fatal cerebral malaria in India. *Malar. J.* 7:83. doi: 10.1186/1475-2875-7-83

Jambou, R., Combes, V., Jambou, M. J., Weksler, B. B., Couraud, P. O., and Grau, G. E. (2010). *Plasmodium falciparum* adhesion on human brain microvascular endothelial cells involves transmigration-like cup formation and induces opening of intercellular junctions. *PLoS Pathog.* 6:e1001021. doi: 10.1371/journal.ppat.1001021

John, C. C., Bangirana, P., Byarugaba, J., Opoka, R. O., Idro, R., Jurek, A. M., et al. (2008a). Cerebral malaria in children is associated with long-term cognitive impairment. *Pediatrics* 122, e92–e99. doi: 10.1542/peds.2007-3709

John, C. C., Panoskaltsis-Mortari, A., Opoka, R. O., Park, G. S., Orchard, P. J., Jurek, A. M., et al. (2008b). Cerebrospinal fluid cytokine levels and cognitive impairment in cerebral malaria. *Am. J. Trop. Med. Hyg.* 78, 198–205. doi: 10.4269/ajtmh.2008.78.198

Kalantari, P., Deoliveira, R. B., Chan, J., Corbett, Y., Rathinam, V., Stutz, A., et al. (2014). Dual engagement of the NLRP3 and AIM2 inflammasomes by *plasmodium*-derived hemozoin and DNA during malaria. *Cell Rep.* 6, 196–210. doi: 10.1016/j.celrep.2013.12.014

Karin, N., and Wildbaum, G. (2015). The role of chemokines in shaping the balance between CD4(+) T cell subsets and its therapeutic implications in autoimmune and cancer diseases. *Front. Immunol.* 6:609. doi: 10.3389/fimmu.2015.00609

Karunaweera, N. D., Grau, G. E., Gamage, P., Carter, R., and Mendis, K. N. (1992). Dynamics of fever and serum levels of tumor necrosis factor are closely associated during clinical paroxysms in *Plasmodium vivax* malaria. *Proc. Natl. Acad. Sci. U.S.A.* 89, 3200–3203. doi: 10.1073/pnas.89.8.3200

Kochar, D. K., Das, A., Kochar, S. K., Saxena, V., Sirohi, P., Garg, S., et al. (2009). Severe *Plasmodium vivax* malaria: a report on serial cases from Bikaner in northwestern India. *Am. J. Trop. Med. Hyg.* 80, 194–198. doi: 10.3410/f.1161230.621714

Kordes, M., Matuschewski, K., and Hafalla, J.C. (2011). Caspase-1 activation of interleukin-1beta (IL-1beta) and IL-18 is dispensable for induction of experimental cerebral malaria. *Infect. Immun.* 79, 3633–3641. doi: 10.1128/IAI.05459-11

Krishnegowda, G., Hajjar, A. M., Zhu, J., Douglass, E. J., Uematsu, S., Akira, S., et al. (2005). Induction of proinflammatory responses in macrophages by the glycosylphosphatidylinositols of *Plasmodium falciparum*: cell signaling receptors, glycosylphosphatidylinositol (GPI) structural requirement, and regulation of GPI activity. *J. Biol. Chem.* 280, 8606–8616. doi: 10.1074/jbc.M413541200

Kwiatkowski, D., Cannon, J. G., Manogue, K. R., Cerami, A., Dinarello, C. A., and Greenwood, B. M. (1989). Tumour necrosis factor production in Falciparum malaria and its association with schizont rupture. *Clin. Exp. Immunol.* 77, 361–366.

Kwiatkowski, D., Hill, A. V., Sambou, I., Twumasi, P., Castracane, J., Manogue, K. R., et al. (1990). TNF concentration in fatal cerebral, non-fatal cerebral, and uncomplicated Plasmodium falciparum malaria. *Lancet* 336, 1201–1204. doi: 10.1016/0140-6736(90)92827-5

Langhorne, J., Ndungu, F. M., Sponaas, A. M., and Marsh, K. (2008). Immunity to malaria: more questions than answers. *Nat. Immunol.* 9, 725–732. doi: 10.1038/ni.f.205

Lennartz, F., Adams, Y., Bengtsson, A., Olsen, R. W., Turner, L., Ndam, N. T., et al. (2017). Structure-guided identification of a family of dual receptor-binding PfEMP1 that is associated with cerebral malaria. *Cell Host Microbe* 21, 403–414. doi: 10.1016/j.chom.2017.02.009

Lepenies, B., Cramer, J. P., Burchard, G. D., Wagner, H., Kirschning, C. J., and Jacobs, T. (2008). Induction of experimental cerebral malaria is independent of TLR2/4/9. *Med. Microbiol. Immunol.* 197, 39–44. doi: 10.1007/s00430-007-0057-y

Liehl, P., and Mota, M. M. (2012). Innate recognition of malarial parasites by mammalian hosts. *Int. J. Parasitol.* 42, 557–566. doi: 10.1016/j.ijpara.2012.04.006

Liehl, P., Zuzarte-Luis, V., Chan, J., Zillinger, T., Baptista, F., Carapau, D., et al. (2014). Host-cell sensors for *Plasmodium* activate innate immunity against liver-stage infection. *Nat. Med.* 20, 47–53. doi: 10.1038/nm.3424

Lopez-Ramirez, M. A., Wu, D., Pryce, G., Simpson, J. E., Reijerkerk, A., King-Robson, J., et al. (2014). MicroRNA-155 negatively affects blood-brain barrier function during neuroinflammation. *FASEB J.* 28, 2551–2565. doi: 10.1096/fj.13-248880

Lucas, R., Juillard, P., Decoster, E., Redard, M., Burger, D., Donati, Y., et al. (1997). Crucial role of tumor necrosis factor (TNF) receptor 2 and membrane-bound TNF in experimental cerebral malaria. *Eur. J. Immunol.* 27, 1719–1725. doi: 10.1002/eji.1830270719

Mai, J., Virtue, A., Shen, J., Wang, H., and Yang, X. F. (2013). An evolving new paradigm: endothelial cells–conditional innate immune cells. *J. Hematol. Oncol.* 6:61. doi: 10.1186/1756-8722-6-61

Mandala, W. L., Msefula, C. L., Gondwe, E. N., Drayson, M. T., Molyneux, M. E., and Maclennan, C. A. (2017). Cytokine profiles in Malawian children presenting with uncomplicated malaria, severe malarial anemia and cerebral malaria. *Clin. Vaccine Immunol.* 24:e00533-16. doi: 10.1128/CVI.00533-16

Mantel, P. Y., Hjelmqvist, D., Walch, M., Kharoubi-Hess, S., Nilsson, S., Ravel, D., et al. (2016). Infected erythrocyte-derived extracellular vesicles alter vascular function via regulatory Ago2-miRNA complexes in malaria. *Nat. Commun.* 7:12727. doi: 10.1038/ncomms12727

Mantel, P. Y., Hoang, A. N., Goldowitz, I., Potashnikova, D., Hamza, B., Vorobjev, I., et al. (2013). Malaria-infected erythrocyte-derived microvesicles mediate cellular communication within the parasite population and with the host immune system. *Cell Host Microbe* 13, 521–534. doi: 10.1016/j.chom.2013.04.009

McCutchan, T. F., Dame, J. B., Miller, L. H., and Barnwell, J. (1984). Evolutionary relatedness of *Plasmodium* species as determined by the structure of DNA. *Science* 225, 808–811. doi: 10.1126/science.6382604

McGilvray, I. D., Serghides, L., Kapus, A., Rotstein, O. D., and Kain, K. C. (2000). Nonopsonic monocyte/macrophage phagocytosis of *Plasmodium falciparum*-parasitized erythrocytes: a role for CD36 in malarial clearance. *Blood* 96, 3231–3240. Available online at: http://www.bloodjournal.org/content/96/9/3231

Medana, I. M., Chaudhri, G., Chan-Ling, T., and Hunt, N. H. (2001). Central nervous system in cerebral malaria: 'Innocent bystander' or active participant in the induction of immunopathology? *Immunol. Cell Biol.* 79, 101–120. doi: 10.1046/j.1440-1711.2001.00995.x

Medana, I. M., and Turner, G. D. (2006). Human cerebral malaria and the blood-brain barrier. *Int. J. Parasitol.* 36, 555–568. doi: 10.1016/j.ijpara.2006.02.004

Medana, I. M., and Turner, G. D. (2007). *Plasmodium falciparum* and the blood-brain barrier–contacts and consequences. *J. Infect. Dis.* 195, 921–923. doi: 10.1086/512089

Miller, J. L., Sack, B. K., Baldwin, M., Vaughan, A. M., and Kappe, S. H. (2014). Interferon-mediated innate immune responses against malaria parasite liver stages. *Cell Rep.* 7, 436–447. doi: 10.1016/j.celrep.2014.03.018

Miller, L. H., Baruch, D. I., Marsh, K., and Doumbo, O. K. (2002). The pathogenic basis of malaria. *Nature* 415, 673–679. doi: 10.1038/415673a

Milner, D. A. Jr., Lee, J. J., Frantzreb, C., Whitten, R. O., Kamiza, S., Carr, R. A., et al. (2015). Quantitative assessment of multiorgan sequestration of parasites in fatal pediatric cerebral malaria. *J. Infect. Dis.* 212, 1317–1321. doi: 10.1093/infdis/jiv205

Milner, D. A. Jr., Whitten, R. O., Kamiza, S., Carr, R., Liomba, G., Dzamalala, C., et al. (2014). The systemic pathology of cerebral malaria in African children. *Front. Cell. Infect. Microbiol.* 4:104. doi: 10.3389/fcimb.2014.00104

Miu, J., Mitchell, A. J., Muller, M., Carter, S. L., Manders, P. M., Mcquillan, J. A., et al. (2008). Chemokine gene expression during fatal murine cerebral malaria and protection due to CXCR3 deficiency. *J. Immunol.* 180, 1217–1230. doi: 10.4049/jimmunol.180.2.1217

Nantakomol, D., Dondorp, A. M., Krudsood, S., Udomsangpetch, R., Pattanapanyasat, K., Combes, V., et al. (2011). Circulating red cell-derived microparticles in human malaria. *J. Infect. Dis.* 203, 700–706. doi: 10.1093/infdis/jiq104

Nie, C. Q., Bernard, N. J., Norman, M. U., Amante, F. H., Lundie, R. J., Crabb, B. S., et al. (2009). IP-10-mediated T cell homing promotes cerebral inflammation over splenic immunity to malaria infection. *PLoS Pathog.* 5:e1000369. doi: 10.1371/journal.ppat.1000369

Oakley, M. S., Gerald, N., Mccutchan, T. F., Aravind, L., and Kumar, S. (2011). Clinical and molecular aspects of malaria fever. *Trends Parasitol.* 27, 442–449. doi: 10.1016/j.pt.2011.06.004

Obermeier, B., Daneman, R., and Ransohoff, R. M. (2013). Development, maintenance and disruption of the blood-brain barrier. *Nat. Med.* 19, 1584–1596. doi: 10.1038/nm.3407

Olivier, M., Van Den Ham, K., Shio, M. T., Kassa, F. A., and Fougeray, S. (2014). Malarial pigment hemozoin and the innate inflammatory response. *Front. Immunol.* 5:25. doi: 10.3389/fimmu.2014.00025

Olotu, A., Fegan, G., Wambua, J., Nyangweso, G., Leach, A., Lievens, M., et al. (2016). Seven-Year efficacy of RTS,S/AS01 malaria vaccine among young African children. *N. Engl. J. Med.* 374, 2519–2529. doi: 10.1056/NEJMoa1515257

Pain, A., Ferguson, D. J., Kai, O., Urban, B. C., Lowe, B., Marsh, K., et al. (2001). Platelet-mediated clumping of *Plasmodium falciparum*-infected erythrocytes is a common adhesive phenotype and is associated with severe malaria. *Proc. Natl. Acad. Sci. U.S.A.* 98, 1805–1810. doi: 10.1073/pnas.98.4.1805

Palomo, J., Fauconnier, M., Coquard, L., Gilles, M., Meme, S., Szeremeta, F., et al. (2013). Type I interferons contribute to experimental cerebral malaria development in response to sporozoite or blood-stage *Plasmodium berghei* ANKA. *Eur. J. Immunol.* 43, 2683–2695. doi: 10.1002/eji.201343327

Parroche, P., Lauw, F. N., Goutagny, N., Latz, E., Monks, B. G., Visintin, A., et al. (2007). Malaria hemozoin is immunologically inert but radically enhances innate responses by presenting malaria DNA to Toll-like receptor 9. *Proc. Natl. Acad. Sci. U.S.A.* 104, 1919–1924. doi: 10.1073/pnas.0608745104

Pasloske, B. L., and Howard, R. J. (1994). Malaria, the red cell, and the endothelium. *Annu. Rev. Med.* 45, 283–295. doi: 10.1146/annurev.med.45.1.283

Pober, J. S., and Cotran, R. S. (1990). Cytokines and endothelial cell biology. *Physiol. Rev.* 70, 427–451.

Pober, J. S., and Sessa, W. C. (2007). Evolving functions of endothelial cells in inflammation. *Nat. Rev. Immunol.* 7, 803–815. doi: 10.1038/nri2171

Ponsford, M. J., Medana, I. M., Prapansilp, P., Hien, T. T., Lee, S. J., Dondorp, A. M., et al. (2012). Sequestration and microvascular congestion are associated with coma in human cerebral malaria. *J. Infect. Dis.* 205, 663–671. doi: 10.1093/infdis/jir812

Prakash, D., Fesel, C., Jain, R., Cazenave, P. A., Mishra, G. C., and Pied, S. (2006). Clusters of cytokines determine malaria severity in *Plasmodium falciparum*-infected patients from endemic areas of central India. *J. Infect. Dis.* 194, 198–207. doi: 10.1086/504720

Renia, L., Howland, S. W., Claser, C., Charlotte Gruner, A., Suwanarusk, R., Hui Teo, T., et al. (2012). Cerebral malaria: mysteries at the blood-brain barrier. *Virulence* 3, 193–201. doi: 10.4161/viru.19013

Riley, E. M., Couper, K. N., Helmby, H., Hafalla, J. C., De Souza, J. B., Langhorne, J., et al. (2010). Neuropathogenesis of human and murine malaria. *Trends Parasitol.* 26, 277–278. doi: 10.1016/j.pt.2010.03.002

Rowe, J. A., Claessens, A., Corrigan, R. A., and Arman, M. (2009). Adhesion of *Plasmodium falciparum*-infected erythrocytes to human cells: molecular mechanisms and therapeutic implications. *Expert Rev. Mol. Med.* 11:e16. doi: 10.1017/S1462399409001082

Sahu, P. K., Satpathi, S., Behera, P. K., Mishra, S. K., Mohanty, S., and Wassmer, S. C. (2015). Pathogenesis of cerebral malaria: new diagnostic tools, biomarkers, and therapeutic approaches. *Front. Cell. Infect. Microbiol.* 5:75. doi: 10.3389/fcimb.2015.00075

Sahu, U., Sahoo, P. K., Kar, S. K., Mohapatra, B. N., and Ranjit, M. (2013). Association of TNF level with production of circulating cellular microparticles during clinical manifestation of human cerebral malaria. *Hum. Immunol.* 74, 713–721. doi: 10.1016/j.humimm.2013.02.006

Schofield, L., and Grau, G. E. (2005). Immunological processes in malaria pathogenesis. *Nat. Rev. Immunol.* 5, 722–735. doi: 10.1038/nri1686

Schofield, L., and Hackett, F. (1993). Signal transduction in host cells by a glycosylphosphatidylinositol toxin of malaria parasites. *J. Exp. Med.* 177, 145–153. doi: 10.1084/jem.177.1.145

Shabani, E., Ouma, B. J., Idro, R., Bangirana, P., Opoka, R. O., Park, G. S., et al. (2017). Elevated cerebrospinal fluid tumour necrosis factor is associated with acute and long-term neurocognitive impairment in cerebral malaria. *Parasite Immunol.* 39:e12438. doi: 10.1111/pim.12438

Sharma, S., Deoliveira, R. B., Kalantari, P., Parroche, P., Goutagny, N., Jiang, Z., et al. (2011). Innate immune recognition of an AT-rich stem-loop DNA motif in the *Plasmodium falciparum* genome. *Immunity* 35, 194–207. doi: 10.1016/j.immuni.2011.05.016

Shrivastava, S. K., Dalko, E., Delcroix-Genete, D., Herbert, F., Cazenave, P. A., and Pied, S. (2017). Uptake of parasite-derived vesicles by astrocytes and microglial phagocytosis of infected erythrocytes may drive neuroinflammation in cerebral malaria. *Glia* 65, 75–92. doi: 10.1002/glia.23075

Sigala, P. A., and Goldberg, D. E. (2014). The peculiarities and paradoxes of *Plasmodium* heme metabolism. *Annu. Rev. Microbiol.* 68, 259–278. doi: 10.1146/annurev-micro-091313-103537

Smith, J. D., Rowe, J. A., Higgins, M. K., and Lavstsen, T. (2013). Malaria's deadly grip: cytoadhesion of *Plasmodium falciparum*-infected erythrocytes. *Cell. Microbiol.* 15, 1976–1983. doi: 10.1111/cmi.12183

Song, L., and Pachter, J. S. (2004). Monocyte chemoattractant protein-1 alters expression of tight junction-associated proteins in brain microvascular endothelial cells. *Microvasc. Res.* 67, 78–89. doi: 10.1016/j.mvr.2003.07.001

Srivastava, K., Cockburn, I. A., Swaim, A., Thompson, L. E., Tripathi, A., Fletcher, C. A., et al. (2008). Platelet factor 4 mediates inflammation in experimental cerebral malaria. *Cell Host Microbe* 4, 179–187. doi: 10.1016/j.chom.2008.07.003

Stamatovic, S. M., Keep, R. F., Kunkel, S. L., and Andjelkovic, A. V. (2003). Potential role of MCP-1 in endothelial cell tight junction 'opening': signaling via Rho and Rho kinase. *J. Cell Sci.* 116, 4615–4628. doi: 10.1242/jcs.00755

Stevenson, M. M., and Riley, E. M. (2004). Innate immunity to malaria. *Nat. Rev. Immunol.* 4, 169–180. doi: 10.1038/nri1311

Storm, J., and Craig, A. G. (2014). Pathogenesis of cerebral malaria–inflammation and cytoadherence. *Front. Cell. Infect. Microbiol.* 4:100. doi: 10.3389/fcimb.2014.00100

Strack, A., Schlüter, D., Asensio, V.C., Campbell, I. L., and Deckert, M. (2002). Regulation of the kinetics of intracerebral chemokine gene expression in murine *Toxoplasma* encephalitis: impact of host genetic factors. *Glia* 40, 372–377. doi: 10.1002/glia.10104

Tachado, S. D., Gerold, P., Mcconville, M. J., Baldwin, T., Quilici, D., Schwarz, R. T., et al. (1996). Glycosylphosphatidylinositol toxin of *Plasmodium* induces nitric oxide synthase expression in macrophages and vascular endothelial cells by a protein tyrosine kinase-dependent and protein kinase C-dependent signaling pathway. *J. Immunol.* 156, 1897–1907.

Takeuchi, O., and Akira, S. (2010). Pattern recognition receptors and inflammation. *Cell* 140, 805–820. doi: 10.1016/j.cell.2010.01.022

Tchinda, V. H., Tadem, A. D., Tako, E. A., Tene, G., Fogako, J., Nyonglema, P., et al. (2007). Severe malaria in Cameroonian children: correlation between plasma levels of three soluble inducible adhesion molecules and TNF-alpha. *Acta Trop.* 102, 20–28. doi: 10.1016/j.actatropica.2007.02.011

Thuma, P. E., Van Dijk, J., Bucala, R., Debebe, Z., Nekhai, S., Kuddo, T., et al. (2011). Distinct clinical and immunologic profiles in severe malarial anemia and cerebral malaria in Zambia. *J. Infect. Dis.* 203, 211–219. doi: 10.1093/infdis/jiq041

Tiberti, N., Latham, S. L., Bush, S., Cohen, A., Opoka, R. O., John, C. C., et al. (2016). Exploring experimental cerebral malaria pathogenesis through the characterisation of host-derived plasma microparticle protein content. *Sci. Rep.* 6:37871. doi: 10.1038/srep37871

Togbe, D., Schofield, L., Grau, G. E., Schnyder, B., Boissay, V., Charron, S., et al. (2007). Murine cerebral malaria development is independent of toll-like receptor signaling. *Am. J. Pathol.* 170, 1640–1648. doi: 10.2353/ajpath.2007.060889

Tripathi, A. K., Sha, W., Shulaev, V., Stins, M. F., and Sullivan, D. J. Jr., (2009). *Plasmodium falciparum*-infected erythrocytes induce NF-kappaB regulated inflammatory pathways in human cerebral endothelium. *Blood* 114, 4243–4252. doi: 10.1182/blood-2009-06-226415

Tripathi, A. K., Sullivan, D. J., and Stins, M. F. (2006). *Plasmodium falciparum*-infected erythrocytes increase intercellular adhesion molecule 1 expression on brain endothelium through NF-kappaB. *Infect. Immun.* 74, 3262–3270. doi: 10.1128/IAI.01625-05

Tripathi, A. K., Sullivan, D. J., and Stins, M. F. (2007). *Plasmodium falciparum*-infected erythrocytes decrease the integrity of human blood-brain barrier endothelial cell monolayers. *J. Infect. Dis.* 195, 942–950. doi: 10.1086/512083

Turner, G. D., Ly, V. C., Nguyen, T. H., Tran, T. H., Nguyen, H. P., Bethell, D., et al. (1998). Systemic endothelial activation occurs in both mild and severe malaria. Correlating dermal microvascular endothelial cell phenotype and soluble cell adhesion molecules with disease severity. *Am. J. Pathol.* 152, 1477–1487.

Turner, G. D., Morrison, H., Jones, M., Davis, T. M., Looareesuwan, S., Buley, I. D., et al. (1994). An immunohistochemical study of the pathology of fatal malaria. Evidence for widespread endothelial activation and a potential role for intercellular adhesion molecule-1 in cerebral sequestration. *Am. J. Pathol.* 145, 1057–1069.

Turner, L., Lavstsen, T., Berger, S. S., Wang, C. W., Petersen, J. E., Avril, M., et al. (2013). Severe malaria is associated with parasite binding to endothelial protein C receptor. *Nature* 498, 502–505. doi: 10.1038/nature12216

Van den Steen, P. E., Deroost, K., Van Aelst, I., Geurts, N., Martens, E., Struyf, S., et al. (2008). CXCR3 determines strain susceptibility to murine cerebral malaria by mediating T lymphocyte migration toward IFN-gamma-induced chemokines. *Eur. J. Immunol.* 38, 1082–1095. doi: 10.1002/eji.200737906

van der Heyde, H. C., Nolan, J., Combes, V., Gramaglia, I., and Grau, G. E. (2006). A unified hypothesis for the genesis of cerebral malaria: sequestration, inflammation and hemostasis leading to microcirculatory dysfunction. *Trends Parasitol.* 22, 503–508. doi: 10.1016/j.pt.2006.09.002

van Hensbroek, M. B., Palmer, A., Onyiorah, E., Schneider, G., Jaffar, S., Dolan, G., et al. (1996). The effect of a monoclonal antibody to tumor necrosis factor on survival from childhood cerebral malaria. *J. Infect. Dis.* 174, 1091–1097. doi: 10.1093/infdis/174.5.1091

Viebig, N. K., Wulbrand, U., Forster, R., Andrews, K. T., Lanzer, M., and Knolle, P. A. (2005). Direct activation of human endothelial cells by *Plasmodium falciparum*-infected erythrocytes. *Infect. Immun.* 73, 3271–3277. doi: 10.1128/IAI.73.6.3271-3277.2005

Villegas-Mendez, A., Greig, R., Shaw, T. N., De Souza, J. B., Gwyer Findlay, E., Stumhofer, J. S., et al. (2012). IFN-gamma-producing CD4+ T cells promote experimental cerebral malaria by modulating CD8+ T cell accumulation within the brain. *J. Immunol.* 189, 968–979. doi: 10.4049/jimmunol.1200688

Viola, A., and Luster, A. D. (2008). Chemokines and their receptors: drug targets in immunity and inflammation. *Annu. Rev. Pharmacol. Toxicol.* 48, 171–197. doi: 10.1146/annurev.pharmtox.48.121806.154841

Wassmer, S. C., and Grau, G. E. (2017). Severe malaria: what's new on the pathogenesis front? *Int. J. Parasitol.* 47, 145–152. doi: 10.1016/j.ijpara.2016.08.002

Wassmer, S. C., Moxon, C. A., Taylor, T., Grau, G. E., Molyneux, M. E., and Craig, A. G. (2011). Vascular endothelial cells cultured from patients with cerebral or uncomplicated malaria exhibit differential reactivity to TNF. *Cell. Microbiol.* 13, 198–209. doi: 10.1111/j.1462-5822.2010.01528.x

WHO (2016). *World Malaria Report 2016*. Geneva: World Health Organisation.

White, M. T., Verity, R., Griffin, J. T., Asante, K. P., Owusu-Agyei, S., Greenwood, B., et al. (2015). Immunogenicity of the RTS,S/AS01 malaria vaccine and implications for duration of vaccine efficacy: secondary analysis of data from a phase 3 randomised controlled trial. *Lancet Infect. Dis.* 15, 1450–1458. doi: 10.1016/S1473-3099(15)00239-X

Wilson, N. O., Jain, V., Roberts, C. E., Lucchi, N., Joel, P. K., Singh, M. P., et al. (2011). CXCL4 and CXCL10 predict risk of fatal cerebral malaria. *Dis. Markers* 30, 39–49. doi: 10.1155/2011/828256

Wu, X., Gowda, N. M., and Gowda, D. C. (2015). Phagosomal acidification prevents macrophage inflammatory cytokine production to malaria, and dendritic cells are the major source at the early stages of infection: implication for malaria protective immunity development. *J. Biol. Chem.* 290, 23135–23147. doi: 10.1074/jbc.M115.671065

Yanez, D. M., Manning, D. D., Cooley, A. J., Weidanz, W. P., and Van Der Heyde, H. C. (1996). Participation of lymphocyte subpopulations in the pathogenesis of experimental murine cerebral malaria. *J. Immunol.* 157, 1620–1624.

Yao, Y., and Tsirka, S. E. (2011). Truncation of monocyte chemoattractant protein 1 by plasmin promotes blood-brain barrier disruption. *J. Cell Sci.* 124, 1486–1495. doi: 10.1242/jcs.082834

Zhu, J., Krishnegowda, G., Li, G., and Gowda, D. C. (2011). Proinflammatory responses by glycosylphosphatidylinositols (GPIs) of *Plasmodium falciparum* are mainly mediated through the recognition of TLR2/TLR1. *Exp. Parasitol.* 128, 205–211. doi: 10.1016/j.exppara.2011.03.010

Zhu, J., Wu, X., Goel, S., Gowda, N. M., Kumar, S., Krishnegowda, G., et al. (2009). MAPK-activated protein kinase 2 differentially regulates plasmodium falciparum glycosylphosphatidylinositol-induced production of tumor necrosis factor-{alpha} and interleukin-12 in macrophages. *J. Biol. Chem.* 284, 15750–15761. doi: 10.1074/jbc.M901111200

Zlotnik, A., and Yoshie, O. (2012). The chemokine superfamily revisited. *Immunity* 36, 705–716. doi: 10.1016/j.immuni.2012.05.008

Permissions

All chapters in this book were first published in PIFEMNS, by Frontiers; hereby published with permission under the Creative Commons Attribution License or equivalent. Every chapter published in this book has been scrutinized by our experts. Their significance has been extensively debated. The topics covered herein carry significant findings which will fuel the growth of the discipline. They may even be implemented as practical applications or may be referred to as a beginning point for another development.

The contributors of this book come from diverse backgrounds, making this book a truly international effort. This book will bring forth new frontiers with its revolutionizing research information and detailed analysis of the nascent developments around the world.

We would like to thank all the contributing authors for lending their expertise to make the book truly unique. They have played a crucial role in the development of this book. Without their invaluable contributions this book wouldn't have been possible. They have made vital efforts to compile up to date information on the varied aspects of this subject to make this book a valuable addition to the collection of many professionals and students.

This book was conceptualized with the vision of imparting up-to-date information and advanced data in this field. To ensure the same, a matchless editorial board was set up. Every individual on the board went through rigorous rounds of assessment to prove their worth. After which they invested a large part of their time researching and compiling the most relevant data for our readers.

The editorial board has been involved in producing this book since its inception. They have spent rigorous hours researching and exploring the diverse topics which have resulted in the successful publishing of this book. They have passed on their knowledge of decades through this book. To expedite this challenging task, the publisher supported the team at every step. A small team of assistant editors was also appointed to further simplify the editing procedure and attain best results for the readers.

Apart from the editorial board, the designing team has also invested a significant amount of their time in understanding the subject and creating the most relevant covers. They scrutinized every image to scout for the most suitable representation of the subject and create an appropriate cover for the book.

The publishing team has been an ardent support to the editorial, designing and production team. Their endless efforts to recruit the best for this project, has resulted in the accomplishment of this book. They are a veteran in the field of academics and their pool of knowledge is as vast as their experience in printing. Their expertise and guidance has proved useful at every step. Their uncompromising quality standards have made this book an exceptional effort. Their encouragement from time to time has been an inspiration for everyone.

The publisher and the editorial board hope that this book will prove to be a valuable piece of knowledge for researchers, students, practitioners and scholars across the globe.

List of Contributors

Totta Ehret
FG16 - Mycotic and Parasitic Agents and Mycobacteria, Robert Koch Institute, Berlin, Germany
Department of Molecular Parasitology, Humboldt-Universität zu Berlin, Berlin, Germany

Francesca Torelli, Christian Klotz and Frank Seeber
FG16 - Mycotic and Parasitic Agents and Mycobacteria, Robert Koch Institute, Berlin, Germany

Amy B. Pedersen
School of Biological Sciences, University of Edinburgh, Edinburgh, United Kingdom

Malgorzata Jennes, Bert Devriendt and Eric Cox
Laboratory for Immunology, Faculty of Veterinary Medicine, Ghent University, Merelbeke, Belgium

Stéphane De Craeye and Katelijne Dierick
National Reference Laboratory for Toxoplasmosis, Operational Direction Communicable and Infectious Diseases, Scientific Institute of Public Health, Security of Food Chain and Environment, Brussels, Belgium

Pierre Dorny
Department of Biomedical Sciences, Institute for Tropical Medicine, Antwerp, Belgium
Laboratory for Parasitology, Faculty of Veterinary Medicine, Ghent University, Merelbeke, Belgium

Che J. Ngwa, Meike J. Kiesow, Olga Papst, Alina N. Rosinski and Gabriele Pradel
Division of Cellular and Applied Infection Biology, RWTH Aachen University, Aachen, Germany
Department of Medical Parasitology and Infection Biology, Swiss Tropical and Public Health Institute, Basel, Switzerland
Department of Chemistry and Huck Center for Malaria Research, The Pennsylvania State University, University Park, PA, United States

Lindsey M. Orchard
Department of Biochemistry and Molecular Biology, The Pennsylvania State University, University Park, PA, United States

Michael Filarsky and Till S. Voss
Department of Medical Parasitology and Infection Biology, Swiss Tropical and Public Health Institute, Basel, Switzerland

Manuel Llinás
Department of Chemistry and Huck Center for Malaria Research, The Pennsylvania State University, University Park, PA, United States
Department of Biochemistry and Molecular Biology, The Pennsylvania State University, University Park, PA, United States

Christina M. Bredtmann, Jürgen Krücken and Georg von Samson-Himmelstjerna
Department of Veterinary Medicine, Institute for Parasitology and Tropical Veterinary Medicine, Freie Universität Berlin, Berlin, Germany

Jayaseelan Murugaiyan
Department of Veterinary Medicine, Institute for Animal Hygiene and Environmental Health, Freie Universität Berlin, Berlin, Germany

Tetiana Kuzmina
Department of Parasitology, I.I. Schmalhausen Institute of Zoology, Kyiv, Ukraine

Maria C. Souza, Denise M. Fonseca, Luciana Benevides, Tiago S. Medina, Murilo S. Dias, Giuliano Bonfá and João S. Silva
Department of Biochemistry and Immunology, Ribeirão Preto Medical School, University of São Paulo, São Paulo, Brazil

Marcondes A. B. Silva, José C. Alves-Filho, Alexandre Kanashiro and Fernando Q. Cunha
Department of Pharmacology, Ribeirão Preto Medical School, University of São Paulo, São Paulo, Brazil

Ricardo T. Gazzinelli and Warrison A. Andrade
Department of Medicine, University of Massachusetts Medical School, Worcester, MA, USA

Aline Gozzi and Marcos C. Borges
Department of Internal Medicine, Ribeirão Preto Medical School, University of São Paulo, São Paulo, Brazil

Martin R. Kraft
Unit 16 Mycotic and Parasitic Agents and Mycobacteria, Robert Koch-Institute, Berlin, Germany
Institute of Clinical Physiology, Charité Campus Benjamin Franklin, Berlin, Germany

Roland Bücker and Jörg-Dieter Schulzke
Institute of Clinical Physiology, Charité Campus Benjamin Franklin, Berlin, Germany

Aindrila Biswas, Timothy French, Henning P. Düsedau, Nancy Mueller and Ildiko Rita Dunay
Institute of Inflammation and Neurodegeneration, Otto-von-Guericke University Magdeburg, Magdeburg, Germany

Monika Riek-Burchardt, Anne Dudeck, Ute Bank and Thomas Schüler
Institute for Molecular and Clinical Immunology, Otto-von-Guericke University Magdeburg, Magdeburg, Germany

Henrique A. L. Ribeiro
Consiglio Nazionale delle Ricerche, Istituto per le Applicazioni del Calcolo, Rome, Italy
Departamento de Nutrição, Universidade Federal de Minas Gerais, Belo Horizonte, Brazil

Tatiani U. Maioli
Departamento de Nutrição, Universidade Federal de Minas Gerais, Belo Horizonte, Brazil

Leandro M. de Freitas
Núcleo de Biointegração, Universidade Federal da Bahia, Vitória da Conquista, Brazil

Paolo Tieri and Filippo Castiglione
Consiglio Nazionale delle Ricerche, Istituto per le Applicazioni del Calcolo, Rome, Italy

Norus Ahmed, Cristin N. Bock, Susanne Hartmann, Katrin Hemminger, Svenja Steinfelder and Sebastian Rausch
Department of Veterinary Medicine, Institute of Immunology, Freie Universität Berlin, Berlin, Germany

Subash Babu
National Institutes of Health-NIRT-International Center for Excellence in Research, Chennai, India
Laboratory of Parasitic Diseases, National Institutes of Allergy and Infectious Diseases, National Institutes of Health, Bethesda, MD, United States

Anuradha Rajamanickam and Yukhti Boothra
National Institutes of Health-NIRT-International Center for Excellence in Research, Chennai, India

Marie-Luise Brunn and Minka Breloer
Section for Molecular Biology and Immunology, Bernhard Nocht Institute for Tropical Medicine, Hamburg, Germany

Anja A. Kühl
Medical Department, Division of Gastroenterology, Infectiology and Rheumatology/Research Center Immuno Sciences, Charité-University Medicine Berlin, Berlin, Germany

Roswitha Merle
Department of Veterinary Medicine, Institute for Veterinary Epidemiology and Biostatistics, Freie Universität Berlin, Berlin, Germany

Max Löhning
Experimental Immunology, Department of Rheumatology and Clinical Immunology, Charité-University Medicine Berlin, Berlin, Germany
Pitzer Laboratory of Osteoarthritis Research, German Rheumatism Research Center (DRFZ), Leibniz Institute, Berlin, Germany

Jayaseelan Murugaiyan and Uwe Roesler
Institute of Animal Hygiene and Environmental Health, Centre for Infectious Medicine, Freie Universität Berlin, Berlin, Germany

Toni Aebischer
Unit 16 Mycotic and Parasitic Agents and Mycobacteria, Robert Koch-Institute, Berlin, Germany

Kai Matuschewski
Department of Molecular Parasitology, Institute of Biology, Humboldt University, Berlin, Germany

Ildiko R. Dunay and Timothy French
Institute of Inflammation and Neurodegeneration, Otto-von-Guericke University, Magdeburg, Germany

Anja Kühl
Division of Gastroenterology, Medical Department, Infection and Rheumatology, Research Center ImmunoSciences, Berlin, Germany

Janaiara A. Cunha, Leonardo J. M. Carvalho, Cesare Bianco-Junior, Lilian R. Pratt-Riccio, Evelyn K. P. Riccio and Cláudio Tadeu Daniel-Ribeiro
Labortorio de Pesquisa em Malária, Instituto Oswaldo Cruz, Fundação Oswaldo Cruz (Fiocruz), Rio de Janeiro, Brazil

Márcia C. R. Andrade
Instiituto de Cireci e Tecnolngi em Biomodelos, Fiocruz, Rio de Janeiro, Brazil

Marcelo Pelajo-Machado and Igor J. da Silva
Laboratório de Patologia, Instituto Oswaldo Cruz, Fiocruz, Rio de Janeiro, Brazil

Pierre Druilhe
Vac4All Initiative, Pepinière Paris Biotech Santé, Paris, France

Josefine Dunst and Faustin Kamena
Institute of Chemistry and Biochemistry, Free University Berlin, Berlin, Germany
Parasitology Unit, Max Planck Institute for Infection Biology, Berlin, Germany

Nahid Azzouz and Peter H. Seeberger
Institute of Chemistry and Biochemistry, Free University Berlin, Berlin, Germany
Department of Biomolecular Systems, Max Planck Institute for Colloids and Interfaces, Potsdam, Germany

Xinyu Liu
Department of Chemistry, University of Pittsburgh, Pittsburgh, PA, USA

Sachiko Tsukita
Department of Frontier Biosciences, Graduate School of Frontier Biosciences, Osaka University, Osaka, Japan

Ankur Midha, Josephine Schlosser and Susanne Hartmann
Department of Veterinary Medicine, Institute of Immunology, Freie Universität Berlin, Berlin

Emanuel Heitlinger
Research Group Ecology and Evolution of Molecular Parasite Host Interactions, Leibniz Institute for Zoo and Wildlife Research, Berlin, Germany
Institute for Biology, Molecular Parasitology, Humboldt University, Berlin, Germany

Susana C. M. Ferreira, Dagmar Thierer, Heribert Hofer and Marion L. East
Department of Evolutionary Ecology, Leibniz Institute for Zoo and Wildlife Research, Berlin, Germany

Josefine Dunst and Faustin Kamena
Parasitology Unit, Max Planck Institute for Infection Biology, Berlin, Germany
Institute of Chemistry and Biochemistry, Free University, Berlin, Germany
Molecular Parasitology, Institute of Biology, Humboldt University, Berlin, Germany

Kai Matuschewski
Parasitology Unit, Max Planck Institute for Infection Biology, Berlin, Germany
Institute of Chemistry and Biochemistry, Free University, Berlin, Germany

Index

www.ingramcontent.com/pod-product-compliance
Lightning Source LLC
LaVergne TN
LVHW081020210926
848485LV00004B/911

9781639874491